Trans Fats
Replacement Solutions

Trans Fats
Replacement Solutions

Editor

Dharma R. Kodali

AOCS PRESS

Urbana, Illinois

AOCS Mission Statement
AOCS advances the science and technology of oils, fats, surfactants and related materials, enriching the lives of people everywhere.

ISBN 978-0-12-810380-7 (print)
ISBN 978-1-6306703-3-7(.epub)
ISBN 978-1-6306703-4-4 (.mobi)

Library of Congress Cataloging-in-Publication Data
Trans fats replacement solutions / editor, Dharma R. Kodali.
pages cm
Includes bibliographical references and index.
ISBN 978-0-12-810380-7 (print) — ISBN 978-1-63067-033-7 (epub)—
ISBN 978-1-63067-034-4 (mobi) 1. Trans fatty acids. 2. Food—Fat content.
3. Food—Labeling. I. Kodali, Dharma R., 1951– editor of compilation.

TX553.U5T73 2014
613.2'84—dc23 2014011130

18 17 16 15 14 5 4 3 2 1

Contents

Preface

In the past two decades, *trans* fats have received a considerable worldwide attention. In the 1990s, many research studies unequivocally demonstrated that *trans* fats are responsible for a higher incidence of coronary heart disease, prompting the Food and Drug Administration (FDA) to regulate *trans* fats in food products. As a result, food manufacturers were required to label the amount of *trans* fats in various food products starting in 2006. The increased public awareness of the harmful effects of *trans* fats through the FDA labeling initiated the removal of *trans* fats from food products. This *trans* fat replacement initiative has created a paradigm shift in the fats and oils industry to find successful alternatives. Never before has such a concerted effort been made to remove an ingredient from the worldwide food chain. After a decade of initial *trans* fat regulation proposals, many *trans* fat replacement solutions were implemented and some countries successfully eliminated industrial *trans* fats from processed food. Buoyed by these successes, the FDA recently proposed the removal of generally recognized as safe (GRAS) status for partially hydrogenated oils (PHOs), the major industrial process responsible for most *trans* fats. If and when this new FDA proposal is implemented, the industrially produced *trans* fats will be entirely eliminated from food chain. This book is an effort to comprehensively document all aspects of *trans* fats and replacement solutions. It will answer questions about *trans* fats, such as how they became part of the food chain in the past century, their chemistry, their functional need, why they remain a health/nutrition issue, and what replacement solutions exist and how they have been adopted around the world.

This book is geared for a general audience as well as for experienced researchers. General readers will not only find the historical perspective of *trans* fats interesting, but also the specific factors that contributed to incorporating *trans* fats into the food chain and their ultimate removal. Experienced scientists will find the literature summaries useful and gain insight into structure–property–functionality relationships of fats and oils, what factors are important for delivering functionality while replacing *trans* fats in food products, and various *trans* fats technologies and solutions used around the world.

The contents of this book can be divided into two parts. The first 11 chapters describe the fundamental aspects of *trans* fats and the strategies, technologies, and solutions for replacing *trans* fats. Chapter 1 provides a comprehensive overview of *trans* fats, including their health effects, chemistry, sources, properties, and functionality. It also provides an in-depth analysis of the structure, properties, and functionality of fats and oils and addresses how this knowledge can provide an insight into finding ideal trans fat replacement solutions. The holy grail of *trans* fats replacement solutions is to find an ideal *trans* fat replacement with an equal or better performance without an increase in saturated fat. Chapter 1 provides background for such solutions and suggests practical solutions of how to create ideal designer fats.

Chapter 2 addresses whether the industrial *trans* fats produced during hydrogenation are different from naturally occurring *trans* fats from ruminant animals. Chapter 3 reviews the nutritional aspects of *trans* fats, and Chapter 4 provides a comprehensive account of their regulatory status. Analytical methods to determine *trans* fats are reviewed in Chapter 5. Chapter 6 provides an overview of *trans* fats replacement solutions with palm-based products by using fractionation and blending, whereas Chapter 7 provides an overview of solutions with high-oleic oils. Chapters 8 and 9 extensively review the interesterification process, a critical technology that offers versatile *trans* fat replacement solutions. Various *trans* fat replacement solutions provided by structuring agents, such as hydrophobic gellators like partial glycerol esters and wax esters, are discussed in Chapter 10. Application-specific *trans* fats replacement solutions for baking and frying are provided in Chapter 11.

The second part of the book, the last 8 chapters, describes *trans* fat regulations and scenarios in different geographies of the world and various practical solutions adopted to replace them. Experts in each region reviewed the regulations and documented the changes in *trans* fat content in various food products, as well as the technologies and solutions responsible for the change. Geographic locations discussed include North and South America, Europe, China, Malaysia, India, Japan, Australia, and New Zealand.

This book would not have been possible without the contributions of the authors. They each readily accepted my request to contribute a chapter, and this is admirable. I am grateful to each one of them for taking the burden of meeting the deadlines in spite of the unexpected interruptions. I thank my colleague Gary List for his contributions and constructive criticism. I also thank my colleague Lucas Stolp for making the figures and for reviewing.

In 2005, Gary List and I edited *Trans Fats Alternatives,* which provided a short account of *trans* fat replacement initiatives. The earlier work was completed in a record seven weeks' time, whereas the current book took more than a year, mainly due to unexpected health issues I faced during this time. Without the support and sustained efforts of the AOCS books and publications staff, this book would not have materialized. I greatly appreciate the expert help of and the extraordinarily long hours spent by Lori Stewart and Janet Brown.

I hope this book will be useful for anyone who wants to know about *trans* fats and will serve as a guide to find *trans* fat replacement solutions. Your suggestions and criticism are welcome.

—Dharma R. Kodali
dkodali@umn.edu

Contributors

AOCS Press extends gratitude and appreciation to the Trans *Fats: Replacement Solutions* chapter authors who helped make this title possible,

Editor

Dharma R. Kodali
Department of Bioproducts and Biosystems Engineering, University of Minnesota, St. Paul, Minnesota, USA

Contributors

Prakash Adhikari
Wilmar Biotechnology Research and Development Center Co., Ltd., Shanghai, China

Toshiharu Arishima
General Manager, Oils and Fats, Processed Foods R&D Center, Fuji Oil Co., Ltd., Tsukubamirai, Japan

Hormoz Azizian
NIR Technologies, Oakville, Ontario, Canada

David J. Baer
Food Components and Health Laboratory, U.S. Department of Agriculture, Agricultural Research Service, Beltsville, Maryland, USA

Jane Mara Block
Universidade Federal De Santa Catarina, Florianopolis SC, Brazil

Ingeborg A. Brouwer
Department of Health Sciences and the EMGO Institute for Health Care Research, Faculty of Earth and Life Sciences, VU University, Amsterdam, The Netherlands

Pierluigi Delmonte
United States Food and Drug Administration, Center for Food Safety and Applied Nutrition, College Park, Maryland, USA

Frédéric Destaillats
Nestlé Research Center, Lausanne, Switzerland

Ali Reza Fardin-Kia
United States Food and Drug Administration, Center for Food Safety and Applied Nutrition, College Park, Maryland, USA

Estelle A. Gaudier
Unilever Foods R&D Vlaardingen, The Netherlands

Véronique Gibon
Desmet Ballestra Group, Zaventem, Belgium

Maria Lidia Herrera
Instituto de Tecnología en Polímeros y Nanotecnología (ITPN), CONICET/University of Buenos Aires, Argentina

Peng Hu
Wilmar Global R&D Center, Pudong, Shanghai, China

Vincent de Jesus
U.S. Food and Drug Administration, Center for Food Safety and Applied Nutrition, College Park, Maryland, USA

Yuanrong Jiang
Wilmar Global R&D Center, Pudong, Shanghai, China

Sivaruby Kanagaratnam
Malaysian Palm Oil Board, and University of Nottingham, Malaysian Campus, Semenyih, Malaysia

Haruyasu Kida
Director and General Manager, Food Science Research Institute, Fuji Oil Co., Ltd., Tsukubamirai, Japan

Mark Kellens
Desmet Ballestra Group, Zaventem, Belgium

John K.G. Kramer
Guelph Food Research Center, Agriculture and Agri-Food Canada, Guelph, Ontario, Canada

Linsen Liu
LS Consulting, Irvine, California, USA

G.R. List
U.S. Department of Agriculture, Peoria, Illinois, USA (Retired)

Amy Logan
CSIRO Animal, Food, and Health Sciences, Werribee, Victoria, Australia

Alejandro G. Marangoni
Department of Food Science, University of Guelph, Guelph, Canada

Kalanithi Nesaretnam
Malaysian Palm Oil Board, No 6, Persiaran Institusi, Selangor, Malaysia

Gerald P. McNeill
IOI Loders Croklaan, Channahon, Illinois, USA

Sergey M. Melnikov
Unilever Foods R&D Vlaardingen, The Netherlands

Magdi M. Mossoba
United States Food and Drug Administration, Center for Food Safety and Applied Nutrition, College Park, Maryland, USA

R.B.N. Prasad
CSIR-Indian Institute of Chemical Technology, Hyderabad, India

Jeanne I. Rader
United States Food and Drug Administration, Center for Food Safety and Applied Nutrition, College Park, Maryland, USA

Teng Kim-Tiu
Malaysian Palm Oil Board, No 6, Persiaran Institusi, Selangor, Malaysia

Cynthia Tyburczy
United States Food and Drug Administration, Center for Food Safety and Applied Nutrition, College Park, Maryland, USA

Anne J. Wanders
Division of Human Nutrition, Wageningen University, Wageningen, The Netherlands

Ye Flora Wang
Metabolic and Cardiovascular Disease Laboratory, Alberta Diabetes Institute, Alberta Institute for Human Nutrition, Alberta, Canada

Leendert H. Wesdorp
Unilever Foods R&D Vlaardingen, The Netherlands

Chakra Wijesundera
CSIRO Animal, Food, and Health Sciences, Werribee, Victoria, Australia

Shuhua Xia
Wilmar Global R&D Center, Pudong, Shanghai, China

Xuebing Xu
Wilmar Global R&D Center, Pudong, Shanghai, China

K.D. Yadav
Kamani Oil Industries, Mumbai, India

Tiankui Yang
Wilmar Global R&D Center, Pudong, Shanghai, China

Alexander K. Zetzl
Department of Food Science, University of Guelph, Guelph, Canada

Hong Zhang
Wilmar Biotechnology Research and Development Center Co., Ltd., Shanghai, China

Jingyi Zhang
Wilmar Global R&D Center, Pudong, Shanghai, China

List of Abbreviations

ABIA	Associação Brasileira das Indústrias de Alimentação (Brazilian Association of Food Industries)
ANIB	Associação Nacional da Indústria de Biscoitos (National Association of Manufacturers of Cookies)
ANPRM	Advance Notice of Proposed Rulemaking
ANVISA	Agência Nacional de Vigilância Sanitária (National Health Surveillance Agency)
AOCS	American Oil Chemists' Society
ATR	Attenuated total reflection
BO	Blend oil
CAA	Código Alimentario Argentino (Argentine Food Code)
CAA	Consumer Affairs Agency
CB	Cocoa butter
CBE	Cocoa butter equivalent
CBS	Cocoa butter substitute
CCFS	Central Committee of Food Standards
CHD	Coronary heart disease
CIE	Chemical interesterification
CLA	Conjugated linoleic acid
CLX	Candelilla wax
CO	Coconut oil
CoA	Coenzyme A
CONAL	Comisión Nacional de Alimentos (Argentinean National Commission of Foods)
CNCD	Control of Chronic Non Communicable Diseases
CSE	Centre for Science and Environment
CSIC	Consejo Superior de Investigaciones Científicas (Spanish National Research Council)
CV AP	CV all-purpose
CVD	Cardiovascular diseases
DAG	Diacylglycerol, Diacylglycerides
DFEH	Director of Food and Enviromental Hygiene
DI	Degree of interesterification
DSC	Differential scanning calorimetry
DV	Daily value

E	Enzyme
EC	Ethylcellulose
ECN	Equivalent carbon number
EEE	Trielaidoylglycerol
EFSA	European Food Safety Authority
EI	Enzymatic interesterification degree
EIE	Enzymatic interesterification
EJCN	European Journal of Clinical Nutrition
EMBRAPA	Empresa Brasileira de Pesquisa Agropecuária (Brazilian Agricultural Research Corporation)
EPA	Eicosapentaenoic acid
FAME	Fatty acid methyl esters
FAO	Food and Agriculture Organization
FDA	Food and Drug Administration
FFA	Free fatty acid
FFDCA	U.S. Federal Food, Drug, and Cosmetic Act
FHSBO	Fully hydrogenated soybean oil
FSC	Food Safety Commission
GC	Capillary gas chromatography
GM	Genetic modification
GMP	Good manufacturing practices
GN	Groundnut oil
HAS	Hydroxystearic acid
HDL	High-density lipoprotein
HDL-C	High-density lipoprotein cholesterol
HEAR	High-erucic acid rapeseed oil
HF	Hydrogenated fat
HME	High melting endotherm
HPLC	High performance liquid chromatography
HSHOSFO	High stearic high oleic sunflower oil
IBGE	Instituto Brasileiro de Geografia e Estatística (Brazilian Institute of Geography and Statistics)
ID	Interesterification degree
IDEC	Institute of Consumer Protection (Instituto de Defesa do Consumidor)
ILSI	International Life Sciences Institute

INDEC	Argentinean National Institute of Statistics and Census (Argentinean National Institute of Statistics and Census)
IS	Internal standard
ISO	International Organization for Standardization
IU	International units
IV	Iodine value
JOCS	Japan Oil Chemists' Society
L	Lauric acid
LDL	Low-density lipoprotein
LDL-C	Low-density lipoprotein cholesterol
LL soy	Low-linolenic soybean
LME	Low melting endotherm
Ln	Linoleic acid
M	Myristic acid
MAFF	Ministry of Agriculture, Forestry and Fisheries
MAG	Monoacylglycerol
MBA	Performance tests in multibatch reaction
MCTM	Method for controlling trans fatty acid in meals
MERCOSUR	Mercado Común del Sur
MF	Milk fat
MHLW	Ministry of Health, Labor and Welfare
MME	Medium melting endotherm
MS	Mass spectrometry
MZ	Maize oil
NIH	National Institute of Health
NIR	Near-infrared
mid NIR	Mid-infrared
NLEA	Nutrition Labeling and Education Act
NMR	Nuclear magnetic resonance
NRV	Nutrition reference value
NSSO	National Sample Survey Organization
O	Oleic acid
OD	Outer diameter
OEO	1,3-dioleoyl-2-elaidoylglycerol
OGL	Open government license

OOO	Trioleoylglycerol
OOP	1,2-dioleoyl-3-palmitoylglycerol
OOS	1,2-dioleoyl-3-stearoylglycerol
OOX	1,2-dioleoyl-3-saturated fatty acylglycerol
OPO	1,3-oleoyl-2-palmitic-triacylglygcerol
OPP	1-oleoyl-2,3-dipalmitoylglycerol
OPS	10oleoyl-2-palmitoyl-3-stearoylglycerol
OSI	Oxidative stability indices
OSO	1,3-dioleoyl-2-stearoylglycerol
OSP	1-oleoyl-2-stearoyl-3-palmitoylglycerol
OSS	1-oleoyl-2,3-distearoylglycerol
OVO	1,3-dioleoyl-2-vaccinoylglycerol
OXO	1,3-dioleoyl-2-saturated fattyacylglycerol
P	Palmitic acid
PAHO	Pan American Health Organization
PCA	Principal component analysis
PFA	Prevention of Food Adulteration Act
PHO	Partially hydrogenated oil
PHVO	Partially hydrogenated vegetable oil
PHS	Partially hydrogenated soybean oil
PMF	Palm mid fraction
POP	1,3-dipalmitoyl-2-oleoylglycerol
POS	1-palmitoyl-2-oleoyl-3-stearoylglycerol
PPP	Tripalmitin
PS	Palm stearin
PUFA	Polyunsaturated fatty acids
PV	Peroxide values
RBO	Rice bran oil
RBX	Rice bran wax
RMSECV	Root mean square error of cross validation
RNI	Recommended nutrient intake
RR	Relative risk
RS	Rapeseed oil
RSPO	Roundtable on Sustainable Palm Oil
S	Stearic acid
SAFA	Saturated fatty acids

SAXS	Small angle X-ray scattering
SB, SBO	Soybean oil
SBOG	Sociedade Brasileira de óleos e Gorduras (Brazilian Society of Fats and Oils)
SSHE	Scraped-surface heat exchanger
SD	Standard deviation
SF	Sunflower oil
SFC	Solid fat content
SFI	Solid fat index
SFX	Sunflower wax
SMP	Slip melting point
SOS	1,3-disteroyl-2-oleoylglycerol
SS	Sesame oil
SSO	1,2-distearoyl-3-oleoylglycerol
SSS	Tristearoylglycerol
SSS	Tristearin
TAG	Triacylglycerol, triacylglycerides
TFA	*Trans* fatty acids
TFFA	*Trans* Fat Free Americas
TLC	Thin layer chromatography
Tp	Highest melt peak temperature
USLP	Unilever Sustainable Living Plan
VLME	Very low melting endotherm
VOP	Vegetable oil product order
VVV	Trivaccinoylglycerol
WHO	World Health Organization
X	Conversion degree

1

Trans Fats: Health, Chemistry, Functionality, and Potential Replacement Solutions

Dharma R. Kodali ■ *Department of Bioproducts and Biosystems Engineering, University of Minnesota, St. Paul, Minnesota, United States*

Introduction

Natural oils and fats are liquids or semisolids consisting primarily of triacylglycerols (TAGs). In the literature, triacylglycerols are often referred to as *triglycerides*, even though this latter term is less accurate in representing the molecular structure of this class of compounds. The distinction between fats and oils is a nuance seen in their physical state at ambient temperature. The major sources of oils and fats are from animals and plants. Greater than 90% of commercial oils and fats used for human consumption are plant-derived vegetable oils. Unrefined natural oils and fats, after extraction from the source, comprise mostly TAGs containing less than 5% of minor components such as sterols, phospholipids, tocopherols, fatty acids, and partial glycerol esters. The minor components and their concentration in the crude oil depend on the origin and method of oil extraction. The crude oils are subjected to various processing steps such as degumming and alkali refining (to remove phospholipids and fatty acids), bleaching (to remove colored pigments and polar matter), and steam stripping or deodorization (to remove volatile components) to make them suitable for human consumption. Oils subjected to these steps are usually referred to as RBD (refined, bleached, and deodorized) oils and contain about 99% TAGs.

The major vegetable oils of commerce are soybean, cottonseed, canola, sunflower, corn, peanut, palm, palm kernel, and coconut. Other vegetable oils like olive, rice bran, safflower, sesame, and other specialty oils are not used extensively due to availability and cost. A typical chemical structure of TAG is shown in Figure 1.1. The TAG contains a glycerol backbone with three hydroxyls esterified to three long linear carboxylic acids called *fatty acids*. The glycerol portion of TAG is constant in all oils and fats. The type of fatty acid structure and the position of esterification on glycerol differ from one TAG to another. Glycerol is a prochiral molecule capable of forming two different TAG stereoisomers, when esterified with different fatty acid chains at the 1 and 3 positions. These stereoisomers, when differentiated from one another, are identified as stereospecifically numbered, *sn*-glycerol derivatives (Kodali et al., 1984, 1989a). Even though biological systems can recognize the isomeric *sn*-glycerol derivatives, the physical and chemical properties of these isomers are very similar. For all functional and practical purposes they are treated as one and the same.

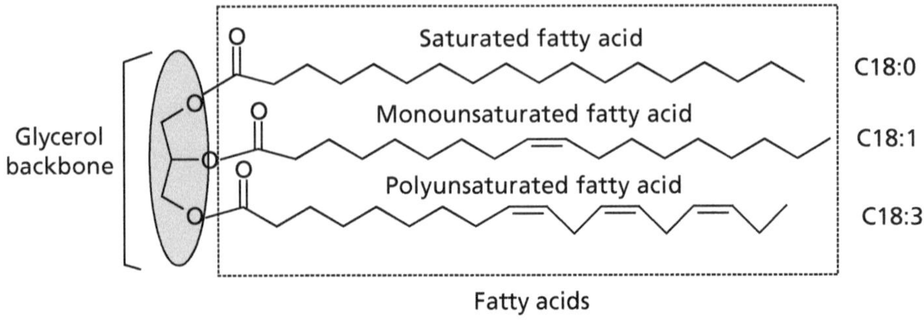

Figure 1.1 A molecular structure of a TAG (fat/oil) showing the glycerol backbone region esterified with three different fatty acids: stearic (C18:0), oleic (C18:1), and linolenic (C18:3) acids.

Vegetable oils contain a mixture of specific TAG molecules of given concentrations. Fatty acid structures differ from each other in carbon chain length and the number of double bonds. Most of the naturally occurring fatty acids are even numbered, 4 to 24 carbon atoms long, because they are synthesized from two-carbon unit acetyl coenzyme A. More prevalent saturated fatty acids with no double bonds that occur in oils and fats are lauric (C12:0), myristic (C14:0), palmitic (C16:0), and stearic (C18:0) acids. The number in parentheses shows the number of carbon atoms corresponding to the fatty acid chain length. A zero after the number indicates that there are no double bonds. The predominant unsaturated fatty acids are oleic (C18:1), linoleic (C18:2), and linolenic (C18:3) acids. The numbers in parentheses show the carbon chain length followed by the number of double bonds. The position of double bonds in the chain and the double-bond configuration are also very important. In oleic acid, the position of unsaturation is at carbon-9, in linoleic it is at C9 and 12, and in linolenic it is at C9, 12, and 15. Most of the unsaturated fatty acids that occur in natural fats and oils, with few exceptions, have the double bonds in *cis* configuration. The fatty acids that contain a single double bond are referred to as *monounsaturated* and others with more than one double bond are *polyunsaturated* fatty acids. Even though there are hundreds of different fatty acids that occur in oils and fats, the fatty acids referred to previously are most common and abundant in natural oils and fats.

The predominant vegetable oils in commerce can be divided into three types based on carbon chain length: lauric, palmitic, and oleic. The lauric oils, mostly coconut and palm kernel oils, contain high levels of 12-carbon lauric acid. The common palmitic oil, palm oil, contains 16-carbon palmitic acid in high concentration. The lauric and palmitic oils are high in saturated fatty acids and are semisolids at ambient temperature. Because coconut, palm, and palm kernel oils are grown in hotter climates closer to the equator, they are referred to as *tropical oils.* Oleic oils predominantly contain 18-carbon fatty acids such as stearic, oleic, linoleic, and linolenic acids. The soybean, sunflower, canola, corn, and cottonseed oils belong in this category. The major types of edible oils that are consumed in North America are soybean, corn, and canola. Palm oil is not extensively used in the United States, but its use has been rising because it provides cost-effective *trans*-free solutions. Palm oil is more extensively used in Asian countries and, to a certain extent, in Europe. Soybean and palm are the two most abundantly available vegetable oils in the world, together accounting for 60% of the total worldwide vegetable oil production of close to 157 million tons per year. The use of various vegetable oils in a given geography mainly depends on what is grown in that area and the cost and availability. Their yields, production volumes, and major production geographies for the four major vegetable oils are given in Table 1.A. Oil palm is a perennial crop with the majority of oil coming from the fruit pericarp and minor quantities from the kernel. Because of the high oil yields and production volumes, palm oil tends to be more cost competitive compared to other oils. However, production of the other vegetable oils yields protein as a byproduct along with the oil, which has nutritional and economic value. Beyond the cost and availability, nutritional and functional characteristics of fats and oils play an important role in their selection and use.

Defining vegetable oil composition by individual TAG molecular structure and concentration, rather than overall fatty acid composition of the oil, is more accurate but very cumbersome. Vegetable oils are identified by gross fatty acid composition (by weight). The fatty acid compositions of most edible oils used in commerce are shown in Table 1.B. The fatty acid compositions of various vegetable oils are determined by plant variety and genetics. In a given variety, the fatty acid composition changes a little due to geography and environmental factors. Because of this variation, the fatty acid composition is often expressed as a range rather than as a single number. The fatty acid compositions in Table 1.B are given in average weight percent.

Table 1.A Major Vegetable Oils, Production Volumes, Yields, and Geography (Estimates 2012–13)

Vegetable Oil	Oil Yield Liters of Oil/ha	Oil Yield from Seed/Fruit %	Production MMT/yr	Major Production Geography
Oil palm	6000	30–32	52	Malaysia, Indonesia
Soybean	450	17–18	43	USA, Brazil, and Argentina
Canola (rapeseed)	1200	42–48	24	Canada, Europe, and Asia
Sunflower	1000	37–40	14	All over the world

Table 1.B Fatty Acid Composition (wt.%) of Conventional and High-Oleic Oils

Oil Type	S.C.[a] C6–10	Lauric C12	Myristic C14	Palmitic C16	Stearic C18	L.C.[b] C20–24	Oleic C18:1	Linoleic C18:2	Linolenic C18:3
Soybean	—	—	—	11	4	—	23	55	7
Cottonseed	—	—	1	22	3	—	19	54	1
Sunflower	—	—	—	7	5	—	19	68	1
Canola	—	—	—	4	2	—	62	22	10
H. oleic canola	—	—	—	4	2	2	75	14	3
V.H.O.[c] canola	—	—	—	4	2	2	80	9	3
Peanut	—	—	—	11	2	7	48	32	—
Corn	—	—	—	11	2	—	28	58	1
Coconut	15	47	18	9	3	—	6	2	—
Palm kernel	8	48	16	8	2	—	15	3	—
Palm	—	—	1	45	4	—	40	10	—

[a]Short chain C6:0 hexanoic (caproic), C8:0 octanoic (caprylic), C10:0 decanoic (capric) fatty acids.

[b]Long chain C20:0 eicosanoic (arachidic), C22:0 docosanoic (behenic), C22:1 *cis* C13 docosenoic (erucic), C24:0 tetracosanoic (lignoceric) fatty acids.

[c]Very high oleic.

Recent developments in biotechnology and plant breeding make it possible to develop new genetic varieties that yield oils with different fatty acid compositions than traditional oils. For example, the oil from regular canola is composed of 62% oleic acid, whereas the high-oleic and very high-oleic canola varieties are composed of about 75% and 84% oleic acid, respectively.

There are numerous review articles that deal with composition, processing, physical and chemical properties, and commercial aspects of oils and fats (Hasenhuettl, 1994; Technical Committee of the ISEO, 2006; Thomas, 2012). More comprehensive and detailed information is provided in *Bailey's* (Hui, 1996). Another source of chemical and physical property information on various specific fatty acids, TAGs, and partial glycerol esters is *The Lipid Handbook* (Gunstone et al., 2007).

The primary purpose of this chapter is to provide comprehensive discussion of most of the aspects of *trans* fats: their health effects, chemistry, sources, properties, and functionality. First, a general overview of fats and oils and their functionality in foods is covered. This is followed by the discussion of the relationship between structure, properties, and functionality of TAG and its constituent fatty acids, leading to the creation of ideal designer fats that can meet the desired functional and nutritional needs. This chapter also provides various strategies to create *trans* fat replacement solutions, including the ideal designer fats with low saturates as a *trans* replacement solution.

Health Effects of *Trans* Fats

Coronary heart disease (CHD)—the narrowing of the inner walls of arteries caused by plaque buildup, thereby reducing the blood flow to the heart—has become the leading cause of death. Around the middle of the 20th century, there were numerous research studies that showed that saturated fat and cholesterol in the blood are major factors in cardiovascular disease. By 1985, the National Institute of Health (NIH) established that lowering the blood levels of low density lipoprotein (LDL), considered "bad cholesterol," would reduce the risk of CHD (NIH, 1985). Based on an inordinate amount of scientific data, it is fairly well established that the reduction of LDL and increase in "good cholesterol" (high density lipoprotein, HDL) reduces the risk of CHD. It has become a common practice in the research investigations to compare the LDL to HDL ratio to assess the CHD risk.

In 1990, the Nutrition Labeling and Education Act (NLEA) provided the Food and Drug Administration (FDA) with the authority to require nutritional labeling. The initial NLEA regulations requiring food products to be labeled with nutrient and health claims became fully effective by 1994. By this time the overall fat consumption—specifically, saturated fats and animal fat–containing foods, and their association with CHD—came under public scrutiny. As a result, food companies replaced the animal fats that contain cholesterol with partially hydrogenated vegetable oils (PHVOs) that provide the necessary solid fat functionality and shelf life. Similarly, tropical oils high in saturated fatty acid, such as palm and palm fractions, have been replaced by PHVO as well. The timeline of the initial NLEA regulations and the consequent changes that influenced the use of PHVO-containing *trans* fats to replace the saturated fat and animal fat in food products and also the subsequent *trans* fat regulations and their replacement solutions are shown in Figure 1.2.

The hydrogenation process to produce PHVO has been in extensive use around the world from the middle of the 20th century. It has been used to functionalize vegetable oils to replace animal fats, which were the most versatile fats used in Western countries at that time. The PHVO technology also provided greater functional versatility for the food manufacturers and increased the shelf life of the food products. The replacement of animal fats and tropical oils containing saturated fats with PHVO was hastened by the NLEA regulations in 1990s because they were perceived to provide the necessary functionality without increasing the saturated fat.

Almost all the unsaturated fats from nature, except ruminant fats, contain a *cis* double bond, which is different from *trans* configuration found in PHVO. PHVO provided better functionality and shelf life, in addition to reduced saturated fat content on the label of food products, which gained greater public acceptance. This hastened the replacement of tropical oils, which contain higher concentrations of saturated fats and animal fats that contain cholesterol, with PHVO, thereby

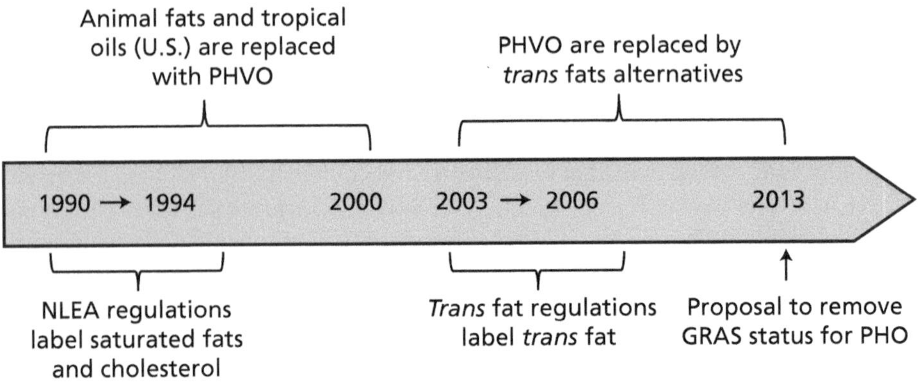

Figure 1.2 Chronology of nutrition and health regulations of saturated fats and *trans* fats and the consequent replacement solutions.

increasing *trans* fat consumption in the population. Before 1990, a few studies showed that *trans* fats behave differently than *cis* fats in elevating the cholesterol levels in blood (Vergroesen, 1975). However, in 1990, Mensink and Katan proved that *trans* fats raise LDL cholesterol and lower HDL cholesterol levels. Thereafter, a number of studies corroborated with these findings (Katan et al., 1995; Mensink et al., 1992). In 1999, Ascherio et al. summarized the nine randomized trials available at that time that directly compared the effects of *trans* fats with those of isocaloric amounts of *cis* fats. The meta-analysis of these trials clearly showed that the *trans* fats increase LDL cholesterol to levels similar to those produced by saturated fats and also decrease the HDL cholesterol levels. The net effect of *trans* fats on the LDL:HDL ratio is approximately double that of saturated fats. The effects of *trans* fats compared to saturated fats on LDL:HDL cholesterol as a percentage of energy intake of these fats are shown in Figure 1.3.

These findings of adverse health effects of *trans* fats on blood cholesterol levels compared to saturated fats were further confirmed by Mozaffarian et al. (2006); replacing saturated fats with *trans* fats up to 5% of energy intake linearly increased LDL cholesterol by 2 mg/dl while decreasing the HDL cholesterol by a similar amount. Later, the adverse effects of *trans* fats, as shown by the increase of the total cholesterol:HDL ratio, were clearly demonstrated by systematically replacing the saturated, monounsaturated, and polyunsaturated fats with *trans* fats (Mozaffarian and Clarke, 2009). Micha and Mozaffarian (2009) have shown the relative risk of *trans* fats and saturated fats on CHD with the consumption of these two fats as a percentage of energy compared to carbohydrates as the reference; this is shown in Figure 1.4. Both *trans* and saturated fats show a positive CHD risk increasing linearly with the consumption, whereas the intake of monounsaturated and polyunsaturated fats have

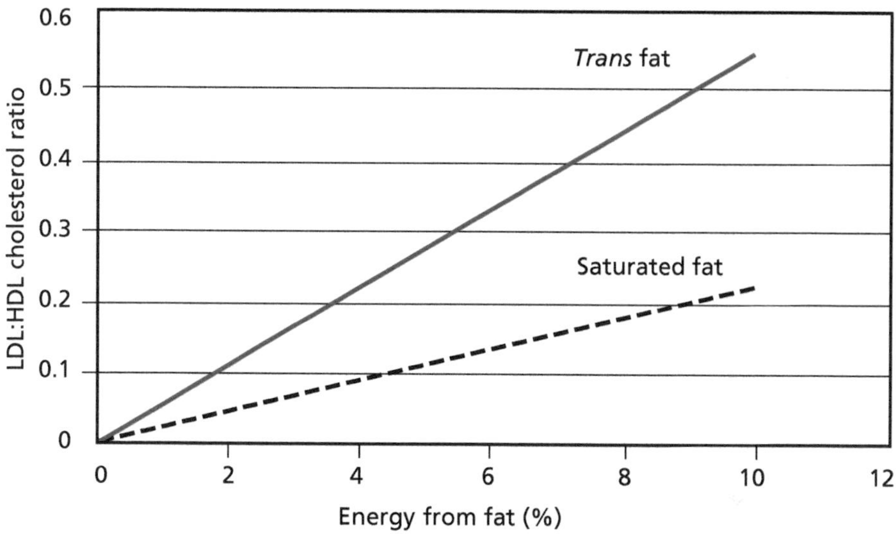

Figure 1.3 The effect of saturated fat and trans fat on the LDL:HDL cholesterol ratio compared to isocaloric amounts of *cis* fat. Based on Ascherio et al. (1999).

a negative CHD risk. According to this study, the CHD risk of *trans* fat is 7 to 8 times greater than that of saturated fat, as shown in Figure 1.4.

Recently, Brouwer et al. (2013) concluded that the detrimental effects of industrial *trans* fatty acids (i.e., PHVO) on heart health are beyond dispute. Considering the overwhelming evidence that *trans* fat consumption increases CHD risk, the FDA initiated *trans* fat labeling regulations. In July 2003, the FDA issued a final rule requiring a mandatory declaration on the nutritional label of the amount of *trans* fat present in foods, including dietary supplements. The declaration of *trans* fat is to be expressed as grams per serving to the nearest 0.5 gram increment below 5 grams and to the nearest gram increment above 5 grams (Moss, 2005). The *trans* fat regulations became effective on January 1, 2006. This development greatly influenced food product manufacturers in various geographical regions to either eliminate or reduce the *trans* fats in their products by adopting various *trans* fats alternatives, as elaborately described in this book. Considering the ill health effects of *trans* fats, Denmark took a more proactive measure and banned any food containing industrially produced *trans* fat at levels greater than 2% of total fat (Stender et al., 2006). This virtually eliminated the consumption of industrially produced *trans* fats in the Danish population very quickly. Beyond the adverse health effects, *trans* fats have virtually no nutritional benefits. Therefore, their removal from the food chain is imperative. On November 8, 2013, based on new scientific evidence and the findings of expert scientific panels,

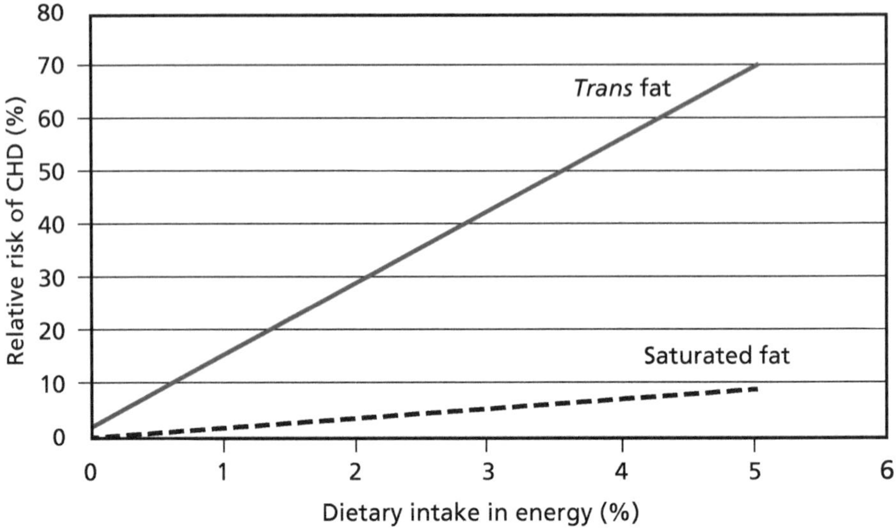

Figure 1.4 Relative risk of CHD as a percentage of energy consumption of saturated fats and *trans* fats, compared to carbohydrate. Based on Micha and Mozaffarian (2009).

the FDA tentatively determined that partially hydrogenated oils (PHOs), which are the primary dietary source of industrially produced *trans* fats, are not generally recognized as safe (GRAS) for any uses in food (FDA, 2013). Here the PHOs include fats and oils derived from plants and animals. If the tentative determination is finalized, oil manufacturers would no longer be permitted to sell PHOs, either directly or as ingredients in other food products.

Extensive coverage of *trans* fats regulations appears in Chapter 3. The nutritional aspects of *trans* fats are discussed in depth in Chapter 4.

Structure, Properties, and Functionality of TAGs

The fats and oils properties and functionality ensue from the TAG structure and the overall TAG composition. Because TAG contains glycerol esterified to different fatty acids, understanding of the fatty acid structure and properties will lead to the influence of various structural features on the properties. The purpose of understanding the relationship between chemical structure and the ensuing properties and functionality is that desired functionality can be created through modification of TAG structure and/or composition. The general relationship between these three features is shown schematically in Figure 1.5.

As shown in Figure 1.5, the properties of a given fat or oil depend on the fatty acid composition and structure. In turn, the properties are responsible for the functionality required for a given application. The molecular origins of functionality can therefore be understood by relating the chemical structure to the molecular packing and physical properties.

Two structural features of fatty acids present in edible fats and oils, chain length and unsaturation, are important. The *cis* unsaturation present in oils plays a big role in the physical properties. The partial hydrogenation converts some of the *cis* unsaturation to *trans,* thereby modifying the properties and functionality.

Cis, Trans Isomers

The double bond (unsaturation) present in the fatty acid inhibits the rotation of carbons on either side and thereby fixes the configuration of atoms present on double-bond carbons. The rest of the chain is free to rotate on C-C single bonds. Because of this fixed geometry, the hydrogen atoms present on double-bond carbons can be on the same side (*cis,* in Latin) or on the opposite side (*trans,* in Latin). The *cis* and *trans* are written in italics to identify their Latin origin and to represent the chemical configuration as shown in Figure 1.6. *Cis* and *trans* isomers are geometric isomers; they differ from one another only in the way that the atoms are oriented in space. The double bond is rigid and creates a kink in the chain. The kink created by the *cis* configuration is a lot more pronounced, whereas the kink created by the *trans* isomer

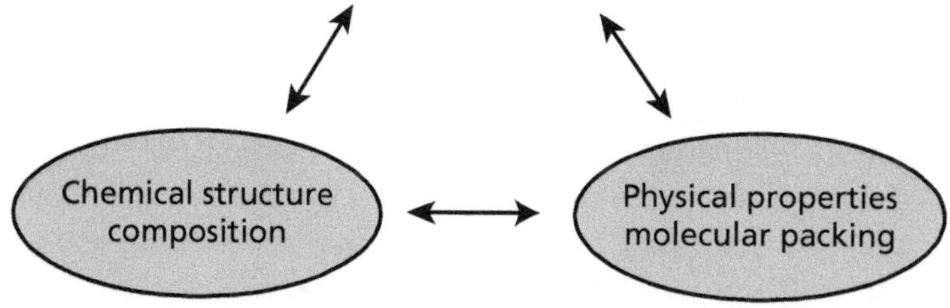

Figure 1.5 Understanding the molecular origins of properties and functionality of TAG will help to manipulate the structure and composition to derive the desired functional fat for a given application.

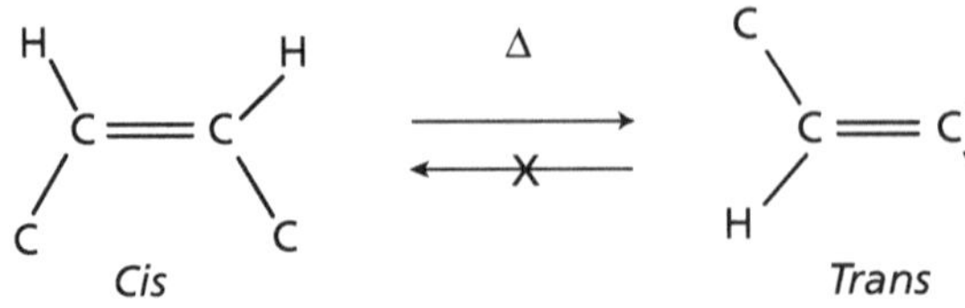

Figure 1.6 *Cis, trans* isomerism of a double bond under thermal conditions.

is relatively symmetrical and closer to a straight chain. *Trans* compounds have higher melting points than the corresponding *cis* isomers, reflecting the greater ease of crystal packing of the somewhat more symmetrical molecules. The interconversion of *cis* and *trans* takes place by the breaking and reformation of the double bond, which requires about 65 kcal/mole of energy. Because of this high energy barrier, the *cis* and *trans* isomerization does not occur easily unless assisted by a catalyst or high temperatures.

The *cis* isomer is more asymmetric than the corresponding *trans* isomer and cannot pack well into a crystal lattice. Because of this, the *trans* isomers have a higher density, lower solubility, and a higher melting point. *Trans* isomers are less sterically hindered and more thermodynamically stable than *cis* isomers. Therefore, the *cis* isomer can be transformed into a *trans* isomer by subjecting it to a high temperature. Very high temperatures provide enough energy to cause rotation about the double bond to convert a *cis* configuration into a thermodynamically more stable *trans* isomer, which is an irreversible process. During vegetable oil refining, the oil is subjected to steam deodorization to remove the volatile compounds. The high temperature conditions of deodorization cause *trans* isomerization. Because of this, most of the refined oils, even though not subjected to hydrogenation, contain as much as 1–2% of *trans* fats.

The unsaturated fatty acids present in the natural oils and fats are in the *cis* configuration. The *cis* isomers are relatively asymmetric and pack poorly in the crystal lattice due to a kink in the middle of the hydrocarbon chain. This kink in the middle of the chain reduces the interchain interactions in the solid state, thereby lowering the melting temperature and enthalpy. The position of the double bond in the middle of the chain most effectively decreases the melting temperature compared to either end of the fatty acid chain. Compared to *cis* double bonds, *trans* double bonds are relatively symmetric and pack better in the crystal lattice, so their melting temperature falls between the melting temperatures of saturated and *cis*-unsaturated fatty acids. A comparison of the molecular structures and melting temperatures of three fatty acids of 18-carbon chain length—oleic acid (*cis*-9 double bond), elaidic acid (*trans*-9 double bond), and stearic acid—illustrate this point. The influence of unsaturation and the type of unsaturation, *cis* versus *trans,* are shown in the space-filling models of stearic acid, oleic acid, and elaidic acid in Figure 1.7A. How

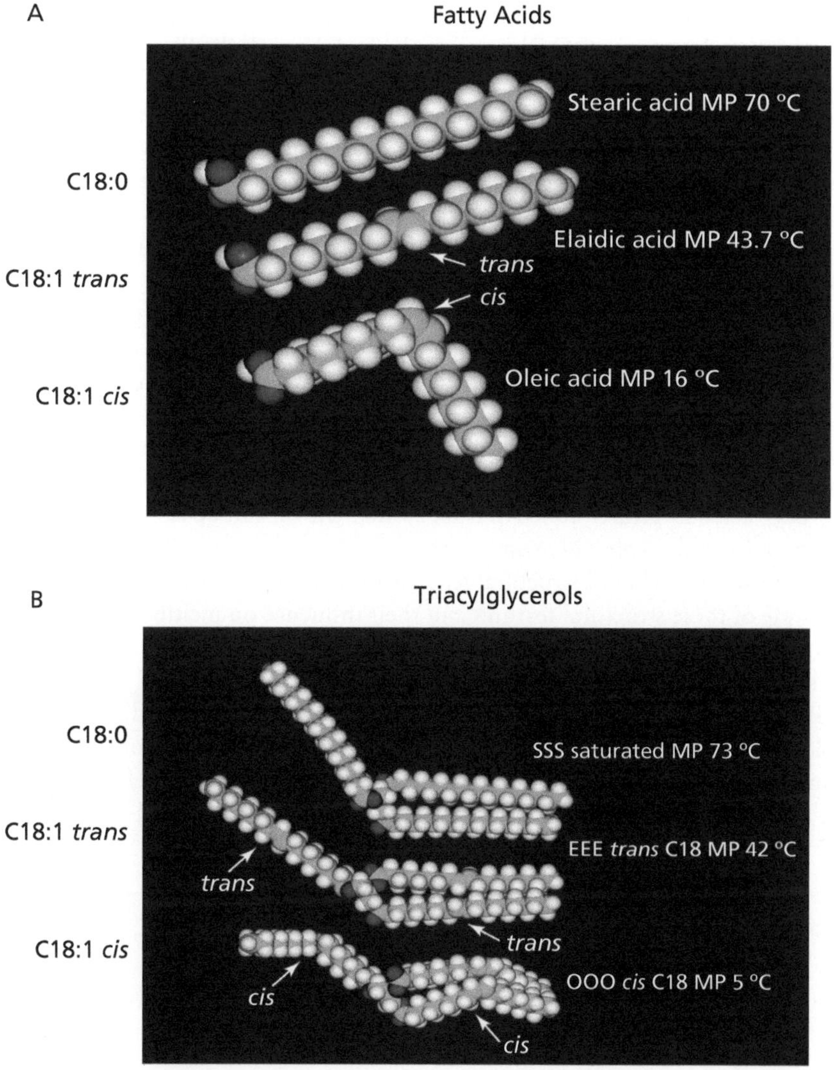

Figure 1.7 The space-filling models of (A) fatty acids, stearic acid (C18:0), elaidic acid (C18:1 *trans* C9), and oleic acid (C18:1 *cis* C9), and (B) the corresponding mono-acid triacylglycerols: tristearoylglycerol (SSS), trielaedoylglycerol (EEE), and trioleoylglycerol (OOO).

the same molecular features influence the corresponding TAG, tristearoylglycerol (SSS), trioleoylglycerol (OOO), and trielaidoylglycerol (EEE) with space-filling models and their melting temperatures are shown in Figure 1.7B. The melting temperatures of fatty acids mimic the melting temperatures of the corresponding TAGs. Even though the molecular packing and crystal structures of fatty acids and their corresponding TAGs are different, the molecular forces responsible for the melting temperatures are similar.

Nature utilized the *cis* configuration to make the high molecular weight TAG molecules as large as 900 Daltons and still keep them in the liquid state at ambient temperature, even though the unsaturated oils contain lower energy content than their corresponding saturated fat. Biological processes occur more efficiently when the TAG molecules are more accessible to the enzymes while in a liquid state. Because of this, the fatty acid compositions of various vegetable oils reflect the climatic and geographic conditions. Tropical oils contain saturated fatty acids in higher concentration, whereas the oleic oils that are grown in temperate climates contain polyunsaturated fatty acids in greater concentration so that the oil can be in liquid state in the corresponding plant's growing conditions.

There are a number of structural features that influence the properties of fats and oils. Some of these structural features and their influence on melting temperature are listed in Figure 1.8. The directionality of the melting temperature with the structural feature is indicated by arrows or greater-than signs.

Based on this information, the fatty acid structural features influence the TAG physical properties and functionality. Even though it is not a one-to-one relationship, the melting temperature of an oil or fat is greatly influenced by the fatty acid structural features and its fatty acid composition. The glycerol-associated factors, such as

- Acyl chain length—longer the chain ↑
- Acyl chain type—
  - Saturated > unsaturated (*trans* > *cis*)
- Number of double bonds ↓
- Position of double bond—middle ↓
- Position of fatty acid on glycerol
  - Symmetrical > Asymmetrical
  - Greater the mismatch (e.g., chain length, type) ↓
  - Partial glycerol esters (MAG/DAG) > TAG

Figure 1.8 Structural features of TAGs that influence the melting temperature.

its configuration and position of fatty acid attachment, which will be discussed later, had smaller influence. The structural features of various fatty acids and their melting temperatures are provided in Table 1.C.

Functional Need for Solid Fat in Food Products

Many fat and oil applications do not require solid fat content. Most of these applications include deep frying, for which thermal and oxidative stabilities are more important. There are some exceptions to this, such as doughnut frying, for which the solid fat content is necessary to provide glaze and crispiness. For frying applications, good oxidative stability is a major requirement that can be met by using high-monounsaturated oils and/or low-linolenic oils. In other applications, such as baked goods, a certain amount of solid fat content (SFC) is crucial. The solid fats provide the pliability to dough and also give layer, spread, or discrete distribution of fat depending

Table 1.C The Fatty Acids That Occur Commonly in the Food Fats and Oils, with Their Structural Features and Their Melting Temperatures

Fatty Acid	Structure[a]	Melting Point (°C)
Caprylic	C8:0	17
Capric	C10:0	32
Lauric	C12:0	44
Myristic	C14:0	54
Palmitic	C16:0	63
Palmitoleic	C16:1, *cis* C9	−0.5
Stearic	C18:0	70
Oleic	C18:1, *cis* C9	16
Elaidic	C18:1, *trans* C9	44
Vaccenic	C18:1, *trans* C11	44
Linoleic	C18:2, *cis* C9,12	−5
Linolenic	C18:3, *cis* C9,12,15	−10
Arachidic	C20:0, *cis* C11	75
Eicosenoic	C20:1, *cis* C13	25
Behenic	C22:0	80
Erucic	C22:1	33
Lignoceric	C24:0	88

[a]The fatty acid chain length is given with carbon number. The position, type, and number of double bonds are indicated for unsaturated fatty acids.

upon the product requirement. Some of the unique properties provided by solid fats in baked goods are flakiness, hardness, volume increase, layer separation, air entrapment while baking, dimensional structure, and freshness (Baldwin et al., 1963).

The oils/fats, proteins, and carbohydrates are the three major classes of building blocks required for living organisms. They are the most concentrated forms of energy (9 cal/g) and, because of this, most living organisms use them as energy storage media for critical functions such as survival during famine and seed germination. In various food applications, oils and fats provide a number of functional benefits. Besides imparting excellent organoleptic properties, they provide lubricity and decrease the interfacial tension of food particles, thereby making the food more palatable and easier to swallow. They supply essential fatty acids and oil-soluble vitamins that are essential for various biological functions.

The chemical composition of a mixture of TAG molecules present in a given vegetable oil is responsible for its physical state at ambient temperature. The oils containing saturated fatty acids in high concentration, like coconut and palm, can provide unique functionality and are more oxidatively stable. In general, the physical state of liquid (oil) or solid (fat) can possess some general and specific characteristics, as is shown in Table 1.D.

There are two primary reasons to use fats instead of oils: oxidative stability and solid fat functionality. The solid fat functionality includes the melting curves, texture, crystal structure, and morphology. These properties are very important depending on the food application. In some frying applications, such as snacks, the oxidative stability is very important but the solid fat content is not. In baking applications, both of these properties are important. Lack of sufficient oxidative stability affects the shelf life of the food product. Oxidation is the cause of off-flavors and rancidity.

Solid fats are preferred in food applications because they are resistant to oxidation and improve texture and sensory attributes. In oxidation, double bonds in unsaturated fatty acids react with molecular oxygen to form hydroperoxides, which in turn break down to create radicals that promote further oxidation. The break-down products formed during oxidation lead to off-flavors. The ease of oxidation depends on the fatty acid structure. The saturated fatty acids are much more stable than unsaturated

Table 1.D General Functional Properties of Oils and Fats

Functional Property	Oils (Liquids)	Fats (Solids)
Oxidative stability	Low	High
Hardness	None	Texture, spreadability, snap
Mouth feel	Good	Better, cooling sensation from enthalpy of melting

fatty acids. The rate of oxidation of monounsaturated oleic acid is about 10 times greater than saturated stearic acid. The polyunsaturated linoleic acid undergoes oxidation 10 times faster than oleic acid and half as fast as linolenic acid (Kodali, 2003). The oxidation rates indicate that saturated fats are more stable than unsaturated fats and will have a longer shelf life. The oils containing polyunsaturated fatty acids are much more susceptible to oxidation than oils containing monounsaturated fatty acids. For this reason, the low-linolenic and high-oleic oils have better functionality for frying applications. The oxidative stability of oils and fats affects the shelf life, process life, and the flavor of a food product.

The solid fat content of a fat imparts certain desirable properties such as hardness, crispiness, snap, and texture to a food product. The composition and individual TAG chemical structure of a fat determines solid content at a given temperature. In fats, liquid oil is entrapped in a solid matrix, giving a solid or semisolid texture. The percentage of solid fat in a fat matrix is quantified by the solid fat index (SFI) or the solid fat content (SFC). Both SFI and SFC measure the percentage of solid fat with the change in temperature using volumetric and NMR methods, respectively. This provides directional information on the functionality of a fat for a given application.

In some formulations, a certain amount of solid fat at ambient temperature is necessary to entrap the liquid oil to prevent oiling-off. In retail popcorn packaging, for example, oiling-off discolors the packaging, giving the consumer a perception of damaged goods. The hardness of fat also provides brittleness or a snap in products like chocolates. If a sufficient amount of solid fat of the formulation melts much above the body temperature of 37 °C, it leaves an undesirable waxy coating in the mouth. For this reason, solid fats that melt above 40 °C may be not used in higher concentration in some food product formulations. On the other hand, if a solid fat has a very high amount of solids at room temperature and melts very quickly at or below body temperature, it creates a smooth cooling sensation in the mouth as it absorbs the energy from the mouth cavity. The cooling sensation is proportional to the enthalpy of melting. Therefore, the fats with higher enthalpy will have the greater effect. The melting of the fat also releases other ingredients responsible for taste and flavor, giving a burst of euphoric sensation of coolness and taste.

Cocoa butter is an excellent example to demonstrate the desirable properties of solid fat. Cocoa butter is a specialty fat mainly used to make chocolate. It has very high solid fat content with suitable melting characteristics, but it is seldom used in food applications due to very high cost and limited availability. However, understanding the cocoa butter structure and functionality provides an insight into the significance of solid fat in food products. Such an understanding might lead to creation of a food fat with right solid fat functionality and without limitations of cost and availability. Cocoa butter is more homogeneous in composition than most natural fats, with only three fatty acids (palmitic, stearic, and oleic) constituting more than 95%

of the composition. The three fatty acids, found in high concentration, lead to the formation of few TAG structures. This relative structural homogeneity and the high amount of saturates provide cocoa butter fat with both high melting temperature and stability. In cocoa butter, the ratio of saturated to unsaturated fatty acids is 2:1; when combined with nature's propensity to attach unsaturated fatty acids at the 2 position of glycerol, symmetrical TAG structures like POP and SOS are favored. In general, symmetrical TAGs have higher melting temperatures than their asymmetrical counterparts. The high melting temperature and steep melting curve of cocoa butter can be observed by measuring the solid fat content of cocoa butter with temperature, as shown in Figure 1.9.

Cocoa butter has a very high solid fat content at or below room temperature (Figure 1.9). Because of this, products containing high concentrations of cocoa butter have good dimensional stability and a snap to the bite below 20 °C. Once in the mouth cavity, the fat melts rapidly by absorbing the surrounding energy. The sharp and high enthalpy of melting of cocoa butter between 20 °C and 35 °C releases the sweet taste and flavor in a very short time, creating a euphoric sensation unique to

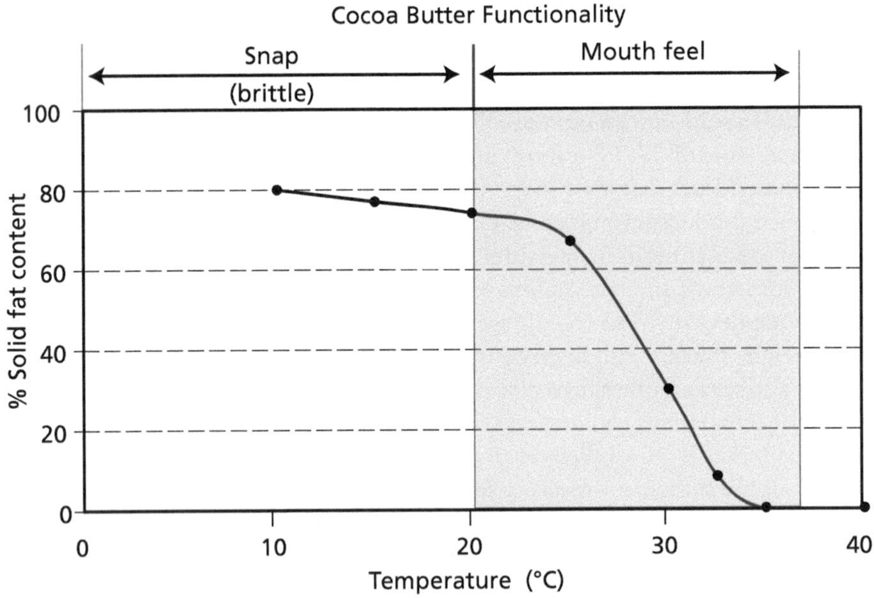

Figure 1.9 Cocoa butter melting curve showing the change in solid fat content with temperature. The shaded portion represents the changes that occur in the mouth temperature range, responsible for the organoleptic properties of chocolate.

solid fat in chocolate. This demonstrates the importance of solid fat content and its valuable functional properties in food.

Sources of *Trans*

The common sources of *trans* fat and the amount of *trans* content in these fats are shown in Table 1.E. Partial hydrogenation of vegetable oils is the major source of *trans* fats in food products. The *trans* fat content of hydrogenated fats varies from 5% to as much as 40%, based on the extent of hydrogenation and hydrogenation conditions. Soybean oil is the one of the most abundant vegetable oil worldwide, accounting for more than 25% of the world's vegetable oil production. It is also the most-consumed vegetable oil in the United States. Soybean oil is composed of more than 60% polyunsaturated fatty acids, which react readily with oxygen and form hydroperoxides. Partial hydrogenation was a common practice used to improve the oxidative stability of soybean oil by reducing the content of polyunsaturated fatty acids. Minor amounts of *trans* fats up to 2% form under the deodorization conditions of vegetable oil processing. The high temperatures employed under the deodorization conditions isomerize the *cis* unsaturation to *trans*. Another source of *trans* fats is of animal origin, from dairy and meat products. The concentration of *trans* fats in dairy and meat fats is usually low, from 3–8%, and these *trans* fats are different from those formed by hydrogenation of vegetable oils. The bacteria present in the ruminants' guts hydrolyze the dietary fat and subject the resulting fatty acids to biohydrogenation. The initial step in this process involves the conversion of a *cis*-12 double bond in polyunsaturated fatty acids to a *trans*-11 configuration, followed by the hydrogenation of a *cis*-9 double bond. Therefore, the fats from ruminant animals contain vaccinic acid, a *trans*-11 fatty acid. Because of this, the *trans* fats of animal origin contain *trans*-11 vaccinic acid in greater concentration, whereas the PHVOs contain a higher concentration of *trans*-9 elaidic acid (Mossoba et al., 2003). The concentration of various *trans* isomers and their relative ratios can help to determine the origin of *trans* fats in the diet. For instance, the examination of adipose fat can reveal the source of dietary *trans* fats from either PHVO or ruminant fats (Combe, 2003).

Table 1.E Common Sources of *Trans* Fat in Food Products.

Source	Amount (wt %)
Refined oils (RBD)	0.5–2
Tallow	5–6
Butter	3–6
Partially hydrogenated vegetable oils (PHVO)	5–45

The health effects of natural *trans* fats from ruminants and whether they are better than or the same as the industrial *trans* fats from PHVO are not fully resolved. Chapter 2 of this book extensively discusses the chemistry, dietary sources, and health impacts of these two classes of *trans* fats. Recent review of *trans* fats by Brouwer et al. (2013) concludes that the detrimental effects of industrial *trans* fats on heart health are beyond dispute and they recommend further research on the effects of natural *trans* fats on CHD.

Trans Fats Replacement Strategies

Trans fat replacement solutions range from simple solutions, such as switching one oil with another, to complex solutions, such as interesterified fat produced from fully hydrogenated fat and native oils. There could be a number of *trans* fat solutions based on the application and the product niche. Some of the common solutions are listed below.

- Fully hydrogenated fats as a source of saturated fat or hard fat for formulation and or interesterification
- Trait-enhanced oils with high oleic and saturated fatty acids
- Stable liquid oils
- Liquid oils with antioxidants
- Liquid oils with texturizers (emulsifiers, encapsulation, structuring agents)
- Liquid oils blended with "hardstock"
- Interesterified fats
- Tropical oils
- Fractionated fats
- Structured fats or designer fats

There are four core strategic technologies that have the ability to eliminate the *trans* fat content in foods. These are formulation, trait-enhanced oils with high oleic and/or saturated fatty acids, tropical oils and their fractionated products, and interesterification. These are enabling technologies that can be used alone or in combination with each other to create *trans* fat solutions. These technologies and their limitations are discussed next.

Formulation

There are a number of *trans* fat solutions that can be created through formulation. Some of these strategies include:

1. Liquid oils can be entrapped in solid fat matrix. A small percentage of completely hydrogenated soybean oil or palm hard stearin can entrap a large amount of

liquid oil. For example, high-oleic oil blends with low saturates have been tested in puff pastry preparation, and their performance is related to TAG composition (Garcia-Macias et al., 2012). Care must be taken not to use large amounts of very high melting fats because they can leave a coating in the mouth cavity and create waxiness. Based on the food product formulation, the entrapment can also be achieved by other components present in the formulation, such as emulsifiers like mono- or diacylglycerols, special starches like maltodextrins, and esters of very long chain linear fatty acid and fatty alcohol such as wax esters (Dassanayake et al., 2011, 2012; Kodali et al., 2011).

2. Blending small amounts of hard fat from fully hydrogenated fat or palm super stearin with stable high-oleic oils can provide structure and oxidative stability with no *trans* fat content.
3. Addition of antioxidants to fats and oils can provide oxidative stability and improve the shelf life of the products. The antioxidants can be natural (such as tocopherols), synthetic, or a combination of both. It has been shown that γ- and δ-tocopherols provide better oxidative stability to liquid oils (Warner, 2007).
4. Use of palm fractions can provide the desired solid fat content without the use of *trans* or hydrogenated fat on the label. However, the trade-off comes from the presence of palm on the label, indicating the use of saturated fat. Formulation with animal fats and their fractions create a similar conundrum of incorporating higher saturates and cholesterol content on the label.

Trait-Enhanced Oils

The vegetable oil traits, such as the fatty acid composition and the minor component composition, can be modified through conventional plant breeding or genetic engineering. For the past three decades, both of these techniques have been used to change oilseed bearing plants to modify their fatty acid composition. This process drastically increased the production of various varieties of specialty oils that provide specific functionality for food and industrial applications (Kodali et al., 2003). In a single crop variety there are a number of genotypes that give specific traits responsible for specific fatty acid compositions. In soybeans, genotypes with special traits have been developed that include low linolenic, high oleic, low palmitic, low saturate, high palmitic, and high stearic varieties (Liu, 1999). Other varieties target enhancement of levels of minor components such as specific tocopherols. A number of high-oleic oils, including canola, sunflower, and safflower, are currently available on the market (Loh, 2000). Performance of a high-oleic, low-linolenic canola in shortenings and deep-fat frying has been discussed by Orthoefer (2005). Genetic modification is also targeted toward the creation of high saturated fatty acid varieties that can replace hydrogenated oils with naturally produced solid fats. These fats could be further fractionated to give value-added cocoa butter substitutes (Kodali, 2004). Most of these crops are in the developmental stage, and some have to overcome penalties like yield lag to become economically successful. Chapters 7 and 11 of this book describe the use of commercially available trait-enhanced oils and their applications.

Tropical Oils and Their Fractionated Products

The process of crystallization under controlled conditions and separation of low-melting liquid and high-melting solid portions of a fat mixture is called *fractionation.* Fractionation can be done with the help of a solvent or without a solvent (dry fractionation). Solvent fractionation done with acetone or hexane is more efficient and gives a cleaner separation of the fractions. Due to greater capital and processing cost involved, however, it is seldom practiced. Dry fractionation is by far the simplest and cheapest fractional crystallization technique with no oil loss and it does not produce effluents or require any chemicals (Kellens et al., 2007). The dry fractionation process is extensively practiced in the palm oil industry (Gibon and Tirtiaux, 2002; Pantzaris, 2000). The solid and liquid thus separated are called *stearin* and *olein,* respectively. To make this a viable process, certain amounts of solids are necessary at ambient temperatures. Because of this, the high saturated or hydrogenated *trans* fatty acid containing oils are good starting feed materials for fractionation. Palm oil is also well suited for fractionation due to its high saturated fatty acid content. The palm fractions are natural and do not contain *trans* fats. Usually the crystallization is effected by cooling the palm oil very slowly to facilitate the nucleation and growth of a desired crystal structure, morphology, and size. The slurry of liquids and solids thus formed is separated by centrifugation or by filtration through a mechanical press by applying pressure. The fractionation process has become very handy in creating different varieties of palm products from very low-melting super olein to very high-melting super stearin from a single source. A typical palm fractionation process with different fractions and their melting ranges are given in Figure 1.10.

A typical fatty acid composition of palm oil and palm fractions is shown in Table 1.F. By varying the crystallization temperature, cooling rate, and amount of pressure applied during the filtration, a number of palm fractions of different compositions and properties can be produced. More than 20 different palm oil fractions are available commercially. A detailed description of palm oil crystallization and fractionation conditions and the properties of the fractionated products is provided by Kellens et al. (2007).

Similar fractional crystallization and filtration is also used on oils that contain small amounts of high-melting TAGs or waxes. This fractionation is usually called *winterization.* Winterization is mostly done to remove the turbidity caused by the high-melting crystals and to improve the oil clarity at room temperature. Chapter 6

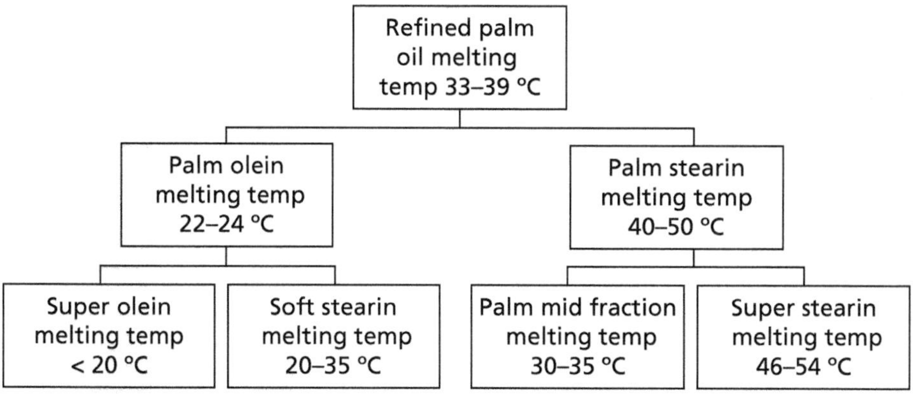

Figure 1.10 Dry fractionation of palm oil into stearins and oleins.

describes the functional characteristics of palm fractions and their blends for various food applications.

Interesterification

In vegetable oils and fats, the distribution of fatty acids on the glycerol backbone is not random. The saturated fatty acids are preferentially esterified to the glycerol primary hydroxyls 1 and 3, and the unsaturated fatty acids are esterified to the 2 position. The interesterification process is used to modify the distribution of fatty acids on glycerol backbone, thus modifying the properties of natural, hydrogenated, or fractionated oils or fats. Interesterification is a transesterification of two or more oils or fats for which the fatty acid arrangement on the glycerol backbone of each of the original TAGs is rearranged. Interesterification is done under chemical or enzymatic conditions. In chemical interesterification, the distribution of fatty acids on the glycerol backbone of

Table 1.F Typical Fatty Acid Composition of Palm Oil and Palm Fractions

Fatty Acid	Palm Oil	Palm Olein	Super Olein	Super Stearin
Myristic (C14:0)	1	1	1	1.5
Palmitic (C16:0)	47	40	35	60
Stearic (C18:0)	4	4	4	4.5
Oleic (C18:1)	41	43	46	28
Linoleic (C18:2)	11	12	14	6
Melting temp.	33–39°C	20–24°C	15°C	46–54°C

the product is rearranged as per the statistical probability at equilibrium. However, in the enzymatic processes, the enzymes are more specific, favoring rearrangement of the fatty acids present at the 1 and 3 positions of glycerol, leaving the 2 position preserved to a greater extent. The enzymatic process is commercially applied to produce more exotic fats like cocoa butter substitutes. However, this is changing rapidly as the cost of the process decreases due to more efficient and less expensive immobilized lipases that are commercially available and continuous processing developments. The chemical interesterification process is simpler and more cost effective but results in oil losses and effluents. However, the enzymatic process, due to positional specificity and improved efficiency, could become more cost effective and beneficial in producing the structured TAG of higher value.

The chemical interesterification of two different base stocks with different melting temperatures that produce an intermediate melting product is shown in Figure 1.11. This process can be affected by heating the components in the presence of a small amount of base catalyst, such as sodium methoxide. Two different fats and oils of different TAG compositions and properties can be transesterified to yield an end product of an entirely different TAG composition.

The interesterified product TAG distribution depends on the initial component concentrations. The interesterification of two pure TAG components is shown in Figure 1.12. Equal parts of tristearoylglycerol (SSS) and trioleoylglycerol (OOO), upon interesterification, produce four new TAG molecules (in addition to starting materials and not counting stereo isomers). In Figure 1.12, the concentration percentage and melting temperatures of each of the six TAGs produced after interesterification is shown, assuming complete randomization without any preferential transesterification

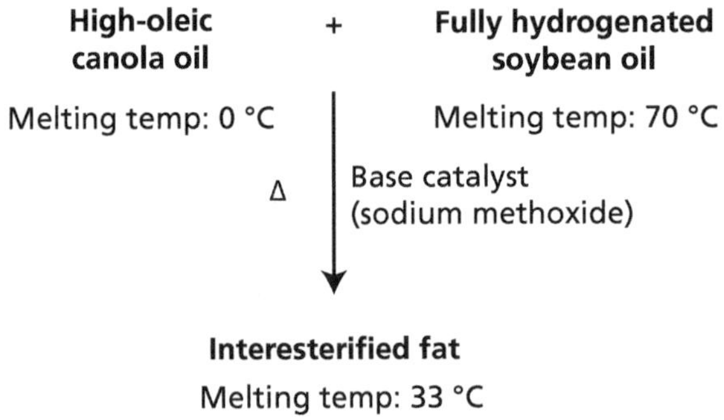

Figure 1.11 Chemical interesterification of high-oleic oil with fully hydrogenated soybean oil gives an interesterified product of intermediate melting temperature.

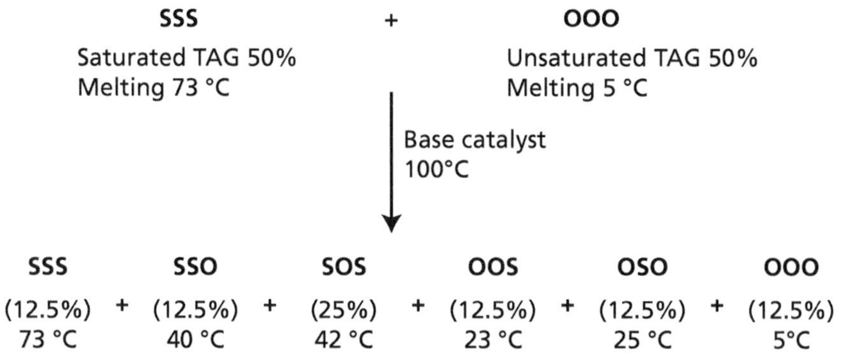

Figure 1.12 Interesterification product composition of equal parts of tristearoylglycerol and trioleoylglycerol.

on the three hydroxyls of glycerol. The interesterified product will have high melting temperature (>50°C), due to the presence of appreciable amount of very high-melting SSS (>10%). For this reason, the product will have a waxy mouth feel and may have limited food applications. The desired physical properties of the end product can be achieved by altering the ratio of starting saturated and unsaturated components. However, the interesterified product can be subjected to fractionation to isolate the intermediate melting fractions, thereby producing a material having desirable melting and solid fat characteristics. Thus, the interesterification combined with fractionation could be a very powerful tool to produce the solid fat with desired functionality by choosing the right starting materials and their relative ratios.

As discussed earlier, cocoa butter's desirable melting characteristics and solid fat functionality arise from its relative homogeneity by having few fatty acids (oleic, palmitic, and stearic acids) in the proportion of 2:1 saturated to unsaturated. If we take the pure TAG of these three fatty acids, namely OOO, PPP, and SSS, and subject them to random interesterification, 11 different new TAG species will be produced (not counting the stereo isomers and the starting materials). The new TAG molecular species produced by this interesterification and their melting temperatures are provided in Table 1.G. As one can see, the melting temperature ranges of these TAGs are very similar to the cocoa butter melting behavior. Due to TAG intersolubility factors and eutectic melting behavior, the higher TAG melting points in the interesterified fat get reduced by a few degrees.

Sometimes the random distribution of fatty acids can be altered by crystallization and separation of higher-melting saturated product from the reaction medium by conducting the transesterification process at temperatures below the crystallization

Table 1.G The New TAG Species Produced by Interesterification of OOO, PPP, and SSS, and Their Melting Temperatures

TAG	Melt Temp. °C	TAG	Melt Temp. °C
OPS	41	SOS	42
OSP	41	OOP	15[a]
OPP	34	OPO	19
POP	37	OOS	23
POS	37	OSO	25
OSS	40[a]		

[a]Predicted

temperature of the high-melting products that form during the reaction. This type of interesterification is called *directed interesterification.*

Specifically, the random chemical interesterification process can be accomplished by drying the base stocks to be interesterified at about 100 °C under vacuum, and then adding a base catalyst of about 0.1 wt% to the heated oil. After the catalyst addition, the oil is kept under vacuum and agitation for 30 minutes to complete the interesterification process. The catalyst can be deactivated by adding bleaching earth or by a water wash. The oil obtained is dried, bleached, and deodorized to produce the final product. Even though the process is simple, care should be taken to prepare the starting oils, as the quality of the feedstock greatly affects the oil losses. The presence of moisture, fatty acids, or peroxides in the feedstock can kill the catalyst and reduce product yield. Starting feedstock of good quality will require lower amounts of catalyst and result in lower oil losses (Kellens, 2000).

The enzymatic and chemical interesterification processes and their applications are extensively covered in Chapters 8 and 9.

Designer Fats

Functional Fat with Nutrition/Health Characteristics

It would be useful to find a solid fat that has ideal functional and nutritional characteristics. The new FDA regulations to ban the *trans* fats, if implemented, will result in the elimination of *trans* fats from food products. The functional void created by the elimination of *trans* can be filled by saturated fats; however, this is not an ideal option because the saturated fats are considered unhealthy as well. Various health organizations recommend that the amount of total dietary fat intake should be 30% of the total daily calories. The recommended saturated fat intake should be less than 10%

of the daily energy (FAO, 2010). This translates to one saturated fatty acid per TAG molecule in the fat, or 33% saturated fat. At the same time, the fat should provide the right solid fat functional properties, such as hardness at room temperature, high and sharp melting characteristics between 20 °C and 35 °C, and high enthalpy of melting. Designing such a functional fat requires an in-depth understanding of the structure–properties–functionality relationship. The discussion of various groups of structurally related pure TAG compounds and their properties in the following section will facilitate the understanding of the concept of such a designer fat.

Molecular Packing and Polymorphism

The physical properties of a fat depend upon the TAG composition and chemical structure. Therefore, to relate the physical properties of a fat to the functionality, it is crucial to understand the connection between the TAG structure and its influence on the molecular packing and ensuing properties. A specific TAG structure and the resulting physical properties have implications in some physiological processes, such as accessibility of molecules in aggregated particles like chylomicrons, enzymatic hydrolysis, and the subsequent metabolism (Redgrave et al., 1988; Small, 1984). Once a fat structure that meets all the functional requirements is identified, it could be produced using the enabling technologies previously discussed.

In addition, fats have the propensity to pack in several different crystal structures of comparable lattice energy with different melting temperatures and molecular packing. These different solid-state crystal structures (crystals) of the same chemical composition are called *polymorphs,* and the phenomenon is called *polymorphism.* Polymorphism of fats and oils has been well-studied and characterized using various techniques like X-ray diffraction and vibrational spectroscopy by different researchers for over 60 years (Chapman, 1962; Kodali et al., 1989a; Larsson, 1964; Sato, 1996). Three distinct polymorphic forms, α, β', and β, have been characterized based on their hydrocarbon chain (subcell) packing. In general, α is the least stable and lowest melting polymorphic form with no specific chain–chain interaction with hexagonal subcell packing, followed by intermediate melting β' with specific chain–chain interaction and orthorhombic perpendicular (O⊥) subcell packing. The most stable and high melting polymorph is β, with very specific chain–chain interaction with triclinic parallel (T∥) subcell packing. These polymorphs are distinguished from each other based on the X-ray diffraction short spacings that characterize the molecular packing on the short axis, called the *hydrocarbon subcell packing.* In reality, most of the fats may have more than three polymorphic forms. For example, a single TAG structure, 1,2-dipalmitoyl-3-decanoyl-*sn*-glycerol, has been shown to form five distinct polymorphs that differ from each other in the molecular packing in the short as well as long axes, resulting in distinct physical properties (Kodali et al., 1989b). Also, when dealing with natural fats having different TAG mixtures, presence of more than one polymorph under given conditions is a common occurrence.

The main factors that contribute to different modes of packing in each of the polymorphic forms are the geometry of the glycerol backbone and the packing of the long hydrocarbon chains along their long and short axes. The packing along the acyl chain length can be identified from the X-ray long spacings, which is also called *layered packing*. Fatty acid chain length, the presence of one or more double bonds, and the position of substitution on the glycerol backbone all influence the layered packing (Kodali et al., 1987, 1989a, 1990).

The molecular structure influences the solid-state behaviors of fats, such as melting temperature, as well as the rates of crystallization and crystal morphology. The understanding of crystal structure, stability, and rates of transformation from one polymorphic form to another can relate to the gross functional properties. For instance, the discoloration or blooming in chocolates is due to transformation of desirable β-crystal form into another higher melting β-form. In margarines and shortenings, crystallization of β-polymorphic form instead of the desirable β'-polymorphic form results in large crystal size and morphology that is responsible for graininess or a sandy feeling in the mouth.

The β' crystals, due to their relatively small crystal size, feel smooth and melt quickly in the mouth. It is known in the industry that oils containing higher concentrations of palmitic acid, like cottonseed oil, stabilize the β'-polymorphic form. For this reason, cottonseed oil is added to soybean oil base stocks that are used to make shortenings and margarines. The mismatch of C16 and C18 chain lengths creates a methyl end chain packing that stabilizes the β'-polymorphic form. The most stable crystal form of the pure TAG with dissimilar chain lengths, 1,2-dipalmitoyl-3-myristoyl glycerol (PPM), is the β'-polymorphic form, and there is no β-form. This provided an opportunity to determine the first single crystal structure of TAG β'-polymorph (Sato et al., 2001a). As described earlier in the case of cocoa butter, the functionality of mouth feel and cooling sensation can be interlinked to the physical properties of melting temperature, melting range, and enthalpy of melting. These properties emanate from the molecular packing of the high-melting β-polymorphic form. In turn, the molecular packing and properties can be related to the relative homogeneity in chemical composition and symmetrical TAG structures present in cocoa butter.

Studying the molecular structure and packing of groups of compounds where the chemical structure is varied systematically will enhance understanding and could lead to the creation of the ideal designer fat with desired functionality. There are a number of systematic studies directed at understanding the chemical structure in relation to the molecular packing (Fahey et al., 1985; Hagemann et al., 1972; Kodali et al., 1987,1989a, 1990; Sato and Ueno, 2001; Yano et al., 1999). A few groups of structurally related TAG, their molecular packing and properties are presented next.

Table 1.H The Melting Temperatures and Enthalpies of 18-Carbon Mono Acid Triacylglycerols

Triacylglycerol, TAG	Abbreviation[a]	Melting Temp. (°C[b])	ΔH of Melt[c] kcal/Mole	Packing Chain Length[d]
Tristearoylglycerol	SSS	73	46	2
Trielaidoylglycerol	EEE	42	36	2
Trivaccinoylglycerol	VVV	42	36	2
Trioleoylglycerol	OOO	5	23	2
Trilinoleoylglycerol	LLL	−13	20	2
Trilinolenoylglycerol	LnLnLn	−24	—	—

[a]S = stearic (C18:0); E = elaidic (C18:1, *trans* C9); V = vaccenoyl (C18:1, *trans* C11); O = oleic (C18:1); L = linoleic (C18:2); Ln = linolenic (C18:3).

[b]The melting temperature is of high-melting polymorphic form.

[c]The enthalpy of melting is from high-melting polymorphic form to melt.

[d]The packing chain length is from powder X-ray diffraction long spacings corresponding to bilayer, two chain length structures (about 45 Å).

Molecular Packing and Properties of Monoacid TAG

The physical properties and molecular packing of single acid TAGs are listed in Table 1.H. As one would expect, the melting temperatures and enthalpies of these TAGs decrease from saturated to monounsaturated to polyunsaturated. Among the monounsaturated, the trielaidoyl (*trans* C9, EEE) and trivaccinoyl (*trans* C11, VVV) glycerols show considerably higher melting temperatures and enthalpies than the monounsaturated *cis* TAG OOO, making them more suitable for solid fat applications.

The comparison of *cis*, *trans*, and saturated monoacid TAGs as space-filling models is shown in Figure 1.7B. The space-filling models clearly show the saturated TAG SSS and *trans-9* TAG, EEE can easily pack due to relative molecular linearity, whereas the *cis*-9 TAG OOO with kinked double bonds cannot. All the single-acid TAGs pack in bilayered structure in the stable β-polymorphic form. However, one notable difference between the *trans* unsaturated EEE and saturated SSS and *cis*-unsaturated OOO is that EEE does not form β'-polymorphic form (Kodali et al., 1987). It is possible that the *trans* unsaturation and the resulting end methyl plane packing may destabilize the orthorhombic subcell packing of β'-polymorphic form. The acyl chain orientation and molecular packing in the layered structure in the stable β-polymorphic form of these TAGs will be similar to the published single-crystal structure of monoacid TAG trilauroyl glycerol (Larsson, 1964). Typical representation of layered packing

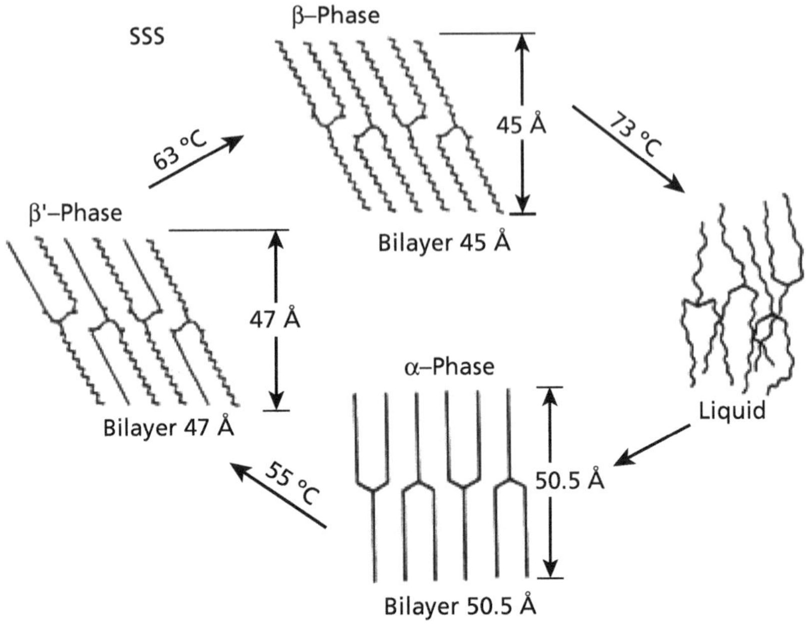

Figure 1.13 Schematic representation of phase behavior of a tristearoylglycerol SSS. Based on Kodali et al. (1987).

and melting behavior of this class of compounds, as represented by SSS, is shown in Figure 1.13.

Molecular Packing and Properties of Symmetric Di-Acid TAGs

A group of symmetrical di-acid triacylglycerols were compared with monoacid TAGs tristearoyl glycerol SSS and trioleoyl glycerol OOO. In this group, all the fatty acid chains have the same carbon chain length, C18, but the unsaturation and position of esterification on glycerol differ from each other (Kodali et al., 1987). In the symmetrical TAG, the nature of the acyl chain at glycerol 2 position influences the melting temperature and enthalpy as shown in Table 1.I. The saturated stearoyl chain has a higher melting temperature and enthalpy than the unsaturated chains. Among the unsaturated, the *trans* acid–containing TAG with the unsaturation in the middle of the chain at C9 (OEO) has higher enthalpy and melting point compared to OVO, where the *trans* double bond is moved to C11 toward the methyl end. This demonstrates that the hydrocarbon chain packing in the methyl end of the chain is more important than the carboxylic acid side. This group of compounds also demonstrates

Table 1.I The Melting Temperatures and Enthalpies of Di-Acid Symmetrical Triacylglycerols in Comparison to Single-Acid Triacylglycerols, SSS and OOO

Triacylglycerol, TAG	Abbreviation[a]	Melting Temp. °C[b]	ΔH of Melt[c] Kcal/Mole	Packing Chain Length[d]
Tristearoylglycerol	SSS	73	46	2
1,3-dioleoyl-2-stearoylglycerol	OSO	25	32	3
1,3-dioleoyl-2-elaidoylglycerol	OEO	9	29	3
1,3-dioleoyl-2-vaccinoylglycerol	OVO	4	23	3
Trioleoylglycerol	OOO	5	23	2

[a]S = stearic (C18:0); E = elaidic (C18:1, *trans* C9); V = vaccenoyl (C18:1, *trans* C11); O = oleic (C18:1)

[b]The melting temperature is of high-melting polymorphic form.

[c]The enthalpy of melting is from high-melting polymorphic form to melt.

[d]The packing chain length is from powder X-ray diffraction long spacings corresponding to bilayer, two chain length structures (about 45 Å) or trilayer, three chain length structures (about 65 Å).

that a single *trans* fatty acid chain in a molecule may not be sufficient to increase the enthalpy and melting temperature appreciably compared to a *cis* fatty acid chain. The molecular packing of these symmetrical TAGs reveals that they pack in trilayered structures. The odd chains at the glycerol 2 position segregate to form a separate layer from the 1 and 3 positions. This acyl chain orientation, namely the 1 and 3 chains of a TAG, pack side by side in one layer, whereas the 2-acyl chain of the same molecule in a separate layer is similar to monoacid triacyl glycerols, even though the latter packs in a bilayered structure. A typical molecular packing of trilayered structure is illustrated by 1,3-dioleoyl-2-stearoylglycerol (OSO) and is shown in Figure 1.14.

Molecular Packing and Properties of Asymmetric Di-Acid TAG

In another systematic study, a set of asymmetric di-acid triacylglycerols with asymmetric chains substituted at *sn*-glycerol-3 position were studied (Fahey et al., 1985). The chain length of this 3-acyl chain is increased 2 carbons at a time from C14, myristic acid, to C24, lignoceric acid. The physical properties and molecular packing of this series of compounds are compared with trioleoyl glycerol and given in Table 1.J. The melting temperatures and enthalpies of these compounds increase with an increasing

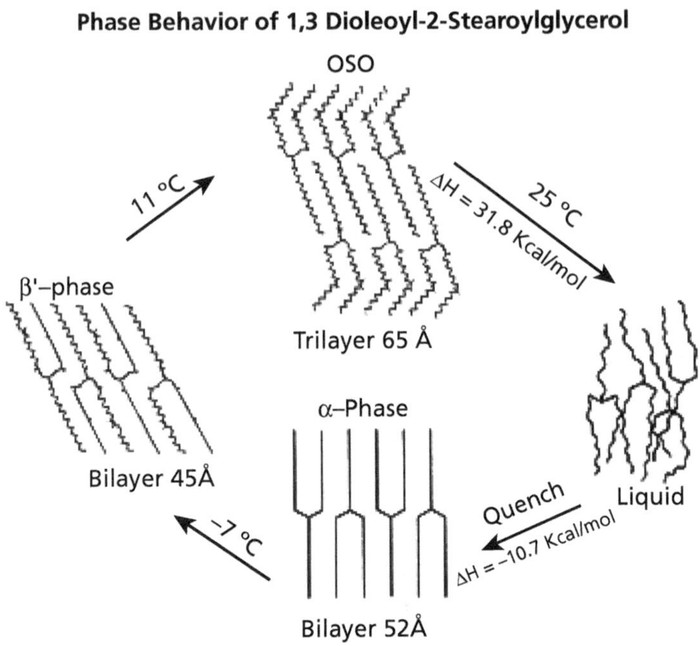

Figure 1.14 A schematic representation of phase behavior of a di-acid triacylglycerol, OSO. Based on Kodali et al. (1987).

chain length. The 3-acyl chain lengths of C18 and above show melting temperatures above 20 °C but below body temperature. The enthalpies of these compounds are similar to or better than trioleoyl glycerol OOO. The molecular packing of all these compounds reveals trilayered structures with the odd 3-acyl chain segregating from the other two chains to form a middle layer. This trilayer structure packs 1- and 2-acyl chains in the same layer, while the 3-acyl chains of two different molecules form the middle layer, which is different from the symmetric TAG packing previously discussed. This type of acyl chain packing forces the glycerol conformation perpendicular to the end methyl layer plane, which is different from the glycerol conformation of single-acid TAG stable crystal structure but similar to diacylglycerols and phospholipids (Goto et al., 1992). The glycerol conformation and the acyl chain packing of the asymmetric di-acid TAG as represented by OOS is shown in Figure 1.15.

Role of Glycerol Conformation in Molecular Packing and Properties

Understanding the stable glycerol conformation in structurally similar TAGs will enable the contribution of glycerol conformation to the stable molecular packing.

Table 1.J The Melting Temperatures and Enthalpies of Asymmetric Di-Acid Triacylglycerols in Comparison to Single-Acid Triacylglycerol OOO

Triacylglycerol, TAG	Abbreviation[a]	Melting Temp. (°C[b])	ΔH of Melt[c] kcal/mole	Packing Chain Length[d]
1,2-dioleoyl-3-myristoylglycerol	OOM	12	18	3
1,2-dioleoyl-3-palmitoylglycerol	OOP	18	21	3
1,2-dioleoyl-3-stearoylglycerol	OOS	23	23	3
1,2-dioleoyl-3-arachidoylglycerol	OOA	29	26	3
1,2-dioleoyl-3-behenoylglycerol	OOB	33	28	3
1,2-dioleoyl-3-lignoceroylglycerol	OOLg	36	26	3
Trioleoylglycerol	OOO	5	23	2

[a]O = oleic (C18:1); M = myristic (C14:0); P = palmitic (C16:0); S = stearic (C18:0); A = arachidic (C20:0); B = behenic (C22:0); Lg = lignoceric (C24:0).

[b]The melting temperature is of high-melting polymorphic form.

[c]The enthalpy of melting is from high-melting polymorphic form to melt.

[d]The packing chain length is from powder X-ray diffraction long spacings corresponding to bilayer, two chain length structures (about 45 Å) or trilayer, three chain length structures (about 65 Å).

The physical properties and packing of OSO and OOS are compared in Table 1.K. The comparison of the molecular packing of symmetric TAG OSO with asymmetric TAG OOS shows that both of them pack in trilayered structures. However, to accomplish this, the oleoyl chains segregate from the stearoyl chains to form different layers, while the stearoyl chains form a separate layer sandwiched in the middle as shown in Figure 1.15. This molecular packing forces the glycerol conformation parallel to the end methyl layer plane in OSO and perpendicular to the same plane in OOS. Except for this difference, the rest of the packing is comparable. The glycerol conformation in these two molecules in relation to the end methyl plane is shown in a circle in Figure 1.15. This change in glycerol conformation influences the enthalpies and melting temperatures of these two compounds. The symmetrical TAG OSO has 2 °C higher melting temperature and 9 kcal/mole higher enthalpy than the asymmetric counterpart, OOS.

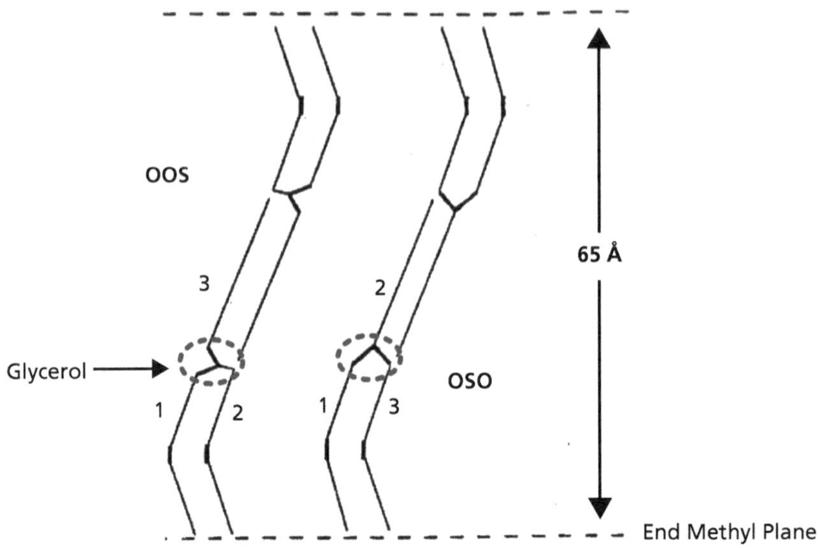

Figure 1.15 The layered packing of symmetric and asymmetric di-acid TAGs OSO and OOS. The 1,2- or 1,3-oleoyl chains of a molecule pack in a layer on either side of stearoyl chains segregated to form a middle layer. This acyl chain arrangement forces the glycerol conformation to be either parallel (OSO) or perpendicular (OOS) to the end methyl layer plane.

Table 1.K The Melting Temperatures and Enthalpies of Di-Acid Symmetric and Asymmetric Triacylglycerols OSO and OOS

Triacylglycerol, TAG	Abbreviation[a]	Melting Temp. (°C[b])	ΔH of Melt[c] kcal/mole	Packing Chain Length[d]
1,3-dioleoyl-2-Stearoylglycerol	OSO	25	32	3
1,2-dioleoyl-3-stearoylglycerol	OOS	23	23	3

[a]O = oleic (C18:1); S = stearic (C18:0).

[b]The melting temperature is of high-melting polymorphic form.

[c]The enthalpy of melting is from high-melting polymorphic form to melt.

[d]The packing chain length is from powder X-ray diffraction long spacings corresponding to trilayer, three chain length structures (about 65 Å).

The glycerol conformation present in OSO is more stable than OOS (Kodali et al., 1987). This is corroborated with the fact that the single-crystal structure of monoacid TAG trilauroylglycerol shows similar glycerol conformation (Larsson, 1964). This indicates that when all the three chains are equal, the glycerol conformation parallel to layer plane orientation is preferred. This also confirms that the symmetric TAG will have higher melting temperatures and enthalpies than the asymmetric isomer.

Ideal Designer Fats for Solid Fat Applications

After evaluating structure–properties–functionality relationships of various TAG molecules and considering the health and nutrition aspects of various fatty acids, one might ask: Can an ideal designer fat having similar or better solid fat functionality to cocoa butter but with half as much saturated fat be created? This challenge, if met, can provide the best *trans* fat replacement solution. To understand the question fully, cocoa butter contains more than 60% saturated fat and melts in the mouth cavity between 20 °C and 37 °C, but also shows the best solid fat functionality at room temperature. These characteristics can fulfill the challenging solid fat food applications like baking, shortenings, and many others. However, to meet all these functional characteristics with half the saturated fat as cocoa butter (about 30% saturates) is a formidable challenge.

From the foregoing structure-properties-functionality discussions so far, one can deduce that the TAG structural features that are desirable and necessary to meet the above challenge include: (1) fat homogeneity to be able to melt in a short range, should contain fewer fatty acids (<4 fatty acids should makeup >90% of the composition); (2) may contain one saturated fatty acid per molecule; (3) should contain no *trans* fatty acids; (4) contain minimum amount of polyunsaturated fatty acids (for optimal melting characteristics and better oxidative stability).

Based on these requirements, the ideal designer fat may contain dioleoyl saturated fatty acid TAG and preferably the saturated fatty acid should be at the glycerol 2 position (symmetrical) to give the high enthalpy and melting characteristics. If the saturated fatty acids are both palmitic and stearic, similar to cocoa butter, they will have the desired functionality but will contain greater than 60% saturated fat. To have the right melting profile with fewer saturated fats, we need longer-chain saturated fatty acids. The symmetrical and asymmetrical dioleoyl saturated fatty acid TAGs containing chain lengths from C16 to C24 with their melting temperatures are listed in Table 1-L. The melting temperatures of these TAGs show that any one of them or all of them together are suitable materials to meet the above challenge. However, the dioleoyl saturated TAGs containing C18, C20, and C22 make the best solid fat that can meet or even exceed the melting characteristics of cocoa butter. The symmetric TAG provides higher melting temperature and enthalpy than its asymmetric isomer.

Table 1.L The Melting Temperatures of Asymmetric 1,2-Dioleoyl-3-saturated TAG (OOX) and Asymmetric 1,3-Dioleoyl-2-saturated TAG (OXO)

Saturated Fatty Acid X	Asymmetrical OOX (°C)	Symmetrical OXO (°C)
C16:0 P	18	20
C18:0 S	23	25
C20:0 A	29	32
C22:0 B	33	36
C24:0 Lg	36	39

To illustrate all the above structural features of ideal TAG molecules, the melting temperatures of 1,3-dioleoyl-2-saturated fatty acyl TAGs are plotted against the carbon number of saturated fatty acid in Figure 1.16. The melting temperature range shaded in the square of the figure represents the mouth cavity melting temperatures, and compounds that melt in this range imitate the cocoa butter functionality. Any single symmetric OXO TAG with carbon numbers from C18 to C24 will provide similar to or superior melting and functional characteristics to cocoa butter as a single molecular structure. Their melting characteristics will also be superior with a short melting range and having higher enthalpy.

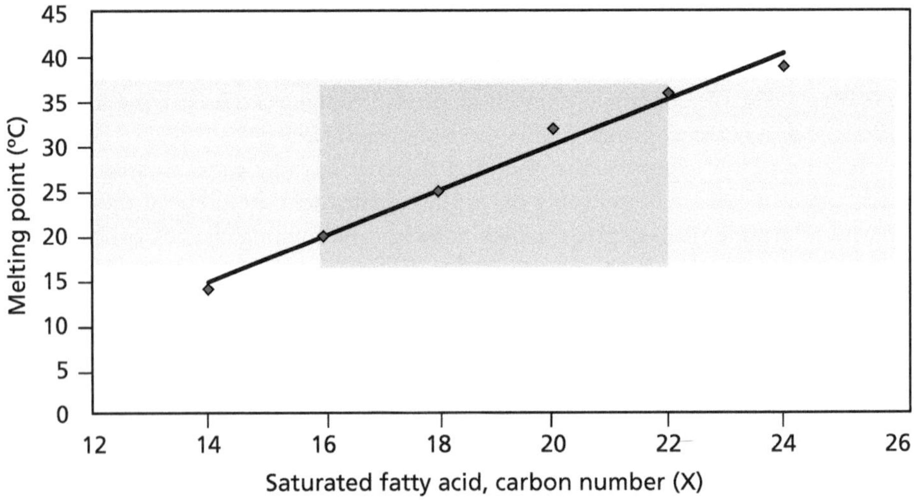

Figure 1.16 The melting temperatures of a symmetrical 1,3-dioleoyl-2-saturated fatty acyl TAG (OXO) plotted against the saturated fatty acid chain length carbon number.

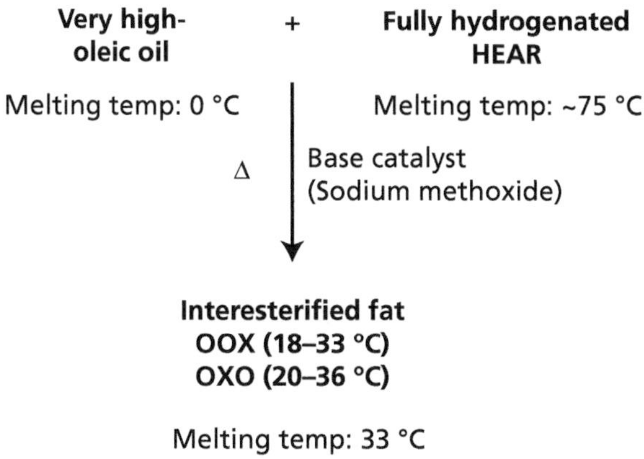

Figure 1.17 Interesterification of very high-oleic oil with fully hydrogenated high-erucic acid rapeseed oil produces the symmetrical and asymmetrical dioleoyl saturated fatty acyl TAG with saturated fatty acid carbon chain lengths from C16 to C24.

The raw materials necessary to create such an ideal designer fat must be readily available to reduce this technology into a practical solution. Fortunately, this is possible. The trait-enhanced very high-oleic oils that are commercially available can provide more than 90% oleic acid containing TAG. The other component that can provide long saturated fatty acids is high-erucic acid rapeseed oil (HEAR). Upon complete hydrogenation, HEAR provides fully saturated TAGs containing C16:0 (<2%), C18:0 (~30%), C20:0 (~10%), C22:0 (45–60%), and C24:0 (<2%). As shown in Figure 1.17, the interesterification of fully hydrogenated HEAR with very high-oleic oil (>90% oleic content) can produce symmetric and asymmetric dioleoyl TAG containing saturated fatty acids C18:0, C20:0, and C22:0 greater than 90%. If needed, further product improvements can be made by using glycerol-2 specific enzymatic interesterification and/or fractionation. In our opinion, the products created by using these technologies will revolutionize the versatility and functionality suitable for all solid fat food applications.

Summary

Fats and oils (TAGs) are a major class of compounds that are essential for various biological functions and also for food functionality. The use of certain oils in the diet around the world is dictated by the cost, availability, production geography, and nutrition/health characteristics. The natural oils and fats contain *cis* double bonds that isomerize into the thermodynamically more stable *trans* form during the industrial processes of hydrogenation and deoderization. *Trans* fats, similar to saturated fats, offer desirable food functionality without being labeled as saturated fat. Because of this, the PHVOs replaced saturated fats in food products in the 1990s. However, in the past 20 years, there have been numerous studies that showed a direct correlation between CHD risk and the consumption of *trans* fats. These studies made it very clear that the *trans* fats are responsible for higher CHD incidence and do not provide any nutritional value. Based on the overwhelming evidence, the FDA proposed to eliminate industrially produced *trans* fat from the food chain by removing the GRAS status of partially hydrogenated oils. When the new FDA regulations are implemented, industrially produced *trans* will disappear from food products.

There are a number of enabling technologies, such as formulation, trait-enhanced oils, tropical oils and their fractions, and interesterified fats, that are available to eliminate *trans* fats in food products. The substitution of saturated fat for *trans* fat is an easy but not healthful solution. However, creating an ideal designer fat with good solid fat functionality and nutritional properties requires an in-depth understanding of TAG structure–properties–functionality relationships. Ideal designer fats with one saturated fatty acid/TAG molecule, such as dioleoyl saturated TAG containing C18 to C22 saturated fatty acids with excellent functional properties, can be produced with the existing knowledge. Producing ideal fats cost effectively requires leveraging enabling technologies and readily available raw materials. Production of an ideal designer fat that can meet the ultimate *trans*-free solution without substituting saturated fat for *trans* fat is shown from the interesterification of very high-oleic oil with fully hydrogenated HEAR.

Acknowledgments

I would like to thank Lucas Stolp for his expert help with the figures and reviewing the manuscript. The editorial help from Gary List, Linsen Liu, and Sithara Kodali is gratefully acknowledged.

References

Ascherio, A.; Katan, M. B.; Zock, P. L.; Stampfer, M. J.; Willett, W. C. *Trans* Fatty Acids and Coronary Heart Disease. *N. Engl. J. Med.* **1999,** *340* (25), 1994–1998.

Baldwin, R. R.; Johansen, R. G.; Keough, W. J.; Titcomb, S. T.; Cotton, R. D. The Role That Fat Plays. *Cereal Science Today* **1963,** *8,* 273–284.

Brouwer, I. A.; Wanders, A. J.; Katan, M. B. *Trans* Fatty Acids and Cardiovascular Health: Research Completed? *European Journal of Clinical Nutrition* **2013,** *67,* 541–547.

Chapman, D. The Polymorphism of Glycerides. *Chem. Rev.* **1962,** *62,* 433–456.

Combe, N. Nutritional Implications of *Trans* Fatty Acids. *Abstracts of 25th World Congress and Exhibition of the International Society of Fat Research (ISF)* **2003,** *2.*

Dassanayake, L. S. K.; Kodali, D. R.; Ueno, S. Formation of Oleogels Based on Edible Lipid Materials. *Current Opinion in Colloid & Interface Science* **2011,** *16,* 432–439.

Dassanayake, L. S. K.; Kodali, D. R.; Ueno, S; Sato, K. Crystallization Kinetics of Organogels Prepared by Rice Bran Wax and Vegetable Oils. *Journal of Oleo Science* **2012,** *61,* 1–9.

Fahey, D. A.; Small, D. M.; Kodali, D. R.; Atkinson, D.; Redgrave, T. G. Structure and Polymorphism of 1,2-Dioleoyl-3-acyl-*sn*-glycerols. Three- and Six-layered Structures. *Biochemistry* **1985,** *24,* 3757–3764.

Food and Drug Administration (FDA). *Tentative Determination Regarding Partially Hydrogenated Oils; Request for Comments and for Scientific Data and Information;* Document Citation 78 FR 67169, Agency/Docket No. FDA-2013-N-1317; Food and Drug Administration, Office of the Federal Register, National Archives and Records Administration: Washington, DC, 2013; pp 67169–67175.

Garcia-Macias, P.; Gordon, M. H.; Frazier, R. A.; Smith, K.; Gambelli, L. Effect of TAG Composition on Performance of Low Saturate Shortenings in Puff Pastry. *Eur. J. Lipid Sci. Technol.* **2012,** *114,* 741–747.

Gibon, V.; Tirtiaux, A. Latest Trends in Dry Fractionation. *Lipid Technology* **2002,** *14,* 33–36.

Goto, M.; Kodali, D. R.; Small, D. M.; Honda, K.; Kozawa, K.; Uchida, T. Single Crystal Structure of a Mixed-chain Triaclyglycerol: 1,2-Dipalmitoly-3-acetyl-*sn*-glycerol. *Proc. Natl Acad. Sci., USA* **1992,** *89,* 8083–8086.

Gunstone, F. D.; Harwood, J. L.; Dijkstra, A. J. *The Lipid Handbook,* 3rd ed.; CRC Press: Boca Raton 2007.

Hagemann, J. W.; Tallent, W. H.; Kolb, K. E. Differential Scanning Calorimetry of Single Acid Triglycerides: Effect of Chain Length and Unsaturation. *J. Am. Oil Chem. Soc.* **1972,** *49,* 118–123.

Hasenhuettl, G. L. Fats and Fatty Oils. In *Kirk-Othmer Encyclopedia of Chemical Technology,* 4th ed.; Howe-Grant, M., Ed.; John Wiley & Sons: New York, 1994; pp 252–287.

Hui, Y. H. (Ed.). *Bailey's Industrial Oil and Fat Products,* 5th ed. New York: John Wiley and Sons, 1996.

Katan, M. B.; Zock, P. L.; Mensink, R. P. *Trans* Fatty Acids and Their Effects on Lipoproteins in Humans. *Annu. Rev. Nutr.* **1995,** *15,* 473–493.

Kellens, M. Interesterification: Process Conditions. *SCI Lecture Papers Series* **2000,** 114, 1–3.

Kellens, M.; Gibon, V.; Hendrix, M.; De Greyt, W. Palm Oil Fractionation. *Eur. J. Lipid Sci. Technol.* **2007,** *109,* 336–349.

Kodali, D. R. Biobased Lubricants—Chemical Modification of Vegetable Oils. *Inform,* **2003,** *14,* 121–123.

Kodali, D. R. Vegetable Oil Having Elevated Stearic Acid Content. U.S. Patent 6,713,117 B1, March 30, 2004.

Kodali, D. R.; Atkinson, D.; Redgrave, T. G.; Small, D. M. Synthesis and Polymorphism of 1,2-Dipalmitoyl-3-acyl-*sn*-glycerols. *J. Am. Oil Chem. Soc.* **1984,** *61,* 1078–1084.

Kodali, D. R.; Atkinson, D.; Redgrave, T. G.; Small, D. M. Structure and Polymorphism of 18-carbon Fatty Acyl Triacylglycerols: Effect of Unsaturation and Substitution in the 2-Position, *Journal of Lipid Research* **1987,** *28,* 403–413.

Kodali, D. R.; Atkinson, D.; Small, D. M. Molecular Packing in Triacyl-*sn*-glycerols: Influence of Acyl Chain Length and Unsaturation. *J. Dispersion Science and Technol.* **1989a,** *10,* 393–440.

Kodali, D. R.; Atkinson, D.; Small, D. M. Molecular Packing of 1,2-Dipalmitoyl-3-decanoyl-*sn* glycerol (PP10): Bilayer, Trilayer, and Hexalayer Structures. *J. Physical Chemistry* **1989b,** *93,* 4683–4691.

Kodali, D. R.; Atkinson, D.; Small, D. M. Polymorphic Behavior of 1,2-Dipalmitoly-3-lauroyl (PP12)- and 3-Myrostoyl (PP14)-*sn*-glycerols. *Journal of Lipid Research* **1990,** *31,* 1853–1864.

Kodali, D. R.; Fan, Z.; DeBonte, L. R. Plants, Seeds, and Oils Having an Elevated Total Monounsaturated Fatty Acid Content. U.S. Patent 6,649,782 B2, Nov 18, 2003.

Kodali, D. R.; Folstad, J. E.; Polzin, M. R.; Haese, T. R.; Narayanaswamy, V.; Lonergan, D. A. *Trans* Fat Replacement System and Method of Making a Baked Good with a *Trans* Fat Replacement System. U.S. Patent 8029847 B2, 2011.

Larsson, K. Solid State Behavior of Glycerides. *Arkiv For Chemie* **1964,** *23,* 35–56.

Liu, K. Soy Oil Modification: Products, Applications. *Inform* **1999,** *10,* 868–877.

Loh, W. Biotechnology and Vegetable Oils: First Generation Products in the Marketplace. In *Physical Properties of Fats, Oils and Emulsifiers;* Widlak, N., Ed.; AOCS Press: Urbana, IL, 2000; pp 247–253.

Mensink, R. P.; Katan, M. B. Effect of Dietary *Trans* Fatty Acids on High-density and Low-density Lipoprotein Cholesterol Levels in Healthy Subjects. *NEJM* **1990,** *323,* 439–445.

Mensink, R. P.; Zock, P. L.; Katan, M. B.; Hornstra, G. Effect of Dietary *Cis* and *Trans* Fatty Acids on Serum Lipoprotein[a] Levels in Humans. *J. Lipid Res.* **1992,** *33* (10), 1493–1501.

Moss, J. S. *Trans* Fat—New FDA Regulations. In Trans *Fat Alternatives;* Kodali, D. R., List, G. R., Eds.; AOCS Press: Urbana, IL, 2005.

Mossoba, M. M.; Kramer, J. K. G.; Delmonte, P.; Yurawecz, M. P.; Rader, J. I. Official Methods for the Detemination of *Trans* Fat; In *AOCS Monograph;* AOCS Press: Urbana, IL, 2003; pp 1–22.

Micha, R.; Mozaffarian, D. Trans Fatty Acids: Effects on Metabolic Syndrome, Heart Disease and Diabetes. *Nat Rev Endocrinol.* **2009,** *5,* 335–344.

Mozaffarian, D.; Clarke, R. Quantitative Effects on Cardiovascular Risk Factors and Coronary Heart Disease Risk of Replacing Partially Hydrogenated Vegetable Oils with Other Fats and Oils. *Eur. J. Clin. Nutr.* **2009,** *63* (Suppl. 2), S22–33.

Mozaffarian, D.; Katan, M. B.; Ascherio, A.; Stampfer, M. J.; Willett, W. C. *Trans* Fatty Acids and Cardiovascular Disease. *N. Engl. J. Med.* **2006,** *354* (15), 1601–1613.

NIH Consensus Development Conference. Lowering Blood Cholesterol to Prevent Heart Disease. *JAMA* **1985,** *253,* 2080–2086.

Orthoefer, F. T. Performance of Trans-free Vegetable Oils in Shortenings and Deep-fat Frying. *Lipid Technology* **2005,** *17,* 101–106.

Pantzaris, T. P. *Pocketbook of Palm Oil Uses,* 5th ed.; Malaysian Palm Oil Board: Perniagaan Rita, Kaula Lampur, 2000.

Redgrave, T. G.; Kodali, D. R.; Small, D. M. The Effect of Triacyl-*sn*-glycerol Structure on the Metabolism of Chylomicrons and Triacylglycerol-rich Emulsions in the Rat. *J. Biol. Chem.* **1988,** *263,* 5118–5123.

Sato, K. Polymorphism of Pure Traiacylglycerols and Natural Fats. In *Advances in Applied Lipid Research,* Vol. 2; Padley, F., Ed.; New York: JAI Press Inc., 1996; pp 213–268.

Sato, K.; Ueno, S. Molecular Interactions and Phase Behavior of Polymorphic fats. In *Crystallization Processes in Fats and Lipid Systems*; Garti, N., Sato, K.. Eds.; Marcel Dekker: New York, 2001; pp 177–209.

Sato, K.; Goto, M.; Yano, J.; Honda, K.; Kodali, D. R.; Small, D. M. Atomic Resolution Structure Analysis of Beta Prime Polymorph Crystal of a Triacylglycerol: 1,2-Dipalmitoyl-3-myristol-*sn*-glycerol, *Journal of Lipid Research* **2001,** *42,* 338–334.

Small, D. M. Lateral Chain Packing in Lipids and Membranes. *Journal of Lipid Research* **1984,** *25,* 1490–1500.

Stender, S.; Dyerberg, J.; Astrup, A. Consumer Protection through a Legislative Ban on Industrially Produced *Trans* Fatty Acids in Foods in Denmark. *Scandinavian Journal of Food and Nutrition* **2006,** *50* (4), 155–160.

Technical Committee of the Institute of Shortening and Edible Oils (ISEO). *Food Fats and Oils,* 9th ed.; Institute of Shortening and Edible Oils Inc.: Washington DC, 2006; pp 1–37.

Thomas, A. Fats and Fatty Oils. In *Ullman's Encyclopedia of Industrial Chemistry,* Wiley-VCH: Weinheim, 2012; pp. 1–71.

Vergroesen, A. J.; Gottenbos, J. J. Introduction. In *The Role of Fats in Human Nutrition;* Vergroesen, A. J., Ed.; Academic Press: New York, 1975; pp 2–41.

Warner, K. Increasing Gamma- and Delta-tocopherols in Oils Improves Oxidative Stability. *Lipid Technology* **2007,** *19,* 229–231.

FAO Food and Nutrition Paper 91. Chapter 2: Summary of Conclusions and Dietary Recommendations on Total Fat and Fatty Acids. In *Fats and Fatty Acids in Human Nutrition: Report of an Expert Consultation* **2010**, 9–19.

Yano, J.; Sato, K.; Kaneko, F.; Small, D. M.; Kodali, D. R. Structural Analysis of Polymorphic Transitions of sn-1,3-Distearoyl-2-Oleoylglycerol (SOS) and sn-1,3-Dioleoyl-2-Stearoyl-glycerol (OSO): Assessment on Steric Hindrance of Saturated Acyl Chain Interactions. *Journal of Lipid Research* **1999,** *40,* 140–151.

2

Natural versus Industrial *Trans* Fatty Acids

Frédéric Destaillats ■ *Nestlé Research Center, Lausanne, Switzerland*

Ye Flora Wang ■ *Metabolic and Cardiovascular Disease Laboratory, Alberta Diabetes Institute, Alberta Institute for Human Nutrition, Alberta, Canada*

David J. Baer ■ *Food Components and Health Laboratory, U.S. Department of Agriculture, Agricultural Research Service, Beltsville, Maryland, USA*

Natural versus Industrial *Trans* Fats: Basic Hypothesis and Background

The objective of this chapter is to guide the reader through the recent literature suggesting that "natural *trans* fatty acids" (TFAs) might have different nutritional values than "industrial TFAs" and review available scientific evidence related to this hypothesis. Such an objective requires accepting the following hypothesis: Consumption of industrial TFAs has no nutritional benefit and may negatively impact human physiology. Several observational and randomized clinical trials have confirmed that the consumption of industrial TFAs increases serum LDL-C and the total:HDL-C ratio relative to saturated and *cis*-unsaturated fatty acid on an isocaloric basis (Mozaffarian et al., 2006). Mechanisms of action still need to be elucidated, but the overall consensus plan to improve health is for the removal of TFAs from the entire food supply chain.

Natural versus Industrial *Trans* Fatty Acids: Chemistry and Dietary Sources

Trans fatty acids are found in almost all food product categories that contain a source of dietary lipids. Their amount and nature differs with the origin and composition of the lipids present in these products. In the recent literature, the term *industrial TFAs* has been used extensively to address the TFAs formed during industrial processes, such as catalytic hydrogenation of vegetable oils, in contrast to the term *natural TFAs*, which is used to describe the TFAs present in lipids from ruminant animal origin. This classification appears to be simple, but the reality is more complex because structural differences between these two categories are subtle. Among the TFAs found in foods, few can exclusively be qualified as industrial TFAs. These TFAs are basically formed from essential fatty acids during the refining process and are known as geometrical isomers of linoleic and α-linolenic acids (structures are provided in Figure 2.1). Similarly, it appears that the only natural TFA that can be exclusively

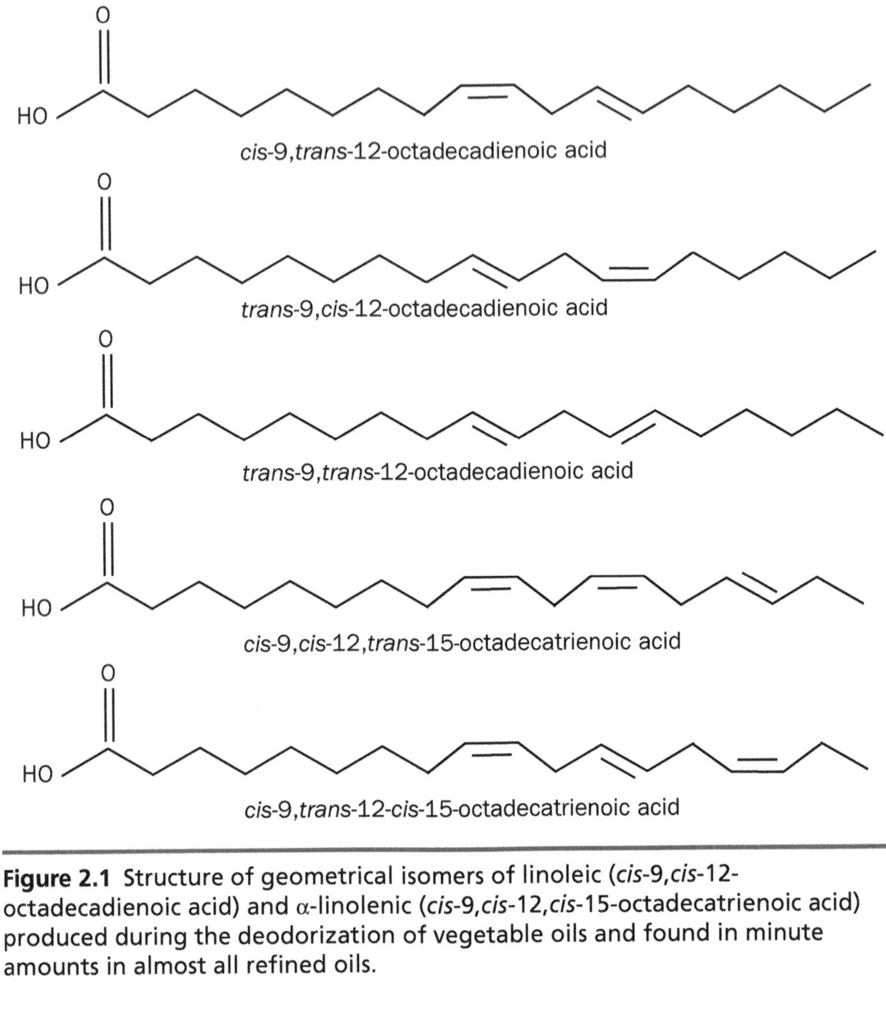

Figure 2.1 Structure of geometrical isomers of linoleic (*cis*-9,*cis*-12-octadecadienoic acid) and α-linolenic (*cis*-9,*cis*-12,*cis*-15-octadecatrienoic acid) produced during the deodorization of vegetable oils and found in minute amounts in almost all refined oils.

found in animal fat is rumenic acid, a conjugated linoleic acid (CLA) isomer (see Figure 2.2).

The majority of TFAs found in food products are *trans*-octadecenoic (*trans*-18:1) acid isomers (see Figure 2.3). *Trans*-18:1 acid isomers can be formed by "natural" and "industrial" processes by partial hydrogenation of linoleic and α-linolenic acids. The isomeric distribution of *trans*-18:1 acids differs between ruminant fats and partially hydrogenated vegetable oils (PHVO) (see Figure 2.4 on page 46). In ruminant animals (e.g., cow, buffalo, goat, and sheep), partial hydrogenation of essential fatty

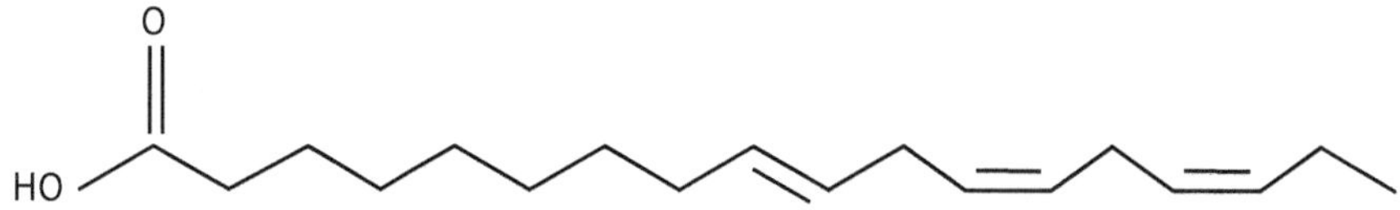

trans-9,*cis*-12-*cis*-15-octadecatrienoic acid

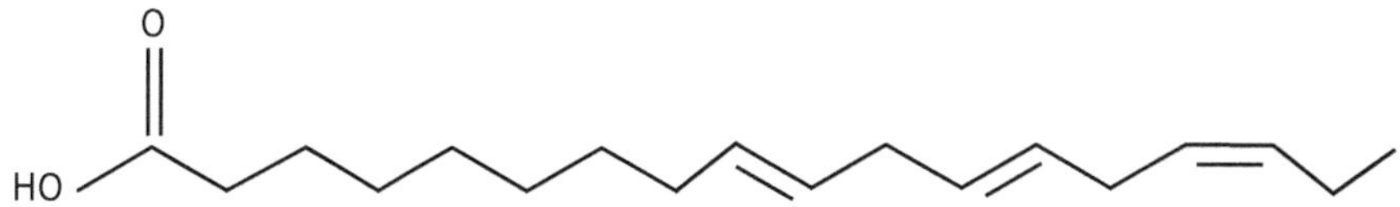

trans-9,*trans*-12,*cis*-15-octadecatrienoic acid

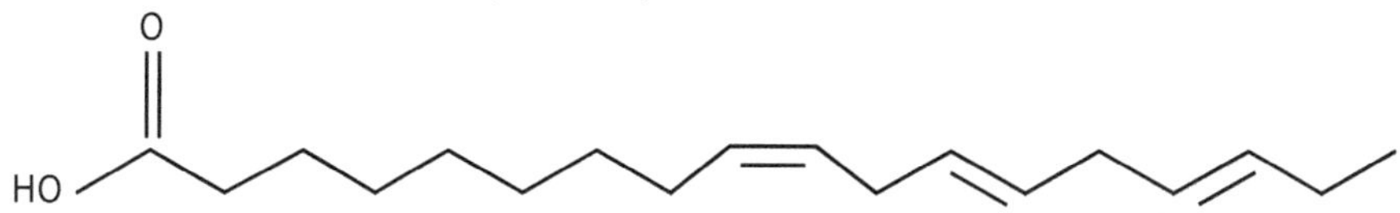

cis-9,*trans*-12,*trans*-15-octadecatrienoic acid

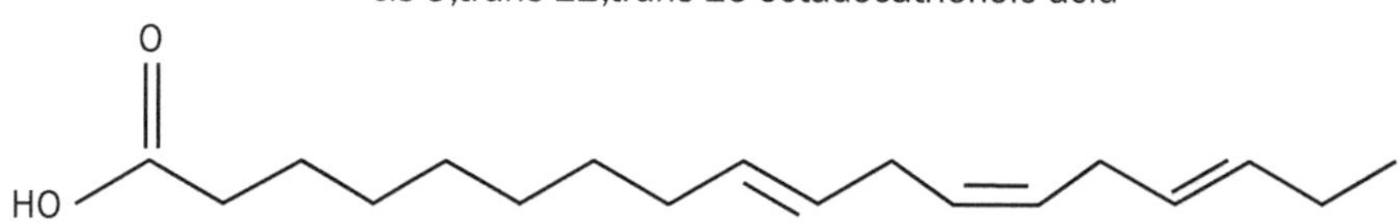

trans-9,*cis*-12,*trans*-15-octadecatrienoic acid

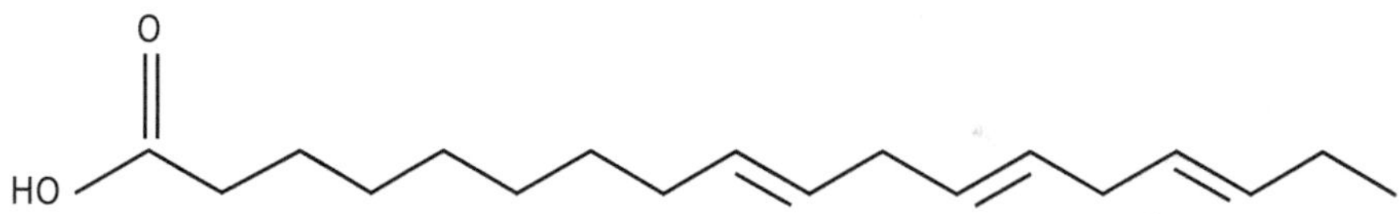

trans-9,*trans*-12,*trans*-15-octadecatrienoic acid

Figure 2.1 *Continued*

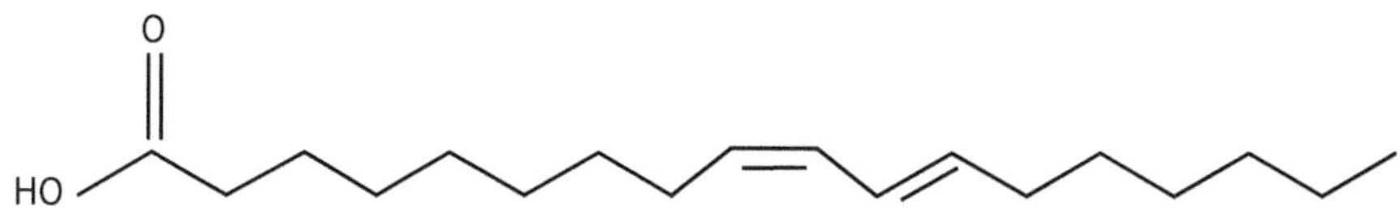

cis-9,*trans*-11-octadecadienoic acid

Figure 2.2 Structure of rumenic acid, a natural conjugated linoleic acid (CLA) isomer, formed either by partial biohydrogenation of essential fatty acids in ruminants or from its dietary precursor vaccenic (*trans*-11 18:1) acid by Δ9-desaturation in animals.

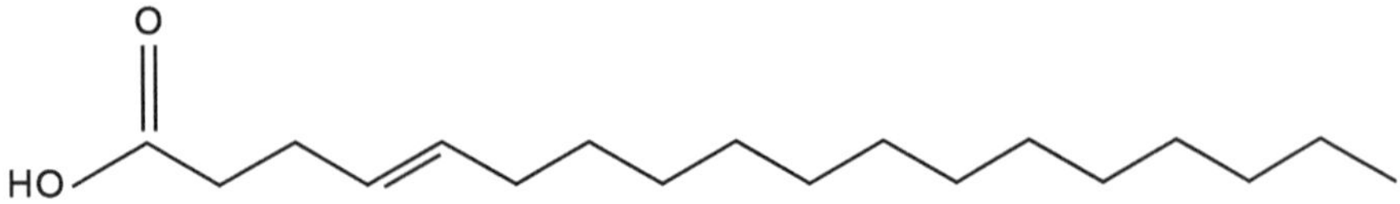

trans-4-octadecenoic acid

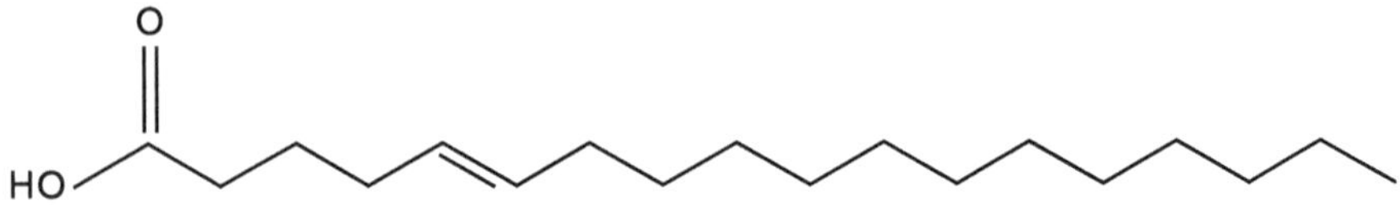

trans-5-octadecenoic acid

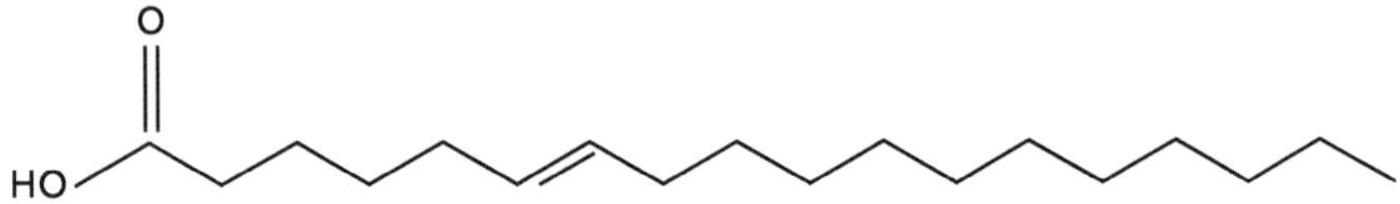

trans-6-octadecenoic acid

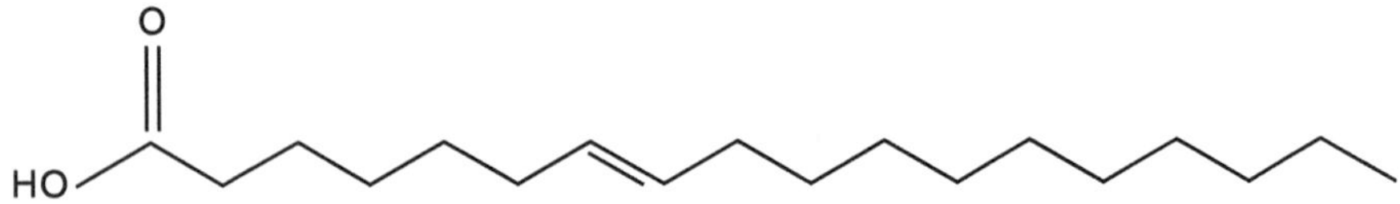

trans-7-octadecenoic acid

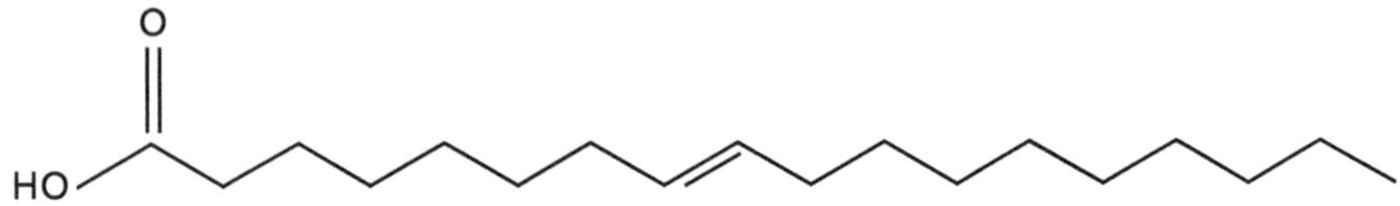

trans-8-octadecenoic acid

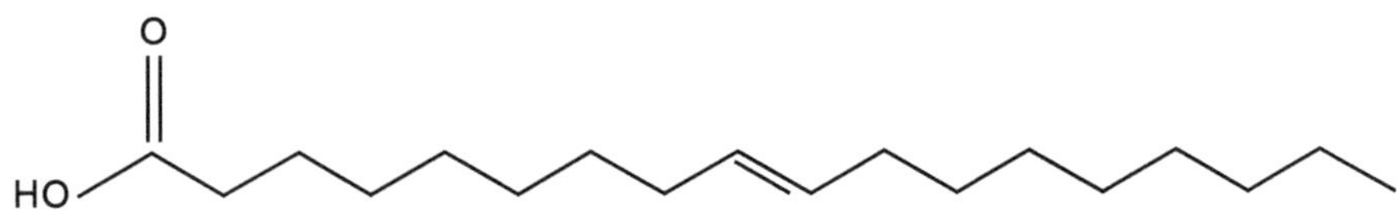

trans-9-octadecenoic acid

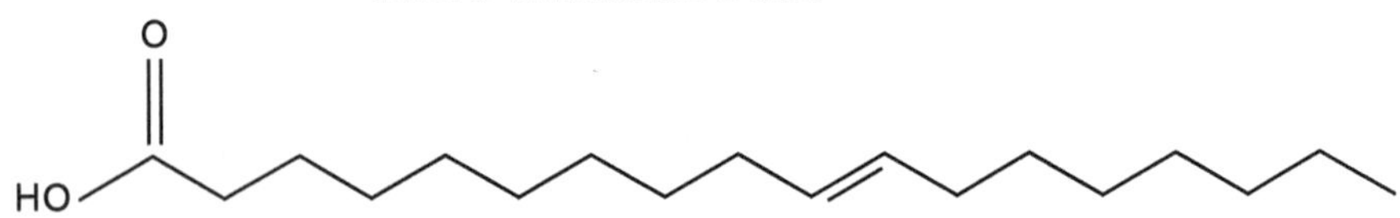

trans-10-octadecenoic acid

Figure 2.3 Structure of the *trans* positional isomers of octadecenoic acids formed either naturally by partial biohydrogenation of essential fatty acids in ruminants (linoleic and α- linolenic acids) or by catalytic (partial) hydrogenation of vegetable oils.

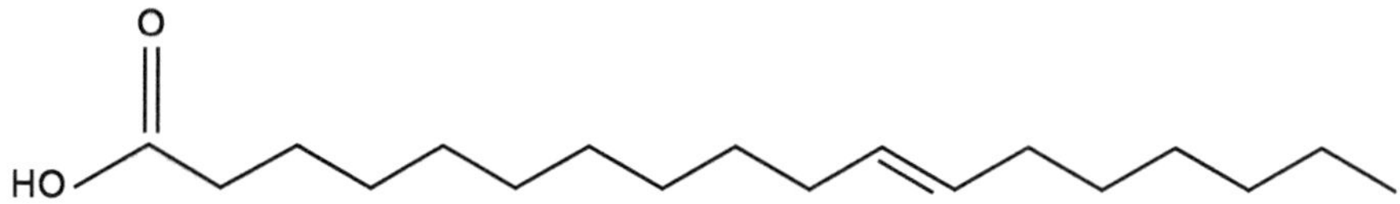

trans-11-octadecenoic acid

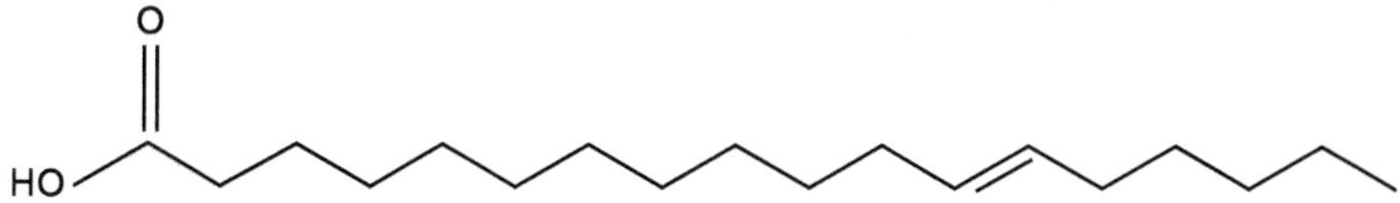

trans-12-octadecenoic acid

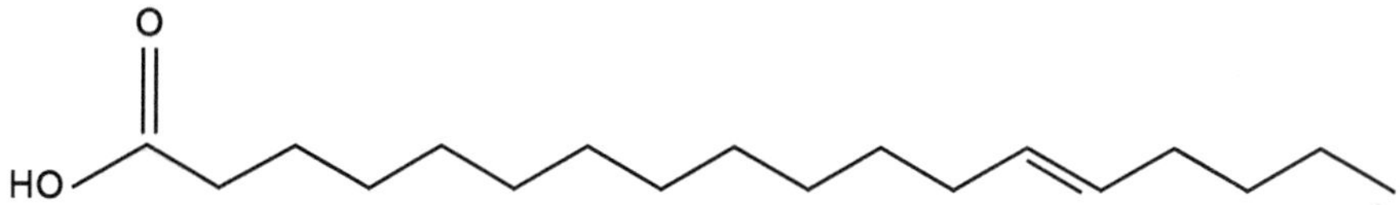

trans-13-octadecenoic acid

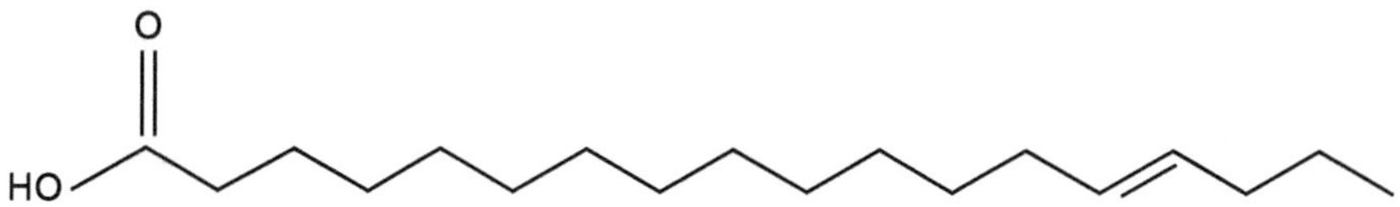

trans-14-octadecenoic acid

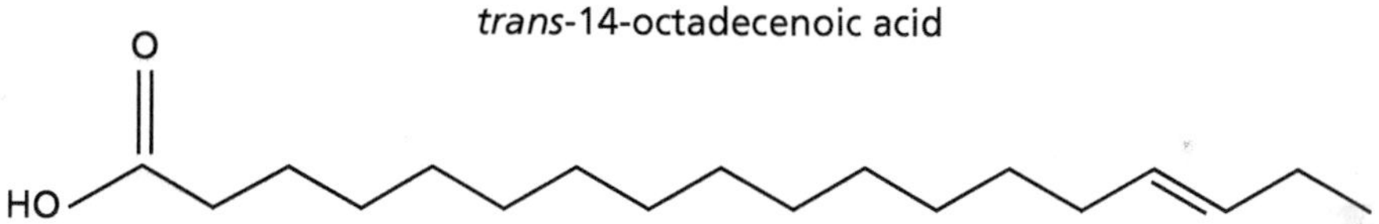

trans-15-octadecenoic acid

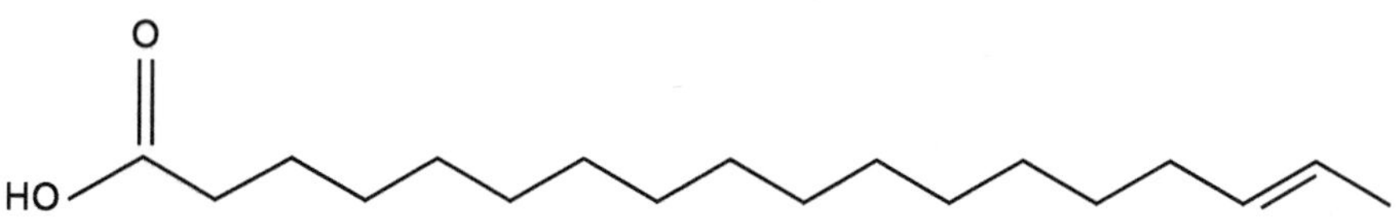

trans-16-octadecenoic acid

Figure 2.3 *Continued*

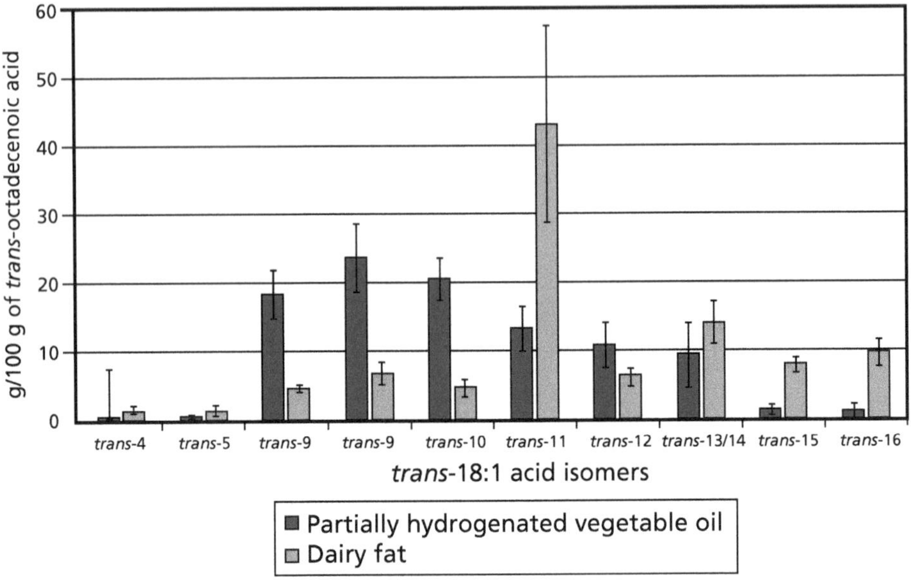

Figure 2.4 Isomeric distribution envelope of *trans*-18:1 acids in dairy fat (n = 1765) and partially hydrogenated vegetable oils (PHVO, n = 46). Data adapted from Precht and Molkentin (1995).

acids occurs in the rumen by bacterial metabolism of dietary lipids. This biological process ends mainly with the formation of stearic (18:0) and vaccenic (*trans*-11 18:1) acids, as well as various amounts of all the other positional isomers and intermediates (see Figure 2.4). In contrast, the partial hydrogenation of vegetable oils results in the formation of mainly elaidic (*trans*-9 18:1), *trans*-10 18:1, and in some cases *trans*-6/8 18:1 acid isomers, depending on the process condition and composition of the starting materials (Bezelgues and Dijkstra, 2009). In addition to the differences in their isomeric distribution, the absolute content of *trans*-18:1 acids in ruminant fats and in PHVO can also substantially differ (Enjalbert and Troegeler-Meynadier, 2009; Lock et al., 2009). Indeed, in PHVO, the amount of TFAs will depend on the extent of the hydrogenation process, which depends on the targeted physical properties after processing. Accordingly, TFA concentration can range from 1% to 60% of total fatty acids, depending on the melting point of the processed fat (Bezelgues and Dijkstra, 2009). However, in animal fats, biohydrogenation in the rumen is tightly regulated and the concentration of *trans*-18:1 acids ranges naturally from 2% to 5% of total fatty acids, and is mainly influenced by the quality and quantity of the lipids consumed by the animals (Enjalbert and Troegeler-Meynadier, 2009).

Analytical Considerations and Biomarkers of Intake

In order to be able to investigate whether TFAs from natural or industrial origins can differentially impact human physiology, it is necessary to understand: (1) whether it is possible to discriminate natural TFAs and industrial TFAs based on their chemical identities in food products, and (2) whether it is possible to distinguish different biomarkers of consumption. The first question relates to the understanding of the chemical composition and ability to quantify the isomeric distribution of the different TFA series in fats and oils from the different origins. Analytical methods are available to quantitatively characterize TFAs in foods, and best practices are now very well-accepted by the scientific communities and regulatory agencies. Therefore, it is possible to claim that the chemical composition of TFAs in foods is known and, by extension, that it is, in principle, possible to evaluate the intake "exposure" of consumers. A lot of data has been published on the TFA content and distribution in fats and oils, and a summary of the sources of different TFAs is provided in Table 2.A.

Although the TFA composition and content in fats, oils, and food products is known, the metabolic fate of the different TFAs in humans following consumption of a variety of food products is far more complex. Indeed, this requires a good understanding of the metabolism of the different TFAs and their dispositions in biofluids and tissues. Important data have been obtained using tracer studies in vivo, as well as using in vitro systems, and this specific topic has been recently reviewed (Sébédio and Christie, 2009). One significant finding that has been obtained is that vaccenic (*trans*-11 18:1) acid is metabolized by animals, including humans (Adlof et al., 2000; Turpeinen et al., 2002) and is converted to rumenic (*cis*-9,*trans*-11 18:2) acid, as depicted in Figure 2.5. The enzyme that is responsible for this step is stearoyl-CoA desaturase or Δ-9-desaturase (Lock et al., 2009). Rumenic acid is therefore present in

Table 2.A Concentration of the Different TFA Classes in Vegetable Oils (Refined but Not Hydrogenated), Partially Hydrogenated Vegetable Oils (PHVO), and Ruminant Fats (Butter Fat)

Trans Fatty Acid	Vegetable Oils	PHVO	Ruminant Fats
trans-18:1	—	1–60%	2–5%
trans-16:1	traces	traces	<0.5%
trans-18:2	0.5–3%	—	0.5–1%
trans-18:3	0.5–3%	—	traces
cis-9,*trans*-11 18:2	—	—	0.5–1%

Source: Data adapted from Precht and Molkentin (1995).

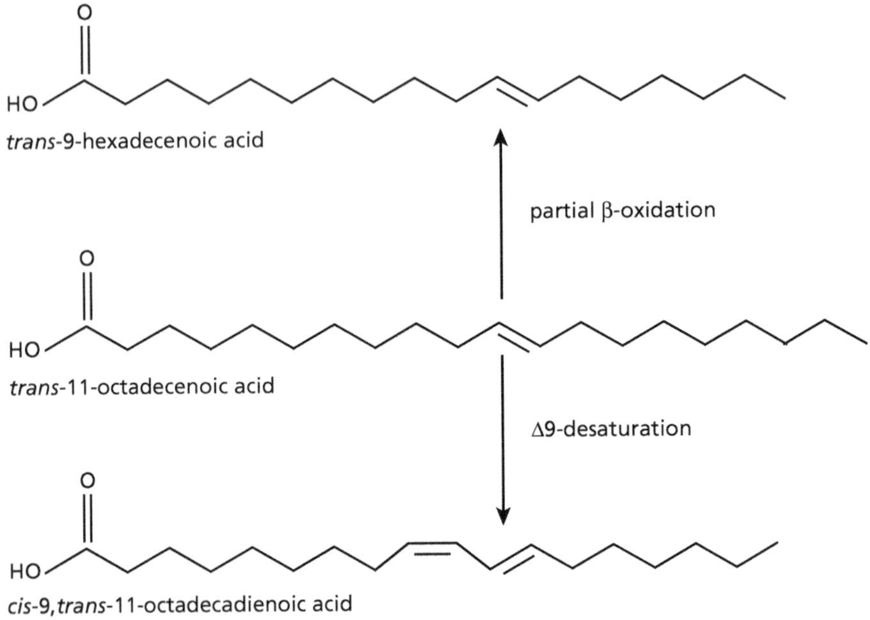

Figure 2.5 Biotransformation of vaccenic (*trans*-11 18:1) acid in humans. Adapted from Adlof et al. (2000).

biofluids and tissues of animals fed with a dietary source of vaccenic acid, such as butter fat or ruminant meat (Lock et al., 2009; Sébédio and Christie, 2009). Similarly, it has been shown that a minor isomer, *trans*-7 18:1 acid, is converted by the same enzyme into another CLA isomer: *trans*-7,*cis*-9 18:2 acid (Lock et al., 2009; Sébédio and Christie, 2009). The extent of the conversion of vaccenic to rumenic acid in humans has been estimated to range between 19% and 25% (Lock et al., 2009); therefore, vaccenic acid is also recovered in tissues and biofluids. It has been reported that *trans*-18:1 acids, such as vaccenic acid, can be partially β-oxidized (chain shortening) (Sébédio and Christie, 2009) and converted into *trans*-9 16:1 acid (see Figure 2.5), which has been reported to be a relevant marker of TFA intake in humans (Micha et al., 2010). The quantification of *trans*-9 16:1 acid is complex because this fatty acid co-elutes with *cis*-16:1 acid or branched chain 17 fatty acids, even on long and polar capillary columns such as 100 m CP-Sil 88 (Precht and Molkentin, 1999). Quantification of total *trans*-18:1 and rumenic acids can be done quite precisely with numerous capillary columns by gas chromatography (Ratnayake and Cruz-Hernandez, 2009). It is, therefore, very important to assess the selectivity of the method used before expressing results and performing complex statistics aimed at associating biomarkers of intake with biological outcomes.

In the course of clinical intervention or observational studies, it is possible to obtain whole blood, plasma, and red blood cells from volunteers. In rare cases, it is possible to sample adipose tissue or breast milk samples. TFAs have been analyzed in all of these types of biological samples, and it has been proposed that the content and profile found in tissues such as adipose tissue (Boué et al., 2000; Castro-Webb et al., 2012; Clifton et al., 2004; Enig et al., 1990; Ohlrogge et al., 1981; Smit et al., 2010) or breast milk (Chardigny et al., 1995; Chen et al., 1995; Li et al., 2009; Mosley et al., 2005, 2006; Mueller et al., 2010; Precht and Molkentin, 1999; Ratnayake and Chen, 1996; Samur et al., 2009; Wolff, 1995) provide a direct reflection of their intake. In addition, the analysis of blood lipids, such as total plasma (Enke et al., 2011), serum (Smedman et al., 1999; Warensjö et al., 2010), plasma phospholipids (Micha et al., 2010; Mozaffarian et al., 2010), plasma cholesteryl esters (Zock et al., 1997), and erythrocyte (Yu et al., 2012) also has been proposed as a good proxy of TFA intake. In large cohort trials, the technical challenge is to identify and use adequate analytical methods with enough sensitivity and resolution to quantify TFA isomers. TFAs found in different human biological samples are listed in Table 2.B.

The quantification of TFAs in adipose tissue has been proposed as a way to evaluate intake of TFAs (Boué et al., 2000). Based on regression analysis, Enig et al.

Table 2.B Specific Biomarkers of Intake of Natural and Industrial TFA in Plasma Phospholipids

	Biomarkers of Intake in Plasma Phospholipids		
TFA	**Natural TFA**	**Industrial TFA**	**Main Dietary Sources**
Total *trans*-18:1		X	Foods made with PHVO, including margarine, and bakery and fried products
trans-18:2		X	Bakery products
trans-9 16:1[a]	X		Red meats, butter, and higher fat dairy products
trans-7 16:1		X	Margarine

[a]Formed by biotransformation of vaccenic (*trans*-11 18:1) acid.

Source: Adapted from Micha et al. (2010).

(1990) proposed that TFA intake can be evaluated by measuring total *trans*-18:1 acids in adipose tissue and by applying the following equation:

$$y = 0.97 + 0.44x$$

where y is the estimated intake and x is the level of *trans*-18:1 acids in adipose tissues expressed as t%.

This equation has been used by Boué et al. (2000) to evaluate the TFA intake of subjects from adipose tissues samples. Similarly, it has been demonstrated that *trans*-18:1 acids accretion in plasma cholesteryl esters provides an accurate measurement of the intake of *trans*-18:1 acids (Zock et al., 1997). The turnover of lipids in plasma is much quicker than in adipose tissue and, therefore, the choice of the type of sample will depend on the duration of the trial. Indeed, to measure the compliance in the framework of a clinical trial, the analysis of TFAs in cholesteryl esters is a preferred option. However, for observational studies aimed at understanding nutritional patterns over a much longer time frame, analysis of adipose tissue might be the preferred tissue sample.

To our knowledge, a method to estimate the relative proportion of TFAs coming from natural or industrial origins by analyzing biological samples has not been developed; therefore, it is very difficult to evaluate the relative intake of both sources of TFAs from biological samples. The prerequisite for such work will be the determination of specific biomarkers of TFA intake representative of natural or industrial TFA sources, or to have extensive and accurate food composition data as well as appropriate validated dietary questionnaires. Micha et al. (2010) conducted an observational study on 3330 adults from the Cardiovascular Health Study and investigated the relationship between the composition of plasma phospholipids and dietary intake of the different sources of TFAs. In this study, population, total *trans*-18:1, *trans*-18:2 (sum of the three geometrical isomers), and *trans*-7 16:1 acids were specific markers of the intake of industrial TFA–containing foods (see Table 2.B). As expected, because of its metabolic origin (see Figure 2.5), *trans*-9 16:1 acid was identified as a specific marker of natural TFA intake (Adlof et al., 2000). This work is extremely valuable and provides information on selective biomarkers.

Impact of Natural and Industrial TFAs on Blood Lipid Profile and Coronary Heart Disease Risk

Consumption of TFAs from PHVO, but not from ruminant sources, has been implicated to contribute significantly to increased risk of cardiovascular diseases (CVD) (Bendsen et al., 2011; Gebauer et al., 2011; Mozaffarian et al., 2009). When specific TFA isomers were studied, nonconjugated *trans*-18:2 have been shown to have a stronger positive relationship with CVD than that for other TFAs (Baylin et al., 2003; Lemaitre et al., 2006; Micha et al., 2010). We hereby present recent evidence from epidemiological, clinical, and mechanistic studies that focused specifically on the impact of natural and industrial TFAs on blood lipid profile, which may explain, in part, their different impacts on cardiovascular health.

Data Available from Epidemiologic and Clinical Studies

A meta-analysis of 12 controlled trials suggested that consuming TFAs mainly from industrial sources increases serum LDL-C and the total:HDL-C ratio relative to saturated and *cis*-unsaturated fatty acid on an isocaloric basis (Mozaffarian et al., 2006). Every 1% energy replacement of carbohydrates by industrial TFAs increased serum LDL-C by 0.04 mmol/L. Every 1% energy replacement of TFA with saturated, *cis*-monounsaturated fatty acids, and polyunsaturated fatty acids, on the other hand, decreased the total:HDL-C ratios by 0.31, 0.54, and 0.67, respectively (Mozaffarian and Clarke, 2009). These changes in blood lipids are consistent with observations from the U.S. National Health and Nutrition Examination Survey (NHANES) cross-sectional data collected in 2000 and 2009, which represents two time periods, one before and one after the U.S. Food and Drug Administration (FDA) mandated the food labeling of TFAs (Vesper et al., 2012). Consistent with the trends shown in the meta-analyses (Mozaffarian and Clarke, 2009), preliminary data from the NHANES dataset showed a reduction in serum LDL-C concentration, which was accompanied by 50–60% reductions in the plasma concentrations of four major TFA isomers (Vesper et al., 2012). Three out of the four TFA isomers studied (elaidic acid, palmitelaidic acid, and geometrical isomers of linoleic acid) were predominantly from partially hydrogenated oils, whereas vaccenic (*trans*-11 18:1) acid may be derived from both natural and industrial sources (Wolff et al., 2000). Unfortunately, a more detailed assessment of the correlations between LDL-C and individual TFA isomers was not feasible in this cohort due to limited information. Using data from another U.S. cohort (the Cardiovascular Health Study), Micah et al. (2010) investigated the association between plasma palmitelaidic (*trans*-9 16:1) acid, a marker for the intake of naturally occurring ruminant TFAs (Micha et al., 2010), and metabolic risk factors (Mozaffarian et al., 2010). Results from this cohort indicated that palmitelaidic acid intake was inversely correlated with total/HDL-C and triglyceride and was independent of adiposity (Mozaffarian et al., 2010). In regions where total TFA intakes were below 0.5% of energy, data remain limited for the impact of TFAs on blood lipid profile. In a recent study in middle-aged and older Chinese individuals (n = 3107), a positive correlation was established between hypertriglyceridemia/high LDL-C concentrations and erythrocyte *trans*-18:2 acid isomers (major industrial TFAs in the Chinese diet) but not with total *trans*-18:1 acid isomers, which are derived primarily from dairy food in this cohort (Yu et al., 2012). However, in a group of Japanese young women (n = 133), no association was found between total/diene TFA intake and serum cholesterol levels (Takeuchi et al., 2012). More robust evidence in support of the differential bioactivities between industrial and ruminant *trans* fat has been presented in a recent meta-analysis of large prospective cohort studies including the Nurses' Health Study, the Zutphen Elderly Study, and the MONICA study, suggesting that dietary consumption of ruminant *trans* fat may be protective against total, as well as fatal, coronary heart disease events (Bendsen et al., 2011).

In addition to observational studies, findings from some randomized controlled trials suggest that natural TFA–enriched dairy fat had neutral effects on serum lipid and lipoprotein profiles in normolipidemic, yet overweight, humans when consumed in moderation (reviewed by Gebauer et al., 2011). Among the few studies that directly compared the health effects of natural and industrial TFAs, dairy fat enriched with natural TFAs appears to be neutral on blood cholesterol profile at moderate consumption levels (1.5% energy), but may be as detrimental as industrial TFAs at extremely high consumption levels (3.6% energy) that would likely be difficult to reach in the general public even with dairy products enriched with TFAs (Motard-Belanger et al., 2008). Recently, the effects of milk naturally enriched with rumenic (*cis*-9,*trans*-11 18:2) acid (1.0 g/day) and vaccenic acid (2.6 g/day) on blood lipids, liver function, and body composition have been examined in overweight humans (Venkatramanan et al., 2010). In this 8-week intervention study, conventional milk (0.3 g vaccenic and 0.2 g rumenic acids/day) was used as the control, and no significant changes were observed in both CLA-supplemented groups on any parameter measured. Similarly, neutral effects of natural TFA (from pasture-fed beef) on blood lipids and body composition were observed in healthy women in a U.S. intervention study at the same dose and duration relative to grain-fed ground beef (Brown et al., 2011). In a group of healthy Canadian women (n = 61), TFA-enriched butter showed a neutral effect on LDL-C relative to regular butter containing one-third of the TFA content in TFA-enriched butter (Lacroix et al., 2012). However, compared to earlier studies, in this Canadian study, the amount of TFA consumed was one-quarter the dose that was used in the other studies, and the length of the intervention was one-half the duration of the earlier studies. Unfortunately, no data have been published thus far using purified preparations of individual TFA isomers in individuals with or without increased CVD risk, which warrants further investigation.

Data Available from Preclinical Studies

The consumption of PHVO, as the major source of industrial TFAs, has been associated with increased serum TAG, total cholesterol, and LDL-C, as compared to oleic acid and fish oil in several animal models of dyslipidemia and cardiovascular disease (Chiang and Lu, 1996; Chiang et al., 1991; Gatto et al., 2001, 2002; Kraft et al., 2011; Park and Park, 2009). On the other hand, there is consistent evidence that natural TFA, either as purified individual isomers or enriched ruminant fat, substantially improves atherogenic lipid profiles (e.g., TAG, LDL-C, and total cholesterol) and hepatic steatosis in a few rodent models of dyslipidemia and metabolic syndrome (Basset et al., 2010; Jacome-Sosa et al., 2010; Meijer et al., 2001; Tyburczy et al., 2009; Wang et al., 2009). In guinea pigs, whose lipid and lipoprotein metabolism largely resembles humans, natural TFA–enriched dairy fat but not industrially produced TFA, raised concentrations of plasma total and small HDL-C (Rice et al., 2010, 2012). It has been further proposed that vaccenic acid binds to and functionally activates peroxisome proliferator-activated receptor (PPAR)-α and -γ, both of which are common targets for lipid-lowering and anti-diabetic medications such as fenofibrates and thiazolidinedoines, respectively (Wang et al., 2012).

A number of recent in vitro cell culture studies have provided an updated perspective in support of the differential bioactivity on cellular metabolic pathways between major TFA isomers. For example, treatment of elaidic acid and palmitic acid, but not vaccenic acid, was associated with impaired cholesterol efflux from mouse and human macrophages (Fournier et al., 2012), which may explain the differences in their effects on cholesterol lipoprotein profiles observed in humans and animal models. The authors credited the changes to reduced long-chain polyunsaturated fatty acid (PUFA) incorporation into membrane phospholipids, and thus altered membrane fluidity in elaidic acid–treated macrophages (Fournier et al., 2012). The negative effect of elaidic acid on n-3 long chain PUFA incorporation is consistent with a recent cross-sectional study assessing maternal TFA intake and corresponding fetal blood fatty acid composition (Enke et al., 2011). The distinctive bioactivity on membrane PUFA incorporation between vaccenic and elaidic acids, and subsequent changes in cell signaling pathways, may be explained by earlier studies that demonstrate elaidic acid (and to a lesser extent linoelaidic acid) is a potent inhibitor of Δ5-desaturation (critical for the biosynthesis of n-3 and n-6 PUFA). No such effect was shown for vaccenic acid (Rosenthal and Doloresco, 1984).

Public Health Implications

Because of the negative health effects of dietary TFAs, there have been public health initiatives around the world to reduce dietary TFA intake. In the United States, the FDA revised food labeling requirements in 2003 to include declaration of TFAs on food labels. These changes took place in 2006, and both the U.S. food industry and the restaurant industry responded by reducing TFAs in ingredients and food products. In 2007, the Canadian Minister of Health called for the food industry to limit TFAs in foods to 2% in vegetable oils and spreads, and to 5% of total fat in other foods. Several European countries, including Denmark, Iceland, Switzerland, and Austria, have laws limiting use of TFAs in foods. In 2004, the World Health Organization (WHO) published a report calling for a shift in fat consumption toward the total elimination of TFAs (WHO, 2004). These initiatives have been primarily focused on industrial sources of TFAs. At this point in time, however, sufficient evidence does not exist to support public health initiatives to limit TFAs from natural sources for several reasons, including lack of clear evidence of negative health effects of natural TFAs, the small dietary contribution that natural TFAs comprises due to very low TFA concentration, and the other essential nutrients that are provided by food ingredients containing natural TFAs, as explained below.

While both observational and intervention studies have suggested associations between industrial TFA intake and increases in risk factors for cardiovascular disease, recent data suggest the association between natural TFAs and cardiovascular disease risk may be less. Studies using vaccenic acid or *trans*-enriched dairy products have shown negative effects on LDL-C and an inconsistent effect on HDL-C (Gebauer et al., 2011). Detrimental health effects of naturally occurring TFAs have been observed to occur only at very high intakes (3.6% of energy), which would be difficult to achieve with the available food supply. Such a level of intake cannot be reached by consuming regular foods; thus, evidence with respect to negative health effects of naturally occurring TFAs at amounts typically consumed does not exist at this time to justify reduction of naturally occurring TFA-containing foods from the diet.

The amount of TFAs consumed from natural sources in the diet is quite low, and thus the window for impacting health through reduction of natural TFAs is quite small. Estimates of natural TFA intakes have been published for Australia, New Zealand, Canada, Denmark, and the United States, and these data suggest that natural *trans* intake is less than 0.5% of total energy intake. Thus, reduction of foods containing natural TFAs to half the current intake would result in reduction of less than a gram of *trans* fat per day, which would likely have no measurable influence on health (Gebauer et al., 2011).

Sources of natural TFAs are derived from ruminant animals and include meat (cow, sheep, goat) and dairy. All of these are excellent sources (providing at least 20% DV) or good sources (providing 10–19% DV) of many shortfall nutrients. Beef is an excellent or good source of nine essential nutrients, including protein, phosphorus, selenium, zinc, iron, niacin, vitamin B6, vitamin B12, and riboflavin. Sheep and goat meat are similarly good sources of these nutrients. Dairy is also an excellent or good source of nine essential nutrients, including calcium, phosphorous, potassium, riboflavin, niacin, vitamin B12, vitamin D, and vitamin A. Thus, public health initiatives discouraging intake of natural TFAs would likely result in a greater proportion of the population not meeting requirements for these essential and shortfall nutrients.

In sum, although consumption of industrial TFAs has been convincingly shown to convey negative impacts on health, the potential health impact of high intakes of natural TFAs is still unclear. However, current evidence suggests consumption of natural TFAs at levels actually found in the diet does not negatively impact health in a measurable way. Moreover, foods containing natural TFAs also provide essential nutrients. Thus, at this point, public health policy should focus on industrial TFAs rather than those from natural sources.

References

Adlof, R. O.; Duval, S.; Emken, E. A. Biosynthesis of Conjugated Linoleic Acid in Humans. *Lipids* **2000,** *35,* 131–135.

Bassett, C. M.; Edel, A. L.; Patenaude, A. F.; McCullough, R. S.; Blackwood, D. P.; Chouinard, P. Y.; Paquin, P.; Lamarche, B.; Pierce, G. N. Dietary Vaccenic Acid Has Antiatherogenic Effects in LDLr-/-mice. *J. Nutr.* **2010,** *140,* 18–24.

Baylin, A.; Kabagambe, E. K.; Ascherio, A.; Spiegelman, D.; Campos, H. High 18:2 *Trans*-Fatty Acids in Adipose Tissue Are Associated with Increased Risk of Nonfatal Acute Myocardial Infarction in Costa Rican Adults. *J. Nutr.* **2003,** *133,* 1186–1191.

Bendsen, N. T.; Christensen, R.; Bartels, E. M.; Astrup, A. Consumption of Industrial and Ruminant *Trans* Fatty Acids and Risk of Coronary Heart Disease: A Systematic Review and Meta-analysis of Cohort Studies. *Eur. J. Clin. Nutr.* **2011,** *65,* 773–783.

Bezelgues, J. B., Dijkstra, A. J. Formation of Trans Fatty Acids During Catalytic Hydrogenation of Edible Oils. In *Trans Fatty Acids in Human Nutrition,* 2nd ed.; Destaillats, F., Sébédio, J. L., Dionisi, F., Chardigny, J. M., Eds.; The Oily Press, P. J. Barnes & Associates: Bridgwater, UK, 2009.

Boué, C.; Combe, N.; Billeaud, C., Mignerot, C.; Entressangles, B.; Thery, G.; Geoffrion, H.; Brun, J. L.; Dallay, D.; Leng, J. J. *Trans* Fatty Acids in Adipose Tissue of French Women in Relation to Their Dietary Sources. *Lipids* **2000,** *35,* 561–566.

Brown, A. W.; Trenkle, A. H.; Beitz, D. C. Diets High in Conjugated Linoleic Acid from Pasture-fed Cattle Did Not Alter Markers of Health in Young Women. *Nutr. Res.* **2011,** 31, 33–41.

Castro-Webb, N.; Ruiz-Narváez, E. A.; Campos, H. Cross-sectional Study of Conjugated Linoleic Acid in Adipose Tissue and Risk of Diabetes. *Am. J. Clin. Nutr.* **2012,** *96,* 175–181.

Chardigny, J. M.; Wolff, R. L.; Mager, E.; Sébédio, J. L.; Martine, L.; Juanéda, P. *Trans* Mono- and Polyunsaturated Fatty Acids in Human Milk. *Eur. J. Clin. Nutr.* **1995,** *49,* 523–531.

Chen, Z. Y.; Pelletier, G.; Hollywood, R.; Ratnayake, W. M. N. *Trans* Fatty Acid Isomers in Canadian Human Milk. *Lipids* **1995,** *30,* 15–21.

Chiang, M. T.; Lu, Y. S. Variation of Plasma Cholesterol Levels in Rats Fed *Trans* Fatty Acids or *Cis* Fatty Acids. *Int. J. Vitam. Nutr. Res.* **1996,** *66,* 263–269.

Chiang, M. T.; Otomo, M. I.; Itoh, H.; Furukawa, Y.; Kimura, S.; Fujimoto, H. Effect of *Trans* Fatty Acids on Plasma Lipids, Platelet Function and Systolic Blood Pressure in Stroke-Prone Spontaneously Hypertensive Rats. *Lipids* **1991,** *26,* 46–52.

Clifton, P. M.; Keogh, J. B.; Noakes, M. *Trans* Fatty Acids in Adipose Tissue and the Food Supply Are Associated with Myocardial Infarction. *J. Nutr.* **2004,** *134,* 874–879.

Enig, M. G., Atal, S., Keeney, M., Sampugna, J. Isomeric *Trans* Fatty Acids in the U.S. Diet. *J. Am. Coll. Nutr.* **1990,** *9,* 471–486.

Enjalbert, F.; Troegeler-Meynadier, A. Biosynthesis of *Trans* Fatty Acids in Ruminants. In Trans *Fatty Acids in Human Nutrition,* 2nd ed., Destaillats, F., Sébédio, J. L., Dionisi, F., Chardigny, J. M., Eds.; The Oily Press, P. J. Barnes & Associates: Bridgwater, UK, 2009; pp 1–42.

Enke, U.; Jaudszus, A.; Schleussner, E.; Seyfarth, L.; Jahreis, G.; Kuhnt, K. Fatty Acid Distribution of Cord and Maternal Blood in Human Pregnancy: Special Focus on Individual *Trans* Fatty Acids and Conjugated Linoleic Acids. *Lipids Health Dis.* **2011,** *10,* 247.

Fournier, N.; Attia, N.; Rousseau-Ralliard, D.; Vedie, B.; Destaillats, F.; Grynberg, A.; Paul, J.-L. Deleterious Impact of Elaidic Fatty Acid on ABCA1-mediated Cholesterol Efflux from Mouse and Human Macrophages. *Biochimica et Biophysica Acta* **2012,** *1821,* 303–312.

Gatto, L. M.; Lyons, M. A.; Brown, A. J.; Samman, S. *Trans* Fatty Acids and Cholesterol Metabolism: Mechanistic Studies in Rats and Rabbits Fed Semipurified Diets. *Int. J. Food Sci. Nutr.* **2001**, *52,* 435–441.

Gatto, L. M.; Lyons, M. A.; Brown, A. J.; Samman, S. *Trans* Fatty Acids Affect Lipoprotein Metabolism in Rats. *J. Nutr.* **2002,** *132,* 1242–1248.

Gebauer, S. K.; Chardigny, J. M.; Jakobsen, M. U.; Lamarche, B.; Lock, A.; Proctor, S. D.; Baer, D. J. Effects of Ruminant *Trans* Fatty Acids on Cardiovascular Disease and Cancer: A Comprehensive Review of Epidemiological, Clinical, and Mechanistic Studies. *Adv. Nutr.* **2011,** *2,* 332–354.

Jacome-Sosa, M. M.; Lu, J.; Wang, Y.; Ruth, M. R.; Wright, D. C.; Reaney, M. J.; Shen, J.; Field, C. J.; Vine, D. F.; Proctor, S. D. Increased Hypolipidemic Benefits of *Cis*-9, *Trans*-11 Conjugated Linoleic Acid in Combination with *Trans*-11 Vaccenic Acid in a Rodent Model of the Metabolic Syndrome, the JCR:LA-cp Rat. *Nutr. Metab.* **2010**, *7,* 60.

Kraft, J.; Spiltoir, J. I.; Salter, A. M.; Lock, A. L. Differential Effects of the *Trans*-18:1 Isomer Profile of Partially Hydrogenated Vegetable Oils on Cholesterol and Lipoprotein Metabolism in Male F1B Hamsters. *J. Nutr.* **2011,** *141,* 1819–1826.

Lacroix, E.; Charest, A.; Cyr, A.; Baril-Gravel, L.; Lebeuf, Y.; Paquin, P.; Choinard, P. Y.; Couture, P.; Lamarch, B. Randomized Controlled Study of the Effect of a Butter Naturally Enriched in *Trans* Fatty Acids on Blood Lipids in Healthy Women. *Am. J. Clin Nutr.* **2012,** *95,* 318–325.

Lemaitre, R. N.; King, I. B.; Mozaffarian, D.; Sotoodehnia, N.; Rea, T. D.; Kuller, L. H.; Tracy, R. P.; Siscovick, D. S. Plasma Phospholipid *Trans* Fatty Acids, Fatal Ischemic Heart Disease, and Sudden Cardiac Death in Older Adults: The Cardiovascular Health Study. *Circulation* **2006,** *114,* 209–215.

Li, J.; Fan, Y.; Zhang, Z.; Yu, H.; An, Y.; Kramer, J. K. G.; Deng, Z. Evaluating the *Trans* Fatty Acid, CLA.; PUFA and Erucic Acid Diversity in Human Milk from Five Regions in China. *Lipids* **2009,** *44,* 257–271.

Lock, A. L.; Kraft, J.; Rice, B. H.; Bauman, D. E. Biosynthesis and Biological Activity of Rumenic Acid: A Natural CLA Isomer. In Trans *Fatty Acids in Human Nutrition,* 2nd ed.; Destaillats, F., Sébédio, J. L., Dionisi, F., Chardigny, J. M., Eds.; The Oily Press, P. J. Barnes & Associates: Bridgwater, UK, 2009.

Meijer, G. W.; van Tol, A.; van Berkel, T. J.; Weststrate, J. A. Effect of Dietary Elaidic versus Vaccenic Acid on Blood and Liver Lipids in the Hamster. *Atherosclerosis* **2001,** *157,* 31–40.

Micha, R.; King, I. B.; Lemaitre, R. N.; Rimm, E. B.; Sacks, F.; Song, X.; Siscovick, D. S.; Mozaffarian, D. Food Sources of Individual Plasma Phospholipid *Trans* Fatty Acid Isomers: The Cardiovascular Health Study. *Am. J. Clin. Nutr.* **2010,** *91,* 883–893.

Mosley, E. E.; Wright A. L.; McGuire M. K.; McGuire, M. A. *Trans* Fatty Acids in Milk Produced by Women in the United States. *Am. J. Clin. Nutr.* **2005,** *82,* 1292–1297.

Mosley, E. E.; McGuire, M. K.; Williams, J. E.; McGuire, M. A. *Cis*-9, *Trans*-11 Conjugated Linoleic Acid Is Synthesized from Vaccenic Acid in Lactating Women. *J. Nutr.* **2006,** *136,* 2297–2301.

Motard-Belanger, A.; Charest, A.; Grenier, G.; Paquin, P.; Chouinard, Y.; Lemieux, S.; Couture, P.; Lamarch, B. Study of the Effect of *Trans* Fatty Acids from Ruminants on Blood Lipids and Other Risk Factors for Cardiovascular Disease. *Am. J. Clin. Nutr.* **2008,** *87,* 593–599.

Mozaffarian, D.; Clarke, R. Quantitative Effects on Cardiovascular Risk Factors and Coronary Heart Disease Risk of Replacing Partially Hydrogenated Vegetable Oils with Other Fats and Oils. *Eur J. Clin. Nutr.* **2009,** *63* (Suppl. 2), S22–33.

Mozaffarian, D.; Katan, M. B.; Ascherio, A.; Stampfer, J. J.; Willett, W. C. *Trans* Fatty Acids and Cardiovascular Disease. *New Engl. J. Med.* **2006,** *354,* 1601–1613.

Mozaffarian, D.; Aro, A.; Willett, W. C. Health Effects of *Trans*-Fatty Acids: Experimental and Observational Evidence. *Eur J. Clin. Nutr.* **2009,** *63* (Suppl. 2), S5–21.

Mozaffarian, D.; Cao, H.; King, I. B.; Lemaitre, R. M.; Song, X.; Siscovick, D. S.; Hotamisligil, G. S. *Trans*-palmitoleic Acid, Metabolic Risk Factors, and New-Onset Diabetes in U.S. Adults: A Cohort Study. *Ann. Intern Med.* **2010,** *153,* 790–799.

Mueller, A.; Thijs, C.; Rist, L.; Simões-Wüst, A. P.; Huber, M.; Steinhart, H. *Trans* Fatty Acids in Human Milk Are an Indicator of Different Maternal Dietary Sources Containing *Trans* Fatty Acids. *Lipids* **2010,** *45,* 245–251.

Ohlrogge, J. B.; Emken, E. A.; Gulley, R. M. Human Tissue Lipids: Occurrence of Fatty Acid Isomers from Dietary Hydrogenated Oils. *J. Lipid. Res.* **1981,** *22,* 955–960.

Park, S.; Park, Y. Effects of Dietary Fish Oil and *Trans* Fat on Rat Aorta Histopathology and Cardiovascular Risk Markers. *Nutr. Res. Pract.* **2009,** *3,* 102–107.

Precht, D.; Molkentin, J. *Trans* Fatty Acids: Implications for Health, Analytical Methods, Incidence in Edible Fats and Intake. *Nahrung* **1995,** *39,* 343–374.

Precht, D.; Molkentin, J. C18:1, C18:2 and C18:3 *Trans* and *Cis* Fatty Acid Isomers Including Conjugated *cis* Δ9,*trans* Δ11 Linoleic Acid (CLA) as well as Total Fat Composition of German Human Milk Lipids. *Nahrung* **1999,** *43,* 233–244.

Ratnayake, N. W. M.; Cruz-Hernandez, C. Analysis of *Trans* Fatty Acids of Patially Hydrogenated Vegetable Oils and Dairy Products. In Trans *Fatty Acids in Human Nutrition,* 2nd ed.; Destaillats, F., Sébédio, J. L., Dionisi, F., Chardigny, J. M., Eds.; The Oily Press, P. J. Barnes & Associates: Bridgwater, UK, 2009.

Ratnayake, W. M.; Chen, Z. Y. *Trans,* n-3, and n-6 Fatty Acids in Canadian Human Milk. *Lipids* **1996,** *31* (Suppl.), S279–282.

Rice, B. H. ; Kraft, J.; Destaillats, F.; Bauman, D. E.; Lock, A. L. Ruminant-Produced *Trans*-Fatty Acids Raise Plasma Total and Small HDL Particle Concentrations in Male Hartley Guinea Pigs. *J. Nutr.* **2010,** *140,* 2173–2179.

Rice, B. H.; Kraft, J.; Destaillats, F.; Bauman, D. E.; Lock, A. L. Ruminant-Produced *Trans*-Fatty Acids Raise Plasma HDL Particle Concentrations in Intact and Ovariectomized Female Hartley Guinea Pigs. *J. Nutr.* **2012,** *142,* 1679–1683.

Rosenthal, M. D.; Doloresco, M. A. The Effects of *Trans* Fatty Acids on Fatty Acyl Delta 5 Desaturation by Human Skin Fibroblasts. *Lipids* **1984,** *19,* 869–874.

Samur, G.; Topcu, A.; Turan, S. *Trans* Fatty Acids and Fatty Acid Composition of Mature Breast Milk in Turkish Women and Their Association with Maternal Diets. *Lipids* **2009,** *44,* 405–413.

Sébédio, J. L.; Christie, W. W. Metabolism of *Trans* Fatty Acid Isomers. In Trans *Fatty Acids in Human Nutrition,* 2nd ed.; Destaillats, F., Sébédio, J. L., Dionisi, F., Chardigny, J. M., Eds.; The Oily Press, P. J. Barnes & Associates: Bridgwater, UK, 2009.

Smedman, A. E.; Gustafsson, I. B.; Berglund, L. G.; Vessby, B. O. Pentadecanoic Acid in Serum as a Marker for Intake of Milk Fat: Relations between Intake of Milk Fat and Metabolic Risk Factors. *Am. J. Clin. Nutr.* **1999,** 69, 22–29.

Smit, L. A.; Willett, W. C.; Campos, H. *Trans*-Fatty Acid Isomers in Adipose Tissue Have Divergent Associations with Adiposity in Humans. *Lipids* **2010,** *45,* 693–700.

Takeuchi, H.; Ito, E.; Tomioka, T.; Tabuchi, E.; Fuhshuku, K.; Asano, Y. *Trans* Fatty Acid Intake and Serum Cholesterol Levels in Young Japanese Women. *Biosci. Biotech, Bioch.* **2012,** *76,* 1627–1632.

Turpeinen, A. M.; Mutanen, M.; Aro, A.; Salminen, I.; Basu, S.; Palmquist, D. L.; Griinari, J. M. Bioconversion of Vaccenic Acid to Conjugated Linoleic Acid in Humans. *Am. J. Clin. Nutr.* **2002,** *76,* 504–510.

Tyburczy, C.; Major, C.; Lock, A. L.; Destaillats, F.; Lawrence, P.; Brenna, J. T.; Salter, A. M.; Bauman, D. E. Individual *Trans* Octadecenoic Acids and Partially Hydrogenated Vegetable Oil Differentially Affect Hepatic Lipid and Lipoprotein Metabolism in Golden Syrian Hamsters. *J. Nutr.* **2009,** *139,* 257–263.

Venkatramanan, S.; Joseph, S. V.; Chouinard, P. Y.; Jacques, H.; Farnworth, E. R.; Jones, P. J. Milk Enriched with Conjugated Linoleic Acid Fails to Alter Blood Lipids or Body Composition in Moderately Overweight, Borderline Hyperlipidemic Individuals. *J. Am. Coll. Nutr.* **2010,** *29,* 152–159.

Vesper, H. W.; Kuiper, H. C.; Mirel, L. B.; Johnson, C. L.; Pirkle, J. L. Levels of Plasma *Trans*-Fatty Acids in Non-Hispanic White Adults in the United States in 2000 and 2009. *J. Am. Med. Assoc.* **2012,** *307,* 562–563.

Wang, Y.; Jacome-Sosa, M. M.; Ruth, M. R.; Goruk, S. D.; Reaney, M. J.; Glimm, D. R.; Wright, D. C.; Vine, D. F.; Field, C. J.; Proctor, S. D. *Trans*-11 Vaccenic Acid Reduces Hepatic Lipogenesis and Chylomicron Secretion in JCR:LA-cp Rats. *J. Nutr.* **2009,** *139,* 2049–2054.

Wang, Y.; Jacome-Sosa, M. M.; Ruth, M. R.; Lu, Y.; Shen, J.; Reaney, M. J.; Scott, S. L.; Dugan, M. E.; Anderson, H. D.; Field, C. J., et al. The Intestinal Bioavailability of Vaccenic Acid and Activation of Peroxisome Proliferator-Activated Receptor-α and -γ in a Rodent Model of Dyslipidemia and the Metabolic Syndrome. *Mol. Nutr. Food Res.* **2012,** *56,* 1234–1246.

Warensjö, E.; Jansson, J. H.; Cederholm, T.; Boman, K.; Eliasson, M.; Hallmans, G.; Johannson, I.; Sgögren, P. Biomarkers of Milk Fat and the Risk of Myocardial Infarction in Men and Women: A Prospective, Matched Case-control Study. *Am. J. Clin. Nutr.* **2010,** *92,* 194–202.

Wolff, R. L. Content and Distribution of *Trans*-18:1 Acids in Ruminant Milk and Meat Fats. Their Importance in European Diets and Their Effect on Human Milk. *J. Am. Oil Chem. Soc.* **1995,** *72,* 259–272.

Wolff, R. L.; Combe, N. A.; Destaillats, F. ; Boué, C.; Precht, D.; Molkentin, J.; Entressangles, B. Follow-up of the Δ4 to Δ16 *Trans*-18:1 Isomer Profile and Content in French Processed Foods Containing Partially Hydrogenated Vegetable Oils during the Period 1995–1999. Analytical and Nutritional Implications. *Lipids* **2000,** *35,* 815–825.

World Health Organization (WHO) Global Strategy on Diet, Physical Activity and Health, 2004. http://www.who.int/dietphysicalactivity/strategy/eb11344/strategy_english_web.pdf.

Yu, D. X.; Sun, Q.; Ye, X. W.; Pan, A.; Zong, G.; Zhou, Y. H.; Li, H. X.; Hu, F. B.; Lin, X. Erythrocyte *Trans*-Fatty Acids, Type 2 Diabetes and Cardiovascular Risk Factors in Middle-aged and Older Chinese Individuals. *Diabetologia* **2012,** *55,* 2954–2962.

Zock, P. L.; Mensink, R. P.; Harryvan, J.; de Vries, J. H.; Katan, M. B. Fatty Acids in Serum Cholesteryl Esters as Quantitative Biomarkers of Dietary Intake in Humans. *Am. J. Epidemiol.* **1997,** *145,* 1114–1122.

3

FDA Food Labeling Regulations for *Trans* Fat

Vincent de Jesus ■ *U.S. Food and Drug Administration, Center for Food Safety and Applied Nutrition, College Park, Maryland, United States*

Introduction

On November 8, 1990, the Nutrition Labeling and Education Act (NLEA) (1990) was signed into law, amending the Federal Food, Drug, and Cosmetic Act (1938) ("the act"). NLEA had a direct bearing on the FDA's revision of nutrition labeling in 1993. NLEA added a section to the act which, in part, specified that (with certain exceptions) a food is to be considered misbranded unless its packaging bears nutrition labeling, and that certain nutrients and food components are to be included in nutrition labeling, although the Secretary of Health and Human Services can add or delete nutrients by regulation if it is found necessary to assist consumers in maintaining healthy dietary practices.

In response to NLEA, the FDA published a proposed rule entitled "Food Labeling; Reference Daily Intakes and Daily Reference Values; Mandatory Status of Nutrition Labeling and Nutrient Content Revision" (U.S. Food and Drug Administration, 1991). In that proposed rule, the agency proposed to require that foods bear nutrition labeling listing certain nutrients and the amount of those nutrients in a serving of the food. Given the scientific knowledge about *trans* fat at the time, the FDA did not propose to require that *trans* fat be listed. However, the FDA requested comments on whether the listing of *trans* fat should be voluntary (U.S. Food and Drug Administration, 1991).

In January 1993, the FDA issued a final rule entitled "Food Labeling; Mandatory Status of Nutrition Labeling and Nutrient Content Revision, Format for Nutrition Label" (U.S. Food and Drug Administration, 1993a) that prescribed how nutrition labeling is to be provided on foods that are regulated by the agency. In that rule, the agency required the declaration of total fat and saturated fat on the nutrition label with the declaration of both monounsaturated fat and polyunsaturated fat required, when claims are made about fatty acids and cholesterol. Based on its review of the comments, the agency stated that it was premature to include *trans* fats in nutrition labeling because of a lack of agreement on the dietary implications of *trans* fat intake. However, the agency acknowledged that it might be necessary to revisit the labeling of *trans* fat in the future (U.S. Food and Drug Administration, 1993a).

Trans Fat in Nutrition Facts

In 1994, the FDA received a citizen petition from a consumer group stating that an increasing body of evidence suggested that dietary *trans* fat raises blood cholesterol levels, thereby increasing the risk of coronary heart disease (CHD) (U.S. Food and Drug Administration, 1994). The petitioner argued that the 1993 final rules on nutrition labeling did not adequately reflect the effect of dietary *trans* fat on CHD and that label values for saturated fat underestimate the total amount of fats that negatively affect the heart because *trans* fat is not declared. The petitioner requested that the FDA amend the regulatory definition of saturated fat in the labeling regulations to include *trans* fat, so the declaration of saturated fat on the nutrition label would provide consumers with complete information on all fatty acids that negatively affect the heart. In addition, the petitioner requested that all nutrient content claims for saturated fat, as well as all other nutrient content claims and health claims that have a threshold for saturated fat as a criteria, be amended to reflect the combined levels of saturated and *trans* fat. The citizen petition was amended by the petitioner in 1998, suggesting options that would leave the current regulatory definition of saturated fat unchanged, while also providing consumers with additional information on the *trans* fat content of the food. Specifically, the amended petition suggested that the FDA: (1) Disclose the sum of *trans* and saturated fats next to the term *saturated fat*, with an asterisk at the bottom of the label that states "contains ___ grams of *trans* fat," or (2) disclose the sum of *trans* and saturated fats next to the term *saturated + trans fat* when *trans* fat was present.

In response to the citizen petition, the FDA issued a proposed rule, "Food Labeling: *Trans* Fatty Acids in Nutrition Labeling, Nutrient Content Claims, and Health Claims" (U.S. Food and Drug Administration, 1999). In that proposed rule, the FDA proposed to amend its nutrition labeling regulations to require that the amount of *trans* fat in a food, including dietary supplements, be included in the amount and percent daily value (%DV) declared for saturated fat, with a footnote indicating the amount of *trans* fatty acids in a serving of the product when the product contains 0.5 or more grams *trans* fatty acids per serving. The FDA reviewed the current research that showed that consumption of diets containing *trans* fat, as with diets containing saturated fats, results in increased serum low-density lipoprotein cholesterol (LDL-C), a major risk factor for CHD. The proposed rule was issued to assist consumers in maintaining healthy dietary practices (U.S. Food and Drug Administration, 1999). The FDA also proposed a definition for the nutrient content claim "*trans* fat free" and proposed limits on the amounts of *trans* fat wherever saturated fat limits are placed on nutrient content claims or health claims.

Due to comments submitted to the proposal, the agency reopened the comment period to also consider "reduced *trans* fat" and "reduced saturated and *trans* fat" claims

(U.S. Food and Drug Administration, 2000). In the notice to reopen the comment period, the agency also proposed requiring an asterisk (or other symbol) in the %DV column for *trans* fat that is tied to a similar symbol at the bottom of the Nutrition Facts label, followed by the statement "Intake of *trans* fat should be as low as possible." In addition, the FDA requested comments on whether "*trans* fat free" claims would help consumers maintain healthy dietary practices and whether they would provide incentive to the food industry to reduce the amount of *trans* fat in the food supply.

The FDA issued a final rule in July 2003 (U.S. Food and Drug Administration, 2003a). The agency's actions were based on an evaluation of comments received in response to the 1999 proposed rule, the 2002 reopening of the comment period, and on the current scientific evidence on *trans* fat. In the final rule, the FDA required mandatory declaration on the nutrition label of the amount of *trans* fat present in the food, but it did not include a %DV that is required for some of the other mandatory nutrients, such as saturated fat. In addition, the agency withdrew the sections of the proposed rule pertaining to the definitions of nutrient content claims for "free" and "reduced" levels of *trans* fatty acids, and limits on the amounts of *trans* fat wherever saturated fat limits are placed on nutrient content claims or health claims. The agency also withdrew the proposed requirement to include the footnote about *trans* fat intake.

As a result of the final rule, the codified language in 21 CFR 101.9(c)(2)(ii) (Office of the Federal Register, 2012) states:

> (ii) "*Trans* fat" or "*Trans*": A statement of the number of grams of *trans* fat in a serving, defined as the sum of all unsaturated fatty acids that contain one or more isolated (i.e., nonconjugated) double bonds in a *trans* configuration, except that label declaration of *trans* fat content information is not required for products that contain less than 0.5 gram of total fat in a serving if no claims are made about fat, fatty acid or cholesterol content. The word "*trans*" may be italicized to indicate its Latin origin. *Trans* fat content shall be indented and expressed as grams per serving to the nearest 0.5 (1/2)-gram increment below 5 grams and to the nearest gram increment above 5 grams. If the serving contains less than 0.5 gram, the content, when declared, shall be expressed as zero. Except as provided for in paragraph (f) of this section, if a statement of the *trans* fat content is not required and, as a result, not declared, the statement "Not a significant source of *trans* fat" shall be placed at the bottom of the table of nutrient values."

In the *trans* fat final rule, the FDA concluded that, based on information and arguments presented in the comments, it was premature to establish new or revised definitions for nutrient content claims or to require the use of the proposed footnote statement in the nutrition label. Instead, the FDA concurrently issued an Advance Notice of Proposed Rulemaking (ANPRM) (U.S. Food and Drug Administration,

2003b) in the same issue of the *Federal Register* that solicited comments and additional consumer research on: (1) an appropriate basis for establishing qualifying criteria for *trans* fat in *trans* fat nutrient content claims and other current nutrient content claims and health claims that include saturated fat criteria; (2) whether such claims mislead consumers about the total fatty acid profile if levels of all cholesterol-raising lipids are not addressed, and if so, whether qualifiers or disclosure statements would remedy this problem; (3) the use of a footnote related to *trans* fat intake in the context of the entire diet; (4) the language that may be appropriate for use in a footnote; and (5) the impact of nutrient content claims, health claims, footnotes, or disclosure statements on consumers' food selections. At the current time, the agency has not yet published any rules addressing the issues described in the *trans* fat ANPRM.

In the 2003 *trans* fat final rule, the FDA estimated that total *trans* fat intake was 5.8 g per day, with the average intake of industrially produced *trans* fat estimated to be 4.6 g per day and naturally occurring *trans* to be 1. 2g per day. The rule went into effect in 2006, but updated estimates of *trans* fat intake after mandatory *trans* fat labeling went into effect were unavailable until the FDA published a study in early 2012 (Doell et al., 2012). According to the FDA study, total *trans* fat intakes had decreased to 2.5 g per day, with the average intake of industrially produced *trans* fat estimated to be 1.3 g per day and naturally occurring *trans* to be 1.2 g per day. Based on the updated estimates, total *trans* fat intake has decreased significantly since the mandatory *trans* fat labeling regulations went into effect.

Nutrient Content Claims

As discussed earlier, the FDA has considered the issues of both establishing nutrient content claims for *trans* fat and establishing *trans* fat criteria for nutrient content claims that include saturated fat criteria. Currently, no nutrient content claims for *trans* fat have been defined. *Trans* fat criteria have also not been added to nutrient content claims that include saturated fat criteria, with the exception of the nutrient content claim "saturated fat free." This nutrient content claim was defined along with most other original nutrient content claims in the 1993 final rules. In January 1993, the FDA issued a final rule entitled "Food Labeling: Nutrient Content Claims, General Principles, Petitions, Definition of Terms; Definition of Nutrient Content Claims for the Fat, Fatty Acid, and Cholesterol Content of Food" (U.S. Food and Drug Administration, 1993b). In that final rule, the agency stated that it did not set a *trans* fat criterion for most claims because the evidence suggesting that *trans* fatty acids raise serum cholesterol was inconclusive at that time (U.S. Food and Drug Administration, 1993b). However, the FDA did set a *trans* fat criterion for the "saturated fat free" claim stating that "because of the uncertainty regarding this issue, the fact that consumers would expect a food bearing a 'saturated fat free' claim to be free of saturated fat and other components that significantly raise serum cholesterol, and the potential importance of a saturated fat free claim, the agency believes that it would be misleading for products that contain measurable amounts of *trans* fatty acids to bear a 'saturated fat free' claim" (U.S. Food and Drug Administration, 1993b). The *trans* fat criterion for the claim "saturated fat free" was set at a level not to exceed 1% of total fat in the food (U.S. Food and Drug Administration, 1993b). The agency stated that 1% was the appropriate threshold because analytical methods for measuring *trans* fatty acids below that level were not reliable (U.S. Food and Drug Administration, 1993b). This action was taken under the authority of section 403(r)(2)(A)(vi) of the act, which prohibits a claim if it is misleading in light of the level of another nutrients in the food.

Some comments that the FDA received after publication of the nutrient content claims final rule objected to the 1% criterion for *trans* fatty acids in the definition of "saturated fat free." One example pointed out that a food product containing 1.5 g of total fat would be allowed to have only 0.015 g of *trans* fatty acids, an amount that could not be accurately measured. In response to these comments, the agency amended the definition of "saturated fat free" to require that a food contain less than 0.5 g of *trans* fatty acids in addition to less than 0.5 g of saturated fat per reference amount customarily consumed and per labeled serving (U.S. Food and Drug Administration, 1993c) to be eligible to bear the claim.

Health Claims

The FDA has not authorized by regulation any health claims that have *trans* fat as the subject of the claim or have had *trans* fat nutrient criteria related to claim eligibility. However, the FDA does permit two health claims that do have *trans* fat criteria that are based on a separate notification process established by the Food and Drug Administration Modernization Act of 1997 (FDAMA) (1997). This notification process is an alternative to the typical petition process and subsequent rulemaking authorizing a nutrient content claim or health claim to be made on a food label. Through this notification process, a manufacturer may submit to the FDA a notification of a health claim based on statements made by certain authoritative bodies on a substance/disease relationship; the claims can be made until either the FDA issues a regulation prohibiting or modifying the claim or finding that the requirements for making the claim have not been met, or a district court in an enforcement proceeding has determined that the requirements for making the claim have not been met. This notification process allows for quicker authorization for claims, but it can only be used under a specific set of conditions and requirements (U.S. Food and Drug Administration, 1998).

In 2003, the FDA received a notification regarding a health claim for whole grain foods and the risk of heart disease. The notification cited information from the

National Academies of Science report "Diet and Health: Implications for Reducing Chronic Disease Risk" as the basis for the claim. Based on the notification, in order for foods to qualify for the claim "Diets rich in whole grain foods and other plant foods, and low in saturated fat and cholesterol, may help reduce the risk of heart disease" the foods must: (1) contain a minimum of 51% whole grains (using dietary fiber as a marker); (2) meet the regulatory definitions for "low saturated fat" and "low cholesterol"; (3) bear quantitative *trans* fat labeling; and (4) contain less than 6.5 g total fat and 0.5 g or less *trans* fat per reference amount customarily consumed (RACC). Beginning 120 days from the date of submission, manufacturers were able to use the claim specified in the notification (U.S. Food and Drug Administration, 2003c).

In 2006, the FDA received a notification regarding a health claim for the relationship between dietary consumption of saturated fat, cholesterol, and *trans* fat, and the risk of heart disease. The notification based the claim on information from the 2005 Dietary Guidelines for Americans (U.S. Department of Health and Human Services and U.S. Department of Agriculture, 2005). As a result of the notification, foods eligible to bear the claim "Diets low in saturated fat and cholesterol, and as low as possible in *trans* fat, may reduce the risk of heart disease" must: (1) meet the FDA regulatory definitions for "low saturated fat" and "low cholesterol"; (2) contain less than 0.5 g of *trans* fat per RACC or must meet any FDA definition of "low" *trans* fat if a definition is established in the future; (3) contain less than 6.5 g total fat per RACC; and (4) be in accordance with all general health claim requirements found in 21 CFR 101.14. One-hundred twenty days after submission, manufacturers were able to use the claim for saturated fat, cholesterol, and *trans* fat and risk of heart disease (U.S. Food and Drug Administration, 2007).

Latest Developments in *Trans* Fats Regulations

On November 8, 2013, the FDA published a notice entitled "Tentative Determination Regarding Partially Hydrogenated Oils; Request for Comments and for Scientific Data and Information" (U.S. Food and Drug Administration, 2013). This notice stated that, based on new scientific evidence and the findings of expert scientific panels, the FDA has tentatively determined that partially hydrogenated oils (PHOs), which are the primary dietary source of industrially produced *trans* fats, are not generally recognized as safe (GRAS) for any use in food based on current scientific evidence establishing the health risks associated with the consumption of *trans* fat and, therefore, that PHOs are food additives. If the tentative determination is finalized, food manufacturers would no longer be permitted to sell PHOs, either directly or as ingredients in other food products, without prior FDA approval for use as a food additive. The notice requested comments, additional scientific data, and information related to this action before a final determination will be made. If the FDA concludes that there is a lack of convincing evidence that the substance is GRAS or is otherwise exempt from the definition of a food additive, the FDA will publish a notice in the *Federal Register*.

Similar International *Trans* Fat Labeling Regulations

Nutrition labeling has been mandatory in the United States since 1994. However, in most countries, nutrition labeling is not required. Consequently, the declaration of the *trans* fat quantity in a food is not common internationally. There are a few countries that do mandate nutrition labeling. Canada has followed the actions in the United States and has had mandatory nutrition labeling since 2005. Since 2001, a number of South American countries, such as Paraguay, Chile, Argentina, Uruguay, and Brazil, have also required nutrition labeling. Various other countries around the globe have also begun to implement mandatory nutrition labeling, mostly in the past decade or so. Examples of these countries include Australia, New Zealand, South Korea, China, India, Malaysia, Hong Kong, Taiwan, and South Korea. Out of the small number of countries that mandate nutrition labeling, an even smaller subset of these specifically require *trans* fat to be included. The United States and Canada require declaration of *trans* fat, as do Paraguay, Chile, Argentina, Uruguay, Brazil, Hong Kong, Taiwan, and South Korea. Most countries that do have mandatory nutrition labeling but do not require mandatory *trans* fat labeling, such as Australia, Malaysia, and China, do, however, allow *trans* fat to be declared voluntarily.

There are continuing efforts internationally for more countries to progress toward mandatory nutrition labeling. For example, in 2011, the European Commission published regulations to implement nutrition labeling in the member states of the European Union (EU) over the course of the next few years. By 2016, most packaged foods sold in the EU will be required to bear nutrition labeling. While the original regulations did not include *trans* fat among the nutrients to be declared, *trans* fat was an issue identified for future labeling discussions.

One of the goals for nutrition labeling of *trans* fat is a reduction of *trans* fat intake through more informed consumer choices regarding food products and by reformulation by food manufacturers to decrease *trans* fat content of individual foods. As an alternative regulatory option to declaration of *trans* fat content on the food label, some countries have instituted limits to *trans* fat levels in oils in order to reach the same goals of reduction of *trans* fat intake. For example, in Denmark, Switzerland, and Austria, legislation has passed that restricts *trans* fat content in oil to no more than 2% of the oil. Other countries have also indicated that they are considering similar legislation to restrict *trans* fat content of oils.

References

Doell, D.; Folmer, D.; Lee, H.; Honigfort, M.; Carberry, S. Updated Estimate of *Trans* Fat Intake by the US Population. *Food Additives and Contaminants: Part A: Chemistry, Analysis, Control, Exposure and Risk Assessment* **2012.** DOI: 10.1080/19440049.2012.664570.

Food and Drug Administration Modernization Act of 1997. Public Law 105-115, 111, Stat. 2296, 1997.

Food, Drug and Cosmetic Act. Public Law 75-717, 52 Stat. 1040, 1938.

Nutrition Labeling and Education Act. Public Law 101-535, 104 Stat. 2353, 1990.

Office of the Federal Register, National Archives and Records Administration. 21 CFR, pt. 101.9, 2012.

U.S. Department of Health and Human Services and U.S. Department of Agriculture. *Dietary Guidelines for Americans,* 6th ed., 2005. (http://www.health.gov/dietaryguidelines/dga2005/document/pdf/ DGA2005.pdf (accessed March 21, 2014).

U.S. Food and Drug Administration. Food Labeling; Reference Daily Intakes and Daily Reference Values; Mandatory Status of Nutrition Labeling and Nutrient Content Revision, Proposed Rule. *Fed Regist.* **1991,** *56,* 60366.

U.S. Food and Drug Administration. Food Labeling; Mandatory Status of Nutrition Labeling and Nutrient Content Revision, Format for Nutrition Label, Final Rule. *Fed Regist.* **1993a,** *58,* 2079.

U.S. Food and Drug Administration. Food Labeling: Nutrient Content Claims, General Principles, Petitions, Definition of Terms; Definition of Nutrient Content Claims for the Fat, Fatty Acid, and Cholesterol Content of Food. *Fed Regist.* **1993b,** *58,* 2302.

U.S. Food and Drug Administration. Food Labeling: Nutrient Content Claims, General Principles, Petitions, Definition of Terms; Definitions of Nutrient Content Claims for Fat, Fatty Acids, and Cholesterol Content of Foods; Food Standards: Requirements for Foods Named by Use of a Nutrient Content Claim and a Standardized Term; Technical Amendment. *Fed Regist.* **1993c,** *58,* 44020.

U.S. Food and Drug Administration. FDA Docket No. FDA-1994-P-0041; 1994.

U.S. Food and Drug Administration. Guidance for Industry: Notification of a Health Claim or Nutrient Content Claim Based on an Authoritative Statement of a Scientific Body., 1998. http://www.fda.gov/food/guidanceregulation/guidancedocumentsregulatoryinformation/labelingnutrition/ucm056975.htm (accessed March 21, 2014).

U.S. Food and Drug Administration. Food Labeling: *Trans* Fatty Acids in Nutrition Labeling, Nutrient Content Claims, and Health Claims, Proposed Rule. *Fed Regist.* **1999,** *64,* 62746.

U.S. Food and Drug Administration. Food Labeling: *Trans* Fatty Acids in Nutrition Labeling, Nutrient Content Claims, and Health Claims, Proposed Rule; Reopening of the Comment Period. *Fed Regist.* **2000,** *65,* 75887.

U.S. Food and Drug Administration. Health Claim Notification for Whole Grain Foods with Moderate Fat Content, 2003. http://www.fda.gov/Food/IngredientsPackagingLabeling/LabelingNutrition/ucm073634.htm (accessed March 21, 2014).

U.S. Food and Drug Administration. Food Labeling; *Trans* Fatty Acids in Nutrition Labeling; Consumer Research to Consider Nutrient Content and Health Claims and Possible Footnote or Disclosure Statements, Final Rule. *Fed Regist.* **2003a,** *68,* 41433.

U.S. Food and Drug Administration. Food Labeling: *Trans* Fatty Acids in Nutrition Labeling; Consumer Research to Consider Nutrient Content and Health Claims and Possible Footnote or Disclosure Statements, Advance Notice of Proposed Rulemaking. *Fed Regist.* **2003b,** *68,* 41507.

U.S. Food and Drug Administration. Health Claim Notification for Saturated Fat, Cholesterol, and *Trans* Fat, and Reduced Risk of Heart Disease, 2007. http://www.fda.gov/Food/IngredientsPackagingLabeling/LabelingNutrition/ucm073631.htm (accessed March 21, 2014).

U.S. Food and Drug Administration. Tentative Determination Regarding Partially Hydrogenated Oils; Request for Comments and for Scientific Data and Information. *Fed Regist.* **2013,** *78,* 67169.

4

Nutritional Aspects of *Trans* Fatty Acids

Ingeborg A. Brouwer ■ *Department of Health Sciences and the EMGO Institute for Health Care Research, Faculty of Earth and Life Sciences, VU University, Amsterdam, The Netherlands.*

Anne J. Wanders ■ *Division of Human Nutrition, Wageningen University, Wageningen, The Netherlands.*

Introduction

Most naturally occurring unsaturated fatty acids have their double bonds in the *cis* configuration. This *cis* configuration makes the molecule bend at the place of that double bond. *Trans* fatty acids (TFAs) are unsaturated fatty acids with at least one double bond in the *trans* configuration instead of the *cis* configuration. The double bond in the *trans* configuration gives the molecule a straighter shape. The straighter shape of the molecules allows them to pack better in solid state. This leads to transformation of oils into semisolid fats (Figure 4.1). There are two sources of TFAs: industrial and ruminant. In this chapter we look at the nutritional aspects of TFAs from various sources. We will only discuss studies in human subjects.

Elaidic acid (9-*trans*-C18:1) is a typical industrial TFA, produced by partial hydrogenation of vegetable oil. Vaccenic acid (11-*trans*-C18:1) is the predominant TFA in milk and meat from ruminant animals, although small amounts are also found in industrially hydrogenated fats. The 9,11 isomer of conjugated linoleic acid, or CLA (9-*cis*, 11-*trans*-C18:2), is found almost exclusively in ruminant fat; industrial production of CLA yields a mixture of 9,11 and 10,12 isomers. Oleic acid (9-*cis* -C18:1) is the predominant *cis*-unsaturated fatty acid in the diet. The location of the *trans* bond(s) in *trans* isomers of α-linolenic acid is not known precisely; for this figure it has been assigned arbitrarily to the 12 or omega-6 location. The same holds for the *trans* bonds in the *trans* isomers of C20:1, C20:2, C22:1, and C22:2 that arise from eicosapentaenoic acid (EPA) and docosahexaenoic acid (DHA) during partial hydrogenation of fish oil.

Characteristics of *Trans* Fatty Acids

Industrial *Trans* Fatty Acids

Industrial TFAs are artificially produced *trans* fats that are formed by partial hydrogenation of vegetable and fish oils with hydrogen gas in the presence of metal catalysts. Industrial TFAs are always formed from *cis*-unsaturated fatty acids, and omega-3 and omega-6 fatty acids may be the original source. Omega-3 and omega-6 fatty acids are

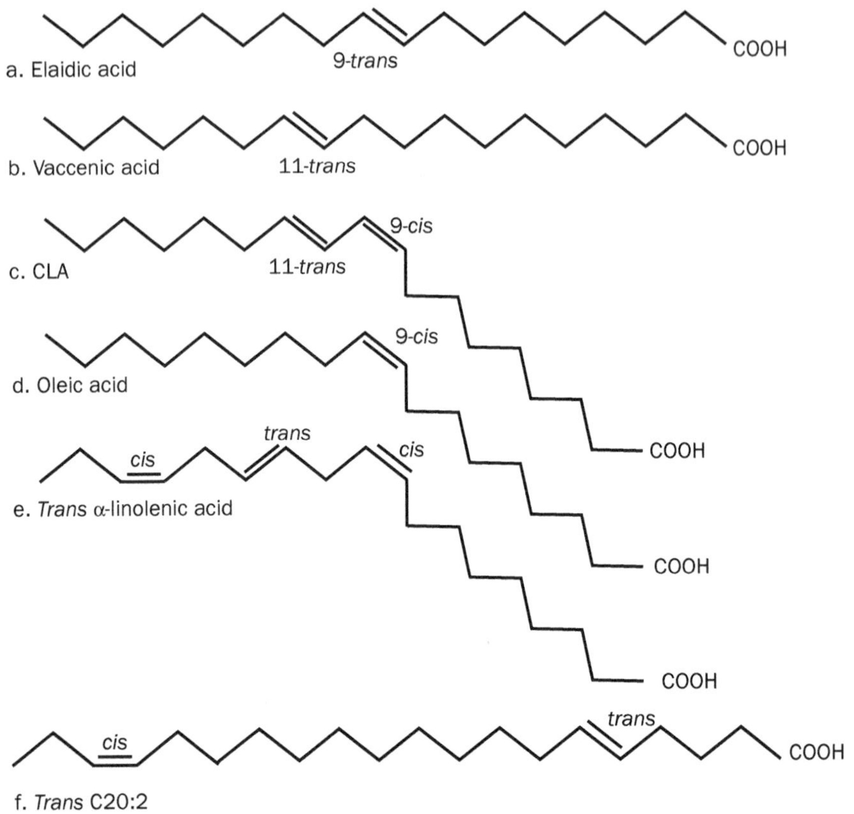

Figure 4.1 Structures of *cis*- and *trans* fatty acids. Adapted from Brouwer, Wanders et al. (2010).

essential fatty acids. However, as soon as these fatty acids have one double bond in the *trans* instead of the *cis* configuration, they lose their vital functions and are no longer considered essential fatty acids. Industry uses TFAs because the semisolid fats that are formed by the TFAs are more functional in the production of food products, such as cookies and pastries, than liquid oil, in addition to increasing shelf life (Parodi, 1976; Precht and Molkentin, 1995).

Ruminant *Trans* Fatty Acids

Ruminant TFAs are produced in the rumens of cows and sheep. Therefore, ruminant TFAs are found in dairy and meat products. Ruminant TFAs arise through biohydrogenation and/or isomerization of *cis*-unsaturated fatty acids from the feed by hydrogen produced during oxidation of substrates with bacterial enzymes as catalysts (Parodi, 1976; Precht and Molkentin, 1995).

Conjugated Linoleic Acids

A special group of TFAs are the fatty acids in the group of conjugated linoleic acids (CLAs). CLA is a *trans* fat that was first discovered in milk. Chemically, CLA is a TFA. CLA has two double bonds, one in the *trans* configuration and one in the *cis* configuration. The double bonds in CLA are conjugated, which results in having only one carbon atom or methylene between the two double bonds instead of the usual two. CLA has several isomers, but the two main isomers are *cis*-9, *trans*-11 CLA and *trans*-10, *cis*-12 CLA. *Cis*-9 *trans*-11 CLA is a component of ruminant *trans* fat. The usual daily intake from the diet is very low. However, nowadays, CLA is also industrially produced and sold in supplements because it is supposed to help people to lose weight. Vegetable oils are the source of supplemental CLA (Ma et al., 1999; Yang and Liu, 2004). Supplemental CLA consists of a mixture of *cis*-9, *trans*-11 CLA and *trans*-10, *cis*-12 CLA. *Cis*-9, *trans*-11 CLA and *trans*-10, *cis*-12 CLA are usually present in a 50:50 ratio, but sometimes also in an 80:20 or other ratio.

Isomers of *Trans* Fatty Acids

Industrial and ruminant C18:1 TFAs consist of the same *trans* isomers, but the distribution of the isomers differs, as shown in Figure 4.2. The isomer profile of industrial TFAs depends on conditions of the hydrogenation process, such as catalysts used and the temperature of hydrogenation. The profile of ruminant TFAs depends on the pH in the rumen and on the composition of oils in the diet of the animals (Parodi, 1976; Precht and Molkentin, 1995). Elaidic acid (C18:1 $\Delta 9t$) is typically the main isomer of industrial *trans* fat, and vaccenic acid (C18:1 $\Delta 11t$) is usually the main component of ruminant *trans* fat. However, industrial *trans* fats also contain a considerable amount of vaccenic acid, usually more than 20% (Hulshof et al., 1999).

Definition

There is some debate about the proper definition of a *trans* fat. The Codex Alimentarius standard and some countries do not consider fats with conjugated double bonds to be *trans* fats. According to that definition, CLA is not a *trans* fat. Also, the government of Denmark has put a ban on *trans* fat, but ruminant *trans* fats are not included in the ban. In this chapter, we use the chemical definition of TFAs and consider all fatty acids that contain one or more double bonds in the *trans* configuration to be TFAs.

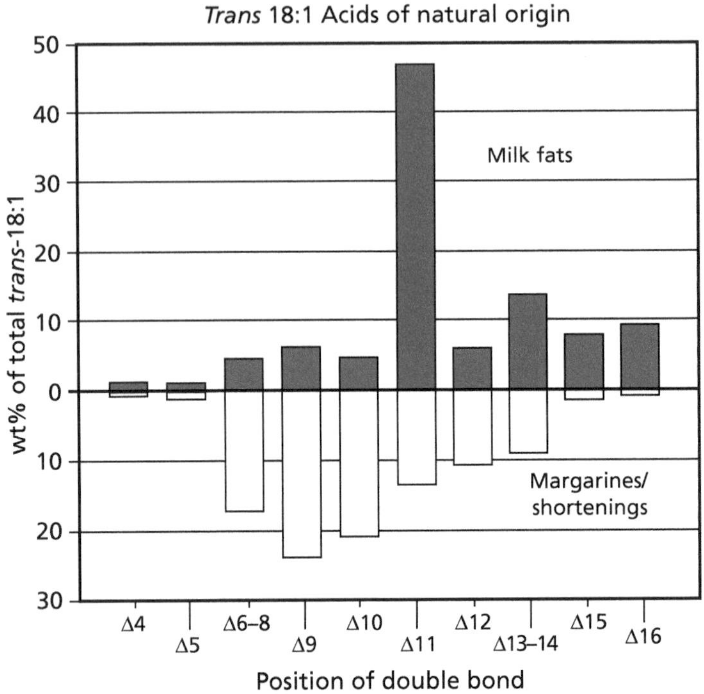

Figure 4.2 Distribution of *trans* fatty acid isomers in industrial and ruminant fats. Reprinted with permission from W. W. Christie, Ed., Trans *Fatty Acids in Human Nutrition;* The Oily Press: Dundee, UK, 1998.

Intake of *Trans* Fatty Acids

TFAs in the diet have various sources, including industrial TFAs from hydrogenated vegetable and fish oils and ruminant TFAs from meat and dairy. There is a wide variety in the consumption of TFAs in various countries. Before 1990, intake in Western countries was high and could be up to 20 g per person per day, whereas intake in Japan and Korea has been estimated to be as low as less than 1 g per person per day. The latter represents less than 0.5% of energy. Intake in the Western world has decreased considerably over the last 20 years because the food industry has changed their production processes and reformulated food products. This has led to much lower amounts of TFAs in food products and thereby a dramatic decrease in the intake (Craig-Schmidt, 2006). Average intakes in European countries have now come down to levels close to 1–2% of energy (Craig-Schmidt, 2006). In the UK, the average intake has decreased to less than 1% of energy (Pot et al., 2012). Similar trends are visible in the United States, although the decrease in intake is lagging behind Europe (Lichtenstein et al., 2006).

CLA is only present in the diet in very small amounts in dairy and meat products. Thus, intake of CLA via the diet is extremely low. However, CLA is also freely available in capsules in many countries. Intake from these commercially produced CLA products can easily mount up to 3 g per day (Brouwer et al., 2010).

Trans Fatty Acids and Cholesterol

Lipoproteins

Since the 1960s, many studies have shown that high concentrations of LDL-C and low concentrations of HDL-C in plasma are associated with an increased risk of cardiovascular disease. Therefore, it is important to know the potential effects of TFAs on cholesterol concentrations. The effect of TFAs on blood cholesterol concentrations is the most investigated health effect of TFAs.

Industrial *Trans* Fatty Acids and Cholesterol

In the beginning of the 1990s, dietary controlled studies were performed to investigate what effect consumption of industrial TFAs would have on lipoprotein concentrations in the blood. It turned out that compared to *cis*-unsaturated fatty acids, industrial TFAs raised LDL-C and decreased HDL-C (Katan et al., 1995; Mensink et al., 1992). Since then several similar studies were performed, and in 1999, Ascherio et al. (1999) summarized the outcomes of all available studies and clearly showed the LDL-C raising and HDL-C lowering potential of industrial TFAs. In 2010 and 2013, we updated and confirmed these findings (Figure 4.3) (Brouwer et al., 2013).

Studies were not weighed by number of subjects or standard error of the estimate because the LDL to HDL ratios were calculated on the basis of mean values of treatment differences within studies without an estimate of variation. Regression lines were forced through the origin because a zero change in diet should produce a zero change in blood lipids. When studies did not use *cis*-monounsaturated fatty acids as their control treatment, effects were recalculated relative to isocaloric amounts of *cis*-monounsaturated fatty acids using the equation of Mensink et al. (2003) (Brouwer et al., 2010).

All studies together showed that the LDL to HDL ratio was higher on a diet rich in industrial *trans* fat than on a *cis* fat diet. Replacement of 1% of energy of control fat by industrial TFAs led to an increase in the plasma LDL to HDL ratio of 0.053 (95% CI 0.042 to 0.063). LDL increased by 0.045 mmol/L (95% CI 0.035 to 0.055) and HDL decreased by –0.01 mmol/L (95% CI –0.013 to –0.007) (Brouwer et al.,

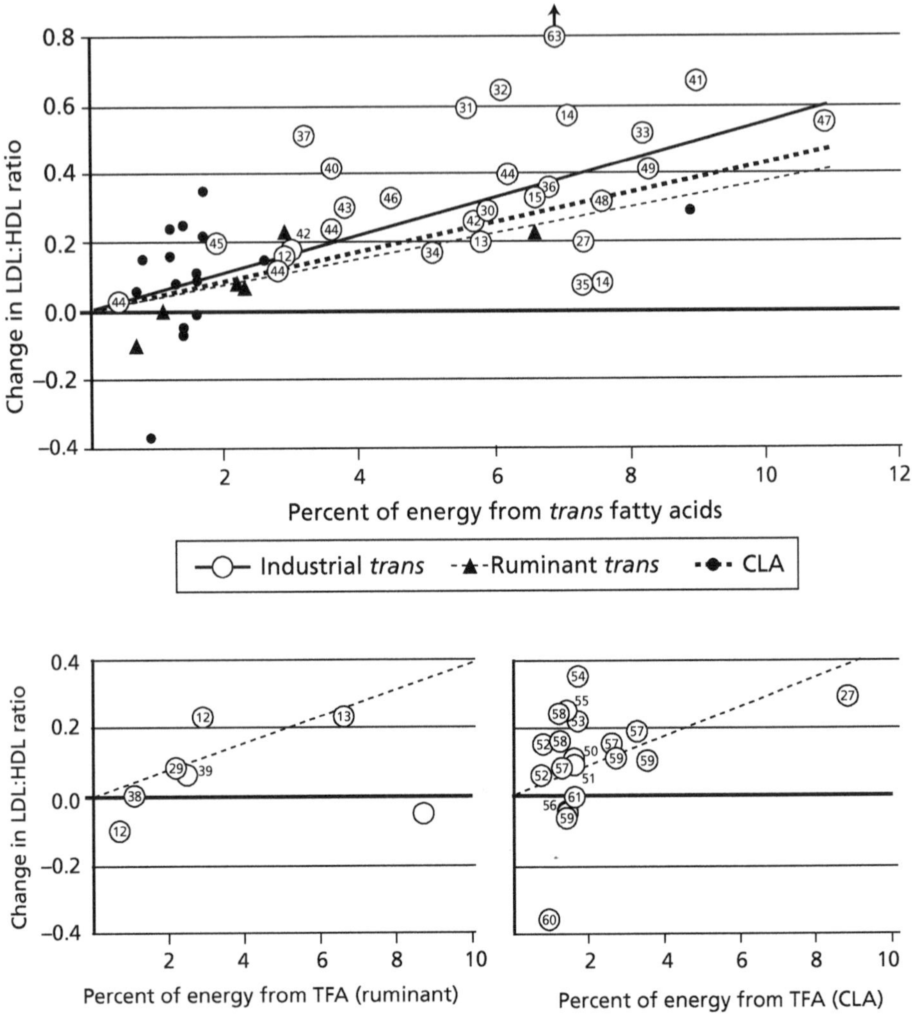

Figure 4.3 Results of randomized studies of the effects of diets high in industrial *trans* fatty acids, ruminant *trans* fatty acids, or CLA compared with *cis*-unsaturated fatty acids on the ratio of LDL to HDL cholesterol. Adapted from Brouwer, Wanders et al. (2010).

2010). Thus, overall, the earlier findings (Ascherio et al., 1999) were confirmed; studies consistently show that industrial TFAs have detrimental effects on blood cholesterol concentrations.

Ruminant *Trans* Fatty Acids and Cholesterol

In contrast to the high number of studies that investigated the effects of industrial TFAs on blood cholesterol concentrations, the number of studies that investigated effects of ruminant TFAs is limited. This is not surprising, as it is much more difficult to isolate ruminant TFAs from other fatty acids, and it is a challenge to create sufficient contrast between the intervention and control treatment to be able to pick up relevant effects.

In the *European Journal of Clinical Nutrition* (EJCN) in 2013, we summarized results of dietary studies available through August 2012. The review included eight published studies and one unpublished study on effects of ruminant TFAs on plasma cholesterol concentrations (Brouwer et al., 2013). Just as in the 2010 paper, we used linear regression analysis to combine the results of the studies and we forced the regression lines through the origin. Again, we recalculated ratios of LDL-C to HDL-C and the ratios of total to HDL-C from the mean LDL, HDL, and total cholesterol levels for all studies, even when ratios had been reported. In contrast to the 2010 publication, we weighed the studies for size using the inverse of the square root of the number of participants, and we used comparisons with the original control treatments in all studies (Brouwer et al., 2013).

The results of 11 comparisons and 672 subjects showed that replacement of 1 g of control fat by 1 g of ruminant TFA led to an increase in the LDL to HDL ratio by 0.014 (95% CI 0.004 to 0.024) per gram. The same replacement led to an increase in LDL by 0.017 mmol/L (95% CI 0.005 to 0.029). HDL did not change (0.0; 95% CI –0.004 to 0.004) (Figure 4.4) (Brouwer et al., 2013).

For comparison with the other TFAs, we also calculated the values per energy percentage. The results of the same 11 comparisons and 672 subjects then showed that replacement of 1% of energy of control fat by 1% of energy of ruminant TFAs led to an increase in the LDL to HDL ratio by 0.034 (95% CI 0.011 to 0.057). The same replacement led to an increase in LDL by 0.042 mmol/L (95% CI 0.014 to 0.071) with no change in HDL (0.00; 95% CI –0.009 to 0.011). The zero change in HDL can be explained because some studies used *cis*-unsaturated fatty acids as their control treatment, whereas other studies used saturated fatty acids as their control treatment. A decrease in HDL can be expected if compared to *cis*-unsaturated fatty acids (Brouwer et al., 2010).

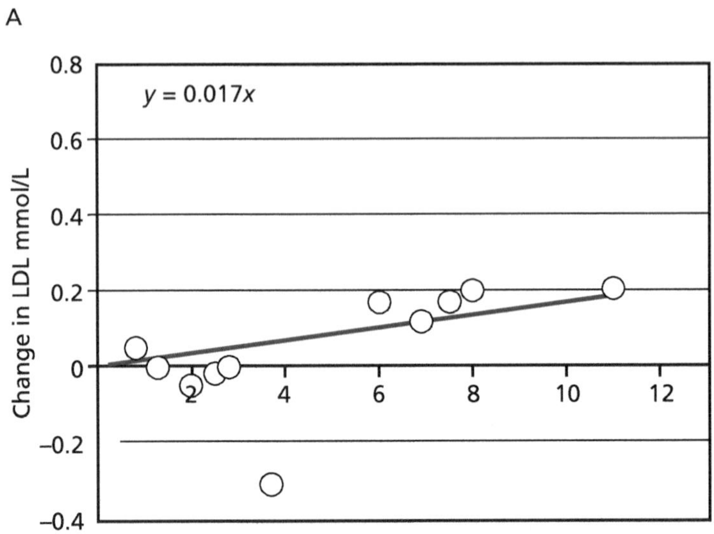

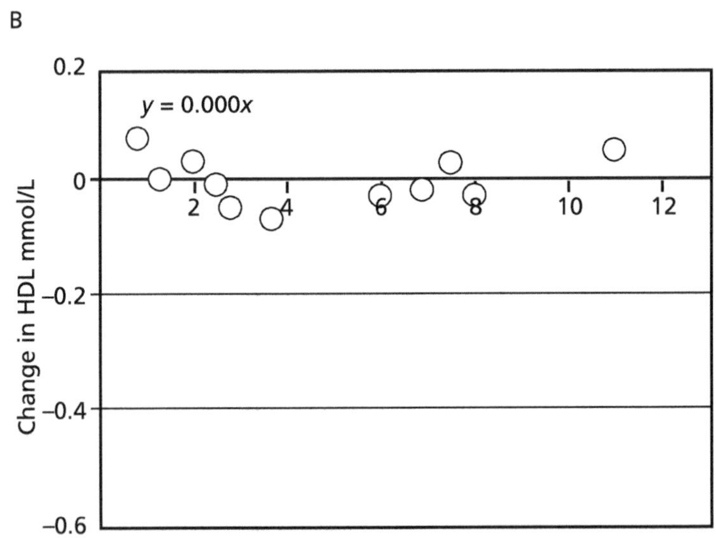

Figure 4.4 Results of randomized studies of the effects in ruminant *trans* fatty acids compared with control fatty acids on lipoproteins. Adapted from Brouwer, et al. (2013).

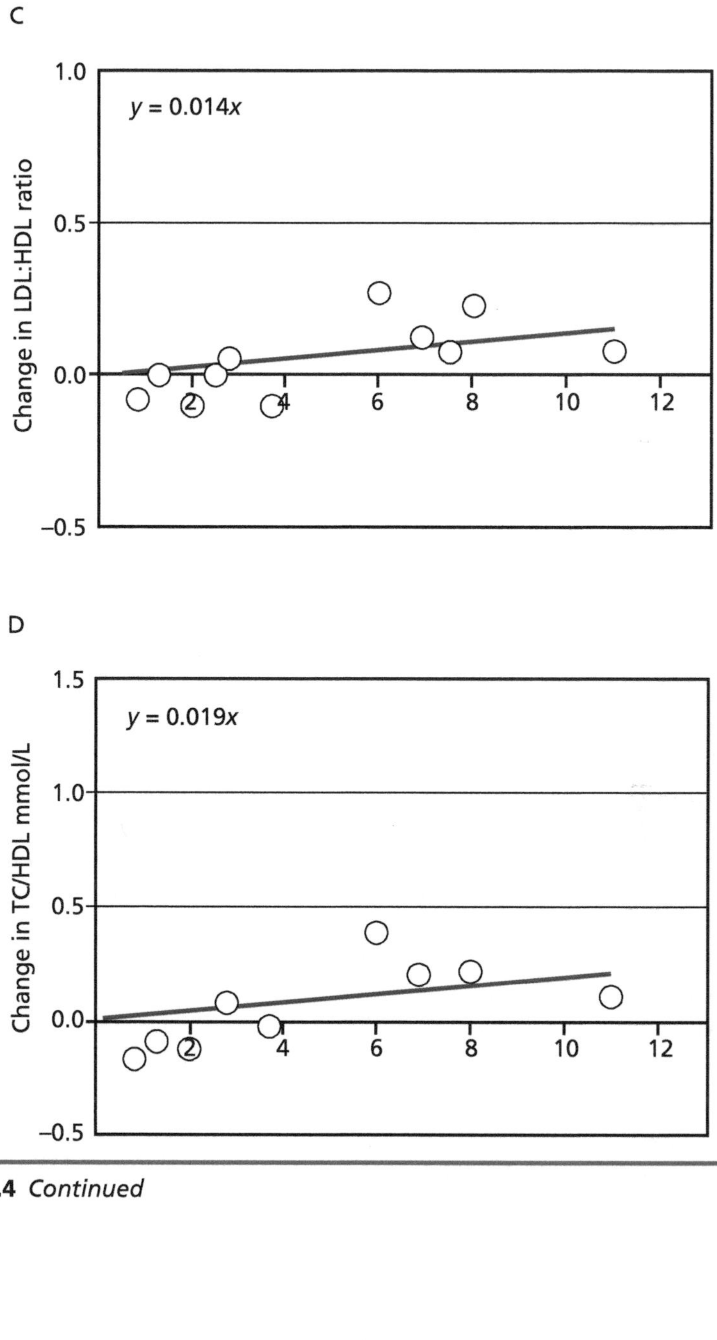

Figure 4.4 *Continued*

Conjugated Linoleic Acid and Cholesterol

Many studies have investigated effects of CLA on blood cholesterol concentrations. These studies differ from the studies on industrial and ruminant TFAs because the vast majority of these studies are not dietary controlled intervention studies, but rather placebo controlled supplement trials. Thus, most studies have investigated effects of supplemental CLA with placebo capsules without taking into account the background diet. This can be expected to lead to slightly more noise around the point estimates than in the case of dietary controlled intervention studies. The CLA used in the trials was usually industrially produced from vegetable oil. Most studies used CLA supplements that contained a 50:50 mixture of *cis*-9, *trans*-11 CLA and *trans*-10 CLA. Some studies used an 80:20 mixture or another ratio.

To summarize all studies on effects of CLA on lipoproteins, we used the same methodological approach as we did for the studies on ruminant TFAs. We identified 33 papers, which included 47 comparisons and 2048 subjects (Brouwer et al., 2013). The results of the CLA trials were quite similar to the results from the dietary intervention studies on ruminant and industrial TFAs. The plasma LDL/HDL ratio increased by 0.018 (95% CI 0.006 to 0.030) and the total cholesterol/HDL ratio increased by 0.027 (95% CI 0.011 to 0.043) when 1 g of control oil was replaced by CLA. CLA increased LDL-C by 0.014 mmol/L (95% CI 0.004 to 0.024) and decreased HDL-C by –0.006 mmol/L (95% CI –0.012 to –0.0001). Because body weight change signficantly influences cholesterol concentrations, we also performed the analysis with only those studies in which the subjects were weight stable during the trial (body weight did not change more than 1.5 kg during the study course). The regression analysis of 24 studies with 30 comparisons showed a somewhat larger increase in the plasma LDL/HDL ratio of 0.022 (95% CI 0.009 to 0.035), and an increase in the total cholesterol/HDL of 0.025 (95% CI 0.007 to 0.043). LDL-C increased by 0.015 mmol/L (95% CI 0.005 to 0.025), and HDL-C decreased by –0.006 mmol/L (95% CI –0.012 to 0.00).

Taking everything together, it is clear that all fatty acids with a double bond in the *trans* configuration have an unfavorable effect on lipoproteins. Effects of ruminant TFAs seem slightly less detrimental than those of industrial TFAs and CLA. However, the ruminant estimate is based on a limited number of studies and the difference between the regression lines was not significant (Brouwer et al., 2010, 2013).

Trans Fatty Acids and Cardiovascular Disease

After publication of the first dietary controlled trials (Katan et al., 1995; Mensink et al. 1992), it became clear that higher intake of TFAs was associated with a higher risk of coronary heart disease in observational studies (Willett and Ascherio, 1994). Pooled analysis of three retrospective control studies using TFA concentrations in adipose tissue resulted in a combined relative risk (RR) of 1.29 (95% CI 1.15 to 1.51; $p < 0.001$). A relative risk, or risk ratio, is the ratio of the risk in the exposed group divided by the risk in the unexposed group. Thus, a relative risk of 1.29 implies that the risk of getting coronary heart disease was 29% higher in the group with the higher intake of TFAs compared to the group with the lower intake. This is an estimate for total TFAs, as it is not possible to make a distinction in the source of fatty acids in adipose tissue samples (Mozaffarian et al., 2006).

Industrial *Trans* Fatty Acids and Cardiovascular Disease

Mozaffarian et al. (2006) summarized the results of observational studies and reported a pooled multivariable adjusted relative risk of 1.23 (95% CI 1.11 to 1.37) for isocaloric replacement of 2% of energy of TFAs by carbohydrate. Based on a meta-analysis of the two U.S. cohorts, Mozaffarian and Clarke (2009) also reported the RRs for replacement by other macronutrients. Replacement of 2% of energy of industrial TFAs by saturated TFAs led to an RR of 1.20 (95% CI 1.07 to 1.34); replacement by monounsaturated fatty acids (MUFA) led to an RR of 1.27 (95% CI 1.14 to 1.42); and replacement by polyunsaturated fatty acids (PUFA) led to an RR of 1.32 (95% CI 1.17 to 1.49) (Mozaffarian et al., 2009).

Bendsen et al. (2011) found very similar results when taking into account seven cohort studies on effects of total TFAs and risk of CHD events (RR = 1.22; 95% CI 1.08 to 1.38; $p = 0.002$) and also on risk of fatal CHD (RR = 1.24; 95% CI 1.07 to 1.43; $p = 0.003$). They also made the distinction between industrial and ruminant TFAs in their meta-analysis. They pooled data of three cohorts on industrial TFAs and four cohorts on ruminant TFA intakes and compared the extreme quintiles of intake. The pooled analysis of the studies on industrial TFAs showed an RR of 1.21 (95% CI 0.97 to 1.50). This finding was not significant, but that might be due to lack of power. The pooled analysis of the four studies on ruminant TFAs showed no association between intake and risk of CHD event (RR = 0.93; 95% CI 0.74 to 1.18).

CLA is only a minor constituent of the usual diet; therefore, not many studies have investigated associations between CLA and cardiovascular disease. As far as we know, only one observational study investigated such an association. In a case-control study in Costa Rica, the concentrations of *cis*-9, *trans*-11-CLA in adipose tissue was associated with a lower risk of myocardial infarction (OR = 1.51; 95% CI 0.36 to 0.71; p-trend < 0.0001) (Smit et al., 2010).

Thus, the observational studies on the association between intake of industrial TFAs and the risk of cardiovascular disease indicate that intake of industrial TFAs has a harmful cardiovascular health effect. Observational studies do not show an association of TFAs from ruminant sources with risk of cardiovascular disease. This could be explained by the fact that ruminant TFAs are usually consumed in dairy products, which may contain other nutrients that protect the heart, or the contrast between the quintiles of intake is too low to show an association, because TFAs from ruminant sources are generally consumed in much lower quantities than TFAs from industrial sources (Warensjo et al., 2010).

There are no dietary intervention trials available on the effect of intake of TFAs on hard endpoints of cardiovascular disease. It is also not expected that such studies will be performed in the future, as the foreseen effect is an increased risk of cardiovascular disease. Therefore, such a trial can be considered unethical.

Trans Fatty Acids and Systemic Inflammation and Endothelial Function

Systemic inflammation, oxidative stress, and endothelial dysfunction are suggested to be pathways by which a higher intake of TFAs could lead not only to a higher risk of cardiovascular disease, but also to other diseases.

Taking all the evidence together, there are indications that industrial TFAs have unfavorable effects on inflammation, although studies do show varying outcomes. For endothelial function, it is unclear whether industrial TFAs have an effect (Wallace and Mozaffarian, 2009). The number of well-designed studies on this topic is extremely limited, and therefore it is difficult to establish whether there is an effect.

The limited number of available studies on ruminant TFAs and CLA and inflammation and endothelial function do not point in the direction of strong effects, but the dosages of ruminant TFAs used in these studies might be too low to pick up an effect (Desroches et al., 2005; Gagliardi et al., 2010; McCrorie et al., 2011; Tholstrup et al., 2006; Tricon et al., 2006).

Trans Fatty Acids and Adiposity and Weight Management

Industrial and Ruminant *Trans* Fatty Acids and Adiposity and Body Weight

No long-term human intervention studies on effects of either industrial or ruminant TFAs to assess effects on adiposity and weight have been published. Some cohort studies have reported associations of intake of TFAs in adults and measurements of adiposity or weight changes. Colditz et al. (1990) reported an association between intake of TFAs and BMI in the Nurses' Health Study. Koh-Banerjee et al. (2003) reported that in the Health Professionals' follow-up study, a 2% increment in energy intake from *trans* fats that were isocalorically substituted for either polyunsaturated fats or carbohydrates was significantly associated with a 0.77-cm waist gain over nine years ($p < 0.001$ for each comparison). In the Nurses' Health Study, intake of TFAs was also associated with increases in body weight in women who were overweight (Field et al., 2007). Thus, there is limited, but consistent, evidence that there is a relation between intake of TFAs and an increase in body weight (Thompson et al., 2011a).

Conjugated Linoleic Acid and Body Weight

In contrast to the limited number of studies on industrial or ruminant TFAs and body weight, many studies have investigated the effect of CLA on body weight. Animal studies showed promising results for the ability of CLA to reduce body weight. However, the studies in humans have shown inconsistent results, as reviewed by McCrorie et al. (2011). In 2010, the European Food Safety Authority (EFSA) decided, based on the then-available evidence, that neither a cause–effect relationship of CLA with maintenance of body weight nor with increase in lean body mass could be established (EFSA, 2010).

Trans Fatty Acids and Diabetes and Insulin Resistance

Part of the effect of TFAs on cardiovascular disease might be through diminished insulin resistance or diabetes. This could specifically be the case for vulnerable groups such as overweight and obese people. However, results of trials and observational studies are not equivocal at the moment (McCrorie et al., 2011; Wallace and Mozaffarian, 2009). Metabolic intervention studies, as well as observational studies on industrial TFAs and glucose-insulin homeostasis, showed mixed results. It is also unclear whether CLA affects diabetes risk or indicators of diabetes (McCrorie et al., 2011). Thompson et al. (2011b) concluded, on the basis of all available evidence, that there is limited evidence for a weak association at high intakes of TFAs, but very little convincing evidence that habitual dietary intake will significantly affect risk of diabetes.

Thus, for the majority of the population, there is no significant risk; however, future research will have to show whether vulnerable groups or people with specific genotypes are at risk. If future research shows that TFAs unfavorably influence insulin resistance and diabetes, or that patients who suffer from this are more sensitive to the effects of TFAs, then the consequences of high intakes of TFAs are higher than when TFAs have no effects on either insulin status or diabetes. This also has consequences for the expected magnitude of effect of TFAs on cardiovascular disease because diabetes gives a higher risk of cardiovascular disease.

Trans Fatty Acids and Cancer

There is limited evidence on the relation between TFAs and cancer. There are studies available on breast cancer, colon/colorectal cancer, prostate cancer, and a few isolated studies on other cancer sites. Thompson et al. (2008) and Smith et al. (2009) have summarized the outcomes of these studies. Overall, there is not enough evidence to state whether intake of TFAs is associated with cancer risk. The studies that have been published vary a lot in design and approach and show conflicting results. Correlations with intake of other nutrients and lifestyle also make it difficult to consider whether the relation is true. Furthermore, none of the studies show very strong associations.

Industrial and Ruminant *Trans* Fatty Acids and Cancer

Laake et al. (2013) made the distinction in the association between TFAs from different sources and risk of cancer. In a large population-based cohort study with 77,568 men and women from Norway, they studied the association between intake from partially hydrogenated vegetable oil, partially hydrogenated fish oil, and ruminant *trans* fat and risk of cancer. The study showed different associations with cancer risk for the different sources. TFAs from partially hydrogenated fish oil showed more unfavorable risks than TFAs from partially hydrogenated plant oils when the highest versus the lowest categories were compared. The hazard ratio for the association of partially hydrogenated fish oil with rectal cancer was 1.43 (95% CI 1.09 to 1.88) and with multiple myeloma was 2.02 (1.24 to 3.28). In contrast, the association with prostate cancer was protective (0.82; 0.69 to 0.96). The hazard ratios for partially hydrogenated vegetable oil were 0.52 (95% CI 0.31 to 0.87) for pancreatic cancer in men and 0.70 (0.50 to 0.98) for non-Hodgkin lymphoma in men and women. Ruminant TFAs showed increased risks for all cancers (1.09; 95% CI 1.02 to 1.16), but the authors speculate that this might be linked to intake of saturated fat.

Up to now, associations are weak and study results are inconsistent, which makes it impossible to determine whether TFAs are associated to risk of cancer.

Conjugated Linoleic Acids and Cancer

Cell and animal studies have suggested that CLA may have anticarcinogenic effects. There are no human studies available that investigated effects of intake of CLA or CLA status on cancer, which is not surprising considering the low dietary intake of CLA (McCrorie et al., 2011). Some observational studies have investigated effects of milk intake on cancer. However, there are so many other ingredients in milk that may influence the association that these studies cannot be considered studies on intake of CLA and cancer. Thus, there is no consistent evidence from human studies suggesting that TFAs are associated with cancer.

Reduction of Intake of *Trans* Fatty Acids

It is clear that all fatty acids with a double bond in the *trans* configuration have unfavorable effects on lipoproteins. Other health effects of TFAs are less clear. However, the effects on lipoproteins already make it worthwhile to reduce intake as much as possible. Since the 1990s, changes in the formulation of foods, labeling of food products, and actions from governments have resulted in a dramatic decrease in the intake of TFAs from industrial sources (Korver and Katan, 2006; L'Abbe et al., 2009). The intake can be further decreased if industrial *trans* fats are avoided in the preparation of fried foods and bakery shortenings (Katan, 2006). Furthermore, there is still a lot of difference between countries with respect to the availability of food products with high contents of TFAs. This has consequences for the intake. For example, popular fast food items in 2009 in Eastern Europe were still high in *trans* fat, whereas *trans* fat had almost disappeared from similar products in Western Europe (Stender et al., 2012).

The exact effect of intake of ruminant TFAs on cardiovascular health is still not known, but it is not a major health problem because the total intake of TFAs from ruminant sources is only about 0.5% of energy, on average. Removal of ruminant TFAs from dairy products and meat is technically not feasible. Therefore, the most sensible advice to consumers is still to consume dairy products that are low in total fat. If consumers follow this advice, they will decrease their intake of ruminant TFAs and of saturated fat, but the intake of the beneficial ingredients in dairy products is assured.

Dietary intake of CLA is low, but CLA is also sold as supplements and those intakes can mount up to several grams per day. The EFSA has denied all health claims on CLA and we conclude that CLA unfavorably affects cholesterol concentrations. Effects on markers of diabetes are also still unclear. Therefore, the Food Standards Australia and New Zealand binational government agency decided not to allow foods enriched with CLA on the market. Thus, CLA supplements have no proven benefit, but regular intake may have unwanted health effects.

Conclusion

It is clear that intake of industrial TFAs has unfavorable health effects. Thus, intake of these fatty acids should be as low as possible, and future research should not focus so much on establishing other health effects but rather should search for technological solutions for replacement of these TFAs in food products. This is specifically a challenge for the bakery industry because of the specific baking properties of TFAs.

Dietary intake of ruminant TFAs and CLA is not a large health problem, because intake is already low. Intake should decrease even further if consumers take the advice to eat low fat dairy and decrease intake of saturated fat.

CLA in the diet is a very minor component, but CLA supplements are sometimes used. Until now, no clear positive health effects are established, and CLA shows similar negative effects on lipoprotein concentrations as other TFAs. Therefore, there is no reason to support intake of CLA supplements at the moment. Future research should show what effects CLA has on inflammatory processes and insulin and other diabetes-related factors.

References

Ascherio, A.; Katan, M. B.; Zock, P. L.; Stampfer, M. J.; Willett, W. C. *Trans* Fatty Acids and Coronary Heart Disease. *N. Engl. J. Med.* **1999,** *340* (25), 1994–1998.

Bendsen, N. T.; Christensen, R.; Bartels, E. M.; Astrup, A. Consumption of Industrial and Ruminant *Trans* Fatty Acids and Risk of Coronary Heart Disease: A Systematic Review and Meta-analysis of Cohort Studies. *Eur. J. Clin. Nutr.* **2011,** *65* (7), 773–783.

Brouwer, I. A.; Wanders, A. J.; Katan, M. J. Effect of Animal and Industrial *Trans* Fatty Acids on HDL and LDL Cholesterol Levels in Humans—A Quantitative Review. *PLoS One* **2010,** *5* (3), e9434.

Brouwer, I. A.; Wanders, A. J.; Katan, M. J. *Trans* Fatty Acids and Cardiovascular Health: Research Completed? *Eur. J. Clin. Nutr.* **2013,** *67* (5), 541–547.

Colditz, G. A.; Willett, W. C.; Stampfer, M. J.; London, S. J.; Segal, M. R. Patterns of Weight Change and Their Relation to Diet in a Cohort of Healthy Women. *Am. J. Clin. Nutr.* **1990,** *51* (6), 1100–1105.

Craig-Schmidt, M. C. World-wide of *Trans* Fatty Acids. *Atheroscler. Suppl.* **2006,** *7* (2), 1–4.

Desroches, S.; Chouinard, P. Y.; Galibois, I.; Corneau, L.; Delisle, J.; Lamarche, B.; Couture, P.; Bergeron, N. Lack of Effect of Dietary Conjugated Linoleic Acids Naturally Incorporated into Butter on the Lipid Profile and Body Composition of Overweight and Obese Men. *Am. J. Clin. Nutr.* **2005,** *82* (2), 309–319.

EFSA Panel on Dietetic Products, Nutrition and Allergies (NDA). *EFSA Journal* **2010**, *8* (10), 1794.

Field, A. E.; Willett, W. C.; Lissner, L.; Colditz, G. A. Dietary Fat and Weight Gain among Women in the Nurses' Health Study. *Obesity (Silver Spring)* **2007,** *15* (4), 967–976.

Gagliardi, A. C.; Maranhao, R. C.; de Sousa, H. P.; Schaefer, E. J.; Santos, R. D. Effects of Margarines and Butter Consumption on Lipid Profiles, Inflammation Markers and Lipid Transfer to HDL Particles in Free-Living Subjects with the Metabolic Syndrome. *Eur. J. Clin. Nutr.* **2010,** *64* (10), 1141–1149.

Hulshof, K. F.; van Erp-Baart, M. A.; Anttolainen, M.; Becker, W.; Church, S. M.; Couet, C.; Hermann-Kunz, E.; Kesteloot, H.; Leth, T.; Martins, I. et al. Intake of Fatty Acids in Western Europe with Emphasis on *Trans* Fatty Acids: The TRANSFAIR Study. *Eur. J. Clin. Nutr.* **1999,** *53* (2), 143–157.

Katan, M. B. (2006). Regulation of *Trans* Fats: The Gap, the Polder, and McDonald's French Fries. *Atheroscler Suppl.* **2006,** *7* (2), 63–66.

Katan, M. B.; Zock, P. L.; Mensink, R. P. *Trans* Fatty Acids and Their Effects on Lipoproteins in Humans. *Annu. Rev. Nutr.* **1995,** *15*, 473–493.

Koh-Banerjee, P.; Chu, N. F.; Spiegelman, D.; Rosner, B.; Colditz, G.; Willett, W.; Rimme, E. Prospective Study of the Association of Changes in Dietary Intake, Physical Activity, Alcohol Consumption, and Smoking with 9-y Gain in Waist Circumference among 16 587 U.S. Men. *Am. J. Clin. Nutr.* **2003,** *78* (4), 719–727.

Korver, O.; Katan, M. B. The Elimination of *Trans* Fats from Spreads: How Science Helped to Turn an Industry Around. *Nutr. Rev.* **2006,** *64* (6), 275–279.

Laake I.; Carlsen M. H.; Pedersen, J. I.; Weiderpass, E.; Selmer, R.; Kirkhus B.; Thune, I.; Veierød, M. B. Intake of *Trans* Fatty Acids From Partially Hydrogenated Vegetable and Fish Oils and Ruminant Fat in Relation to Cancer Risk. *Int. J. Cancer.* **2013** *132* (6):1389–1403.

L'Abbe, M. R.; Stender, S.; Skeaff, C. M.; Ghafoorunissa; Tavella, M. Approaches to Removing *Trans* Fats from the Food Supply in Industrialized and Developing Countries. *Eur. J. Clin. Nutr.* **2009,** *63,* S50–S67.

Lichtenstein, A. H.; Appel, L. J.; Brands, M.; Carnethon, M.; Daniels, S.; Franch, H. A.; Franklin, B.; Kris-Ehterton, P.; Harris, W. S.; et al. Diet and Lifestyle Recommendations Revision 2006: A Scientific Statement from the American Heart Association Nutrition Committee. *Circulation* **2006,** *114* (1), 82–96.

Ma, D. W.; Wierzbicki, A. A.; Field, C. J.; Clandinin, M. T. Conjugated Linoleic Acid in Canadian Dairy and Beef Products. *J. Agric. Food Chem.* **1999,** *47* (5), 1956–1960.

McCrorie, T. A.; Keaveney, E. M.; Wallace, J. M.; Binns, L.; Livingstone, M. B. Human Health Effects of Conjugated Linoleic Acid from Milk and Supplements. *Nutr. Res. Rev.* **2011,** *24* (2), 206–227.

Mensink, R. P.; Zock, P. L.; Katan, M. B.; Hornstra, G. Effect of Dietary *Cis* and *Trans* Fatty Acids on Serum Lipoprotein[a] Levels in Humans. *J. Lipid Res.* **1992,** *33* (10), 1493–1501.

Mensink, R. P.; Zock, P. L.; Kester, A.; Katan, M. B. Effects of Dietary Fatty Acids and Carbohydrates on the Ratio of Serum Total to HDL Cholesterol and on Serum Lipids and Apolipoproteins: A Meta-analysis of 60 Controlled Trials. *Am. J. Clin. Nutr.* **2003,** *77* (5), 1146–1155.

Mozaffarian, D.; Clarke, R. Quantitative Effects on Cardiovascular Risk Factors and Coronary Heart Disease Risk of Replacing Partially Hydrogenated Vegetable Oils with Other Fats and Oils. *Eur. J. Clin. Nutr.* **2009,** *63* (Suppl. 2), S22–33.

Mozaffarian, D.; Katan, M. B.; Ascherio, A.; Stampfer, M. J.; Willett, W. C. *Trans* Fatty Acids and Cardiovascular Disease. *N. Engl. J. Med.* **2006,** *354* (15), 1601–1613.

Mozaffarian, D.; Aro, A.; Willett, W. C. Health Effects of Trans-Fatty Acids: Experimental and Observational Evidence. *Eur. J. Clin. Nutr.* **2009,** *63* (Suppl. 2), S5–21.

Parodi, P. W. Distribution of Isomeric Octadecenoic Fatty Acids in Milk Fat. *J. Dairy Sci.* **1976,** *59* (11), 1870–1873.

Pot, G. K.; Prynne, C. J.; Roberts, C.; Olson, A.; Nicholson, S. K.; Whitton, C.; Teacher, B.; Bates, B.; Henderson, H.; Pigott, S.; et al. National Diet and Nutrition Survey: Fat and Fatty Acid Intake from the First Year of the Rolling Programme and Comparison with Previous Surveys. *Br. J. Nutr.* **2012,** *107* (3), 405–415.

Precht, D.; Molkentin, J. *Trans* Fatty Acids: Implications for Health, Analytical Methods, Incidence in Edible Fats and Intake (A Review). *Nahrung* **1995,** *39* (5–6), 343–374.

Smit, L. A.; Baylin, A.; Campos, H. Conjugated Linoleic Acid in Adipose Tissue and Risk of Myocardial Infarction. *Am. J. Clin. Nutr.* **2010,** *92* (1), 34–40.

Smith, B. K.; Robinson, L. E.; Nam, R.; Ma, D. W. *Trans*-fatty Acids and Cancer: A Mini-Review. *Br. J. Nutr.* **2009**, *102* (9), 1254–66.

Stender, S.; Astrup, A.; Dyerberg, J. A. *Trans* European Union Difference in the Decline in *Trans* Fatty Acids in Popular Foods: A Market Basket Investigation. *BMJ Open.* **2012,** *17,* 2–5.

Tholstrup, T.; Raff, M.; Basu, S.; Nonboe, P.; Sejrsen, K.; Straarup, E. M. Effects of Butter High in Ruminant *Trans* and Monounsaturated Fatty Acids on Lipoproteins, Incorporation of Fatty Acids into Lipid Classes, Plasma C-reactive Protein, Oxidative Stress, Hemostatic Variables, and Insulin in Healthy Young Men. *Am. J. Clin. Nutr.* **2006,** *83* (2), 237–243.

Thompson, A. K.; Minihane, A. M.; Williams, C. M. *Trans* Fatty Acids and Weight Gain. *Int. J. Obes. (Lond)* **2011a,** *35* (3), 315–324.

Thompson, A. K.; Minihane, A. M.; Williams, C. M. *Trans* Fatty Acids, Insulin Resistance and Diabetes. *Eur. J. Clin. Nutr.* **2011b,** *65* (5), 553–564.

Thompson, A. K.; Shaw, D. I.; Minihane A. M.; Williams, C. M. *Trans*-fatty Acid and Cancer. The Evidence Reviewed. *Nutr. Res. Rev.* **2008**, 21(2), 174–88.

Tricon, S.; Burdge, G. C.; Jones, E. L.; Russell, J. J.; El-Khazan, S.; Moretti, E.; Hall, W. L.; Gerry, A. B.; Leake, D. S.; Grimble, R. F.; et al. Effects of Dairy Products Naturally Enriched with *Cis*-9,*trans*-11 Conjugated Linoleic Acid on the Blood Lipid Profile in Healthy Middle-aged Men. *Am. J. Clin. Nutr.* **2006,** *83* (4), 744–753.

Wallace, S. K.; Mozaffarian, D. *Trans*-Fatty Acids and Nonlipid Risk Factors. *Curr. Atheroscler. Rep.* **2009,** *11* (6), 423–433.

Warensjo, E.; Jansson, J. H.; Cederholm, T.; Boman, K.; Eliasson, M.; Hallmans, G.; Johannson, I.; Sjögren, P. Biomarkers of Milk Fat and the Risk of Myocardial Infarction in Men and Women: A Prospective, Matched Case-Control Study. *Am. J. Clin. Nutr.* **2010,** *92* (1), 194–202.

Willett, W. C.; Ascherio, A. *Trans* Fatty Acids: Are the Effects Only Marginal? *Am. J. Public Health* **1994,** *84* (5), 722–724.

Yang, T. S.; Liu, T. T. Optimization of Production of Conjugated Linoleic Acid from Soybean Oil. *J. Agric. Food Chem.* **2004,** *52* (16), 5079–5084.

5

Application of Gas Chromatography and Infrared Spectroscopy for the Determination of the Total *Trans* Fatty Acid, Saturated Fatty Acid, Monounsaturated Fatty Acid, and Polyunsaturated Fatty Acid Contents in Edible Fats and Oils

Magdi M. Mossoba, Cynthia Tyburczy, Pierluigi Delmonte, Ali Reza Fardin-Kia, and Jeanne I. Rader ■ *United States Food and Drug Administration, Center for Food Safety and Applied Nutrition, College Park, Maryland, United States*

Hormoz Azizian ■ *NIR Technologies, Oakville, Ontario, Canada*

John K.G. Kramer ■ *Guelph Food Research Center, Agriculture and Agri-Food Canada, Guelph, Ontario, Canada*

Introduction

Labeling Regulations

The U.S. Food and Drug Administration (FDA) is the federal agency charged with protecting public health by ensuring, among other things, the safety of foods. Specifically, the FDA is responsible for ensuring the public has accurate, science-based information that they need to plan a healthy diet. The FDA is currently updating the nutrition facts label and implementing new rules for restaurant menus and vending machines (FDA, 2011). Optimized and validated analytical methods are needed to ensure high rates of compliance with new food safety and labeling regulations. Recent advances in three chromatographic and spectroscopic methodologies—capillary gas chromatography (GC), mid-infrared (mid-IR), and near-infrared (NIR)—needed to meet this challenge are presented and discussed.

The FDA is responsible for ensuring that food products sold in the United States are properly labeled (FDA, 1993). The agency's mandate applies to foods, including dietary supplements, produced both domestically and in foreign countries. It has jurisdiction over approximately 80% of all food products sold in the United States; meat, poultry, and processed egg products, however, fall under the jurisdiction of the U.S. Department of Agriculture. The primary statutes governing the labeling requirements for foods under the FDA's jurisdiction are the U.S. Federal Food, Drug, and Cosmetic Act (FFDCA) and its amendments.

In response to a citizen petition and the increasing body of literature associating *trans* fat intake and risk of coronary heart disease, the FDA issued a proposed rule on food labeling in 1999 (FDA, 1999, 2000, 2002) and a corresponding final rule in 2003 (FDA, 2003a). In this final rule, the declaration of the amount of *trans* fat present in food products became mandatory on the nutrition facts label, effective

January 1, 2006. The final rule required that the declaration of the amount of *trans* fat be expressed as grams per serving to the nearest 0.5 g increment below 5 g, and to the nearest gram increment above 5 g. There was no requirement to list a percent daily value for *trans* fat on the nutrition facts label, as required for saturated fat and other mandatory nutrients (FDA, 2003a).

In the final rule (FDA, 2003a), *trans* fats are defined as unsaturated fatty acids that contain one or more isolated (i.e., nonconjugated) double bonds in a *trans* configuration. This definition identifies *trans* fat by its chemical structure regardless of its origin (i.e., industrially produced through partial hydrogenation or processing, or derived from dairy or meat products by biohydrogenation in ruminants). The FDA's definition of *trans* fat as unsaturated fatty acids with isolated double bonds is consistent with that of *cis* isomers of polyunsaturated fatty acids. However, *trans* conjugated linoleic acid isomers are excluded from the definition of *trans* fat because they do not meet the FDA's regulatory chemical definition of *trans* fat (FDA, 2003a).

The FDA has not stated how a company should determine the nutrient content of its products for labeling purposes. While FDA policy recommends that nutrient values for labeling be based on product composition as determined by laboratory analysis, there is no prohibition from using average values for a product derived from databases if a manufacturer is confident that the values obtained meet FDA compliance criteria (FDA, 2003b). Regardless of source, a company is responsible for the accuracy and compliance of the information on the label (FDA, 2003b; Health Canada, 2006).

Current Dietary Intake of *Trans* Fat from Partially Hydrogenated Oils

Mandatory *trans* fat labeling provides consumers with the ability to compare information provided on nutrition facts labels and select foods that are low in *trans* fat. *Trans* fat labeling also led to increased interest among food manufacturers in reformulating foods with the aim of reducing the amount of *trans* fat (Eckel et al., 2007; Mossoba et al., 2005). The food industry has been researching and implementing alternatives to *trans* fats that will eliminate or greatly reduce *trans* fat in food products. Current industry reformulation efforts focus on many new and original solutions, including use of trait-enhanced oils, modification of the hydrogenation process, use of interesterification, and use of natural oils and/or fractions high in solids (Eckel et al., 2007).

The *trans* fat content of many foods was assessed by the FDA prior to and after the mandatory labeling became effective. In a 2003 report (Federal Register, 2003), the mean intake by adults of *trans* fat from products containing partially hydrogenated oils was estimated to be 4.6 g/person/day (g/p/d) (2.0% of energy based on a 2,000 calorie diet). At that time, total *trans* fat intake from products containing partially hydrogenated oils and from animal products containing *trans* fat (1.2 g/p/d) was estimated to be 5.8 g/p/d for adults (2.6% of caloric energy). In 2010, an estimate of the current intake of industrially produced *trans* fat was prepared using available food consumption data, market share information, *trans* fat levels based on label declarations, and analytical data for products that were identified as containing partially hydrogenated oils (Doell et al., 2012). The reported mean *trans* fat intake for the U.S. population aged two years or more who consumed one or more of the processed foods identified as containing partially hydrogenated oil was estimated to be 1.3 g/p/d (0.6% of caloric energy). For high-level consumers (represented by the 90th percentile), the corresponding intake was estimated to be 2.6 g/p/d (1.2% of caloric energy). Based on these estimates, it was determined that the mean dietary intake of industrially produced *trans* fat for the U.S. population aged two years or more had decreased significantly since 2003. The data also showed that many food products, such as frozen potato products and most frozen breaded products, had been reformulated to eliminate partially hydrogenated oil. However, several products formulated with partially hydrogenated oil are still available on the market today and fall into two categories: foods that could be produced with lower levels of *trans* fat (e.g., cookies, baked goods, microwave popcorn, frozen pizza, frozen pies, shortening) and foods for which alternative choices for consumers are currently limited or unavailable (e.g., ready-to-use frostings, stick margarines) (Doell et al., 2012).

In addition, some U.S. jurisdictions, such as the state of California (State of California, 2010), New York City (City of New York, 2006), the city of Baltimore (Mayor and City Council of Baltimore City, 2009), and Montgomery County, Maryland (Montgomery County Board of Health, 2007), have imposed restrictions on the use of *trans* fat in food service establishments. These regulations do not permit food service establishments to sell or distribute foods or use food ingredients that contain more than 0.5 g *trans* fat per serving. As a result, by 2008, an estimated 98% of restaurants in New York City, compared with 50% in 2005 (Doell et al., 2012), were no longer using ingredients containing industrially produced *trans* fat.

Structure of Isolated and Conjugated TFAs and Their Sources

Fatty acids occur with different chain lengths and degrees of unsaturation. The naturally occurring unsaturated fatty acids with *cis* double bond configurations have double bonds that are found at specific positions along the fatty acid hydrocarbon chain. If two or more double bonds in a fatty acid are separated by a single methylene ($–CH_2$) group, the molecule is referred to as a *methylene-interrupted fatty acid.* If the double bonds are separated by more than one methylene group, they are referred to as non-methylene-interrupted fatty acids. An "isolated" double bond occurs in monounsaturated fatty acid, and double bonds are also considered "isolated" in methylene-interrupted and non-methylene-interrupted fatty acids.

The position of a double bond is defined by one of two methods: relative to the carboxyl group carbon atom (at C1) using the systematic Δ nomenclature, or relative to the terminal end methyl group of the hydrocarbon chain using the "n-" nomenclature. The latter is preferred for the designation of polyunsaturated fatty acids, and is also currently favored in the scientific literature, although the synonymous "omega" notation is commonly used in the popular media (e.g., for omega-3 polyunsaturated fatty acids in fish oils). According to the n- nomenclature, naturally occurring polyunsaturated fatty acids are designated as follows: [chain length]:[number of double bonds] n-[position of first double bond from the methyl end of the molecule]. For instance, oleic acid contains a single *cis* double bond between C9 and C10 along the C18 hydrocarbon chain. This fatty acid is commonly designated as 18:1n-9, but may also be referred to as *cis*-9-18:1 or *c*9-18:1. Most naturally occurring polyunsaturated fatty acids, such as those found in many edible fats and oils, have the first double bond located at the third, sixth, or ninth position from the methyl end of the molecule, as given for 18:3n-3 (or *cis*-9,*cis*-12,*cis*-15-18:3); 18:2n-6 (or *cis*-9,*cis*-12-18:2); or 20:3n-9 (or *cis*-5,*cis*-8,*cis*-11-20:3).

Geometric isomers are fatty acids with the same chain length and position of double bonds but differ in double bond configuration (i.e., *cis* or *trans*), while positional isomers are fatty acids that have the same chain length and number of double bonds but differ in the position of the unsaturation site along the fatty acid hydrocarbon chain.

TFAs are carboxylic acids that contain at least one double bond in the *trans* configuration, such as elaidic and vaccenic acids. These *trans* monounsaturated fatty acids are abbreviated as *trans*-9-18:1 (*trans*-9-18:1) and *trans*-11-18:1, respectively. *Trans* polyunsaturated fatty acids, such as *cis*-9,*trans*-12-18:2 or *trans*-9,*cis*-12,*cis*-15-18:3, may contain one or more *trans* double bonds per molecule. *Trans* "conjugated" fatty acids, such as *cis*-9,*trans*-11-18:2 or *cis*-9,*trans*-11,*cis*-15-18:3, are defined as fatty acids in which any two adjacent double bonds along the hydrocarbon chain are separated only by a carbon-carbon single bond rather than a methylene group.

TFAs can be produced through processes that involve catalytic hydrogenation and/or heating and can also occur naturally. *Trans* fat produced industrially by the partial hydrogenation of vegetable oils is the major contributor to TFA in the human diet, while smaller amounts are derived from processed (fully refined, bleached, and deodorized) vegetable oils and from frying operations. Other contributors are TFAs that are naturally produced in ruminants and those that are naturally found in some plant lipids.

Industrially Produced *Trans* Fatty Acids

For decades, the majority of *trans* fatty acids (TFAs) in the human diet were those industrially produced during the partial hydrogenation of vegetable oils (Ackman and Mag, 1998; Craig-Schmidt, 1998; List and Reeves, 2005; Wolff et al., 2000). Levels of *trans* fat of up to 50% of total fat have been reported in products containing partially hydrogenated vegetable oils. Prior to 2006, when the new TFA regulations became effective in the United States (Craig-Schmidt, 1998), Canada, and elsewhere (Ratnayake et al., 2007), similarly high levels could still be found in some food products. The peaks for *trans*-18:1 isomers in partially hydrogenated vegetable oils observed by gas chromatography (GC) generally exhibit a bell-shape abundance distribution (Mossoba et al., 2005). Using GC official methods, this distribution starts with the co-eluting mixture of three positional isomers, *trans*-6-*trans*-8-18:1, and ends with the co-eluting pair of isomers *trans*-13-/*trans*-14-18:1 (Cruz-Hernandez et al., 2004; Molkentin and Precht, 1995; Ratnayake et al., 2002, 2006). The content of *trans* polyunsaturated fatty acid is a function of the linoleic and linolenic acid contents of the oil that was partially hydrogenated and on the extent of hydrogenation. A greater extent of partial hydrogenation leads to a correspondingly lower level of *trans* polyunsaturated fatty acid and higher yields of *trans* monounsaturated fatty acid and saturated fatty acid (Hunter, 2006).

TFAs are produced during the partial hydrogenation and deodorization of vegetable oils as a result of the formation of geometric and positional isomers from the corresponding polyunsaturated fatty acid of the same chain length. The presence of TFA isomers in processed vegetable oils is usually limited to C18 *trans* containing fatty acid isomers because vegetable oils consist mainly of C18 polyunsaturated fatty acid and only small amounts of C16 or C20 polyunsaturated fatty acid. By contrast, the TFAs derived from ruminant fats contain more *trans* 16:1 and 20:1 isomers. These isomers are generated during the biohydrogenation of their corresponding polyunsaturated fatty acid in the animals' diets and by chain shortening to 16:1 and chain elongation to 20:1 of their 18:1 precursors (Kramer et al., 2008). Ruminant fats also contain branched chain fatty acids that often co-elute by GC in the same retention time region as that for the *cis* and *trans* monounsaturated fatty acids.

The deodorization of vegetable oils at temperatures above 200 °C was shown to yield up to 3% TFA (as percentage of total fat) due mainly to geometric isomerization of the all-*cis* linoleic and linolenic acids (Ackman, 1974; Buchgraber and Ulberth, 2002; Wolff, 1992). Similarly, deep frying at temperatures that exceeded 200 °C also led to the isomerization of these acids (Sebedio et al., 1996). Heating vegetable oils at such elevated temperatures resulted in approximately 14 times more products of isomerization of *cis* linolenic acid (i.e., *cis*-9,*cis*-12,*trans*-15-18:3 and *trans*-9,*cis*-12,*cis*-15-18:3 with minor quantities of *cis*-9,*trans*-12,*cis*-15-18:3, *cis*-9,*trans*-12,*trans*-15-18:3) than those of *cis* linoleic acid (i.e., *trans*-9,*trans*-12-18:2, and *cis*-9,*trans*-12-18:2 and *trans*-9,*cis*-12-18:2) (Sebedio et al., 1996; Wolff and Precht, 2002).

Capillary Gas Chromatography

Use of a single GC run for the determination of fatty acid composition, including total TFA content, has been the industry standard as evidenced by the various GC official methods of international scientific associations such as AOAC International, the American Oil Chemists' Society (AOCS), the International Organization for Standardization (ISO), and the Japan Oil Chemists' Society (JOCS). GC determinations, while time-consuming, have become increasingly more accurate with the availability of very long (100 m) and highly polar polysiloxane capillary columns (Buchgraber and Ulberth, 2001; Golay et al., 2007; Hunter, 2006; Kramer and Zhou, 2001; Kramer et al., 2002; Precht and Molkentin, 1999, 2000b, 2000c; Ratnayake, 2004; Ratnayake et al., 2002, 2006; Wolff and Precht, 2002; Wolff et al., 1998). New ionic liquid capillary columns, such as the SLB-IL111 column, have recently become available on the market. However, to date, no official method has yet recommended the use of these extremely high polarity GC columns (Delmonte et al., 2011).

GC requires derivatization to fatty acid methyl esters (FAME) and expertise particularly in identification of several *trans*-containing fatty acids and their isomers. Some FAME isomers may exhibit unresolved and overlapping GC peaks (Cruz-Hernandez et al., 2004, 2006; Hunter, 2006; Precht and Molkentin, 1996, 1999, 2000a, 2000b, 2000c; Wolff and Precht, 2002). At very low TFA levels (<2% of total fat) and under certain conditions (i.e., injection of less than optimal amounts of analytes), this overlapping may lead to underestimation of the content of an analyte. When the 100 m highly polar polysiloxane columns were first introduced over a decade ago, their use led to a significant improvement in GC performance over that of shorter capillary columns (Golay et al., 2007; Sebedio et al., 1996). Improved resolution and accuracy could also be obtained through procedures that entailed the prior separation of *trans* from *cis* geometric isomers by application of silver-ion chromatographic techniques—thin layer chromatography (TLC), high performance liquid chromatography (HPLC), or solid phase extraction (SPE) (AOCS, 2005; Cruz-Hernandez et al., 2006; Henninger and Ulberth, 1994; Hunter, 2006; Kramer and Zhou, 2001; Precht and Molkentin, 1999, 2000c; Wolff and Precht, 2002; Wolff et al., 1998). GC analysis of each isolated fraction could subsequently be carried out under significantly lower GC isothermal conditions (and requiring much longer separation times) and all individual TFA isomers could be resolved (Cruz-Hernandez et al., 2006; Hunter, 2006; Kramer et al., 2002; Precht and Molkentin, 2000c; Wolff et al., 1998). GC official methods [e.g., AOCS Ce 1h-05 (AOCS, 2005)] do not declare lower limits of detection and quantification, but total *trans* levels as low as 0.06% of total fat have been reported. However, the precision of the method was reported to be unsatisfactory at very low (<2% of total fat) levels (AOCS, 2005; Mossoba et al., 2005, 2009b). Comprehensive reviews on the determination of *trans* fat by GC have recently been published (Mossoba et al., 2005, 2009b).

Determination of Total Saturated, *Trans*, Monounsaturated, and Polyunsaturated Fatty Acid Contents of Representative Fast Foods by GC

In a recent GC study (Tyburczy et al., 2012a), the levels of *trans* fat, including the content of *trans* polyunsaturated fatty acids, in representative fast food samples from U.S.-based chain retail food establishments were quantified using the extraction and transmethylation procedure of AOAC Official Method 996.06 (AOAC, 2005) and the chromatography of GC Official Method AOCS Ce 1j-07 (AOAC, 2009). This GC method recommends the use of 100 m cyanopropyl polysiloxane columns, such as the SP-2560 column, for the separation and determination of FAME content and composition. The prepared FAME were also analyzed (Tyburczy et al., 2012a) using the 200 m SLB-IL111 ionic liquid column. The aim of this comparison was to evaluate whether the quantification of total, *trans*, saturated, and *cis*-unsaturated fat contents using the 200 m SLB-IL111 GC column was comparable to that obtained using official method Ce 1j-07 (AOAC, 2009) while also allowing for the determination of *trans* 18:1, *trans* 18:2, and *trans* 18:3 fatty acid isomeric content.

For that study, products from five fast food categories were selected, namely hamburgers, cheese pizza, chicken tenders/nuggets, french fries, and apple pie/turnovers (Tyburczy et al., 2012a). Few differences were found between the two GC columns for the quantitation of total fat and total saturated fatty acids, monounsaturated fatty acids, and polyunsaturated fatty acids contents in 32 fast food products. The content of total TFAs in these food products is presented in Table 5.A. Notably, ruminant-derived foods (i.e., hamburgers, cheese pizza) showed higher levels of total TFAs when samples were analyzed using the 200 m SLB-IL111 column than when the SP-2560 column was used. This difference between columns could be attributed to the improved separation of several TFA isomers, including *trans* 15-18:1 and the *trans* 18:3 fatty acid isomers, achieved with the 200 m SLB-IL111 column. Figure 5.1 presents the mean content of *trans* fat in the five fast food categories and shows that current levels ranged from 0.0 to 3.1 g of *trans* fat per serving. Foods with the highest levels had a *trans* fat content that was nearly 1.5 times the recommended maximum daily intake of 1% daily energy for *trans* fat (Lichtenstein et al., 2006; Mossoba et al., 2005).

The findings of Tyburczy et al. (2012a) verified the importance of AOCS Official Method Ce 1j-07 for the determination of total *trans*, saturated, monounsaturated, and polyunsaturated fatty acid contents of fats extracted from ruminant food products, and also demonstrated the advantage of the complementary analysis with the 200 m SLB-IL111 column (Delmonte et al., 2012) for the determination of *trans* monounsaturated fatty acid and *trans* polyunsaturated fatty acid isomeric compositions. As the restaurant industry continues to explore reformulation options for oils used in the production and preparation of menu items, with an emphasis on lowering total *trans* fat levels, the importance of the contribution of *trans* 18:2 and *trans* 18:3 fatty acids to the total *trans* fat content and the need for the accurate GC determination of these *trans* polyunsaturated fatty acids will be increasingly important.

Mid-Infrared Spectroscopy

A number of mid-IR spectroscopic procedures (Mossoba et al., 1996, 2005, 2009a, 2009b) and official methods (AOAC, 2000; AOCS, 2009c, 2009d) for quantifying

Table 5.A. Content of Total *Trans* Fat (% Total FA) in Fast Food Samples Determined by GC Analysis According to AOCS Official Method Ce 1j-07 or with the 200 m SLB IL111 Ionic Liquid Column[a-c]

Sample	Total *trans* FA	
	Ce 1j-07	SLB-IL111
Hamburger-1	4.81 ± 0.03[B]	5.00 ± 0.01[A]
Hamburger-2	5.35 ± 0.03	5.57 ± 0.07[A]
Hamburger-3	4.59 ± 0.02[B]	4.82 ± 0.01[A]
Hamburger-4	5.70 ± 0.02[B]	5.92 ± 0.03[A]
Hamburger-5	2.79 ± 0.01[B]	3.02 ± 0.00[A]
Hamburger-6	3.23 ± 0.03[B]	3.52 ± 0.01[A]
Pizza-1	5.69 ± 0.06[B]	5.90 ± 0.02[A]
Pizza-2	4.49 ± 0.02[B]	4.78 ± 0.00[A]
Pizza-3	4.12 ± 0.02[B]	4.43 ± 0.03[A]
Pizza-4	3.65 ± 0.03[B]	3.94 ± 0.02[A]
Pizza-5	3.93 ± 0.11	4.06 ± 0.02
Pizza-6	3.86 ± 0.04[B]	4.12 ± 0.02[A]
Chicken tenders-1	0.71 ± 0.00[B]	0.74 ± 0.00[A]
Chicken tenders-2	1.69 ± 0.00	1.71 ± 0.00
Chicken tenders-3	0.87 ± 0.00	0.84 ± 0.01
Chicken tenders-4	11.69 ± 0.01[B]	11.88 ± 0.02[A]
Chicken tenders-5	0.89 ± 0.01[A]	0.84 ± 0.01[B]
Chicken tenders-6	1.12 ± 0.00	1.12 ± 0.01
Chicken tenders-7	6.05 ± 0.07	6.15 ± 0.01
French fries-1	0.63 ± 0.02	0.70 ± 0.02
French fries-2	0.63 ± 0.01[B]	0.70 ± 0.00[A]
French fries-3	0.51 ± 0.00[B]	0.56 ± 0.00[A]
French fries-4	12.51 ± 0.53	12.62 ± 0.02
French fries-5	1.21 ± 0.01	1.25 ± 0.02
French fries-6	0.91 ± 0.01	0.92 ± 0.00
French fries-7	6.54 ± 0.04	6.64 ± 0.05
Apple pie-1	0.39 ± 0.00[B]	0.42 ± 0.00[A]
Apple pie-2	0.84 ± 0.00	0.85 ± 0.06
Apple pie-3	1.42 ± 0.00	1.41 ± 0.02
Apple pie-4	1.75 ± 0.01	1.78 ± 0.01
Apple pie-5	0.74 ± 0.03	0.84 ± 0.02
Apple pie-6	4.73 ± 0.02[B]	4.81 ± 0.02[A]

[a]Method Ce 1j-07 (AOAC, 2009) utilized the 100 m SP 2560 cyanopropyl polysiloxane column; chromatographic conditions with the 200 m SLB IL111 column were according to Delmonte et al. (Delmonte et al., 2012).

[b]Values (FA, % total FA) represent the means ± SD of two determinations for each food item.

[c]One-way analysis of variance was used to determine the effect of method on the mean content of *trans* FA; mean comparisons were performed using the Student's *t*-test, $\alpha = 0.05$. Superscript letters for pairwise comparisons indicate the significantly higher value, A>B.

Adapted from (Tyburczy et al., 2012a).

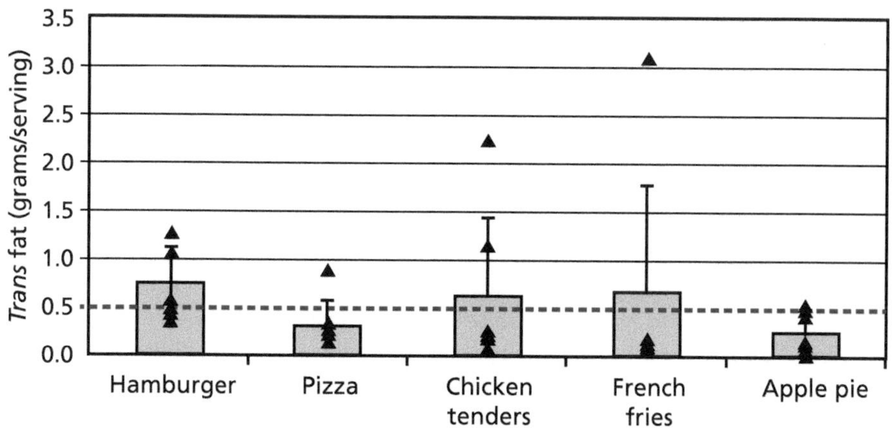

Figure 5.1 Grams/serving of *trans* fat in fast food samples. Bars represent the means ± SD of all determinations for each food category analyzed according to AOCS GC official method Ce 1j-07 (AOAC, 2009). Individual points represent the mean of two determinations for each food item (n = 6–7 per food category). The cutoff value of 0.5 g/serving, below which foods may be labeled as containing zero gram of *trans* fat, is depicted by a dashed line. Adapted from Tyburczy et al. (2012a).

total TFAs have been published as interest in an accurate and rapid methodology has steadily increased. Several procedures have been validated through national and international multilaboratory collaborative studies and approved as official methods (AOAC, 2000; AOCS, 2009c, 2009d).

The IR determination of total *trans* fats in edible oils is based on the measurement of the C–H out-of-plane deformation band height or area observed at 966 cm^{-1} that is uniquely characteristic of isolated (nonconjugated) double bonds with *trans* configuration. In partially hydrogenated oils, these *trans* double bonds are found primarily in *trans*-18:1 positional isomers, and often at much lower levels in minor hydrogenation products such as *cis*/*trans* and *trans*/*trans* methylene-interrupted (e.g., *cis*-9,*trans*-12-18:2 and *trans*-9,*trans*-12-18:2, respectively) and non-methylene-interrupted (e.g., *cis*-9,*trans*-13-18:2 and *trans*-9,*trans*-13-18:2, respectively) fatty acids. These minor components are also found in nonhydrogenated, processed edible oils. These and other more complex *trans*-containing polyunsaturated fatty acids may also occur in processed marine oils.

IR methodology has been extensively used in the edible fats and oils industry. The more recently validated attenuated total reflection (ATR) Fourier transform infrared (FT-IR) official methods can be applied directly to triacylglycerols (TAG). By contrast, while FAME derivatives are required for GC analysis, they could be measured as easily as TAG by IR spectroscopy in the internal reflection mode.

A major limitation of the IR methodology has been that the highly characteristic *trans* absorption at 966 cm^{-1} occurs on an elevated and sloping baseline. Thus, the measurement of its height or area becomes increasingly inaccurate as the TFA levels decrease, particularly below 5% of total fat. Although many modifications have been proposed to improve accuracy, only some transmission (AOCS, 2009d) and more recently ATR (AOAC, 2000; AOCS, 2009c) FT-IR official methods have succeeded in partially improving the accuracy of this determination. This is because several previously undetected interferences (for instance, those due to saturated or conjugated fatty acids or minor oil matrix components) adversely impacted accuracy and precision. However, most of these issues were overcome when the negative second derivative ATR-FT-IR spectroscopic procedure was proposed (Mossoba et al., 2009a) and validated as AOCS Official Method Cd 14e-09 in 2009 (AOCS, 2009b).

Another minor limitation of this IR methodology has been the assumption that the vast majority of unknown mono-*trans* fat components (mono-*trans* monoenes, mono-*trans* dienes, and mono-*trans* trienes) or their positional and geometrical (e.g., *cis,trans* and *trans,cis*) isomers have the same absorptivity as that of mono-*trans* trielaidin (*trans* double bond at C9) used for calibration. Although the absorptivity of these various mono-*trans* products has not been measured because commercial standards are not available, their absorptivities are presumed to be fairly similar. By contrast, significant differences in absorptivity would be expected between mono-*trans* monoenes, di-*trans* dienes, and tri-*trans* trienes. However, these products are usually found in fats and oils at extremely low levels (<0.1%) and would most probably not have any significant adverse impact on quantification.

ATR-FTIR Official Methods AOCS Cd 14d-99 and AOAC 2000.10

In the late 1990s, a new ATR-FT-IR procedure was developed, validated in a collaborative study, and identified as AOCS Official Method Cd 14d-99 (AOCS, 2009c) and AOAC Official Method 2000.10 (AOAC, 2000). Lower reproducibility relative standard deviation, RSD(R), values (Adam et al., 2000; AOCS, 2009b; Mossoba et al., 2005, 2009b) were obtained in comparative studies by ATR-FT-IR (AOAC, 2000; AOCS, 2009c) relative to transmission FT-IR methods (AOCS, 2009c, 2009d).

This ATR method was successfully used to rapidly (<5 min) measure the 966 cm^{-1} *trans* band as a symmetric feature on a nearly horizontal baseline. The experimental aspects of this ATR-FT-IR official method were simpler than those involving transmission measurements. This method required the measurement of the *trans* fat single-beam spectrum relative to that of a reference *trans*-free oil. This reference material was found by GC to contain a very low level, approximately 0.03%, *trans* fat as a percentage of total fat. The ATR approach avoided issues from earlier IR methods, such as the need to weigh test portions and their quantitative dilution in the volatile CS_2 solvent, which was also used as the reference background material. When this *trans*-free oil reference background material was used (instead of CS_2), the sloping baseline of the 966 cm^{-1} *trans* band became approximately horizontal (Adam et al., 2000; AOAC, 2000; AOCS, 2009c; Mossoba et al., 1996, 2001a). Therefore, the contributions of the TAG absorptions that led to an elevated and sloping baseline in the first place were removed. The fairly horizontal baseline reduced the uncertainty in measuring the band area at low *trans* levels.

In the ATR mode, calibration is achieved by accurately preparing quantitative *trans* fat standards in the range of interest. This is accomplished by weighing varying amounts of neat (without any solvent) trielaidin (*tr*ans-9-18:1) and adding them to a neat *trans*-free reference oil. A small volume of each standard is then placed on the top of the preheated (65 °C) horizontal surface of the internal reflection zinc selenide or diamond element of a single- or multiple-reflection ATR accessory. The larger the number of internal bounces of the IR beam inside an ATR crystal, the proportionately greater the sensitivity (Mossoba et al., 2012).

Depending on the size of the internal reflection element, the volume of test sample used can range from 50 μL to as little as 1 μL. The surface of the crystal must be completely covered with the test portion during data collection. In addition, cross contamination must be avoided and careful cleaning of the ATR element with ethanol after each measurement is essential. Single-beam spectra of *trans* reference *tr*ans-9-18:1 TAG standards are measured by FT-IR spectroscopy and referenced relative to the single beam spectrum of a *trans*-free reference oil to obtain absorbance spectra. These spectra exhibit the 966 cm^{-1} *trans* band as a symmetric feature on a nearly horizontal baseline. The areas under the *trans* band can then be integrated electronically between fixed limits, (e.g., 990 and 945 cm^{-1}) and used to generate a calibration function. The resulting linear regression function relating the integrated area of the absorption band and the amount of *tr*ans-9-18:1 TAG (as percent of total fat) has a negligible *y*-intercept and a high regression coefficient R^2 value of 0.999 (Adam et al., 2000; AOAC, 2000; AOCS, 2009c; Mossoba et al., 1996, 2001a). Single beam spectra of unknown test samples are similarly measured relative to the single beam spectrum of the same *trans*-free reference oil used for calibration. The *trans* fat content (as percentage of total fat) is then calculated by substituting the value of the integrated area of the *trans* band in the linear regression function. This ATR method also assumes that the major component to be determined in any test sample is trielaidin.

During evaluation of the applicability of ATR-FT-IR for matrices of low *trans* fat and/or low total fat content (e.g., milk), it was found that the presence of low levels (<1%) of conjugated *cis*/*trans* dienes absorbing near 985 cm^{-1} and 947 cm^{-1} interfered with the determination of total isolated TFAs and that use of spectral subtraction techniques did not provide a satisfactory solution (Mossoba et al., 2001b). To overcome this limitation of the ATR-FT-IR method, Mossoba et al. (2001b) added known amounts of trielaidin to *trans* fat test portions, measured the resulting ATR-FT-IR *trans* bands, and calculated the *trans* content of the product using a linear regression equation. This standard addition modified ATR-FT-IR procedure was more time-consuming than the original ATR-FT-IR procedure, but eliminated adverse effects on accuracy resulting from interferences near 966 cm^{-1}. Mossoba et al. recommended that the modified method be applied to the determination of total isolated *trans* fat in ruminant-derived products (Mossoba et al., 2001b).

ATR-FTIR Spectroscopy Negative Second Derivative Method

One limitation of the ATR-FT-IR method (AOAC, 2000; AOCS, 2009c) has been that the composition of every unknown *trans* fat–containing fat or oil sample under investigation should match that of the *trans*-free reference oil as closely as possible. This condition is often hard to meet, especially for milk fat matrices (Kramer et al., 1997), and has led to unsatisfactory quantification, particularly for *trans* fat levels below 5% of total fat (Adam et al., 2000; AOAC, 2000; AOCS, 2009c; Mossoba et al., 1996, 2001a). However, this limitation was overcome with the negative second derivative ATR-FT-IR method (AOCS, 2009b).

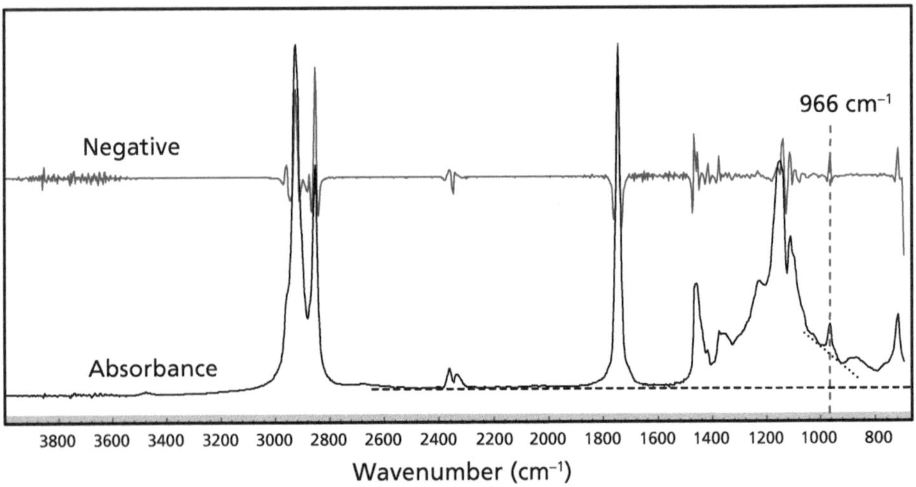

Figure 5.2 Negative second derivative (top) and absorption (bottom) spectra for a test sample consisting of trielaidin in tripalmitin with a *trans* level of 12.58% (as percentage of total fat). A vertical line indicates the position of the unique band due to isolated *trans* double bonds at 966 cm^{-1}. The second derivative spectrum was multiplied by −1 to orient the bands in an upward position that facilitates analysis. Adapted from Mossoba et al. (2011).

A novel ATR-FT-IR spectroscopic procedure that measures the height of the negative second derivative of the *trans* absorption band relative to an open beam (instead of a *trans*-free reference oil) was recently reported (Milosevic et al., 2004; Mossoba et al., 2007a, 2007b, 2009a). This procedure eliminated both the baseline offset and slope of the *trans* IR band (966 cm^{-1}) and the need for a *trans*-free reference fat (Figures 5.2 and 5.3). Due to the narrow width observed for second derivative bands, it became possible, for the first time, to detect the presence of weak interference bands close to the *trans* absorption band, specifically near or below 960 cm^{-1}. The latter bands were subsequently confirmed to be due to saturated fat components (Mossoba et al., 2007a). The saturated TAG standards trilaurin (12:0), trimyristin (14:0), tripalmitin (16:0), and triarachidin (20:0) were all found to exhibit weak absorption bands with varying degrees of interferences (Mossoba et al., 2007a). Therefore, for fats and oils with a high content of saturated fats and only a trace amount of *trans* fat (≤0.1% of total fat), such as coconut oil and cocoa butter, the weak bands observed at wavenumbers slightly lower than 966 cm^{-1} must not be erroneously reported as *trans*

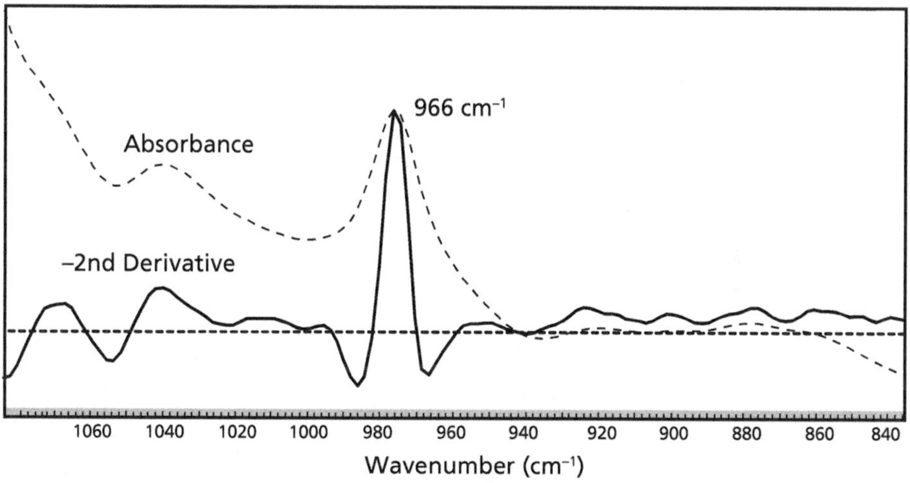

Figure 5.3 The region of the spectra that exhibit the deformation band for isolated *trans* double bonds at 966 cm^{-1} is expanded for the negative second derivative (solid line) and absorption (dotted line) spectra for a test sample consisting of trielaidin in tripalmitin with a *trans* level of 12.58% (as percentage of total fat). The height of the negative second derivative band can be accurately measured from a horizontal baseline. It is noted that several weak bands observed in the same spectral region are also more pronounced in the negative second derivative spectrum (narrower bandwidths) than in the absorption spectrum. Adapted from Mossoba et al. (2011).

fat bands. This recognition of potential interferences from saturated fats (Mossoba et al., 2007a) led to more accurate interpretations of IR spectra for unknown fats and oils and improved the accuracy of the IR spectroscopic determination at low *trans* fat levels (<5% of total fat). In addition, the second derivative approach allowed the spectral resolution of the 966 cm^{-1} feature from interferences attributed to conjugated *trans, trans* (near 990 cm^{-1}) and/or *cis*/*trans* (near 990 and 950 cm^{-1}) double bonds in fatty acids found in products such as milk fat.

This negative second derivative ATR-FT-IR procedure was subsequently validated in an international collaborative study (Mossoba et al., 2011) and adopted as Official Method AOCS Cd 14e-09 in 2009 (AOCS, 2009b).

Evaluation of a Portable FT-IR Spectrometer

Recently, the performance of a novel, portable FT-IR system equipped with a heated, nine-bounce diamond ATR crystal was evaluated and compared to that of a conventional benchtop single-bounce ATR-FT-IR spectrometer (Mossoba et al., 2012). For comparison, unknown fat and oil test samples containing varying levels of TFAs were analyzed by both systems. The total *trans* fat levels for all of the unknown test samples fell within the range of 0.5% to 54% of total fat. When the two sets of *trans* fat values for unknown test samples were plotted, good agreement was found (slope of 1.04, $R^2 = 0.999$) between the results obtained with the two ATR-FT-IR systems. The introduction of the nine-bounce diamond ATR crystal resulted in the lowering of the limit of quantification for *trans* fat in gravimetrically prepared TAG standards from approximately 2% to 0.34% of total fat. This study indicated that the application of the negative second derivative ATR-FT-IR official method AOCS Cd 14e-09 and the use of the new nine-bounce portable ATR-FT-IR instrumentation could lead to a five-fold enhancement in sensitivity relative to that of single-bounce systems.

Evaluation of Low *Trans* Fat Edible Oils by ATR-FT-IR and GC Methods

Tyburczy et al. (2012b) recently evaluated the quantitation of *trans* fat in 25 edible fats and oils, all labeled as containing 0 g *trans* fat, by current ATR-FT-IR and GC Official Methods. A comparative ATR-FT-IR analysis was also performed using (1) a benchtop instrument equipped with a heated seven-reflection diamond ATR crystal and a high-sensitivity cryogenically cooled detector, and (2) on a portable instrument equipped with a heated nine-reflection diamond ATR crystal and a detector that operates at room temperature. Consistent with the findings of Mossoba et al. (2012), the two ATR-FT-IR instruments yielded comparable quantitations of *trans* fat in the gravimetric standards (trielaidin added to triolein) over the range of 0.33–4.83% of total fat (Figure 5.4). The quantitation of *trans* fat in the edible oils differed significantly between the ATR-FT-IR and GC methods at *trans* fat levels that were less than

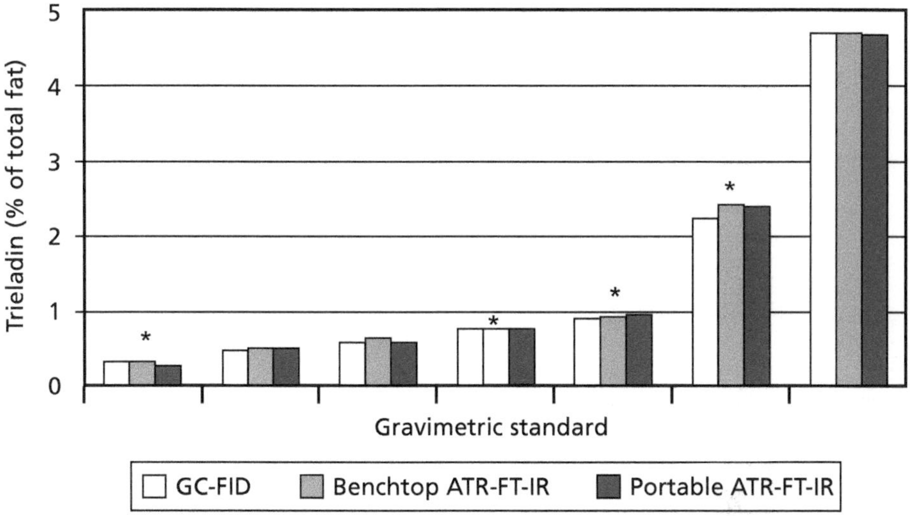

Figure 5.4 Evaluation of the content of *trans* fat in gravimetrically-prepared TAG standards by GC and ATR-FT-IR methods. Gravimetric standards were prepared by adding trielaidin (*trans* 9-18:1) to triolein (*cis* 9-18:1) at 0.33%, 0.51%, 0.59%, 0.78%, 0.92%, 2.30%, and 4.73% of total fat. Values represent the means ± SD for two independent determinations. One way analysis of variance was used to compare mean values (*$P < 0.05$). Adapted from Tyburczy et al. (2012b).

2% of total fat (Figure 5.5). Differences between these two analytical approaches were especially pronounced for oils that were processed by cold or expeller pressing, which is known to preserve the content of many non–fatty acid constituents, including vitamins, polyphenols, and nonsaponifiable lipids (e.g., squalene) (Koski et al., 2002; Parker et al., 2003). Unlike GC methods, which require substantial sample preparation (that selectively removes many of these non-FA components during the extraction, methylation, and chromatographic procedures), analysis by IR is performed directly on the neat oils and little to no sample preparation is required. Thus, the amplified ATR-FT-IR signal at 966 cm^{-1} was suspected to be related to the presence of non–fatty acid constituents in the edible oils. Further investigation by Tyburczy et al. (2012b) revealed that certain non–fatty acid constituents with one or more *trans* double bonds (e.g., β-carotene, retinol) when added to a low *trans* fat oil (e.g., 0.03% *trans* fat as percentage of total fat) increased the response at 966 cm^{-1} and the apparent *trans* fat content when measured by ATR-FT-IR spectroscopy (Figure 5.6). It is noted that only low levels of β-carotene are usually found in olive oils by liquid chromatography. For example, Koski et al. (2002) reported 1.5–3.6 ppm of β-carotene in virgin olive oils.

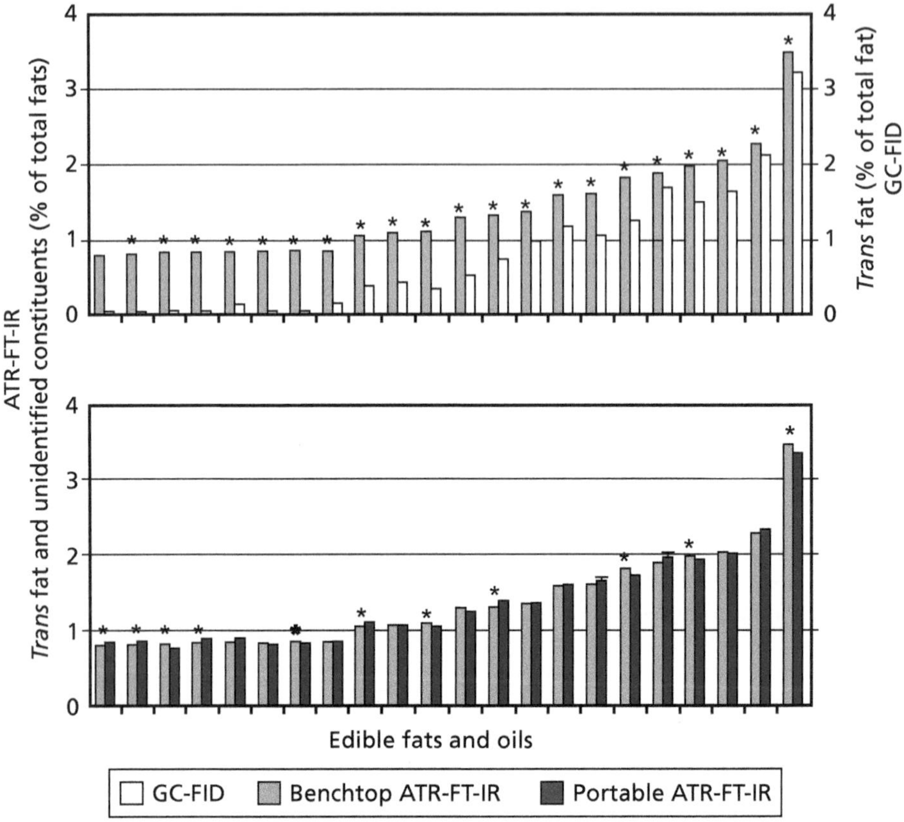

Figure 5.5 Comparisons of the quantitation of *trans* fat in 25 edible fats and oils, all labeled as containing zero grams *trans* fat, by ATR-FT-IR and GC methods. In the top panel, the right *y*-axis represents the quantitation of *trans* fat (as percentage of total fat) by GC analysis according to AOCS Official Method Ce 1j-07. The left *y*-axes represent the ATR-FT-IR quantitation of *trans* fat or unidentified oil constituents (as percent of total fat) based on the response at 966 cm^{-1} in the IR spectrum. Benchtop ATR-FT-IR analysis was performed using a heated seven-reflection diamond ATR accessory while for the portable instrument (bottom panel) a heated, nine-reflection diamond ATR accessory was used. Values represent the means ± SD for two independent determinations. One way analysis of variance was used to compare mean values ($*P < 0.05$). Adapted from Tyburczy et al. (2012b).

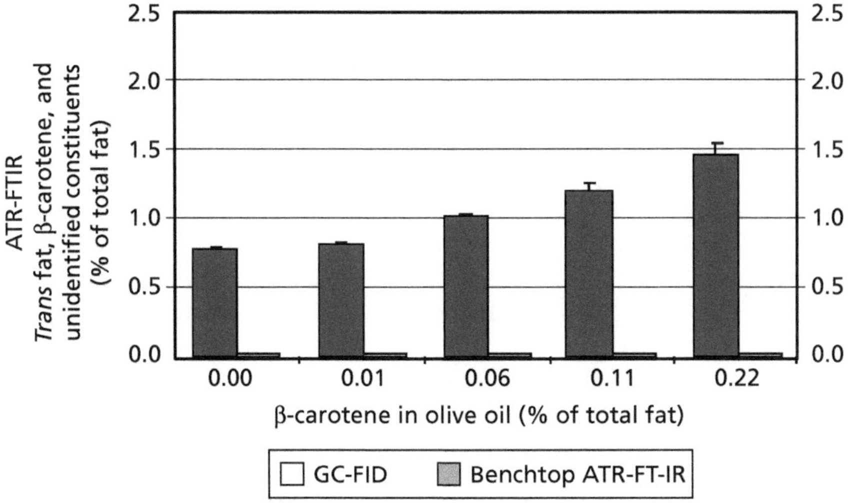

Figure 5.6 Evaluation of standard additions of β-carotene spiked in olive oil by benchtop ATR-FT-IR and GC analyses. The left *y*-axis represents the ATR-FT-IR quantitation of *trans* fat or unidentified oil constituents (as percentage of total fat) based on the response at 966 or 964 cm^{-1}, depending on the band maximum, in the IR spectrum. The right *y*-axis represents the quantitation of *trans* fat (as percentage of total fat) by GC analysis according to AOCS Official Method Ce 1j-07. Values represent the means ± SD for two independent determinations. One way analysis of variance was used to compare mean values (*$P < 0.05$). Adapted from Tyburczy et al. (2012b).

Near-Infrared Spectroscopy

NIR spectroscopy entails the measurement of broad combinations and overtones of fundamental mid-infrared stretching vibrations from X–H vibrations (where X = C, O, and N). For fatty acid profiling, the most important bands are those attributed to $-CH$, $-CH_2$, and $-CH_3$ groups that originate from either the fatty acid chain or the glycerol moiety of TAG and phospholipid molecules, or other oil constituents. Therefore, the correlation of the fatty acid concentrations to the overall NIR spectral fingerprint represents the contribution of individual fatty acids, which in turn is due to combinations and overtones of $-CH$, $-CH_2$, and $-CH_3$ stretching vibrations of the various fatty acid components.

The rapid determination of moisture, lipid, protein, carbohydrates, and fiber in cereals, grains, feeds, meats, and dairy products has been accomplished by use of NIR reflectance spectroscopy for many years (Dunmire and Williams, 1990). In the last two decades, there has been a significant increase in the development of various applications of NIR for the analysis of fats and oils (Pasquini, 2003; van de Voort et al., 2001). Bewig et al. (1994) performed discriminant analysis of cottonseed, peanut, soybean, and canola oil types by NIR spectroscopy. Second derivative spectra of these oils were subjected to discriminant analysis and results showed that all four groups could be successfully differentiated. Sato (1994) showed that nine varieties of vegetable oils (soybean, corn, cottonseed, olive, rice bran, peanut, rapeseed, sesame, and coconut oil) could all be successfully differentiated when the full NIR spectral data in the range of 1600–2200 nm were subjected to principal component analysis (PCA). Wesley et al. (1995) reported an NIR method for predicting the level of adulteration in a set of virgin and extra-virgin olive oils adulterated with corn oil, sunflower oil, and raw olive residue oil. Their results suggested that PCA may offer a means to identify the adulterant, but that additional work was needed to provide an acceptable level of accuracy (Wesley et al., 1995). Li et al. (1999) reported a rapid FT-NIR procedure for the determination of total *cis* and *trans* content, iodine value (IV), and saponification number of a range of edible oils and successfully correlated the NIR predictions to those obtained from mid-FT-IR spectroscopy for IV and *cis* and *trans* fat contents. The results of their international collaborative study of the methodology fo r determination of IV with a FT-NIR global calibration using disposable vials (Cox et al., 2000) was adopted as standard procedure AOCS Cd 1e-01 for the determination of IV (AOCS, 2009a). FT-NIR has also been applied to the determination of conjugated TFA in the presence of isolated TFA (Christy et al., 2003).

Recent advances in FT-NIR spectroscopy have made it possible to rapidly (<5 min) determine the total TFA content, as well as the fatty acid composition of neat fats or oils (Azizian and Kramer, 2005), without the need for derivatization to volatile FAME as required for GC analysis. These determinations have not been attempted previously because of the assumption that the FT-NIR spectral information of fatty acids present at low concentrations in a fat or oil was below the detection limit of the technique (Christy et al., 2003). However, in the last decade, advances in instrumentation and computing power, combined with advances in chemometric analysis, have made it possible to develop calibration models to analyze FT-NIR spectral features based on characteristic overtones and combination bands of any given chemical compound (Christy et al., 2003).

Development of PLS Calibration Models for FT-NIR Using GC as the Primary Reference Method

The first step in FT-NIR determinations entails the development of calibration models. Calibration is the process of constructing a mathematical model to relate the spectral response from an analytical instrument to the properties of test samples characterized by a primary reference method. Prediction is then the process of using the developed calibration model to predict properties of an unknown test sample given the output from the analytical instrument. Approaches to the generation of calibration models can be univariate or multivariate. Univariate calibrations, in which a single response (i.e., one specific wavenumber) from the analytical instrument is related to the concentration of a single component in the sample, are most common in mid-infrared spectroscopy; these are used, for example, for the determination of total *trans* fat content by ATR-FT-IR analysis. In multivariate calibrations, which are commonly used in near-infrared spectroscopy, multiple responses (spectral ranges) from the spectrometer are related to the properties of the sample. Partial least squares (PLS) regression is a quantitative tool performed using both concentration (obtained from a primary reference method) and spectral data. Chemometric techniques such as PLS regression have found applications in quality control and assurance measurements in, among others, the food, agricultural, and pharmaceutical industries (Anonymous, 2003).

Quantitative FT-NIR PLS calibration models based on GC primary reference data have now been developed and used for the rapid analysis of fatty acids in edible fats and oils (AOCS, 2009a; Azizian and Kramer, 2005, 2006; Azizian et al., 2004, 2007, 2010b; Christy et al., 2003; Cox et al., 2000). In addition, non–fatty acid components that may be present in a given oil matrix are usually not measured directly by GC, but need to be determined using a primary reference method and incorporated into the calibration models. Reliance on the accuracy of the GC determinations is absolutely crucial during the model development stage. Once reliable calibration models are created and validated, the subsequent analysis of test samples by FT-NIR is fully automated and can be accomplished in less than a minute without the need for additional GC analysis. Several factors are considered in the development of the calibration models because these variables strongly influence the quantitation of fatty acids in unknown samples. The most important factors to consider when GC data are used in the time-consuming development of FT-NIR calibration models include: (1) reporting of all GC peaks (including those attributed to unknown FAME components and non–fatty acid analytes); (2) maximizing the resolution of all components; and (3) providing accurate quantification. In addition, while generating these models, it was assumed that the position of a fatty acid on the glycerol moiety (at stereospecific number sn-1, sn-2, or sn-3) has only a minimal effect on the NIR spectrum; also, the quantitative GC data obtained for FAME were used without conversion to TAG equivalent (Azizian and Kramer, 2005).

Reporting of All GC Peaks

While reporting all GC peaks is critically important for the development of accurate FT-NIR calibration models, this requirement is generally neither essential for GC determinations themselves nor recommended by official GC methods (AOAC, 2005, 2009; AOCS, 2005). In fact, GC peaks for unknown FAME are generally not included in a detailed fatty acid composition of the test sample, and non–fatty acid components (e.g., squalene) are usually ignored in GC reports unless their identities can be confirmed.

NIR spectra and calibration models are matrix dependent. Thus, the vibrations of each molecule in a mixture will contribute to the overall NIR spectrum and influence the outcome of the analysis. Therefore, all unknown FAME peaks should be resolved and incorporated into FT-NIR calibration models. The identifications of the unknown FAME peaks are not essential, but they must be accounted for and listed as "unknown 1," "unknown 2," and so forth. On the other hand, identification of the non–fatty acid peaks is critical to the development of accurate FT-NIR calibration models. Appropriate supplementary analyses, such as GC mass spectrometry (MS), mid-IR spectroscopy, high performance liquid chromatography, silver-ion chromatography, and/or classical chemical methods, are needed to determine the identity and abundance of the unknown non–fatty acid peaks. Non–fatty acid peak components such as sterols may be naturally present in a fat or oil, but are not measured by the GC methods used for the determination of fatty acid composition. These should be incorporated into the FT-NIR PLS models as background signals as long as their concentrations remain below the levels incorporated into the model (Azizian et al., 2007). If non–fatty acid peaks are due to artifacts generated during the preparation of FAME derivatives, they should be removed from the total fatty acid composition (Azizian et al., 2004) because these artifacts would not have been present in the natural neat fat or oil matrix measured by FT-NIR. In some cases, non–fatty acid peaks could arise due to processing intermediates (e.g., during the preparation of fish oil fractions [Azizian et al., 2010a]). Building FT-NIR calibration models for such diverse mixtures is difficult unless the processing intermediates remain similar between samples. A careful examination of all artifacts and processing intermediates would result in the development of robust models for quantitative analysis.

Maximizing the Resolution of All Components

GC has generally been accepted as the chromatographic method of choice for the determination of the fatty acid composition of fats and oils. Improvements in GC technology, related to the reproducibility of injections and fine control of temperature programs and flow rates, have contributed to its success. One of the greatest advances is related to developments in the nature of column stationary phases that significantly enhance the resolution of many FAME components. The use of very long (100 m) flexible fused silica capillary columns coated with highly polar stationary phases has now made it possible to maximize the resolution of most FAME, including those of *trans* FAME and their isomers.

The potential impact of the overlap of some GC peaks on FT-NIR spectroscopic determinations must be considered. The reporting of co-elution of some GC FAME peaks (i.e., 13-*trans*-18:1 and 14-*trans*-18:1, 16-*trans*-18:1 and 14-*cis*-18:1, or 21:0 and 10-*trans*-12*cis*-CLA) is acceptable and common under specific experimental conditions. However, when developing an FT-NIR model based on GC reference data, this practice will lead to significant errors. Two (or more) overlapping components with their unique NIR spectra are unlikely to be present in the same proportion in all test samples subsequently analyzed by FT-NIR. To overcome this problem, GC procedures have been developed to resolve as many FAME peaks as possible. As an example, the same test samples can be separated on the same GC instrument using the same column, but by using two different temperature programs (Kramer et al., 2008). This can be achieved because the highly polar cyanopropyl polysiloxane columns recommended for TFA analysis are sensitive to temperature variations (Castello et al., 1997), which affect the relative elution sequence of different groups of FAME under different column temperatures (Kramer et al., 2008). The success of such a GC experiment depends on selecting two temperature settings that are sufficiently different to produce marked changes in the relative elution of different FAME types. This can be carried out in such a way that the same pair of isomers that co-elute under one set of temperature conditions do not co-elute again under the conditions of the second temperature program.

Recently, two types of GC columns for the analysis of fish oil FAME were successfully used in combination for the development of an FT-NIR calibration model for fish oil fatty acid (Azizian et al., 2010a). A 30 m Carbowax™ (polyethylene glycol) column was helpful in the identification of the polyunsaturated fatty acids in fish oils, but did not resolve most of the *trans* fat isomers of mono- and polyunsaturated FAME. The latter were resolved by use of a 100 m cyanopropyl polysiloxane column. Data from the complementary GC separations were used to develop an FT-NIR calibration model for the determination of FA from fish oil (Azizian et al., 2010a).

Providing Accurate Quantitation

The accuracy of quantitation of FAME by GC with flame ionization detection is another important consideration when FT-NIR calibration models are under development. The response of individual FAME at the flame ionization detector is proportional to the number of carbon atoms in the FA molecule and the degree of unsaturation (Bannon et al., 1986). To account for these variable responses, theoretically derived correction factors may be applied to individual GC peak areas. Theoretical correction factors are recommended in some but not all of the official GC methods [see AOCS Official Methods Ce 1h-05 (AOCS, 2009a) and Ce 1j-07 (AOAC, 2009)], and are available for most FAME. Empirical correction factors derived from gravimetrically prepared mixtures of pure individual FAME are recommended for long chain FAME (>20 carbon atoms) and for FAME for which no theoretical correction factors are available. Determinations of the empirical correction factors are strongly dependent on the purity of standards used and their chromatographic resolution and accurate quantitation (Altman and Bland, 1983). For example, accurate response factors can only be obtained if the purity of individual FAME in the standard mixture is assessed with at least the power of resolution equal to that of the 100 m cyanopropyl polysiloxane GC columns that are recommended for use with the official methods.

Matrix Dependence of NIR Spectroscopy

Azizian et al. (2007, 2010b) have shown that structural changes in the fatty acids of TAG have a significant impact on the observed FT-NIR spectra. The observed second derivative spectra for soybean and canola oils exhibited significant fingerprint differences between the two native vegetable oils. A primary difference between these two oils was a content of almost 57% oleic acid in canola oil and 52% linoleic acid in soybean oil. Their compositions changed after both oils were subjected to partial hydrogenation. The partial hydrogenation of soybean and canola oils led increasingly to more similar TAG products containing higher concentrations of TFA. As a result, the FT-NIR spectral fingerprints were no longer significantly different due to the increasing similarities in their *trans* fat isomeric profiles (Azizian et al., 2007).

Another significant factor has been the impact of residual solvent on the observed FT-NIR spectra for oils, which was demonstrated by analyzing the oil extracted from French fries (Azizian and Kramer, 2006; Azizian et al., 2004, 2010b). The observed spectra changed continually as the residual solvent was removed. This is critical for the determination of fats and oils that have been extracted from food products using a solvent extraction method.

Vegetable oils, especially the cold pressed oils such as olive oil, would naturally contain non–fatty acid constituents (e.g., β-sitosterol), and unless these constituents are incorporated in the calibration models, they would have an adverse impact on the accuracy of the FT-NIR determination. One method to overcome this limitation is by spiking several test samples with low concentrations of a specific minor constituent (e.g., β-sitosterol) and incorporating the spectra into the calibration model. More accurate determinations of fatty acid composition were obtained when the resultant spectra that accounted for some minor constituents were incorporated into the quantitative calibration models (Azizian et al., 2007). Alternatively, these non–fatty acid components could be measured independently by a primary reference method and incorporated into the models.

Finally, to make the calibration models temperature independent, all reference test samples were measured by FT-NIR at various temperatures between 15 and 50 °C and results were included in the development of the models (Azizian and Kramer, 2005; Azizian et al., 2007, 2010b). Hence, there was no need to specify a temperature (within this calibrated range) for collecting FT-NIR data for oil and fat test samples.

Table 5.B Total SFA, *Trans* FA, MUFA, and PUFA Contents for Six Fats and Oils Determined by GC and FT-NIR

Product	Method[a]		Σ SFA	Σ *trans* FA	Σ MUFA	Σ PUFA
Partially hydrogenated soybean oil	GC		18.7	28.6	27.9	20.4
	FT-NIR	Mean	18.3	28.0	29.6	22.1
		SD	0.6	1.5	1.9	0.5
		RMSECV	1.6	1.6	3.0	1.4
Soybean oil	GC		16.0	1.6	21.5	61.6
	FT-NIR	Mean	16.7	1.5	22.7	60.5
		SD	0.7	0.2	1.8	0.8
		RMSECV	1.0	1.3	2.3	2.0
Canola oil	GC		8.0	1.7	63.3	25.8
	FT-NIR	Mean	8.4	1.2	63.3	25.5
		SD	1.0	1.3	2.3	2.0
		RMSECV	1.6	1.6	3.0	1.4
Sunflower oil	GC		11.7	0.8	24.5	62.7
	FT-NIR	Mean	11.5	1.1	24.3	62.8
		SD	0.3	0.2	1.0	1.6
		RMSECV	1.0	1.3	2.3	2.0
Coconut oil	GC		89.1	1.5	7.3	1.8
	FT-NIR	Mean	89.4	1.7	7.3	1.7
		SD	0.7	0.5	0.4	0.2
		RMSECV	1.2	0.6	2.3	0.6
Palm oil	GC		52.9	2.1	36.4	8.9
	FT-NIR	Mean	53.0	3.2	37.1	8.9
		SD	0.8	0.5	1.4	0.1
		RMSECV	1.2	0.6	2.3	0.6

[a]GC: gas chromatography. All oils were analyzed using a 100 m SP 2560 column.

FT-NIR: Fourier transform near-infrared spectroscopy.

Mean of 9 independent measurements (5 instruments, 2 modes, 3 different path lengths).

SD: standard deviation; RMSECV: root mean square error of cross validation.

Adapted from Azizian et al. (2012).

Table 5.C Method Comparison

Methodology	**GC**	**Mid-IR**	**Near-IR**
Scope of determination	fatty acid profile	total *trans* fatty acids only	Fatty acid profile
Allows determination of total SFA, *trans* FA, MUFA, PUFA needed for food labeling	Yes	No	Yes
Calibration requirements	Use of an internal standard	Generation of a univariate calibration function	Development of multivariate calibration model(s)
Sample preparation	Yes	No	No
Matrix	Fame	Neat oil, melted fat, or fame	Neat oil, melted fat, or fame
Time needed for data collection and analysis	2–3 Hrs per analysis	5 Min per analysis	5 Min per analysis
Chemicals needed	Yes	No	No
Solvent disposal	Yes	No	No
Nondestructive	No	Yes	Yes
Data interpretation	Complex	Simple	Simple

Limited Collaborative Validation FT-NIR Study

In general, once a calibration model for an NIR method is developed, validated, and applied in an electronic form as part of an instrument/software package, it would not be transferrable to another instrument of a different make unless calibration transfer procedures and criteria are applied to demonstrate that the model remains valid on the second or subsequent instruments. In a recent three-laboratory limited collaborative study (Azizian et al., 2012), the transferability of pre-developed PLS calibration models to four other FT-NIR spectrometers from the same manufacturer was evaluated. The neat edible fats and oils investigated consisted of one partially hydrogenated fat and five commercially available edible oils. These samples were selected because they contained a wide concentration range of total saturated fatty acids, TFAs, monounsaturated fatty acids, and polyunsaturated fatty acids contents. The results of this study indicated that the available calibration models were transferable to all four same-make FT-NIR spectrometers operating in either the transflection mode with 2 or 4 mm pathlength fiber optic probes, or in the transmission mode with tubes having 5 mm outer diameter (OD) [3 mm internal diameter (ID)], but not with the 8 mm OD (6 mm ID) tubes. Hence, the latter tube size was not recommended. The fatty acid composition of the various oils determined on all spectrometers fell within the accepted limits of agreement between FT-NIR and GC analyses according to the statistical analysis by Bland and Altman (Altman and Bland, 1983; Bland and Altman, 1986) (Table 5.B). The application of these pre-developed calibration models gave satisfactory precision and accuracy. The FT-NIR repeatability and reproducibility precision data were consistent with those previously reported in AOCS GC Official Method Ce 1h-05 (AOCS, 2005). The FT-NIR protocol for determining fatty acid composition offers the advantage of being fully automated and independent of analyst skill or bias because calibration models are pre-developed and cannot be subjectively modified. Lately, we have applied this precalibrated FT-NIR procedure to the rapid (<5 min) determination of the total saturated fatty acid, monounsaturated fatty acids, polyunsaturated fatty acids, and TFA contents of 30 commercial edible fats and oils (Mossoba et al., 2013). Table 5.C provides a brief comparison of gas chromatographic and infrared spectroscopic approaches.

Conclusions

Trans fat labeling and other regulations in many countries prompted the food industry to accelerate food reformulation to reduce the amount of total *trans* fat in most products. It also increased interest in the development of rapid yet reliable methods for the accurate determination of the fatty acid composition and for monitoring the declarations of total *trans* and saturated fatty acid contents on food labels.

Current nutrition labeling requirements to declare the total *trans* fat content in edible fats and oils with *trans* levels greater than 2% of total fat can be met conveniently and rapidly (<5 min) by using mid-infrared spectroscopic official methods in the internal reflection mode.

Recent findings of enhanced ATR-FT-IR signals attributed to the presence of minor non–fatty acid constituents with one or more *trans* double bonds (e.g., beta-carotene, retinol) in edible oils demonstrate that GC methods remain the analytical approach of choice for determination of *trans* fat content in edible fats and oils with a *trans* fat content less than 2% of total fat.

FT-NIR spectroscopy in the transmission or transflection modes may potentially offer a novel and rapid (<5 min) alternative methodology to GC for the determination of fat and fatty acid composition. Under carefully defined conditions and the use of appropriate calibration models, FT-NIR may match the capability of GC in providing the fatty acid composition of fats and oils without the need to dilute or derivatize fats and oils to FAME. At this time, the FT-NIR procedure has yet to be fully validated in a collaborative study although transferability of FT-NIR calibration models among five same-make spectrometers has been reported (Azizian et al., 2012).

References

Ackman, R. Linolenic Acid Artifacts from the Deodorization of Oils. *J. Am. Oil Chem. Soc.* **1974,** *51,* 42–49.

Ackman, R.; Mag, T. *Trans* Fatty Acids and the Potential for Less in Technical Products. In *Trans Fatty Acids in Human Nutrition*, Sébédio, J. L., Christy, W. Eds.; Oily Press: Dundee, Scotland, **1998;** pp 35–38.

Adam, M.; Mossoba, M. M.; Lee, T. Rapid Determination of Total *Trans* Fat Content by Attenuated Total Reflection Infrared Spectroscopy: An International Collaborative Study. *J. Am. Oil Chem. Soc.* **2000,** *77* (5), 457–462.

Altman, D. G.; Bland, J. M. Measurement in Medicine: The Analysis of Method Comparison Studies. *The Statistician* **1983,** *32,* 307–317.

Anonymous. In *Near Infrared Spectroscopy,* Proceedings of the 11th International Conference, Davies, A. M. C.; Garrido-Varo, A., Eds.; NIR Publications: Chichester, U.K., 2003.

AOAC. Official Method 2000.10: Determination of Total Isolated *Trans* Unsaturated Fatty Acids in Fats and Oils by ATR-FTIR, 2000. In *Official Methods of Analysis,* 18th ed.; AOAC: Gaithersburg, MD, 2005.

AOAC. Official Method 996.06: Fat (Total, Saturated, and Unsaturated) in Foods. In *Official Methods of Analysis,* 18th ed.; AOAC: Gaithersburg, MD, 2005.

AOAC. Official Method Ce 1j-07: Determination of *Cis-, Trans-*, Saturated, Monounsaturated, and Polyunsaturated Fatty Acids in Extracted Fats by Capillary GLC. In *Official Methods and Recommended Practices of the AOCS,* 6th ed.; AOCS Press: Urbana, IL, 2009.

AOCS. Official Method Cd 14d-95, Isolated *Trans* Isomers Infrared Spectroscopic Method. In *Official Methods and Recommended Practices of the AOCS*, 6th ed., 2nd printing; Firestone, D., Ed.; AOCS Press: Urbana, IL. 1995.

AOCS. Official Method Cd 1h-05, Determination of of *Cis-*, *Trans-*, Saturated, Monounsaturated and Polyunsaturated Fatty Acids in Vegetable or Non-ruminant Animal Oils and Fats by Capillary GLC. In *Official Methods and Recommended Practices of the AOCS*, 6th ed., 2nd printing; Firestone, D., Ed.; AOCS Press: Urbana, IL, 2005.

AOCS. AOCS Standard Procedure Cd 1e-01: Determination of Iodine Value by Pre-calibrated FT-NIR with Disposable Vials. In *Official Methods and Recommended Practices of the AOCS*, 6th ed., 2nd printing; Firestone, D., Ed.; AOCS Press: Champaign, IL, 2009a.

AOCS. Official Method Cd 14e-09 Negative Second Derivative Infrared Spectroscopic Method for the Rapid (5 min) Determination of Total Isolated *Trans* Fat. In *Official Methods and Recommended Practices of the AOCS*, 6th ed., 2nd printing; Firestone, D., Ed.; AOCS Press: Urbana, IL, 2009b.

AOCS. Official Method Cd 14d-99 Rapid Determination of Isolated *Trans* Geometric Isomers in Fats and Oils by Attenuated Total Reflection Infrared Spectroscopy. In *Official Methods and Recommended Practices of the AOCS*, 6th ed., 2nd printing; Firestone, D., Ed. AOCS Press: Urbana, IL, 2009c.

AOCS. Official Method Cd 14-954, Isolated *Trans* Isomers in Margarine and Shortenings. In *Official Methods and Recommended Practices of the AOCS*, 6th ed., 2nd printing; Firestone, D., Ed.; AOCS Press: Urbana, IL, 2009d.

Azizian, H.; Kramer, J. K. A Rapid Method for the Quantification of Fatty Acids in Fats and Oils with Emphasis on *Trans* Fatty Acids Using Fourier Transform Near Infrared Spectroscopy (FT-NIR). *Lipids* **2005,** *40* (8), 855–867.

Azizian, H.; Kramer, J. K. Application of FT-NIR for Rapid Determination of the *Trans* Fatty Acid Composition in Fats and Oils. In *Lipid Analysis and Lipidomics—New Techniques and Applications*; Mossoba, M. M., Kramer, J. K., Brenna, J. T., McDonald, R. E., Eds.; AOCS Press: Urbana, IL, 2006; pp 303–334.

Azizian, H.; Kramer, J. K.; Kamalian, A. R.; Hernandez, M.; Mossoba, M. M.; Winsborough, S. Quantification of *Trans* Fatty Acids in Foods by GC, ATR-FTIR and FT-NIR Methods. *Lipid Technology* **2004,** *16*, 229–231.

Azizian, H.; Kramer, J. K. G.; Winsborough, S. Factors Influencing the Fatty Acid Determination in Fats and Oils Using Fourier Transform Near-infrared Spectroscopy. *Eur. J. Lipid Sci. Tech.* **2007,** *109* (9), 960–968.

Azizian, H.; Kramer, J. K. G.; Ehler, S.; Curtis, J. M. Rapid Quantitation of Fish Oil Fatty Acids and Their Ethyl Esters by FT-NIR Models. *Eur. J. Lipid Sci. Tech.* **2010a,** *112* (4), 452–462.

Azizian, H.; Kramer, J. K. G.; Mossoba, M. M. Progression to Fatty Acid Profiling of Edible Fats and Oils Using Vibrational Spectroscopy. In *Handbook of Vibrational Spectroscopy*, Li-Chan, E. C.; Griffiths, P. R.; Chalmers, J. M., Eds.; John Wiley & Sons, Chichester, West Sussex, U.K., 2010b.

Azizian, H.; Kramer, J. G.; Mossoba, M. Evaluating the Transferability of FT-NIR Calibration Models for Fatty Acid Determination of Edible Fats and Oils among Five Same-make

Spectrometers Using Transmission or Transflection Modes with Different Pathlengths. *J. Am. Oil Chem. Soc.* **2012,** *89* (12), 2143–2154.

Bannon, C.; Craske, J.; Hilliker, A. Analysis of Fatty Acid Methyl Esters with High Accuracy and Reliability. V. Validation of Theoretical Relative Response Factors of Unsaturated Esters in the Flame Ionization Detector. *J. Am. Oil Chem. Soc.* **1986,** *63* (1), 105–110.

Bewig, K.; Clarke, A.; Roberts, C.; Unklesbay, N. Discriminant Analysis of Vegetable Oils by Near-infrared Reflectance Spectroscopy. *J. Am. Oil Chem. Soc.* **1994,** *71* (2), 195–200.

Bland, J. M.; Altman, D. G. Statistical Methods for Assessing Agreement between Two Methods of Clinical Measurement. *Lancet* **1986,** *1* (8476), 307–310.

Buchgraber, M.; Ulberth, F. Determination of *Trans* Octadecenoic Acids by Silver-ion Chromatography-gas Liquid Chromatography: An Intercomparison of Methods. *Journal of AOAC International* **2001,** *84* (5), 1490–1498.

Buchgraber, M.; Ulberth, F. Determination of Low Level *Trans* Unsaturation in Physically Refined Vegetable Oils by Capillary GLC—Results of 3 Intercomparison Studies. *Eur. J. Lipid Sci. Tech.* **2002,** *104* (12), 792–799.

Castello, G.; Vezzani, S.; D'Amato, G. Effect of Temperature on the Polarity of Some Stationary Phases for Gas Chromatography. *J. Chrom. A* **1997,** *779* (1–2), 275–286.

Christy, A. A.; Egeberg, P. K.; Østensen, E. T. Simultaneous Quantitative Determination of Isolated *Trans* Fatty Acids and Conjugated Linoleic Acids in Oils and Fats by Chemometric Analysis of the Infrared Profiles. *Vibrational Spectroscopy* **2003,** *33* (1–2), 37–48.

City of New York. New York City Health Code Subsection 81.08. 2006.

Cox, R.; Lebrasseur, J.; Michiels, E.; Buijs, H.; Li, H.; Voort, F. R.; Ismail, A. A.; Sedman, J. Determination of Iodine Value with a Fourier Transform–Near Infrared Based Global Calibration Using Disposable Vials: An International Collaborative Study. *J. Am. Oil Chem. Soc.* **2000,** *77* (12), 1229–1234.

Craig-Schmidt, M. Consumption of *Trans* Fatty Acids. In *Trans Fatty Acids in Human Nutrition*; Sébédio, J., Christy, W., Eds.; Oily Press: Dundee, Scotland, 1998; pp 59–114.

Cruz-Hernandez, C.; Deng, Z.; Zhou, J.; Hill, A. R.; Yurawecz, M. P.; Delmonte, P.; Mossoba, M. M.; Dugan, M. E.; Kramer, J. K. Methods for Analysis of Conjugated Linoleic Acids and *Trans*-18:1 Isomers in Dairy Fats by Using a Combination of Gas Chromatography, Silver-ion Thin-layer Chromatography/Gas Chromatography, and Silver-ion Liquid Chromatography. *Journal of AOAC International* **2004,** *87* (2), 545–562.

Cruz-Hernandez, C.; Kramer, J. K.; Kraft, J.; Santercole, V.; Or-Rashid, M.; Deng, Z.; Dugan, M. E.; Delmonte, P.; Yurawecz, M. P. Systematic Analysis of *Trans* and Conjugated Linoleic Acids in the Milk and Meat of Ruminants. In *Advances in Conjugated Linoleic Acid Research*; Yurawecz, M. P., Kramer, J. K., Gudmundsen, O., Pariza, M., Banni, S., Eds.; AOCS Press: Urbana, IL, 2006; Vol. 3, pp 45–93.

Delmonte, P.; Fardin Kia, A. R.; Kramer, J. K.; Mossoba, M. M.; Sidisky, L.; Rader, J. I. Separation Characteristics of Fatty Acid Methyl Esters Using SLB-IL111, a New Ionic Liquid Coated Capillary Gas Chromatographic Column. *Journal of Chromatography. A* **2011,** *1218* (3), 545–554.

Delmonte, P.; Fardin-Kia, A. R.; Kramer, J. K. G.; Mossoba, M. M.; Sidisky, L.; Tyburczy, C.; Rader, J. I. Evaluation of Highly Polar Ionic Liquid Gas Chromatographic Column for the Determination of the Fatty Acids in Milk Fat. *Journal of Chromatography A* **2012,** *1233*, 137–146.

Doell, D.; Folmer, D.; Lee, H.; Honigfort, M.; Carberry, S. Updated Estimate of *Trans* Fat Intake by the U.S. Population. *Food Additives & Contaminants. Part A, Chemistry, Analysis, Control, Exposure & Risk Assessment* **2012,** *29* (6), 861–874.

Dunmire, D. L.; Williams, R. C. Automated Qualitative and Quantitative NIR Reflectance Analyses. *Cereal Foods World* **1990,** *35* (9), 913.

Eckel, R. H.; Borra, S.; Lichtenstein, A. H.; Yin-Piazza, S. Y. Understanding the Complexity of *Trans* Fatty Acid Reduction in the American Diet: American Heart Association *Trans* Fat Conference 2006: Report of the *Trans* Fat Conference Planning Group. *Circulation* **2007,** *115* (16), 2231–2246.

Federal Register, Vol. 68, Issue 133 (July 11, 2003) Food Labeling: *Trans*. In *FR DOC # 03-17525*, 68 ed.; National Archives and Records Administration: Washington, DC, Vol. 21 CFR 101, pp 41434–41506.

Food and Drug Administration (FDA). *Food Labeling: Nutrient Content Claims, General Principles, Petitions, Definition of Terms; Definition of Nutrient Content Claims for Fat, Fatty Acid, and Cholesterol Content of Food: Final Rule.* Department of Health and Human Services. Federal Register, 1993; Vol. 58, p 2302.

Food and Drug Administration (FDA). *Food Labeling:* Trans *Fatty Acids in Nutrition Labeling, Nutrient Content Claims, and Health Claims: Proposed Rule.* Department of Health and Human Services. Federal Register, 1999; Vol. 64, p 62746.

Food and Drug Administration (FDA). *Food Labeling:* Trans *Fatty Acids in Nutrition Labeling, Nutrient Content Claims and Health Claims: Proposed Rule, Reopening of Comment Period.* Department of Health and Human Services. Federal Register, 2000; Vol. 65, p 75887.

Food and Drug Administration (FDA). *Food Labeling:* Trans *Fatty Acids in Nutrition Labeling, Nutrient Content Claims and Health Claims: Proposed Rule, Reopening of Comment Period.* Department of Health and Human Services. Federal Register, 2002; Vol. 67, p 69171.

Food and Drug Administration (FDA). *Food Labeling:* Trans *Fatty Acids in Nutrition Labeling, Nutrient Content Claims and Health Claims: Final Rule.* Department of Health and Human Services. Federal Register, 2003a; Vol. 68, p 41433.

Food and Drug Administration (FDA). Guidance for Industry: *Trans* Fatty Acids in Nutrition Labeling, Nutrient Content Claims, Health Claims; Small Entity Compliance Guide, 2003b. http://www.fda.gov/Food/GuidanceComplianceRegulatoryInformation/GuidanceDocuments/FoodLabelingNutrition/ucm053479.htm (accessed December 17, 2012).

Food and Drug Administration (FDA). Food Labeling; Nutrition Labeling of Standard Menu Items in Restaurants and Similar Retail Food Establishments; Proposed Rule. Federal Registrar 2011, 29:6, 861–874.

Golay, P.-A.; Dionisi, F.; Hug, B.; Giuffrida, F.; Destaillats, F. Direct Quantification of Fatty Acids in Dairy Powders with Special Emphasis on *Trans* Fatty Acid Content. *Food Chem.* **2007,** *101* (3), 1115–1120.

Health Canada. (2006). TRANSforming the food supply. Report by Canada's *Trans* Fat Task Force (ISBN 0-662-43689-X). Online: http://www.hc-sc.gc.ca/fn-an/nutrition/gras-Trans-fats/tf-ge/tf-gt_rep-rap-eng.php.

Henninger, M.; Ulberth, F. *Trans* Fatty-Acid Content of Bovine-Milk Fat. *Milchwissenschaft-Milk Science International* **1994,** *49* (10), 555–558.

Hunter, J. E. Dietary *Trans* Fatty Acids: Review of Recent Human Studies and Food Industry Responses. *Lipids* **2006,** *41* (11), 967–992.

Koski, A.; Psomiadou, E.; Tsimidou, M.; Hopia, A.; Kefalas, P.; Wahala, K.; Heinonen, M. Oxidative Stability and Minor Constituents of Virgin Olive Oil and Cold-Pressed Rapeseed Oil. *Eur. Food Res. Technol.* **2002,** *214* (4), 294–298.

Kramer, J. K.; Blackadar, C. B.; Zhou, J. Evaluation of Two GC Columns (60-m supelcowax 10 and 100-m cp sil 88) for Analysis of Milkfat with Emphasis on CLA, 18:1, 18:2 and 18:3 Isomers, and Short- and Long-chain FA. *Lipids* **2002,** *37* (8), 823–835.

Kramer, J. K.; Hernandez, M.; Cruz-Hernandez, C.; Kraft, J.; Dugan, M. E. Combining Results of Two GC Separations Partly Achieves Determination of All *Cis* and *Trans* 16:1, 18:1, 18:2 and 18:3 except CLA Isomers of Milk Fat as Demonstrated Using AG-ION SPE Fractionation. *Lipids* **2008,** *43,* 3, 259–273.

Kramer, J. K. G.; Fellner, V.; Dugan, M. E. R.; Sauer, F. D.; Mossoba, M. M.; Yurawecz, M. P. Evaluating Acid and Base Catalysts in the Methylation of Milk and Rumen Fatty Acids with Special Emphasis on Conjugated Dienes and Total *Trans* Fatty Acids. *Lipids* **1997,** *32* (11), 1219–1228.

Kramer, J. K. G.; Zhou, J. Conjugated Linoleic Acid and Octadecenoic Acids: Extraction and Isolation of Lipids. *Eur. J. Lipid. Sci. Tech.* **2001,** *103* (9), 594–600.

Li, H.; Voort, F. R.; Sedman, J.; Ismail, A. A. Rapid Determination of *Cis* and *Trans* Content, Iodine Value, and Saponification Number of Edible Oils by Fourier Transform Near-infrared Spectroscopy. *J. Am. Oil Chem. Soc.* **1999,** *76* (4), 491–497.

Lichtenstein, A. H.; Appel, L. J.; Brands, M.; Carnethon, M.; Daniels, S.; Franch, H. A.; Franklin, B.; Kris-Etherton, P.; Harris, W. S.; Howard, B.; et al. Diet and Lifestyle Recommendations Revision 2006—A Scientific Statement from the American Heart Association Nutrition Committee. *Circulation* **2006,** *114* (1), 82–96.

List, G.; Reeves, R. Dietary Guidelines, Processing and Reformulation for *Trans* Reduction. In *Trans Fats Alternatives;* Kodali, D. R., List, G. R., Eds.; AOCS Press: Urbana, IL, 2005; pp 71–86.

Mayor and City Council of Baltimore City. *Health Code of Baltimore City.* Baltimore City Department of Legislative Practice: Baltimore, MD, 2009; Vol. Section 6-507, Ordinance 08-001, pp 83–84.

Milosevic, M.; Milosevic, V.; Kramer, J. K.; Azizian, H.; Mossoba, M. M. Determining Low Levels of *Trans* Fatty Acids in Foods by an Improved ATR-FTIR Procedure. *Lipid Technology* **2004,** *16,* 229–231.

Molkentin, J.; Precht, D. Optimized Analysis of *Trans*-octadecenoic Acids in Edible Fats. *Chromatographia* **1995,** *41* (5–6), 267–272.

Montgomery County Board of Health. Artificial *Trans* Fats in Eating and Drinking Establishments. In *Resolution 16-34,* Clerk of Council: Montgomery County, MD, 2007.

Mossoba, M.; Yurawecz, M.; McDonald, R. Rapid Determination of the Total *Trans* Content of Neat Hydrogenated Oils by Attenuated Total Reflection Spectroscopy. *J. Am. Oil Chem. Soc.* **1996,** *73* (8), 1003–1009.

Mossoba, M.; Seiler, A.; Kramer, J. K. G.; Milosevic, V.; Milosevic, M.; Azizian, H.; Steinhart, H. Nutrition Labeling: Rapid Determination of Total *Trans* Fats by Using Internal Reflection Infrared Spectroscopy and a Second Derivative Procedure. *J. Am. Oil Chem. Soc.* **2009a,** *86* (11), 1037–1045.

Mossoba, M.; Azizian, H.; Tyburczy, C.; Kramer, J. K.; Delmonte, P.; Kia, A. R. F.; Rader, J. I. Rapid FT-NIR Analysis of Edible Oils for Total SFA, MUFA, PUFA, and *Trans* FA with Comparison to GC. *J. Am. Oil Chem. Soc.* **2013,** *90* (4), 757–770.

Mossoba, M. M.; Adam, M.; Lee, T. Rapid Determination of Total *Trans* Fat Content—An Attenuated Total Reflection Infrared Spectroscopy International Collaborative Study. *Journal of AOAC International* **2001a,** *84* (4), 1144–1150.

Mossoba, M. M.; Kramer, J. K. G.; Fritsche, J.; Yurawecz, M. P.; Eulitz, K. D.; Ku, Y.; Rader, J. I. Application of Standard Addition to Eliminate Conjugated Linoleic Acid and Other Interferences in the Determination of Total *Trans* Fatty Acids in Selected Food Products by Infrared Spectroscopy. *J. Am. Oil Chem. Soc.* **2001b,** *78* (6), 631–634.

Mossoba, M. M.; Kramer, J. K.; Delmonte, P.; Yurawecz, M. P.; Rader, J. Determination of *Trans* Fats by Gas Chromatography and Infrared Methods. In *Trans Fats Alternatives;* Kodali, D., List, G., Eds; AOCS Press: Urbana, IL, 2005; pp 47–70.

Mossoba, M. M.; Kramer, J. K. G.; Milosevic, V.; Milosevic, M.; Azizian, H. Interference of Saturated Fats in the Determination of Low Levels of *Trans* Fats (below 0.5%) by Infrared Spectroscopy. *J. Am. Oil Chem. Soc.* **2007a,** *84* (4), 339–342.

Mossoba, M. M.; Milosevic, V.; Milosevic, M.; Kramer, J. K. G.; Azizian, H. Determination of Total *Trans* Fats and Oils by Infrared Spectroscopy for Regulatory Compliance. *Anal. Bioanal. Chem.* **2007b,** *389* (1), 87–92.

Mossoba, M. M.; Kramer, J. K.; Delmonte, P.; Yurawecz, M. P.; Rader, J. I. *Official Methods for the Determination of Trans Fat*, 2nd ed.; AOCS Press: Urbana, IL, 2009b.

Mossoba, M. M.; Seiler, A.; Steinhart, H.; Kramer, J. K. G.; Rodrigues-Saona, L.; Griffith, A. P.; Pierceall, R.; van de Voort, F. R.; Sedman, J.; Ismail, A. A.; et al. Regulatory Infrared Spectroscopic Method for the Rapid Determination of Total Isolated *Trans* Fat: A Collaborative Study. *J. Am. Oil Chem. Soc.* **2011,** *88* (1), 39–46.

Mossoba, M. M.; Kramer, J. K. G.; Azizian, H.; Kraft, J.; Delmonte, P.; Kia, A. R. F.; Bueso, F. J.; Rader, J. I.; Lee, J. K. Application of a Novel, Heated, Nine-reflection ATR Crystal and a Portable FTIR Spectrometer to the Rapid Determination of Total *Trans* Fat. *J. Am. Oil Chem. Soc.* **2012,** *89* (3), 419–429.

Parker, T. D.; Adams, D. A.; Zhou, K.; Harris, M.; Yu, L. Fatty Acid Composition and Oxidative Stability of Cold-pressed Edible Seed Oils. *J. Food Sci.* **2003,** *68* (4), 1240–1243.

Pasquini, C. Near Infrared Spectroscopy: Fundamentals, Practical Aspects and Analytical Applications. *J. Braz. Chem. Soc.* **2003,** *14,* 198–219.

Precht, D.; Molkentin, J. Rapid Analysis of the Isomers of *Trans*-octadecenoic Acid in Milk Fat. *International Dairy Journal* **1996,** *6* (8–9), 791–809.

Precht, D.; Molkentin, J. C18:1, C18:2 and C18:3 *Trans* and *Cis* Fatty Acid Isomers Including Conjugated *Cis* Delta 9, *Trans* Delta 11 Linoleic Acid (CLA) as well as Total Fat Composition of German Human Milk Lipids. *Die Nahrung* **1999,** *43* (4), 233–244.

Precht, D.; Molkentin, J. Identification and Quantitation of *Cis/Trans* c16:1 and c17:1 Fatty Acid Positional Isomers in German Human Milk Lipids by Thin-layer Chromatography and Gas Chromatography/Mass Spectrometry. *Eur. J. Lipid. Sci. Tech.* **2000a,** *102* (2), 102–113.

Precht, D.; Molkentin, J. Overestimation of Linoleic Scid and *Trans*-c18:2 Isomers in Milk Fats with Emphasis on *Trans* δ9, *Trans* δ12-octadecadienoic Acid. *Milchwissenschaft* **2000b,** *58*, 30–34.

Precht, D.; Molkentin, J. Recent Trends in the Fatty Acid Composition of German Sunflower Margarines, Shortenings and Cooking Fats with Emphasis on Individual c16:1, c18:1, c18:2, c18:3 and c20:1 *Trans* Isomers. *Die Nahrung* **2000c,** *44* (4), 222–228.

Ratnayake, W. M. Overview of Methods for the Determination of *Trans* Fatty Acids by Gas Chromatography, Silver-ion Thin-layer Chromatography, Silver-ion Liquid Chromatography, and Gas Chromatography/Mass Spectrometry. *Journal of AOAC International* **2004,** *87* (2), 523–539.

Ratnayake, W. M.; Plouffe, L. J.; Pasquier, E.; Gagnon, C. Temperature-sensitive Resolution of *Cis*- and *Trans*-Fatty Acid Isomers of Partially Hydrogenated Vegetable Oils on sp-2560 and cp-sil 88 Capillary Columns. *Journal of AOAC International* **2002,** *85* (5), 1112–1118.

Ratnayake, W. M.; Hansen, S. L.; Kennedy, M. P. Evaluation of the CP-sil 88 and SP-2560 GC Columns Used in the Recently Approved AOCS Official Method Ce 1h-05: Determination of *Cis-, Trans-*, Saturated, Monounsaturated, and Polyunsaturated Fatty Acids in Vegetable or Non-ruminant Animal Oils and Fats by Capillary GLC Method. *J. Am. Oil Chem. Soc.* **2006,** *83* (6), 475–488.

Ratnayake, W. M. N.; Gagnon, C.; Dumais, L.; Lillycrop, W.; Wong, L.; Meleta, M.; Calway, P. *Trans* Fatty Acid Content of Canadian Margarines Prior to Mandatory *Trans* Fat Labelling. *J. Am. Oil Chem. Soc.* **2007,** *84* (9), 817–825.

Sato, T. Application of Principal-component Analysis on Near-infrared Spectroscopic Data of Vegetable Oils for Their Classification. *J. Am. Oil Chem. Soc.* **1994,** *71* (3), 293–298.

Sebedio, J. L.; Catte, M.; Boudier, M. A.; Prevost, J.; Grandgirard, A. Formation of Fatty Acid Geometrical Isomers and of Cyclic Fatty Acid Monomers during the Finish Frying of Frozen Prefried Potatoes. *Food Res. Int.* **1996,** *29* (2), 109–116.

State of California. California Codes: Health and Safety Codes Section 114377, 2010.

Tyburczy, C.; Delmonte, P.; Fardin-Kia, A. R.; Mossoba, M. M.; Kramer, J. K.; Rader, J. I. Profile of *Trans* Fatty Acids (FAs) Including *Trans* Polyunsaturated FAs in Representative Fast Food Samples. *J. Ag. Food Chem.* **2012a,** *60* (18), 4567–4577.

Tyburczy, C.; Mossoba, M. M.; Fardin-Kia, A. R.; Rader, J. I. Evaluation of Low *Trans* Fat Edible Oils by Attenuated Total Reflection-Fourier Transform Infrared Spectroscopy and Gas Chromatography: A Comparison of Analytical Approaches. *Anal. Bioanal. Chem.* **2012b,** *404* (3), 809–819.

van de Voort, F. R.; Sedman, J.; Russin, T. Lipid Analysis by Vibrational Spectroscopy. *Eur. J. Lipid. Sci. Tech.* **2001,** *103* (12), 815–826.

Wesley, I. J.; Barnes, R. J.; McGill, A. E. J. Measurement of Adulteration of Olive Oils by Near-infrared Spectroscopy. *J. Am. Oil Chem. Soc.* **1995,** *72* (3), 289–292.

Wolff, R. L. *Trans*-Polyunsaturated Fatty Acids in French Edible Rapeseed and Soybean Oils. *J. Am. Oil Chem. Soc.* **1992,** *69* (2), 106–110.

Wolff, R. L.; Precht, D. A Critique of 50-m cp-sil 88 Capillary Columns Used Alone to Assess *Trans*-Unsaturated FA in Foods: The Case of the Transfair Study. *Lipids* **2002,** *37* (6), 627–629.

Wolff, R. L.; Precht, D.; Molkentin, J. Occurence and Distribution Profiles of *Trans*-18:1 Acids in Edible Fats of Natural Irigin. In *Trans Fatty Acids in Human Nutrition*; Sébédio, J., Christie, W., Eds.; Oily Press: Dundee, Scotland, 1998; pp 1–34.

Wolff, R. L.; Combe, N. A.; Destaillats, F.; Boue, C.; Precht, D.; Molkentin, J.; Entressangles, B. Follow-up of the Delta4 to Delta16 *Trans*-18:1 Isomer Profile and Content in French Processed Foods Containing Partially Hydrogenated Vegetable Oils during the Period 1995–1999. Analytical and Nutritional Implications. *Lipids* **2000,** *35* (8), 815–825.

6

Processing Solutions: Fractionation and Blended Oils

Gerald P. McNeill ■ *IOI Loders Croklaan, Channahon, Illinois, USA*

Introduction

In the beginning of the 20th century, the majority of cooking, baking, and frying was carried out using animal fats—mainly lard, beef tallow, and butter. These fats are semisolid at room temperature and resistant to oxidation during frying. Animal fats are semisolid due to a relatively high content of heat-stable saturated fat ranging from 40% to 65% (see Table 6.A) (U.S. Department of Agriculture, 2011). In animals (including humans), saturated fat is predominantly palmitic acid with varying amounts of stearic acid. The remainder is composed mostly of stable monounsaturated fat and small amounts of easily oxidizable polyunsaturated fat. The combination of high melting point saturated fatty acids and low melting point unsaturated fat gives rise to many individual triacylglycerols (TAGs) with varying melting points. As a result, this type of fat will have a smooth texture at room temperature that helps blend these fats with other food ingredients, such as flour and sugar, to produce a wide range of baked goods. Low levels of polyunsaturated fat ensure stability for long shelf life and long fry life.

In the 1950s, lard was the ideal shortening for baked goods because it naturally possessed a soft texture, a desirable flavor, and was the lowest-cost fat available. It also had excellent aerating properties that were essential for the creaming process in many baked goods (Knightly, 1981). The source of the air cell stabilization was the presence of many small beta-prime crystals, which are still critical for preparation of many baked goods today (Baldwin et al., 1963). Beef tallow was also available, but due to its firmer texture it was less useful in many bakery applications. This drawback was

Table 6.A Fatty Acid Composition of Natural Semi-Solid Fats and Soybean Oil (wt%)

Fat/Oil	*Trans*	Saturates	Monounsaturates	Polyunsaturates
Coconut oil	0	92	7	1
Palm kernel	0	82	14	2
Butterfat	3	65	31	2
Beef tallow	3	53	43	2
Palm oil	0.2	51	39	10
Soybean oil	0.5	15	23	61

overcome by pressing a high melting point *stearin* "fraction" from beef tallow (oleostearin) and blending it with 80% liquid vegetable oil. In the 1970s, a new vegetable oil called *palm oil,* which was naturally semisolid, started to become commercially available around the world; it had physical properties similar to animal fats.

Early in the 19th century, large quantities of liquid polyunsaturated vegetable oils became available as byproducts from cottonseeds and later from soybeans. Other sources of liquid oils became commercially available around the world, including sunflower and canola (rapeseed). Direct use of liquid oils in baked goods was limited because they did not naturally possess a semisolid texture. They also had limited use in deep-fat frying due to high levels of polyunsaturated fat. The commercial application of a chemical process called *hydrogenation* converted vegetable oils into semisolid fats that had a low polyunsaturated fat content and a high *trans* fat content. Partially hydrogenated vegetable oil (PHVO) was resistant to oxidation and had a texture and functionality similar to animal fats due to the presence of the *trans* fat. By varying the reaction conditions of the hydrogenation process, a broad range of different stable products with different physical characteristics could be made from liquid oils. This technological breakthrough resulted in a surge in innovation within the modern baking and snack food industries. Benefits not available from animal fats ranged from the creation of novel products for ever more sophisticated consumers, to manufacturing innovations and efficiencies for reduction of processing costs. The use of animal fat started to decline, and its use was almost completely eliminated starting in 1988, mostly due to a media campaign to reduce saturated fat in the diet. An American multimillionaire, Phil Sokolof, funded the "Poisoning of America" campaign to reduce or eliminate consumption of animal fats and palm oil. His proposal was that saturated fat was the main dietary cause of heart disease, an idea that has subsequently been shown to be inaccurate. An informal House of Representatives Agriculture Committee hearing on the topic (U.S. House of Representatives, 1987) led to a media frenzy that caused widespread substitution of natural semisolid fats with PHVO, not only in the United States but also in Europe and other countries (Schleifer, 2012). *Trans* fat was also promoted as a healthy alternative for saturated fat, even though hardly any studies on the long term effects of PHVO on human health had been performed. Ultimately, PHVO was found to be much worse than saturated fat (Mensink and Katan, 1990).

After 1990, additional research convinced the government of Denmark to effectively ban PHVO on Jan. 1, 2004, by limiting the content of artificial *trans* fat to no more than 2% of all vegetable oils used for food preparation (Stender, et al., 2006). In order to reduce *trans* fat (and PHVO) consumption in the United States, the FDA introduced mandatory labeling for *trans* fat on the nutrition facts panel of all retail food products on January 1, 2006 (U.S. Food and Drug Administration, 2003). Negative media coverage of "hidden" *trans* fat convinced much of the food industry around the world to search for *trans* fat alternatives. By the end of 2013, the

FDA had completed a review of *trans* fat consumption in the United States and announced a proposal to ban partially hydrogenated oils (PHOs) from food (Food and Drug Administration, 2013). PHOs include any partially hydrogenated edible fat or oil, including animal fat and vegetable oils. This chapter outlines the pros and cons of the main fat- and oil-based *trans* fat alternatives available, focusing on the versatility of palm oil fractionation.

Sources of Solid Fat Alternatives for Partially Hydrogenated Vegetable Oils

Fat can only be semisolid if it contains a significant content of fatty acids that have a melting point above room temperature. Only saturated fat and *trans* fat have high melting points; therefore, saturated fat is the only practical option for fat products that are free of *trans* fat. The source of saturated fat can be natural (Table 6.A) or derived from fully hydrogenated vegetable oil.

Natural Sources of Saturated Fat

In nature, fats and oils are used as dense, long-term storage sources of energy. Animals store fat in the adipose tissue for use in times of food scarcity, and plants utilize oil as a dense energy source in seeds for use during germination. The most efficient form of fat is saturated fat, with a slightly higher energy content per gram than either mono- or polyunsaturated fat. Fat in living things must be present in liquid form in order to be accessible as an energy source by the plant or animal (Linder, 2000). Therefore, warm-blooded animals (including humans) can have a relatively high content of high melting point saturated fat in their body fat and maintain it in a liquid state.

Plants cannot directly control body temperature and instead rely on the ambient temperature, determined by climate, as their source of heat. Plants that grow in hot climates within 20 degrees of the equator, such as Africa, South East Asia, and South America, often produce seeds that have a high content of saturated fat. Analogous to warm-blooded animals, the high ambient temperature allows the seed oil to remain liquid while containing relatively high levels of saturated fat (Linder, 2000). Plants that produce oils that are solid at room temperature include the oil palm tree, coconut tree, shea tree, and the cacao tree. These oils are contained in the fruit, kernel, bean, or nut and all are high in saturated fat (50–90%) and are solid or semisolid at room temperature (Table 6.A). Palm fruit oil, with a natural mixture of 50% saturated fat and 50% unsaturated fat, is relatively soft and possesses a similar texture and stability to animal fats and PHVO. The other highly saturated plant oils, including the kernel of the palm fruit, are hard and brittle in texture and are traditionally useful in the manufacture of chocolate and chocolate alternatives.

In contrast, plants that grow in temperate climates produce seeds with a low content of saturated fat (<30%) in order to remain liquid at ambient temperatures; this allows proper germination (Linder, 2000). Temperate climate seeds are, therefore, high in oleic and/or polyunsaturated fat and remain liquid at room temperature. Efforts to significantly increase the saturated fat content in temperate seed oils using genetic modification techniques have resulted in unintended effects that adversely affect plant seed germination. The maximum saturated fat content in commercial oilseeds produced in temperate climates is 30%, including cottonseed oil and Nutrisun, a new variety of sunflower oil.

Saturated Fat from Fully Hydrogenated Vegetable Oil

During the process of hydrogenation, conditions can be selected that result in the conversion of almost all the unsaturated fat in vegetable oils into saturated fat, while maintaining a low level of residual *trans* fat (<5%). The majority of the newly created saturated fat is stearic acid, the highest melting point fatty acid commonly found in food oils and fats and a useful source of saturated fat. Due to the high content of saturated fat, fully hydrogenated fat has limited functionality because it is a hard, waxy fat that does not melt at body temperature, but it can be made useful in frying and bakery applications after interesterifying with liquid oils.

Essential Characteristics for Successful Alternatives to Partially Hydrogenated Vegetable Oils

- *Saturated fat.* Saturated fat is the only kind of fat that provides a similar texture or functionality to *trans* fat. In order to substitute a partially hydrogenated product, it is reasonable to assume that the content of saturated fat in the substitute should approximate the sum of the *trans* fat plus the saturated fat content in the original partially hydrogenated product. From a pure labeling perspective, this results in an increase in saturated fat content, potentially raising concerns for consumer acceptance in developed countries. An ideal substitute should provide little or no increase in saturated fat compared to partially hydrogenated products, while maintaining functionality.
- *Versatility.* Partial hydrogenation is a very versatile technique that has resulted in many new, tailor-made shortening products fulfilling diverse functional and process needs not available from animal fats. Therefore, any suitable replacement must also deliver a multitude of products for a broad range of food applications and processing demands. The functionality of substitutes should closely mimic their partially hydrogenated counterparts to minimize reformulation time and costly research and development efforts.

- *Oxidative stability.* The process of hydrogenation eliminated most of the polyunsaturated fat in PHVO, resulting in highly stable products that provided a long shelf life in finished goods and frying. Maintaining that long shelf life is necessary for any substitute because a long shelf life is a standard requirement for most modern baked and fried goods and snack foods. A low level of polyunsaturated fat is essential to avoid oxidative rancidity and off-flavor development.
- *Cost.* The cost of any substitute should be neutral to PHVOs to prevent loss of sales revenue or reduced sales volume.
- *Commercial availability.* A reliable, large supply of oil is required to support food manufacturing around the world.

Performance Characteristics of Natural Commercial Sources of Semisolid Fats

- *Animal fats.* A logical substitute for PHVOs is animal fat. From its origination, fats such as lard, tallow, and butter were used for baking, and animal fat was an ingredient in baked goods for centuries. Those fats have not been completely substituted by PHVO. Lard is occasionally used on a commercial scale to make pie crusts and butter is used in high quality applications such as puff pastries, croissants, and other laminated products. In general, however, there are several barriers to prevent the widespread industrial use of tallow and lard in baking today:

    1. Many food manufacturing facilities are kosher certified and therefore cannot utilize tallow and lard.
    2. These products have relatively high levels of saturated fat, which is still considered a risk factor for heart disease by regulatory bodies in developed countries.
    3. These fats are not versatile with respect to physical properties and functionality. Only natural lard and interesterified lard were traditionally used in baking. Use of beef tallow was limited to a blend of a fraction of tallow stearin with vegetable oil (Knightly, 1981).

    Butter or anhydrous milk fat continues to be perceived as a high quality natural product in contrast to other animal fats. It can be fractionated, but only offers a limited range of functional options. It has the highest level of saturated fat of the animal fat options (65%), which can be a barrier for healthy food product lines. The characteristic desirable natural flavor, color, and odor of butter makes it an attractive choice for artisanal and high quality products. Perhaps the biggest barrier to widespread use of butter in industrial applications is a persistently high cost.

- *Naturally semisolid vegetable oils.* Temperate climate seeds contain low levels of saturated fat (7–30%). Because they are liquid at room temperature, they are not suitable for use on their own as a *trans* fat replacement solution where a solid fat is required. They may be included as a component in other more functional solutions (see below).

  Several plants that grow in hot climates produce oils that are high in saturated fat and low in polyunsaturated fat, which results in a semisolid texture at room temperature (Table 6.A). All of these oils have been produced commercially since the 1970s and have been shown to be suitable for use in baked goods, frying, and in confectionery products. Palm oil is widely available and has the highest annual production of any other vegetable oil, with 54 million t produced in 2013, 23% more than global soybean oil production (U.S. Department of Agriculture, 2012/13). This oil tends to crystallize in the preferred small beta-prime form, providing small crystals that effectively stabilize air cells and entrap liquid oil (Yap et al., 1989).
- *Fully hydrogenated vegetable oil.* Fully hydrogenated vegetable oil has limited use directly in food applications because of its very high melting point and unacceptable waxy mouth feel. To overcome this problem, small amounts (~10%) can be blended with liquid oils to form a viscous liquid that can be used in limited applications, such as bread. The approach is limited because the lack of a semisolid structure does not find widespread use in baking and snack foods. An undesirable waxy mouth feel becomes evident at relatively low levels of incorporation in products. The range of use of fully hydrogenated oil can be extended by interesterifying (randomizing) it with liquid oil instead of blending. This results in a less waxy product that can be used in some bakery applications. From a practical point of view, this approach requires a hydrogenation step and an interesterification step that contribute to cost.

  In general, the natural fats and oils traditionally used in making baked goods are mostly high in palmitic acid. Fat products made with high levels of stearic acid will potentially have different effects on the finished products. Compared to fats that have a high content of palmitic acid (the most common saturated fatty acid present in natural fats), fats that have a high content of stearic acid tend to form larger beta crystals that can be less effective in bakery applications (Garcia-Macias et al., 2012).

Palm Oil: The Most Versatile Solution to *Trans* Fat Reduction in Processed Foods

Widespread commercial cultivation of palm oil began in the 1970s, and today it has the largest production of all other edible oils (U.S. Department of Agriculture,

2012/13). Grown within 10 degrees of the equator, mainly in Malaysia and Indonesia, palm fruit is produced all year round. Productivity is by far the highest of any commercial oil crop, producing 10 times more oil per acre than soybean oil. With continuous improvements in palm tree cultivation, it is likely to produce double the current yield of oil per acre in the coming decades. Extraction of palm oil is carried out by softening the fibrous palm fruit with steam, followed by expelling the oil in a high pressure press. No organic solvents are required.

Palm oil has a soft semisolid texture at room temperature and is composed of a natural balance of 50% saturated fat and 50% unsaturated fat. Containing just 10% of polyunsaturated fat as linoleic acid and no linolenic acid, it is inherently resistant to oxidation. Natural antioxidants called *tocotrienols* are present in the oil and provide additional protection against oxidative damage. Tocotrienols are closely related in composition to the tocopherol antioxidants widely found in commercial vegetable oils.

Palm oil is well-suited for bakery applications because it tends to form small beta-prime crystals (Baldwin et al., 1963). These small crystals impart a smooth texture to the fat and effectively entrap air cells during the creaming process. Air entrapment is needed to impart a desirable light texture and high volume to the food after baking. Palm oil can be used without further processing as an all-purpose shortening. Due to its resistance to oxidation, it also has a naturally long shelf life.

Taking Palm Oil Functionality to the Next Level: Fractionation

The food industry today needs many different fats and shortening products that are tailor made to match the complexities of PHVOs. Palm oil is comprised of many structurally unique TAGs, each with different melting points and physical properties. Many of these components can be separated from the original oil by a physical process called *fractionation* (Kellens et al., 2007). In the fractionation process, palm oil is first melted then cooled to crystallize slowly under controlled conditions to maximize the formation of large crystals of the highest melting components. A high pressure press is used to separate the suspension of crystals, forcing the liquid oil though a filter. The crystals are retained on the filter and collected separately. In this way, the original palm oil has been converted into two completely different fats, one that is a liquid at room temperature, called *olein,* and the second a hard waxy solid called *stearin.*

The new palm olein and stearin fractions are still composed of many different TAGs. Each new fraction can then be further fractionated after they are crystallized under new conditions to generate two new fractions. When stearin is fractionated, a double stearin is generated that is more saturated and is significantly harder than the original stearin. The new olein fraction is called a *palm mid fraction* (PMF). Mid fractions tend to be hard at lower temperatures, but have a low solid fat content at higher temperatures and a corresponding low melting point, similar to chocolate fat.

The physical characteristics of fats can be quickly determined by measuring the solid fat content at different temperatures, typically ranging from 10 °C to 40 °C. This procedure is routinely carried out by a rapid NMR technique (Madison and Hill, 1978). A plot of solid fat content versus temperature, called a *melting curve,* is generated. The melting curve quickly indicates the key physical characteristics of the fat and is a critical tool for formulating fat-based products. Typical commercially available palm fractions are compared by their melting curves in Figure 6.1. The solid

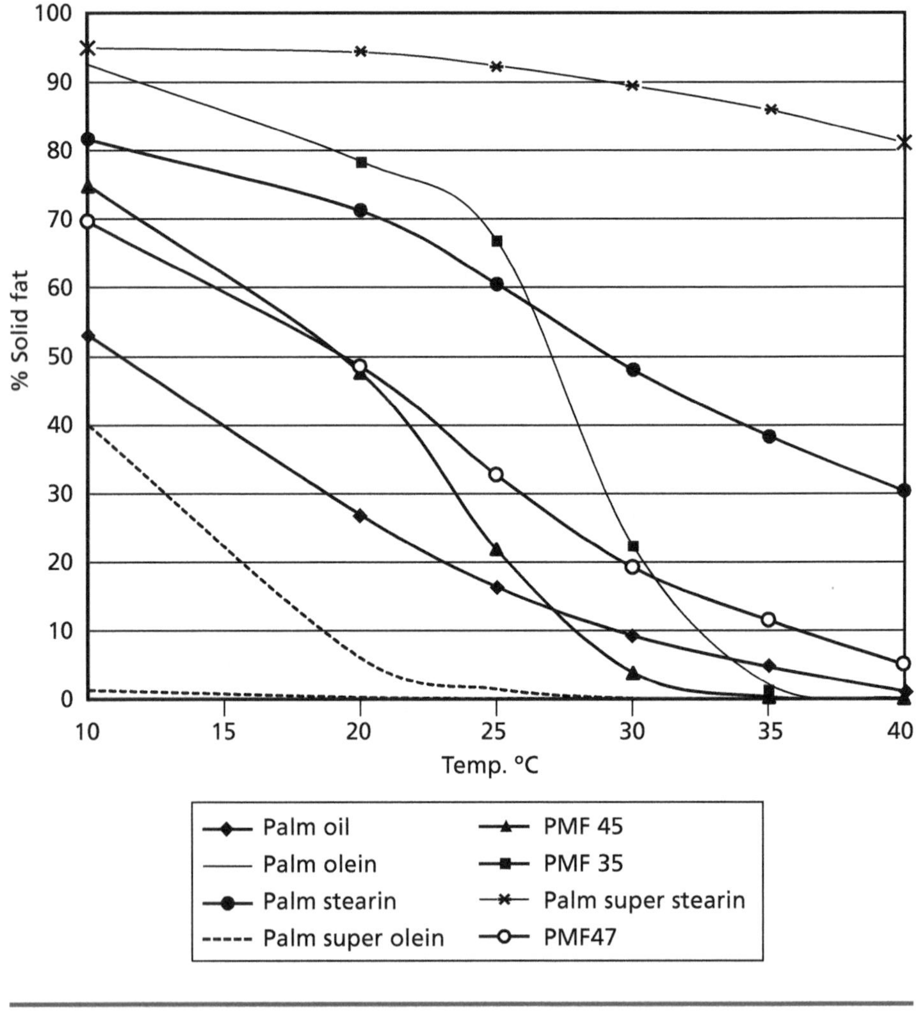

Figure 6.1 Melting curves of palm oil fractions.

fat content at 20–25 °C indicates the hardness of the product at room temperature, while the solid fat content at 40 °C predicts the mouth feel or waxiness of the product at body temperature. Stearins have a high solid fat content at all temperatures and can impart a waxy mouth feel, whereas the oleins have a low content of solid fat at all temperatures and are liquid or viscous at room temperature. Mid fractions have intermediate functionality, with a high content of solid fat at room temperature and low solid fat at body temperature.

Application of Palm Kernel Oil to Extend the Versatility of Palm Oil

After extracting the oil from the palm fruit, a hard kernel is left behind. The kernel is related to a coconut, but with a diameter of about 1 inch. Yield of palm kernel oil per acre is approximately 8% of palm oil yield, with global production of about 4 million t. With approximately 82% saturated fat, it is very hard and brittle at room temperature but melts quickly at body temperature (Table 6.A). This is explained by the presence of 48% lauric acid, a low melting point saturated fat. Palm kernel oil or fractionated palm kernel stearin are popular components of confectionery products, often used in chocolate-type coating for baked goods.

Palm Oil Interesterification

In contrast to fractionation, in which purer TAG components of palm oil are continually enriched, interesterification is a process that seeks to reduce the fatty acid distribution of the TAG components to a fully randomized or "rearranged" state. Using a catalyst or an enzyme, the fatty acids in relatively pure mixtures of TAG are redistributed completely randomly, resulting in a large number of different new TAGs. The effect of creating more random TAGs is to increase the content of the desirable small beta-prime crystals compared to pure palm oil fractions. The melting curve of interesterified palm oil fractions typically has a moderate solid fat content at both low and high temperatures.

Component Blending to Match PHVO High *Trans* Shortenings and Fats

Palm oil and palm kernel oil, single natural products, can be readily transformed into several components and products using fractionation and interesterification. The final step in formulation of a comprehensive set of products that substitute PHVO is component blending. Palm oil–based formulas are developed by determining the physical and chemical properties of specific PHVO products, followed by empirically matching these properties with blends of palm oil and/or palm kernel oil components. In addition to palm oil and palm kernel oil fractions, other liquid vegetable oils are used as components, further extending the range and functionality of the different finished products that can be made.

In order to make a large number of finished products on a commercial scale from a collection of individual components, any production facility must possess a component blending capability. This requires dedicated tanks for each component, with the ability to accurately deliver each type and proportion required for each component to the blend tank. An analogous approach was previously used for PHVO products, in which large-volume base stocks of commonly used partially hydrogenated components were blended to generate a large number of finished shortenings (Latondress, 1981). By combining fractions of palm oil, IOI Loders Croklaan has already produced more than 100 *trans*-free products based on palm oil that are available around the world as substitutes for PHVO products. Figure 6.2 shows a range of melting

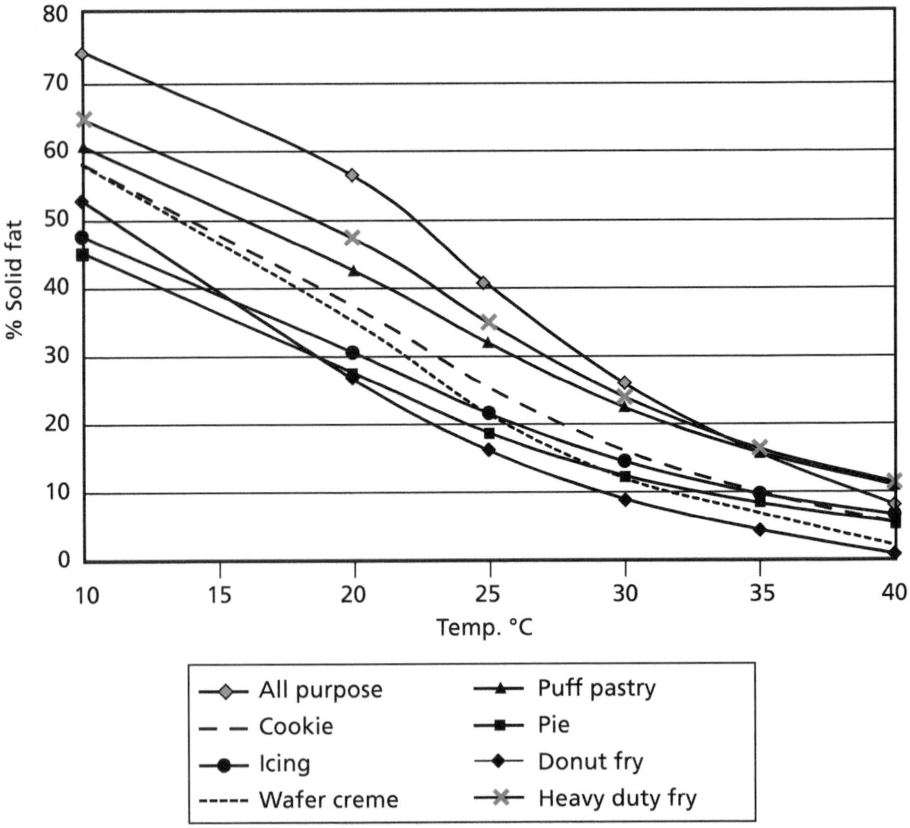

Figure 6.2 Melting curves of palm oil–based shortenings.

curves for several categories of bakery shortenings. The differences in the melting curves indicate the wide variation in formulations that enable the fats to be tailor made for a large number of applications. Although the fraction/component blending approach will continue to provide solutions for *trans* fat replacement, this approach is equally valid to support the innovation needs of the bakery industry in the future.

Formulating Palm Oil and Its Fractions for a Diverse Range of Functional Products

Using melting curves, this section will describe a small selection of product categories in more detail that showcase the existing and future potential for palm oil as an essential and versatile *trans*-free ingredient for the U.S. baking and snack food industries.

Icings

Aerated icings (often called buttercream icing) is a rich, uncooked frosting made by creaming powdered sugar and shortening together to form a light aerated mass (using nitrogen). Specialized semisolid shortenings that assist in entrapping small air bubbles provide a functional source of fat (Figure 6.3). Functional attributes of buttercream

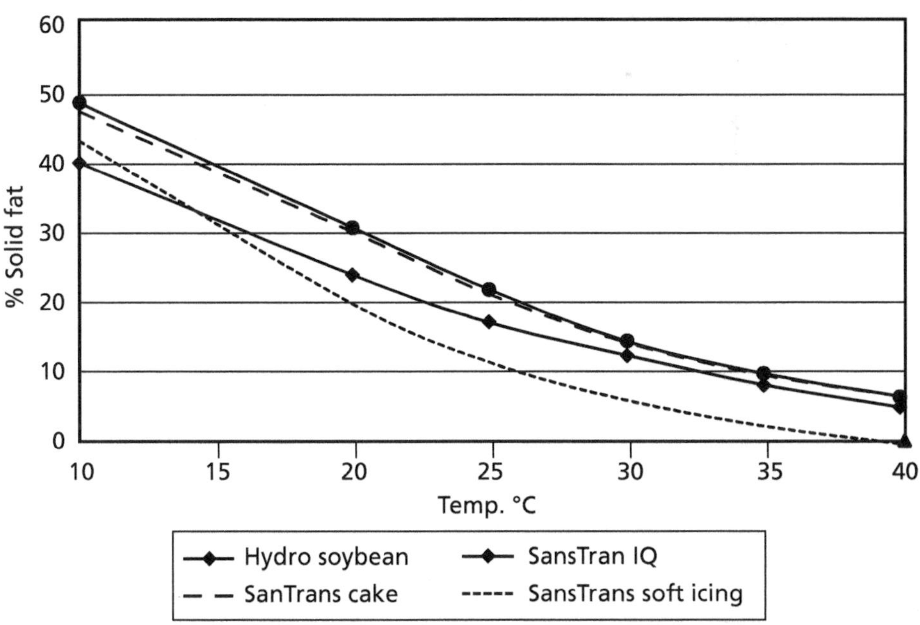

Figure 6.3 Melting curves of icing shortenings.

icings include the hardness of the icing, which is affected by the fat hardness. The icing should not have a waxy texture but should remain heat stable and nonoily. In the case of food service applications, icing pails can remain for months in the supply chain. In this case, the fat should not become harder over time, making it difficult to spread the icing on cakes.

Puff Pastry

Laminated pastries are manufactured by first making a thin layer of dough and spreading a thin layer of fat over the dough. The double layer is folded back and forth over itself many times until it forms a block of dough with up to 100 layers of fat layered with dough. When the dough is baked, the thin dough layers start to harden and begin to rise up. The result is many thin, hard, crispy flakes with large spaces in between.

Figure 6.4 shows the melting curves of various palm oil–based laminating fats. The shortenings need to be very flexible (or “plastic”) so that they withstand the layering process. Any damage to the fat can cause defects, resulting in poor lift or distorted

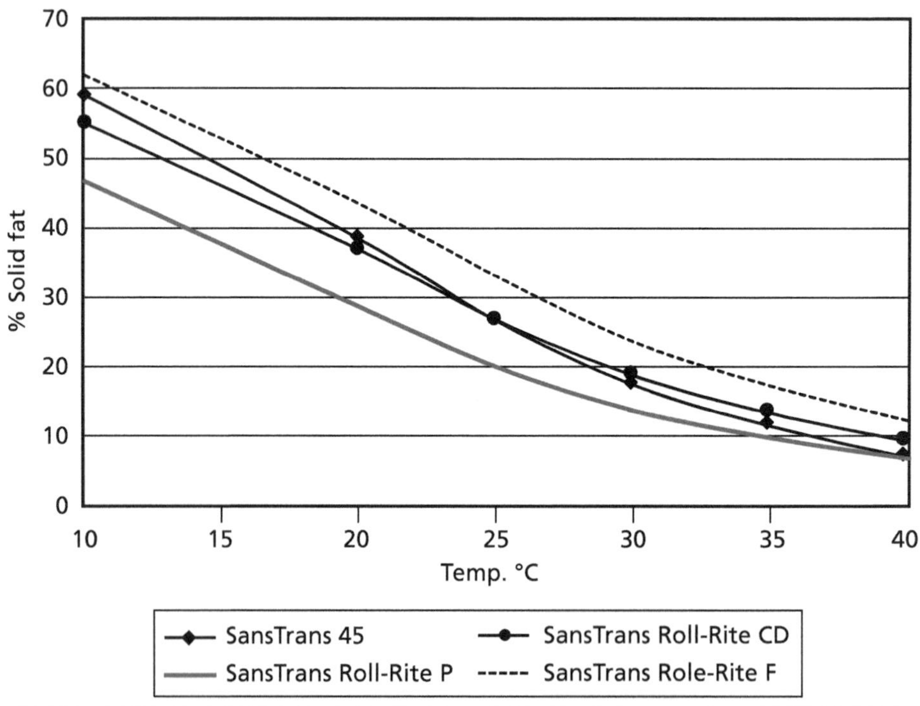

Figure 6.4 Melting curves of palm-based puff pastry shortenings.

shapes in the final product. In addition, they must be "temperature tolerant" and not become too hard or too soft as the temperature of the product or the bakery decreases or increases as part of the dough preparation process. Different applications require different hardnesses, so each shortening is designed to specifically match different types of laminated products, including puff pastry, croissants, and other pastries (Figure 6.4).

Doughnut Frying Oil

The majority of doughnuts produced in the United States are made with a solid fat. If liquid oil is used, the doughnut can be soggy and oil will leak out of the doughnut, causing unacceptable stains in the packaging. Another common defect is oil migration into doughnut coatings. Popular coatings include chocolate and sugar coatings. Frying oil can migrate into chocolate, making it soft and tacky and causing it to slide off the doughnut and smear on the plastic windows of packaging. Palm oil makes an excellent doughnut frying fat because it is naturally semisolid. It is also extremely versatile and can be tailored to meet the diverse needs of the complex doughnut frying industry. Doughnuts fried in palm oil do not exhibit the oil migration problems mentioned. In addition, the oil can deliver heat-resistant doughnuts in hot climates and reduced waxy flavor in more temperate climates. Reduced saturated fat doughnut shortenings based on palm oil are also available. A combination of liquid vegetable oil and high melting point components will adequately fry the doughnut, but freezing or refrigeration of the doughnut during storage is recommended to limit oil migration due to a high content of liquid oil. If polyunsaturated liquid oil is chosen, there is a risk of off-flavor development (Figure 6.5).

Coating Fats

Many food products are coated with a layer of chocolate. The traditional cocoa butter in the chocolate is often replaced with lower cost alternatives, and the main types in use today are lauric (hydrogenated palm kernel and coconut oils), nonlauric (blends of palm oil fractions), and blends of palm oil with palm kernel oil.

Palm oil fractions provide a similar texture and mouth feel to cocoa butter but at lower cost. Melt-out is slower compared with palm kernel, but is similar to cocoa butter. These products are nonhydrogenated and lower in saturated fat (~70%). Palm oil is relatively slow crystallizing and generally runs slower on production lines compared to palm kernel.

Blends of palm oil and palm kernel oils provide the benefits of both individual oils. Crystallization rates are high, hydrogenation is eliminated, and cost is lower than palm kernel alone. The combination retains some of the hardness and the melting properties of pure palm kernel and is usually a cost-effective solution (Figure 6.6).

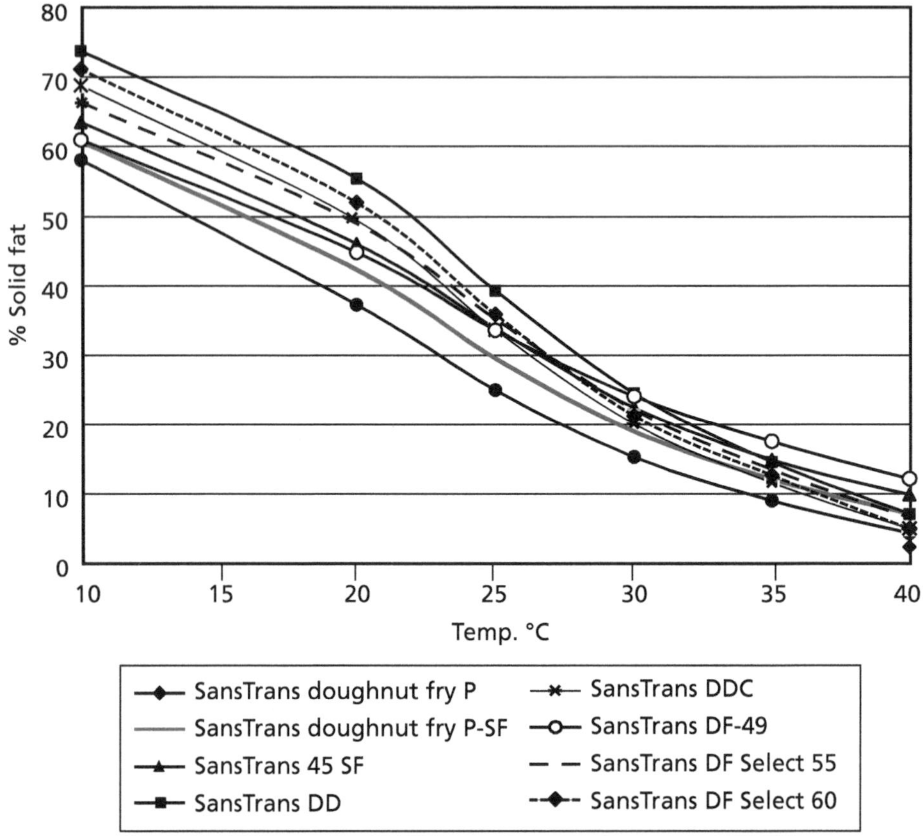

Figure 6.5 Melting curves of palm oil doughnut frying fats.

Summary and Conclusions

Beginning in 2006, many food manufacturers began to reduce the content of *trans* fat in their products. In 2013, the FDA estimated that about 75% of *trans* fat had been eliminated from the U.S. diet (Food and Drug Administration, 2013). The proposal by the FDA in 2013 to revoke GRAS status (Generally Regards As Safe) for PHO was designed to eliminate the remaining *trans* fat in the diet. Following the lead of the FDA in the United States, other countries that have high levels of *trans* fat in their diets, such as Eastern Europe and China, may implement similar measures to protect their populations. Natural palm oil has emerged as a versatile, cost-effective solution for elimination of *trans* fat in any product that requires a solid fat for functionality. The few product examples presented here indicate that palm oil will continue to deliver innovative solutions to the needs of the food industry long after *trans* fat has

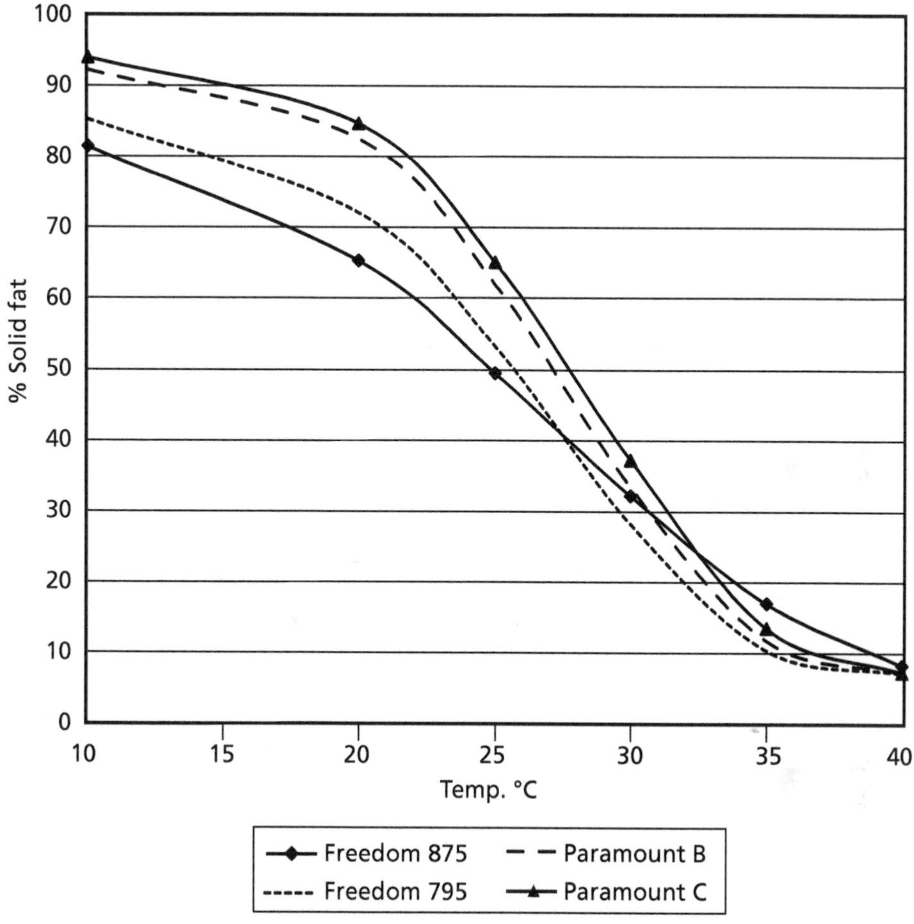

Figure 6.6 Melting curves of palm oil bakery coatings.

been forgotten as a food ingredient. Based on the ever bigger demands of the growing world population, palm oil will be a critical source of oil to meet those needs well into the future.

References

Baldwin, R. R.; Johansen, R. G.; Keough, W. J.; Titcomb, S. T.; Cotton, R. D. The Role That Fat Plays. *Cereal Science Today* **1963,** *8,* 273.

Food and Drug Administration. *Tentative Determination Regarding Partially Hydrogenated Oils; Request for Comments and for Scientific Data and Information;* Document Citation 78

FR 67169, Agency/Docket No. FDA-2013-N-1317; Washington, DC: Food and Drug Administration, Office of the Federal Register, National Archives and Records Administration, 2013; pp 67169–67175.

Garcia-Macias, P.; Gordon, M.; Frazier, R.; Smith, K.; Gambelli, L. Effect of TAG Composition on Performance of Low Saturate Shortenings in Puff Pastry. *European Journal of Lipid Science and Technology* **2012,** *114* (7), 741–747.

Kellens, M.; Gibon, V.; Hendrix, M.; De Greyt, W. Palm Oil Fractionation. *European Journal of Lipid Science and Technology,* **2007,** *109* (4), 336–349.

Knightly, W. H. Shortening Systems: Fats, Oils, and Surface-Active Agents—Present and Future. *Cereal Chem.* **1981,** *58* (3), 171–174.

Latondress, E. G. Formulation of Products from Soybean Oil. *J. Am. Oil Chem. Soc.* **1981,** *53,* 185–187.

Linder, R. Adaptive Evolution of Seed Oils in Plants: Accounting for the Biogeographic Distribution of Saturated and Unsaturated Fatty Acids in Seed Oils. *Am. Nat.* **2000,** *156,* 442–458.

Madison, B. L.; Hill, R. C. Determination of the Solid Fat Content of Commercial Fats by Pulsed Nuclear Magnetic Resonance. *J. Am. Oil Chem. Soc.* **1978,** *55,* 328–331.

Mensink, R.; Katan, M. Effect of Dietary *Trans* Fatty Acids on High-Density and Low-Density Lipoprotein Cholesterol in Healthy Subjects. *New England Journal of Medicine* **1990,** *323,* 439–445.

Schleifer, D. The Perfect Solution. How *Trans* Fats Became the Healthy Replacement for Saturated Fats. *Technology and Culture* **2012,** *53* (1), 94–119.

Stender, S.; Dyerberg, J.; Astrup, A. Consumer Protection Through a Legislative Ban on Industrially Produced Trans Fatty Acids in Foods in Denmark. *Scandanavian Journal of Food Nutrition* **2006,** *50,* 155-60.

U.S. Department of Agriculture. *Nutrient Database, Release 24.* U.S. Department of Agriculture.

U.S. Department of Agriculture. Appendix Table 47. In *Oil Crops Yearbook (89002);* Ithaca, NY: Cornell University.

U.S. Food and Drug Administration. *Food Labeling; Trans Fatty Acids in Nutrition Labeling; Consumer Research to Consider Nutrient Content and Health Claims and Possible Footnote or Disclosure Statements; Final Rule and Proposed Rule;* Regulation: 21 CFR 101.9 (c)(2)(ii). Food and Drug Administration (2003-07-11). 21 CFR Part 101; Washington, DC: 2007. U.S. Government Printing Office (GPO).

U.S. House of Representatives. *Labeling of Meat Food Products to Reflect the Inclusion of Imitation or Alternate Cheese; and the Effects of Consumption of Tropical Oils on the Soybean Program (10 September 1987);* Committee on Agriculture Serial Number 100-44, Hearing ID: HRG-1987-HAG-0038; Committee on Agriculture, Subcommittee on Livestock, Dairy, and Poultry, 1987.

Yap, P. H.; deMan, J. M.; deMan, L. Polymorphism of Palm Oil and Palm Oil Products. *J. Am. Oil Chem. Soc.* **1989,** *66,* 693–697.

7

High-Oleic Oils and Their Uses for *Trans* Fats Replacement

Linsen Liu ■ *LS Consulting, Irvine, California, United States*

Introduction

Commodity vegetable oils, such as soybean and canola oils, are not stable enough for most shelf-stable food manufacturing and restaurant frying because they are rich in polyunsaturated fatty acids (PUFAs), such as linolenic and linoleic acids. Linoleic and linolenic acids have a 10- and 25-fold higher oxidation rates, respectively, than oleic acid; therefore, stability improvement on commodity oils can be achieved through their reduction by hydrogenation or biotechnology. Partially hydrogenated oil had been preferred by the food industry for many decades mainly due to its high stability, which is contributed by *trans* fat. In the past two decades, however, concerns regarding the health implications of *trans* fat have been forcing partially hydrogenated oil out of the food supply chain. Instead, high stability oils rich in oleic acid developed through breeding have been introduced to replace *trans* fat and have been become the healthy alternative to *trans* fat in food formulation and industrial frying. A recent proposal by the FDA to ban *trans* fat will certainly accelerate replacement of *trans* fat with healthy oils.

Linolenic and linoleic acids are PUFAs and are prone to oxidation. Their oxidative degradation leads to short-chain ketones and aldehydes that present as unpleasant off-flavors described by consumers as painty, grassy, fishy, beany, or rancid. Oleic acid is the precursor to biosynthesis of linoleic and linolenic acids in oilseeds; therefore, selectively limiting the biosynthetic pathway from oleic to linoleic acid and to linolenic acid can lower either or both of them. Simple reduction in linolenic acid can produce low-linolenic oil, and dual reduction of linolenic and linoleic acids can result in high-oleic oil, which can be achieved through breeding or genetic modification (GM). Low-linolenic and high-oleic oils are both relevant in product development and in *trans* fat replacement; we will discuss them together in this chapter. In general, oxidative stability is in order of high-oleic oils > low-linolenic oils > commodity oils. Hydrogenated *trans* fat typically has higher stability than commodity oils and its stability increases with the degree of hydrogenation. Those high-oleic or low-linolenic oils with stability equal to or better than *trans* fat are suitable for *trans* fat replacement without sacrificing product stability performance and shelf life. *Trans* fat in this article refers to a group of unsaturated fatty acids generated during industrial hydrogenation that contain at least one double bond in *trans* configuration. The most common forms of *trans* fats from hydrogenation are isomers of oleic acid and they are solid at room temperature.

Soybean is a major oilseed crop for producing soy meal, and its oil is mostly a byproduct of meal production. Soybean breeding has been undergoing changes since linolenic acid was identified as the root cause for flavor reversion in refined soybean oil in the 1950s, and it primarily focused on lowering linolenic acid content until recently. Reducing linolenic acid from 7–10% in commodity soybean oil down to 3.5% or lower results in low-linolenic or ultra-low-linolenic soybean oils, which give limited improvement in oxidative stability because low-linolenic soybean oils still contain over 50% linoleic acid. Low-linolenic soybean oils are not oxidatively stable enough to replace *trans* fat in most food applications without sacrificing product quality. As a result, low-linolenic soybean oils have not achieved market acceptance and meaningful market share after about 20 years in the test market. High-oleic soybean is technically challenging to breed and currently relies on GM technology. Because oil is a byproduct of soybean meal production, it is difficult to justify crop value simply by improving oil stability alone. Current high-oleic soybean varieties in testing are GM crops, and their full-scale commercial production may be decades away because their market acceptance depends on oil performance in food applications, global deregulation, yield improvement, supply chain development, and cost competitiveness. Similarly, high-oleic corn was also developed but not commercialized because corn oil is a byproduct of cornstarch and feed production.

High-oleic peanuts were commercialized in the 1990s, mainly to improve shelf life of peanuts and their products. Because the majority of peanuts are directly used in manufacturing peanut butters and food products, high-oleic peanut oil is not significantly important for *trans* fat replacement due to limited supply. Safflower oil has been typically classified as industrial oil due to its high linoleic acid content (80%). Breeding successfully introduced high-oleic safflower with 80% oleic acid. However, both safflower and high-oleic safflower oils are not widely available due to their limited growing regions. Similarly, sunflower oil, containing 70% linoleic acid, is notoriously unstable against oxidation. Mid- and high-oleic sunflower oils have been successfully introduced through breeding and contain about 50% and 80% (or higher) oleic acid, respectively. Sunflowers also have limited growing regions in North America; therefore, sunflower oils are very volatile in production, quality, and price. Sunflowers are recognized as non-GM crops and play an important role in markets where GM crops are rejected by consumers or government regulations. High-oleic palm oil, containing more than 54% oleic acid and less than 31% saturated fatty acid and developed in South America as a result of breeding for disease-resistant varieties, may be used also as alternative to *trans* fat.

Canola was the first oilseed purposefully selected for breeding high-stability oil as a healthy solution to *trans* fat in the 1980s. Canadian scientists bred canola from traditional rapeseed in the 1950s to improve meal and oil quality by reducing glucosinolates and erucic acid contents. Canola oil is considered healthy due to its lowest saturated fatty acid content and it is widely used for general cooking. Containing 7–10% linolenic acid, canola oil is not stable enough for commercial frying and manufacturing of shelf-stable foods. Canola is a perfect candidate for development of high-oleic oil because it is an oil crop, is widely grown in North America, and is naturally low in linoleic acid in its seed oil. Those advantages made canola a good candidate for developing and producing healthy and high-oleic oil in large scale. Simple reduction of linolenic acid can result in low-linolenic canola that has higher oxidative stability than commonly used *trans* fat. Further reduction of linoleic acid can result in high-oleic canola oil that has extraordinary oxidative stability to replace *trans* fat in most food formulations. Low-linolenic canola has slightly higher oleic content than canola and is often referred to as high-oleic oil also. After more than 20 years of commercialization, the high-oleic canola industry has established a sustainable supply chain and has achieved a dominant market share in food and food service industries. High-oleic canola oils, including low-linolenic canola, have dominated other oils as healthy solutions to *trans* fat for over 20 years in North America. Major varieties of high-oleic canola have been achieved through breeding, but may incorporate the GM herbicide-tolerant gene. Over 90% of the canola crop in North America is GM due to incorporation of the GM herbicide-tolerant gene. Consumers in North America generally embrace GM crops well because they understand the associated benefits in reduction of agricultural chemical usage and environmental pollution. Non-GM high-oleic canola oils are commercially available and in production in regions in which they are in demand.

After decades of efforts, the edible oil industry has commercialized high-oleic and mid-oleic sunflower oils, high-oleic canola oils, and high-oleic safflower oils, and is testing high-oleic soybean oils. High-oleic canola oils are the most widely used high-stability oils and dominate the high-oleic oil market due to their high stability, clean flavor, lowest saturated fat content, sustainable supply chain, and large crop production scale in North America. With implementation of a regulatory requirement to label *trans* fat on packaged foods in the United States since 2006, the demand for high-oleic canola oils has been steadily growing and is expected reach 1.3 billion pounds (590,000 t) in 1–2 years (DeBonte et al., 2012; Liu and Iassonova, 2012). A recent proposal to ban *trans* fat by the FDA will certainly accelerate production of high-oleic oils.

Compositions and Properties

Table 7.A lists common commodity oils and higher stability oils (low linolenic and high oleic) developed in the past several decades, along with their fatty acid compositions and oxidative stability indices (OSI) for comparison. Commodity oils are not

Table 7.A Fatty Acid Composition, Oxidative Stability, and Availability of Commodity and High-Oleic Oils[a]

Oils	Commercial Availability	Oleic	Linoleic	Linolenic	Sat	OSI Typical
Sunflower, regular	Limited	20	65	<1	8	6
Sunflower, mid oleic	Limited	57	33	<1	8	12
Sunflower, high oleic	Limited	82	9	<1	8	24
Soybean, commodity	Large	23	54	7	15	6
Soybean, low linolenic	Limited	26	56	3	15	8
Soybean, high oleic	Testing	75	15	3	7	25
Canola, commodity	Large	60	20	10	7	9
Canola, low linolenic	Large	63	24	3	7	15
Canola, high oleic	Large	80	9	3	7	26
Safflower, regular	Limited	13	75	0	10	5
Safflower, high oleic	Limited	80	12	0	7	14
Corn, commodity (6)	Limited	24	63	<1	13	9
Corn, high oleic (6)	No	65	23	<1	11	14

[a]Sat: saturated fatty acids; OSI: oxidative stability index measured at 110 °C.

suitable to replace *trans* fat because they are rich in either linoleic acid and linolenic acid (or both) and their OSIs are typically below 10 hours. Because the ratio of oxidative stability of oleic, linoleic, and linolenic acids is in the order of 1:10:25, reduction in linolenic and linoleic acids can significantly improve oil oxidative stability. For instance, sunflower oil stability improvement is achieved by progressive reduction of linoleic acid because linolenic acid is nearly absent in sunflower oil. Reduction of linoleic acid results in a corresponding increase in oleic acid. For instance, with reduction of linoleic acid from 65% to 33% in mid-oleic and to 9% in high-oleic oils, oxidative stability of sunflower oil increases as shown by the OSI from 6 to 12 and 24 hours, respectively. In comparison, soybean oil's OSI only improves by 2 hours by reducing linolenic acid from 7% to 3%. Therefore, low-linolenic soybean oils are not high-stability oils. Further reduction of linoleic acid from 54% to 15% results in high-oleic soybean oil with 25 or more OSI hours, which is an improvement of four-fold over commodity soybean oil or three-fold over low-linolenic soybean oil. Canola is naturally high in oleic and linolenic acids and low in saturated and linoleic acids. Therefore, a simple reduction in linolenic acid can significantly improve oxidative stability from 9 hours to 15 hours as shown by low-linolenic canola, which is comparable to or better than commonly used *trans* fat. Further reduction of linoleic acid results in high-oleic canola that can have an OSI as high as 26 hours. High-oleic safflower oil is about three-fold higher in OSI than high-linoleic safflower oil, but much lower than other high-stability oils with a similar oleic content to high-oleic canola and sunflower oils. High-oleic corn oil, having a 5-hour OSI improvement over corn oil, is similar in fatty acid profile and stability to low-linolenic canola.

Fatty acid composition is a very important criterion for selecting the right oil for applications in order to achieve target oxidative stability and flavor profiles. For instance, linolenic acid easily develops fishy, painty, or grassy off-flavors, and should ideally be limited to below 4% to maintain or improve oil flavor stability and food shelf life. Linoleic acid at high concentrations can develop similar off-flavors upon oxidation. However, studies have shown that oils with 20–30% linoleic acid are ideal for best fried flavors and product shelf stability (Liu and Iassonova, 2012; Warner et al., 1994, 1997, 2013). Among those oils listed in Table 7.A, low-linolenic canola oil is the only commercial oil that naturally meets the ideal fatty acid profile for frying (<4% linolenic and 20–30% linoleic acids). In fact, low-linolenic canola has been the dominant and preferred no-*trans* frying oil in food services for over 20 years in North America. The higher oleic oils having over 20 OSI hours are ideal for manufacturing shelf-stable foods because they provide clean flavors and higher oxidative stability required for long product shelf life. Table 7.B lists thermal properties including smoking point, flash point, and fire points of the high-oleic oils in comparison to commodity oils (ISEO, 2014). Although those thermal properties also depend on oil refining quality and oil sample age, it is very interesting that high-oleic and low-linolenic canola oils not only

Table 7.B Thermal Properties of Commodity and High-Oleic Oils

	Smoke Point		Flash Point		Fire Point	
Oils	**(°C)**	**(°F)**	**(°C)**	**(°F)**	**(°C)**	**(°F)**
Sunflower, regular	240	464	—	—	—	—
Sunflower, mid oleic	211	412	319	607	359	678
Sunflower, high oleic	244	471	319	606	360	680
Soybean, commodity	240	464	330	626	360	680
Soybean, low linolenic	237	458	331	628	362	684
Hydrogenated soya oil (IV 70)	230	446	330	626	360	680
Canola, commodity	236	457	326	619	350	662
Canola, low linolenic	240	464	340	644	360	680
Canola, high oleic	246	468	—	—	—	—
Safflower, regular	230	446	—	—	—	—
Safflower, high oleic	242	468	—	—	—	—
Corn, commodity	235	455	325	617	354	670

consistently outperform commodity canola oils with higher smoke points, but also outperform other high-oleic and mid-oleic or low-linolenic oils, respectively. Because the samples analyzed are commercially produced, it is acceptable to assume the results represent average thermal properties of commercial high-oleic and commodity oils. Those data provide further proof that high-oleic canola oils would perform better at high temperatures than other high-oleic oils and are preferred in *trans* replacement, particularly for frying.

High-oleic oils are liquid at room and refrigeration temperatures and have thermal properties, such as melting and solidification, comparable to commodity oils. Therefore, high-oleic oils can be processed with regular equipment and production lines and used for frying, food manufacturing, and salad dressing formulation.

Food Applications

Selection of frying oil is based on target flavor profile and product stability, including shelf life and fry life (pot life). Overall, food operators want to achieve the best flavors and longest shelf life at the lowest cost. Good frying oil should contain no more than 4% linolenic acid to prevent fishy off-flavors and premature foaming after a few days of frying. Warner et al. recommended that linoleic acid in a frying oil should be maintained within 20–37% to balance flavor and shelf stability based on a series of studies using high-oleic canola and high-oleic sunflower, high-oleic corn, and high-oleic soybean oils (Warner and Knowlton, 1997; Warner et al., 1994, 1997). Oil with linoleic acid below 20% produces a bland taste in fried foods, while oil with more than 37% of linoleic acid breaks down too soon during frying. Because high-oleic canola and sunflower oils are the two major commercial products, we will focus on these two oils and their applications in this chapter.

Table 7.C lists the major commercial high-oleic canola oils on the North American market, along with their typical fatty acid profiles and OSIs. As shown, reduction of linolenic acid alone, from 10% in canola oil to 3% in Clear Valley® 65 (CV65),

Table 7.C Commercial High-Oleic Canola Oils

Oils	Features	Fatty Acid Profile (%)				OSI (hrs)
		Sat	Oleic	Linoleic	Linolenic	
Canola	Commodity	7	60	20	10	9
Clear Valley® 65 (CV65)	Low linolenic	7	65	24	3	15
Clear Valley® 75 (CV75)	High oleic	7	75	14	3	19
Omega-9 canola oils	High oleic	7	73	15	<3	17
Clear Valley® 80 (CV80)	Highest oleic	7	80	9	3	26

results in a significant increase of OSI from 9 to 15 hours. It is interesting to note that linoleic acid increases from 20% to 24% at the same time. The reduction in linolenic acid improves oil stability, while the increased level of linoleic acid provides a balanced flavor profile ideal for frying. Indeed, as shown in Figure 7.1, CV65, with 23–25% linoleic acid, delivers the best "overall liking" in the french fries study compared to CV75 (high-oleic canola), HoSun (high-oleic sunflower), and commodity soybean oil. In the test, overall liking was evaluated as part of acceptance testing using a 9-point hedonic scale in which 9 is equal to "like extremely" and 1 is equal to "dislike extremely" (Lawless and Heymann, 2010). This result is consistent with the findings by Warner et al. (1994, 1997, 1997).

Figure 7.2 compares OSIs of various canola and soybean oils, including a commonly used partially hydrogenated soybean oil (PHS). PHS has an OSI value of 10 hours, which is typically a minimum requirement for frying and food manufacturing. As shown, all high-oleic canola oils have OSI values greater than 10 hours and are able to replace *trans* fat in those food applications. In comparison, soybean, canola, and low-linolenic soybean (LL soy) oils have relatively lower OSI values than PHS and, therefore, have limited market acceptance as *trans* replacements. The true test of stability is obtained from sensory analysis of the food products, but OSI is a common stability measure for screening. Figure 7.3 compares Schaal Oven stability of three CV high-oleic canola oils, which clearly shows both CV65 and CV80 have much higher resistance to oxidation, which is consistent with the OSI results shown in Figure 7.2 (Liu and Iassonova, 2012).

As previously discussed, desirable frying oil should be low in linolenic acid and adequate in linoleic acid for high stability and high intensity of fried flavors.

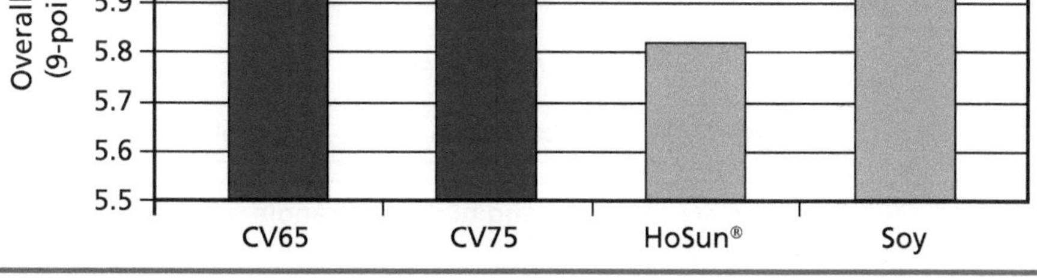

Figure 7.1 Overall liking scores of french fries with various oils.

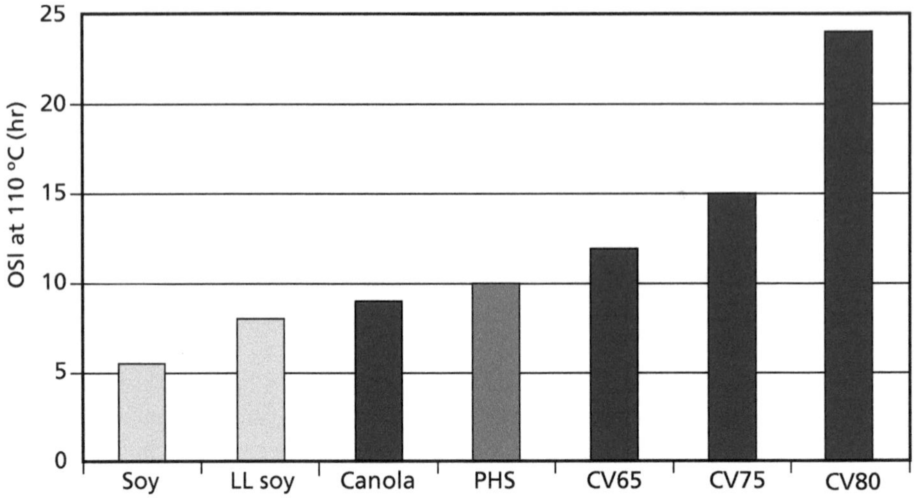

Figure 7.2 Oxidative stability index comparison of canola and soybean oils.

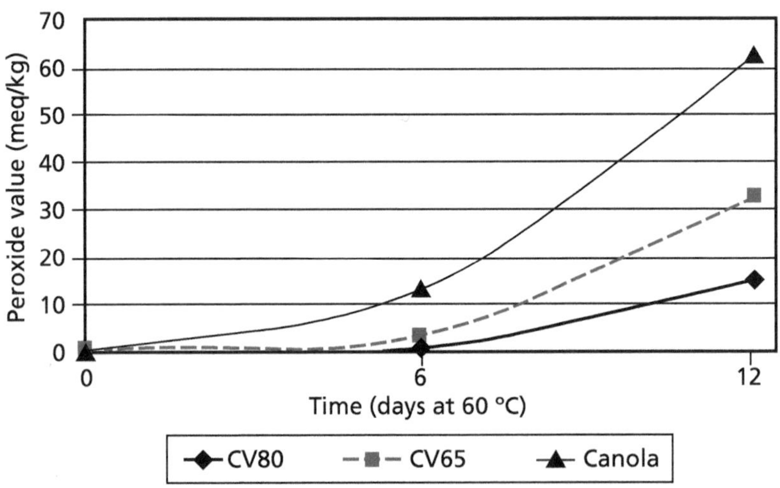

Figure 7.3 Oxidative stability of canola and high oleic canola oils in Schaal Oven test.

Generally, commodity oils such as soybean and canola oils can generally last three to five days in restaurant frying, while CV65 can last two to three weeks as measured by food quality. With over several-fold longer frying life than commodity oils, CV65 not only provides better food quality, but also can lower overall fry cost.

High-oleic sunflower oil is not suitable for frying because it contains an inadequate amount of linoleic acid to develop preferred fried flavors. To improve frying performance, mid-oleic acid sunflower was developed to improve frying performance. However, mid-oleic sunflower oil is relatively low in stability because it contains around 33% linoleic acid and is low in total tocopherols (509–741 ppm) with mainly α-Tocopherol (488–668 ppm) (Warner and Knowlton, 1997). α-Tocopherol has lower antioxidant efficacy than other tocopherol isomers commonly found in soybean and canola oils. Development of new varieties high in γ- and Δ-tocopherols are in progress to improve oxidative stability of mid- and high-oleic sunflower oils (Warner et al., 2008). Because sunflower crop has a limited growing region compared to canola, and high-oleic and mid-oleic sunflower oils are significantly behind high-oleic and low-linolenic canola oils in market supply and penetration, they mainly play niche roles in non-GM applications in North America.

High-oleic oils are majorly used as ingredient oils by food manufactures to formulate or process retail food products. Their resistance to flavor deterioration is the foundation to support long shelf life and fry life. Requiring identity-preserve conditions or a dedicated supply chain for production, high-oleic canola and similar specialty crops have higher production costs than commodity oils. Desirable ingredient oil should be low in linolenic and linoleic acids to deliver high flavor stability for shelf-stable foods. Clear Valley® 80 (CV80) is the newest generation of high-oleic canola oil, which can deliver up to 26 OSI hours with 80% oleic acid and less than 10% linoleic and 3% linolenic acids. Its extraordinarily high stability can maintain preferred flavors in storage, extend shelf life, reduce packaging, and even enable new applications. Generally, oleic acid content can be used as the mark for canola oil stability because it correlates positively and linearly with OSI (Liu and Iassonova, 2012). CV80, having the highest oleic acid content, is particularly useful for shelf-stable product formulations that deliver long shelf life and reduce packaging cost. Figure 7.4 compares CV80 and CV65 with commodity soybean and canola oils in cereals packed in plastic bags without oxygen barrier and aged at 60 °C for 12 days. The results show that, not surprisingly, soybean oil has the least stability. Both soybean and canola oils developed unacceptable high peroxide values (PV) and sensory scores, while CV65 only developed 6.8 PV with acceptable sensory scores and CV80 demonstrated the highest stability with nearly no PV development. This result not only demonstrates the usefulness of CV65 and CV80 for shelf-stable formulations, but also suggests the potential of CV80 in reducing packaging cost or extending product shelf life.

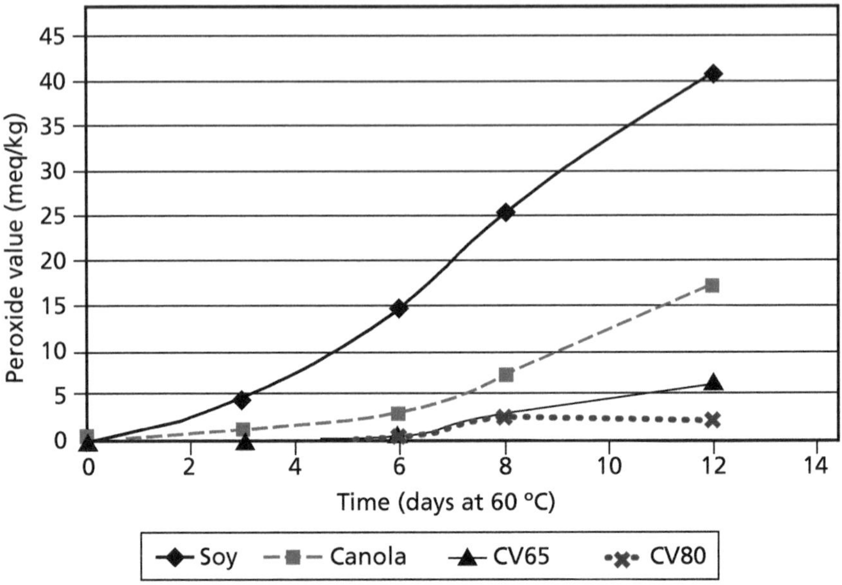

Figure 7.4 Oil stability of cereals packed in plastic packaging.

In summary, high-oleic canola oils, including low linolenic, have been widely used in North America to replace *trans* fat in frying and food manufacturing mainly due to their better functionality and availability in large scale. CV65 is optimal for frying, owing to its low linolenic acid content for oxidative stability and ideal linoleic acid level for fried flavor. CV80 is optimal as an ingredient oil for shelf-stable food formulations and its highest oxidative stability can potentially reduce packaging cost and extend product shelf life. High- and mid-oleic sunflower oils play a niche role in non-GM applications due to their limited supply and high cost. Table 7.D summarizes the typically applications of commercial canola and high-oleic canola oils.

High-oleic canola oils can be used in many baking applications to replace *trans* fat, or further formulated into low-saturate shortenings for broad baking applications when combined with solid fats such as fully hydrogenated fats or stearins. Tables 7.E and 7.F compare the nutrition of CV all-purpose (CV AP) shortening with palm and *trans* shortenings and doughnuts cooked in those shortenings (Bordi et al., 2009). The data show that saturated fat can increase dramatically when palm oil is used to replace *trans* shortening. In comparison, CV AP can eliminate *trans* fat without increasing saturated fat, which is ideal in *trans* fat replacement and is preferred by food manufactures and health-conscious consumers. In any food product or reformulation, due to *trans* fat regulations, the *trans* and saturated fat contents are important

Table 7.D Preferred Food Applications of Canola and High-Oleic Canola Oils

Categories	Applications	Function/Properties	Application Examples
Canola	Cooking oil	Short shelf life, low cost	Retail bottled oil
CV65	Frying Ingredient Shortening	Fry flavors; to enrich flavors	Restaurant and industrial frying Shelf-stable formulation, baking, top spraying Baking, frying
CV75	Ingredient Shortening	Clean food flavors	Shelf-stable formulation, baking, top spraying
CV80	Ingredient Shortening	Clean food flavors; lower packaging cost	Shelf-stable formulation, baking, top spraying, low cost packaging

Table 7.E Nutrition Comparison of High-Oleic Canola Shortening with Palm and Hydrogenated Shortenings

	Nutrition per Serving (13 g fat)			
Commercial Shortenings	**Sat**	***Trans***	**Total Sat + *Trans***	**Ingredients**
Bunge VFD	3	5	8	Partially hydrogenated soybean oil
Loders Croklaan DDA	8	0	8	Palm and cottonseed oils
Cargill CV AP	3	0	3	High-oleic canola, soybean, and fully hydrogenated cottonseed oils

Table 7.F Nutrition of Doughnuts Cooked in *Trans*, Palm, and CV AP Shortenings

Commercial Shortenings	Doughnut Serving Size	Sat	*Trans*	Sat + *Trans*
Bunge VFD	50 g	1.5	1.5	3
Loders Croklaan DDA	50 g	2.5	0	2.5
Cargill CV AP	50 g	1.5	0	1.5

because they appear on the label of the product and determine whether certain health claims can be used.

Supply Chain

Like other trait-enhanced products, high-oleic oils are specialty agricultural products produced under identity preservation. Among all high-oleic oilseeds, canola is the only one that has established a large-scale and sustainable supply chain in North America. After over 20 years of commercialization, high-oleic canola oils have become the dominant healthy replacement for *trans* fat. Customers with high-volume demand for high-oleic oil need to contract crop production with suppliers for reliable oil supply. There are many unpredictable factors impacting crop production, and suppliers must be carefully screened for their technical and commercial capabilities in risk control, crop varieties with disease and drought resistance, diversity in genetics, and crop production regions. A supplier with a fully integrated closed-loop production system—from trait development to plant breeding to oil production and formulation technology—may be an ideal option because this supplier can provide one-stop shopping for supply, quality, and product development from seed genetics to crop and oil production. Sustainability and ensured supply are essential to food manufacturers.

Outlook

After 20 years of commercialization, high-oleic canola oils have been proven very successful and have become the main working oils in *trans* fat replacement for food processing and frying. New varieties for high yield, disease resistance, and specialty uses are continuously coming out of the development pipeline. Cargill announced that they would develop low saturated fat and high-oleic canola oil (Gelski, 2011). Specialty oils beside high-oleic are also in development. For instance, Cargill and BASF are developing omega-3 canola containing DHA and EPA for commercialization in 2020, and Monsanto is developing soybean oil containing stearidonic acid.

References

Bordi, P. L.; Hack, D. M.; Cocci, S. J.; Rager, M. D; Hessert S. W. Comparing *Trans*-Fat and *Trans*-Fat-Free Doughnut Shortenings Based on Sensory Evaluation and Oil Degradation. *Journal of Sensory Studies* **2009**, *24,* 41–57.

DeBonte, L.; Iassonova, D.; Liu, L.; Loh, W. Commercialization of High Oleic Canola Oils, *Lipid Technology* **2012**, *24,* 175–177.

Gelski, J. Cooking Oils Evolution. *Food Business News.* **2011.** http://www.foodbusinessnews.net/News/News%20Home/Features/2011/10/Cooking%20oils%20evolution.aspx?cck=1.
Institute of Shortening and Edible Oils. Typical Smoke, Flash & Fire Points of Commercially Available Edible Fats and Oils. http://iseo.org/httpdocs/Publications/Smoke-Fire_Chart_0310.pdf (accessed March 6, 2014).

Lawless, H. T.; Heymann H. *Sensory Evaluation of Food: Principles and Practices.* Springer: New York, 2010; 149–174.

Liu, L.; Iassonova, D. High-oleic Canola Oils and Their Food Applications. *Inform* **2012**, *23,* pp. 491–496.

Warner, K.; Knowlton, S. Frying Quality and Oxidative Stability of High-Oleic Corn Oils. *J. Am. Oil Chem. Soc.* **1997**, *74,* 1317–1322.

Warner, K.; Orr, P.; Parrott, L.; Glynn, M. Effect of Frying Oil Composition on Potato Chip Stability. *J. Am. Oil Chem. Soc.* **1994**, *74,* 1123–1128.

Warner, K.; Orr, P.; Glynn, M. Effect of Fatty Acid Composition of Oils on Flavor and Stability of Fried Foods. *J. Am Oil Chem. Soc.* **1997**, *74,* 347–356.

Warner K.; Miller J.; Demurin Y. Oxidative Stability of Crude Mid-Oleic Sunflower Oils from Seeds with High γ- and δ-Tocopherol Levels. *J. Am Oil Chem. Soc.* **2008**, *85,* 529–533.

Warner, K.; Vick, B.; Kleingartner, L.; Isaak, R.; Doroff, K. Compositions of Sunflower, NuSun (Mid-oleic Sunflower) and High-Oleic Sunflower Oils. http://www.sunflowernsa.com/uploads/resources/51/warner_.pdf (accessed March 6, 2014).

8

Latest Developments in Chemical and Enzymatic Interesterification for Commodity Oils and Specialty Fats

Véronique Gibon and Marc Kellens ■ *Desmet Ballestra Group, Zaventem, Belgium*

Introduction

Today there is a specific demand for optimizing the industrial processes and for improving the quality of the fat food products in accordance with strict criteria related to oil, to health, and to environmental concerns (Figure 8.1). Until recently, the standards mainly covered organoleptic properties of the refined oil: odorless and bland taste, light and brilliant color, good oxidation parameters, and optimal shelf life. Due to health concerns and environmental issues, extra factors now come into play. The nutritional aspects of oils and fats have always raised many discussions. Whereas in the past scientists focused on a reduction of the saturated fat level in food products only, more attention is now paid to the *trans* fatty acid (TFA) content, a more balanced fatty acid composition, and on high retention of the natural vitamins in the refined oils. Focus is also on removal of the majority of the contaminants of various origins (environmental, crop protection, transport, storage, and production processes) and also on the reduction of fat degradation, in the case of highly sensitive oils. In addition, there are strong commitments for lowering the oil losses, for reducing effluent and waste, and for avoiding the use of chemicals and solvents. Fats are normally processed to have a wide range of physicochemical properties, enabling their use in most formulations; several processing technologies, including fractionation, interesterification, hydrogenation, and blending, allow the refiner to supply tailor-made products that will meet requirements of the food manufacturers. Among these, partial hydrogenation is particularly criticized because it generates excessive amounts of TFAs. The negative health effects of these fatty acids are clearly identified, and this comes with strict legislation and labeling requirements regarding the maximal content allowed in fat foods (<5% fat base in the low-*trans* products; <0.5% fat base in the zero-*trans* products). Formulation based on fractionated, interesterified, and/or fully hydrogenated fats is the only alternative to meet these requirements. In previous years, chemical interesterification was principally used for the elaboration of commodity products, while enzymatic interesterification was reserved for the production of specialty fats. Today, enzymatic interesterification is becoming a cost-effective process for commodity fats as well, and is intensively developed for the elaboration of a number of new specialty products. This chapter will focus on the interesterification process that can be carried out chemically or enzymatically for commodity oils and enzymatically for specialty fats. Whatever the option, the basic principle of

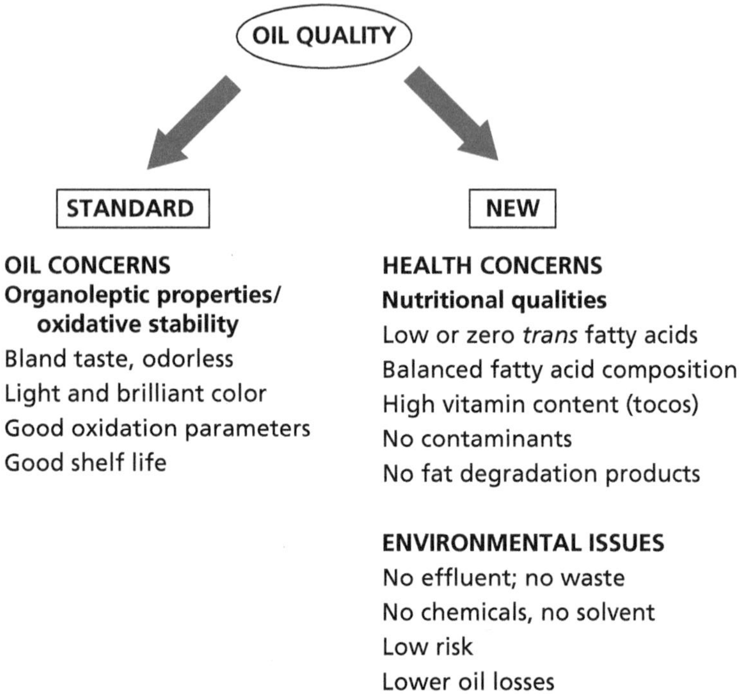

Figure 8.1 Quality criteria for food products containing fats and oils.

interesterification is to modify, selectively or not, the position of fatty acids on the glycerol backbone of triacylglycerol (TAG) molecules.

Random Interesterification for Commodity Oils

The easiest way to modify the composition of a fat used in margarine or shortening formulation is to allow random chemical or enzymatic migration of the fatty acids on the glycerol backbone. Applied to oils and fats, the term *interesterification* refers to a reaction in which a rearrangement of the acyl groups within and between the TAG molecules is allowed. This process is used to modify the physicochemical properties of fatty materials and can be applied directly to natural or to already fractionated and/or hydrogenated oils. The main objectives of this process are to change the overall melting profiles, to improve the compatibility of the different triacylglycerols in the solid state, to modify the plasticity of a product by changing its crystallization behavior, and to combine properties of mixed products.

Chemical Interesterification

To alter the natural distribution of fatty acids on TAGs by chemical interesterification, heat and traces of alkaline catalysts are required. In the past, chemical interesterification was regarded as a risky process due to the use of quite unstable catalysts, and it was also characterized by high oil losses (up to 5%). Thanks to major technological improvements and deeper mastering of the reaction mechanism, chemical interesterification can now be conducted in a more secure way and with significantly reduced oil losses (1% max).

Reaction Mechanism

The best known catalysts are alkali metals such as sodium, potassium, or their alloys and alkoxides such as sodium ethoxide. Alkali hydroxides such as sodium hydroxide are also occasionally used, but they are less active and therefore require higher temperatures. One of the most popular catalysts is sodium methylate or, optionally, sodium ethylate. During chemical interesterification, the actual catalytic material presumably consists of anions formed in the fat after addition of the alkaline precursor (sodium methylate). It is generally admitted that the anion involved is a glycerolate. However, mechanistic anomalies of the glycerolate mechanism were reported and a new theory, referred as an *enolate mechanism,* was recently proposed (De Greyt and Dijkstra, 2008). Whatever the hypothesis (glycerolate or enolate mechanism), the reaction takes place in two steps, with the initial formation of a fatty catalyst followed by propagation of the reaction. Considering the glycerolate mechanism, the slightly negative diacylglycerol ion will attack the slightly positive carbon atom of the carbonyl group of another fatty acid ester, resulting in a transition complex that decomposes in order to form a new TAG together with a new active catalyst ion (Figure 8.2). The reaction continues (fatty acid interchange) until the equilibrium governed by the law of probability is reached.

Oil Quality Criteria

The ingoing oil quality has a strong impact on the catalyst, which can be inactivated by a number of impurities. In order to enable the catalytic reaction to proceed properly, certain quality standards need to be satisfied. Care must be taken with the moisture content, the free fatty acid level, and the peroxide value, all of which will inactivate the catalyst (Table 8.A). In contact with water, sodium methylate decomposes into methanol and sodium hydroxide; methanol will react with TAGs to form methyl esters and sodium hydroxide will make soaps. The free fatty acids will destroy the catalyst activity by also forming methyl esters and soaps. To ensure perfect conduct of the process with optimal activity of the catalyst and formation of a minimum of byproducts, the oil must be fully neutralized and perfectly predried. Prebleaching of the oil also reduces the peroxides and reinforces the catalytic activity. Partially (NB)

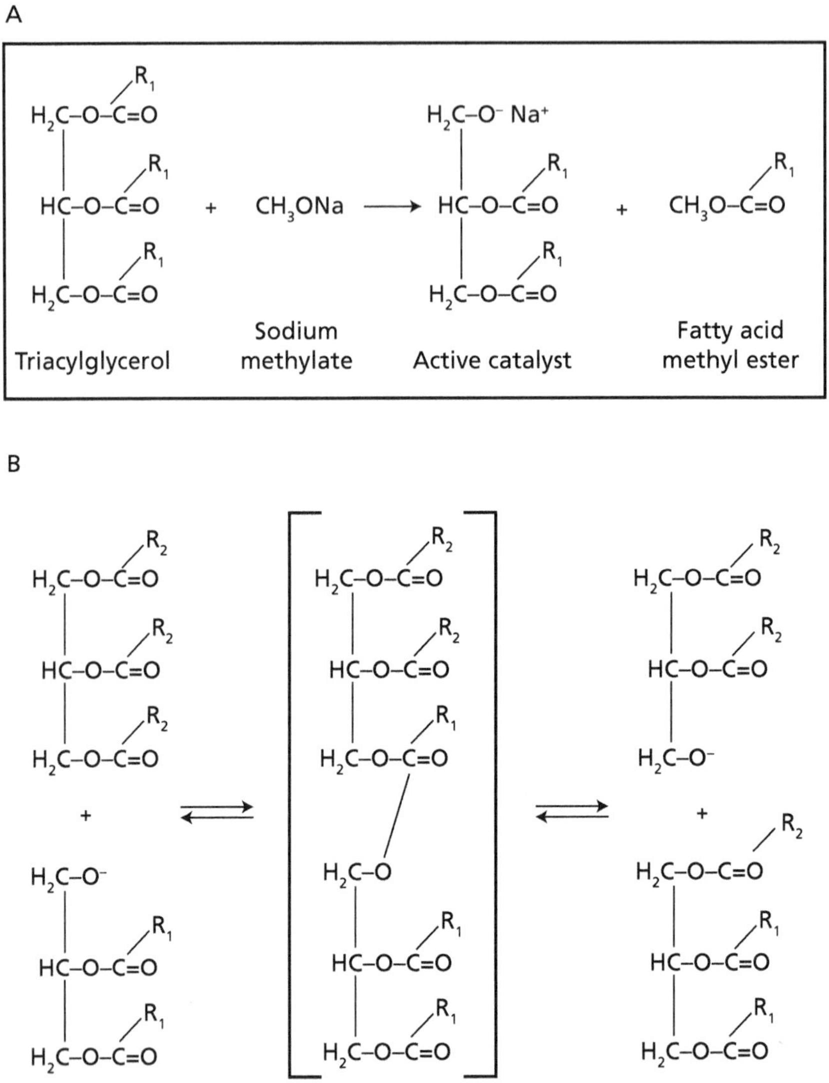

Figure 8.2 Initiation (A) and propagation (B) mechanisms during chemical interesterification; R_1 and R_2: fatty alkyl chains.

Table 8.A Quality Criteria of the Oil before Chemical Interesterification

FFA (%): 0.1 max
Peroxide Value (meqO_2/kg): 1.0 max.
Moisture (ppm): 100 max

Parameters		Ch_3ONa	Na	Na
FFA (%)	0.05	0.01	0.004	0.007
Peroxide value (meqO_2/kg)	1.0	0.0054	0.0023	0.004
Moisture (ppm)	100	0.03	0.013	—
Total inactivated catalyst (% on oil)		0.0454	0.0193	0.044

or fully refined (NBD or RBD) oils can be processed as long as the moisture content, free fatty acid level, and peroxide value are kept sufficiently low.

Catalytic Reaction

Every mole of sodium methylate added to the oil usually generates one mole of methyl esters and one mole of soaps; the reaction mechanism also induces the formation of diacylglycerols, which are found in some proportions in the chemically interesterified oil. When the reaction is finished, the catalyst must be deactivated. This can be done by adding water (wet deactivation) or acid (dry deactivation). When water is added, soaps and extra methyl esters are formed. Because soaps make it difficult to separate water from oil by decantation (formation of emulsions), salts or acids are usually added. Soap formation can be minimized by using sufficient quantities of acids to allow conversion back into free fatty acids. During dry deactivation, one mole of phosphoric acid, for example, is theoretically sufficient to convert three moles of catalyst into methanol and phosphate salts without soap formation. In practice, because soaps are also formed during the interesterification reaction (reaction of the catalyst with water and free fatty acids in oil), an acidic solution (typically 20% of citric acid solution with some excess) is frequently used to favor conversion of soaps into fatty acids. Catalyst deactivation is also possible by adding special adsorptive silica, the most commonly used being Trisyl (Grace Silica). The high moisture content of Trisyl permits catalyst deactivation concurrent with soap removal in the chemically interesterified oil.

Post-Treatment

The chemical interesterification process can be described as an operation in six steps. When necessary, the oil is first neutralized to decrease its free fatty acid content at acceptable levels. It is then dried until there is preferably 50 ppm of water, and the catalyst is added at a 0.05–0.10% dosage. In practice, the reaction is visualized by coloring of oil, which usually starts after 10–30 minutes; the mixture is kept another period (30–60 min.) to ensure completeness of the reaction (too long reaction times can darken the oil and fix the color). Once the catalyst is destroyed and the water phase is removed, the oil is post-bleached, typically with 0.2–0.5% of bleaching earth, and post-deodorized, typically at 230–240 °C. Bleaching allows complete removal of soaps and colored bodies, while deodorization enables the stripping of the extra free fatty acids and methyl esters.

Oil Losses and Byproducts

The oil losses can be expressed as losses due to the catalytic reaction and losses due to post-treatments (post-bleaching and post-deodorization). Every 0.1 kg of catalyst will generate 5.6 kg of soaps, which correspond to 5.2 kg of free fatty acids assuming full conversion during deactivation. In addition, methyl esters will be formed at a level of 5.5 kg, or 5.2 kg when expressed in free fatty acids. In total, the oil losses due to catalyst inactivation can reach about 1%. The formation of substantial amounts of diacylglycerols during the reaction also has an impact on the oil loss calculation. Counting the need of 0.5% bleaching earth and of post-deodorization, the overall oil losses of the chemical interesterification process can be estimated at 1.5% minimum. An accurate monitoring of oil quality, as well as a proper operation of the interesterification plant during the successive steps (neutralization, drying, catalytic reaction, deactivation, post-bleaching, and post-deodorization), allow reduction of oil losses and therefore improve the profitability of the process. The byproducts created during chemical interesterification are summarized in Figure 8.3. As previously described, soaps, color bodies, free fatty acids, and methyl esters can easily be removed during post-bleaching and post-deodorization. However, it is obvious that few colored materials may sometimes remain fixed in the chemically interesterified oil, even after an appropriate bleaching, and that the diacylglycerol content is often significantly increased. On the other side, it was shown that the unsaponifiable fraction can also be affected as part of the tocopherols and tocotrienols are degraded or transformed into the ester forms. The main consequence of this is a reduction of the oxidative stability of the chemically interesterified oil compared to the native oil. The formation of substantial amounts of long-chain dialkylketones not removable by any of the post-treatments is also reported (Verhe et al., 2006). These are molecules whose toxicity should be avoided, especially in infant formulation products. Dialkylketones can be formed at high amounts (up to 750 ppm) during chemical interesterification, but the quantity can be reduced below 25 ppm by properly adapting the catalyst dosage (Loders Crokland, 2009).

Batch versus Continuous Process

Industrial-scale chemical interesterification is generally a batch process, but it can also easily be conducted in a continuous way. In a batch operation, and when the initial

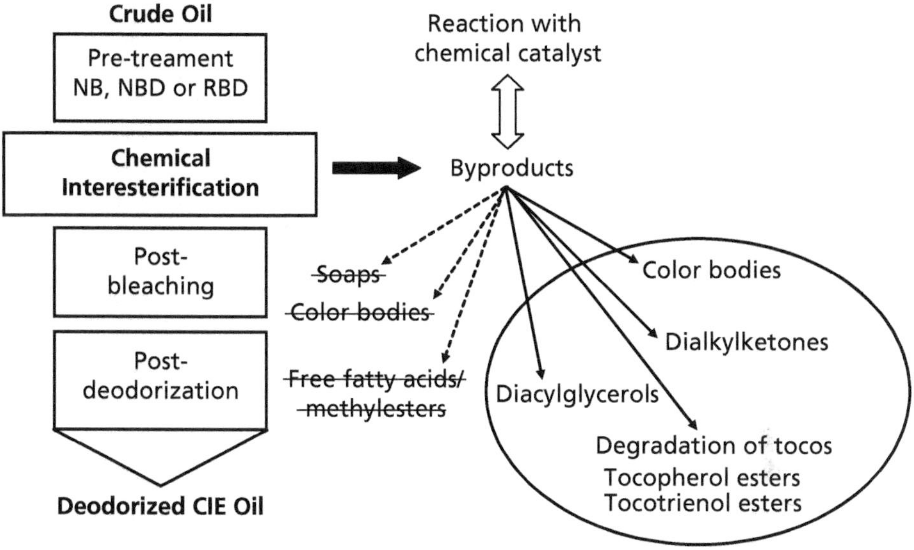

Figure 8.3 Byproducts formed during chemical interesterification; the crossed out byproducts are removed by post-bleaching and post-deodorization.

amount of free fatty acids is above 0.1%, the oil or blend of oils is mixed with a caustic soda solution for neutralization and heated to 120–130 °C under reduced pressure (~80 mbar) for drying. After this, the neutral oil is sprayed slowly in the reaction vessel and kept about 30 minutes at approximately 10 mbar to remove as much water as possible. The oil is subsequently cooled down at the reaction temperature (90 °C) and the catalyst is introduced as dry powder or as slurry mixed with some direct oil. The whole is intensively mixed for about 30–60 minutes. Once the reaction is completed, the catalyst must be deactivated, and the remaining soaps that were formed during the reaction must be eliminated by post-treatment. The oil is pumped to the acid reactor/bleacher and water and/or acid is added to stop the reaction. In the case of wet deactivation, the water phase is first decanted. When acid deactivation is used, a small excess is added and the mixture is subsequently dried and post-bleached. The bleached oil passes through one hermetic leaf filter and safety filters before being sent to the post-deodorization section. Figure 8.4 presents a flow diagram of a batch chemical interesterification plant (Desmet Ballestra Group, 2014).

Continuous operation is considered for larger capacities. The oil or the different components of the blend are dosed continuously by metering pumps together with diluted caustic soda in the neutralizing tank and properly mixed to neutralize the free fatty acids. The neutralized oil is then heated by heat exchanger and sprayed continuously in a vacuum drying tank operating at low pressure. The dried oil is

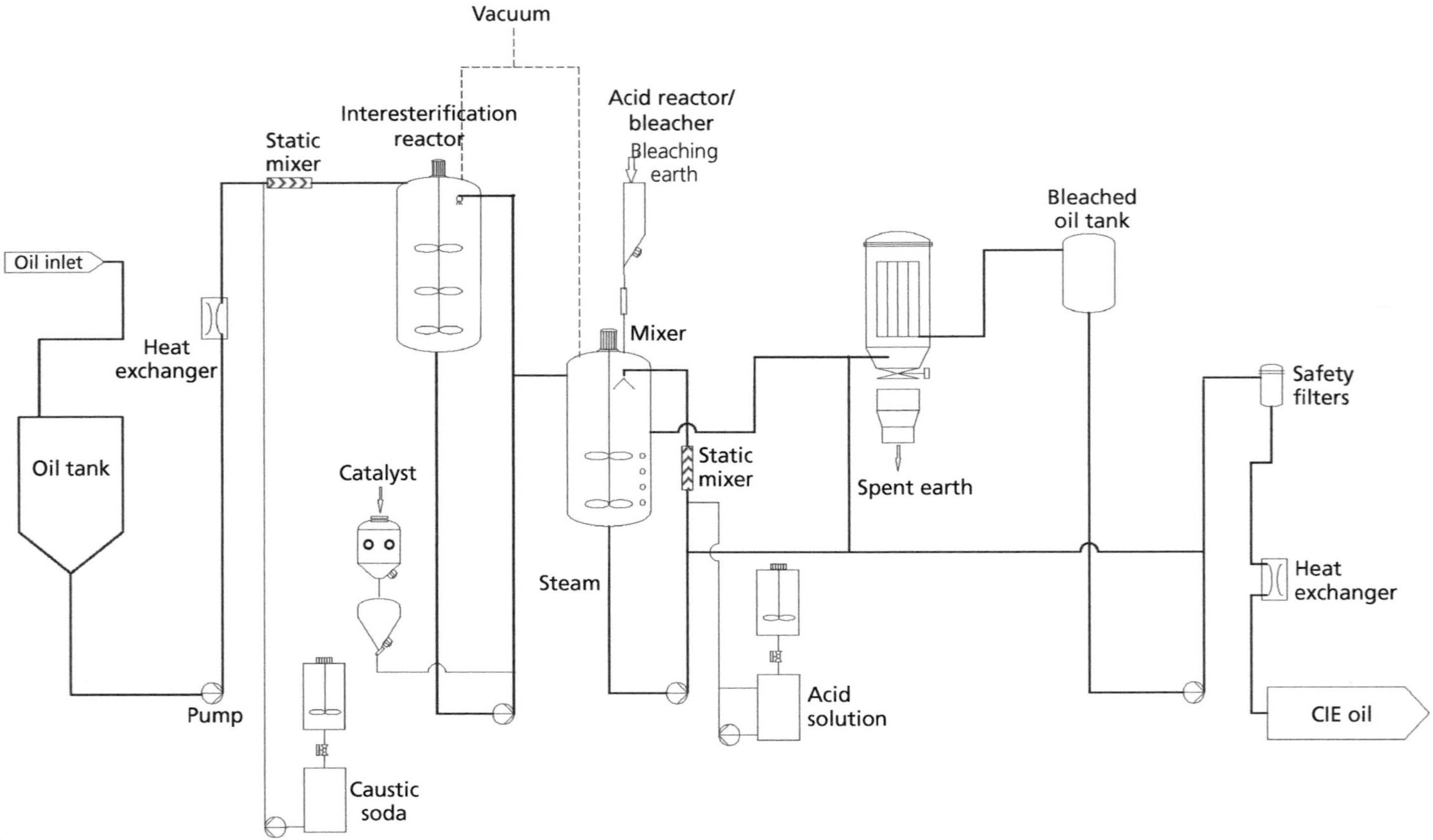

Figure 8.4 Flow diagram of a batch chemical interesterification process.

cooled down by means of a heat exchanger to reaction temperature and the catalyst is dosed. The mixture is sent to a multicompartment reaction vessel where the whole is kept for about 30–60 minutes; then it goes to a separate reactor for catalyst deactivation. For wet deactivation, the water phase is first separated before the drying step prior to post-bleaching and post-deodorization. Although a continuous process offers a number of real advantages, most of the chemical interesterification plants today are batch, due to the relatively low plant capacities.

Directed Chemical Interesterification

In random chemical interesterification, the fatty acids are redistributed nonselectively throughout the different positions on the glycerol backbone. In some cases, chemical interesterification can also, to a certain extent, be directed by segregation of the newly formed high melting point TAGs from the reaction mixture. The interesterification is directed away from randomness because the oil is maintained at a temperature below the melting point of the highest melting components. This results in selective crystallization of the most trisaturated TAGs with the effect of removing them from the reaction mixture. Directed chemical interesterification proceeds without the formation of more trisaturated TAGs that would have otherwise occurred. As trisaturated TAGs are formed, they crystallize from the solution and the fatty acid composition of the remaining liquid phase keeps changing. The reaction equilibrium in the liquid phase is pushed toward increased production of trisaturated TAGs. The process continues until most of the trisaturates in the oil have precipitated from the reaction medium. Compared to random chemical interesterification, the reaction temperature is lower (20–60 °C), the reaction time is longer (6–24 h), and the catalyst consumption is generally higher (0.1–0.3%). Being highly active at a low temperature, sodium-potassium alloy is more suitable and continuous directed process is usually required.

Enzymatic Interesterification

The current trends in edible oil processing are to develop, modify, and improve the existing technologies with the objective of preserving the maximum nutritional qualities of the original fat; to avoid chemicals and organic solvents; and to generate less waste and reduce the oil losses. This can explain why replacement of chemicals by enzymes is desired today. In oils and fats processing, specific enzymes are commercially available for degumming crude oils; other enzymes have also been developed with the objective of modifying the composition of the original fats to extend their applications as commodity oils and as specialty fat products. An enzyme is a protein that plays the role of a biocatalyst to facilitate a reaction; it lowers the activation energy and is found intact at the end of the reaction. Function is related to presence in the structure of the enzyme of an active site, in which the substrates will bind through weak chemical bonds. Once bound at the active site, the substrates will react and turn into product. Active sites may be sensitive to the presence of impurities that have the adverse effect of reducing the sites' potential activity.

Enzyme: Free versus Immobilized

Enzymatic reactions in organic media are actually divided into two systems: reactions performed in organic solvent systems and in solvent-free systems. The solvent-free system comprises only liquid organic substrates, such as liquid oil, and has high volumetric performance and economical advantages, especially for large-scale productions. It is also desirable for the synthesis of food-grade products due to stricter regulations regarding the use of organic solvents. Contrary to liquid enzymes, the immobilized form is defined as a biocatalyst that is restrained or localized in a microenvironment, yet retains its catalytic properties. Immobilization often increases the enzyme stability and makes it easily recovered and reused, allowing continuous processes to be carried out. Since it is not in liquid form, the immobilized enzyme does not contaminate the food product; therefore, there is no need for purification. However, immobilized enzymes are most of the time less active compared to liquid forms because they do not mix freely with the substrate. For example, the lipozyme TL IM is a commercially available immobilized enzyme manufactured by Novozymes A/S Denmark that can be used for random enzymatic interesterification; this immobilized enzyme allows modifications of the position of the fatty acids on the glycerol backbone according to the law of probability. TL IM is produced by immobilization of a microbial lipase from *Thermomyces lanuginosus* on a granular silica carrier and is mostly not positional specific (Novozymes A/S, 2011). After reaction, the TAG composition and the melting profile of the oil are modified in a similar way to the chemical process.

Enzyme Specificity

Lipases are known as being possibly positional or fatty acid specific. In terms of positional specificity, they can be placed into two groups: nonpositional specific and *sn*-1,3 positional specific. However, it should be noted that the positional specificity of lipases is not strictly divided into the two categories, but rather it varies widely in the range of very specific, weakly specific, or nonspecific. Moreover, a nonenzymatic acyl migration phenomenon from *sn*-2 to *sn*-1 and *sn*-3 positions makes this categorization a bit more complicated to establish. Fatty acid specificity comes from the difference in the reaction rate of the ester functional groups with different types of fatty acids; again, lipases seem not to have fully strict fatty acid specificity.

Reaction Mechanism

Enzymatic modifications can be categorized in four main groups: (1) the ester–ester exchange, which operates within oils or between oils and fatty acid esters; (2) the acidolysis, which is the reaction of an ester group and a fatty acid; (3) the alcoholysis, during which an ester group is reacting with an alcohol; and (4) the glycerolysis, in which an ester group is reacting with glycerol. Enzymatic interesterification for the formulation of zero- and low-*trans* margarines and shortenings consists of an ester–ester exchange reaction within oils or blends of oils that takes place at the active sites of the enzyme. The enzymatic interesterification currently carried out on the industrial scale is a continuous operation: The feedstock (oil or blend of oils) is pumped through a number of fixed-bed reactors filled with the immobilized enzyme. Depending on the plant capacity, the reactors may contain tens to hundreds of kilograms of immobilized enzymes. They are placed in series and kept at a constant and relatively low temperature (typically 70 °C); the oil is generally flowing from the top to the bottom of the reactors. An enzymatic interesterification industrial plant is presented in Figure 8.5. The oil flow rate (kg interesterified oil/kg enzyme • h) is regulated in order to ensure full conversion of the oil at the outlet of the plant. The enzymatically interesterified oil is generally gently post-deodorized in order to reduce the final free fatty acid content.

Continuous versus Batch Process

As mentioned before, immobilized enzymes are particularly suitable and economical for a continuous process and, therefore, contrary to chemical interesterification, the majority of the industrial enzymatic interesterification plants are working continuously. The batch process is reserved for laboratory investigations; this is generally

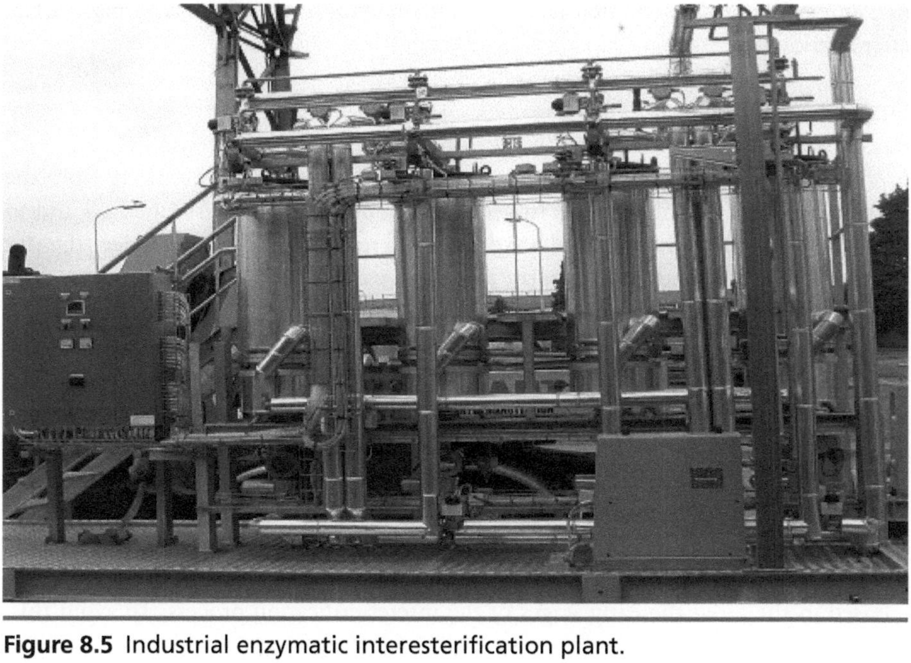

Figure 8.5 Industrial enzymatic interesterification plant.

performed for small-scale production of oils and blends with the objective of evaluating the compositional and melting properties of specific products and assessing the suitability for final use in the formulated products. Table 8.B summarizes some data collected during a batch laboratory scale enzymatic interesterification experiment with palm oil. The enzyme load was 4% (w/w) and the batch operation was conducted during a full period of 22 hours with regular sample withdrawal. The TAG composition was progressively modified and regularly evolved to a final equilibrium composition with a significant increase in trisaturated (StStSt) and triunsaturated (UUU) TAGs, a decrease in monounsaturated (StUSt) TAGs, and small modifications in diunsaturated (StUU) TAGs. The final composition was similar to the one of the chemically interesterified palm oil. However, more diacylglycerols were formed during the chemical interesterification process. The solid fat content profile of the 22-hour enzymatically interesterified palm oil was also similar to the one of the chemically interesterified palm oil; the interesterified palm oil was harder on the whole temperature range. A more detailed examination showed that during the first hours of reaction (4 h), the solid fat content was continuously decreased at temperatures below 5 °C and only later increased to reach the final equilibrium values; however, above 5 °C, the solid fat content profile was regularly increased up to final equilibrium. Such behavior is observed in the majority of oils and oil blends during interesterification, and was explained by some authors (Danthine et al., 2014; De Clercq et al., 2012) as being related to a multiphase structural modification mechanism involving positional *sn*-2 migration of the saturated fatty acids at the latest stage of the enzymatic interesterification process.

Enzyme Conditioning

Before being used for interesterification, the enzyme must be preconditioned. This preconditioning is necessary in order to remove air and excessive humidity from the enzyme particles; the objective is to avoid oxidation of the interesterified oil and to limit the losses due to oil hydrolysis during interesterification. In practice, the dry enzyme is first suspended in a slurry tank and wetted with a quantity of oil (feed or interesterified oil). A vacuum is created in the tank and the enzyme suspension is agitated for a period; after returning to atmospheric pressure, the suspension is transferred by gravity from the slurry tank to the enzyme reactor and recirculation starts from the enzyme reactor back to the slurry tank. When the conditioning time is elapsed, the conditioning oil is pumped back to storage. This conditioning oil will contain higher amounts of free fatty acids, as well as sodium soaps resulting from the first contact of the dry enzyme with oil. In the majority of the industrial plants, the enzyme conditioning is a single batch operation; however, because the wet enzyme will retain about 50% of the conditioning oil, some free fatty acids and soaps are still released in the oil at the early stages of the interesterification process. To avoid this,

Table 8.B Changes in Composition and Melting Properties of RBD Palm Oil with Time during Batch Laboratory-Scale Enzymatic Interesterification and after Chemical Interesterification

	RBD Palm Oil	EIE 1 hour	EIE 2 hours	EIE 4 hours	EIE 6 hours	EIE 8 hours	EIE 22 hours	CIE
DAG (% by HPLC)	7.7	7.7	7.6	7.6	7.7	7.8	7.9	8.8
TAG (% by HPLC)[a]								
StStSt	6.9	7.9	8.5	9.9	10.6	11.1	12.0	12.1
StUSt	46.5	43.7	42.5	40.9	39.7	39.0	38.1	38.1
StUU	39.7	39.6	39.3	38.7	38.4	38.2	37.7	37.6
UUU	6.9	8.8	9.7	10.5	11.3	11.7	12.2	12.2
SFC profile (°C)[b]								
0	55.4	51.3	48.8	50.0	55.9	58.4	62.9	62.8
5	58.4	56.2	56.0	54.7	58.5	60.7	64.4	64.6
10	50.8	50.7	52.3	52.6	55.2	56.2	59.2	59.6
15	39.9	41.6	43.0	43.2	44.6	46.1	48.7	48.7
20	28.0	29.8	31.2	32.7	34.6	36.5	39.4	39.1
25	16.9	19.2	20.4	22.0	24.2	25.5	28.0	27.9
30	10.0	11.9	12.9	14.4	16.2	17.6	19.1	18.6
35	5.0	6.9	7.7	9.2	10.3	11.8	12.6	12.2
40	1.1	2.7	3.9	4.3	6.6	7.9	8.5	8.6
45	0.0	0.9	1.0	2.0	2.8	3.6	4.1	4.1
50		0.0	0.0	0.0	0.9	1.0	1.5	1.6

[a]Reported to 100% TAG.

[b]According to IUPAC serial non tempering method. St: saturated fatty acids; U: unsaturated fatty acids; EIE: enzymatic interesterification; CIE: chemical interesterification.

multistep enzyme batch conditioning may be considered, each extra step allowing more efficient washing of the wet enzyme by assuring more complete removal of water from the enzyme granules and less free fatty acid and soap in the conditioning oil (Figure 8.6). Continuous conditioning through the enzyme-packed bed is an option that allows less conditioning oil consumption for better conditioning efficiency. The conditioning oil is ideally bleached or silica treated and mixed in some proportion with the fully interesterified oil before post-deodorization.

Degree of Interesterification

During a continuous enzymatic interesterification process, the degree of interesterification (DI) is typically calculated using the solid fat content profile of the interesterified oil. This calculation is useful to optimize the flow rate, the objective being to ensure full conversion under the operating conditions used. Based on the solid fat content profile (SFC) of the native and of the fully interesterified oil, the largest SFC difference (ΔSFC_{ref}) is used to calculate the degree of interesterification. In practice, a sample is regularly withdrawn at the outlet of each enzymatic reactor and the SFC is measured at the temperature of the ΔSFC_{ref}. The SFC difference is measured

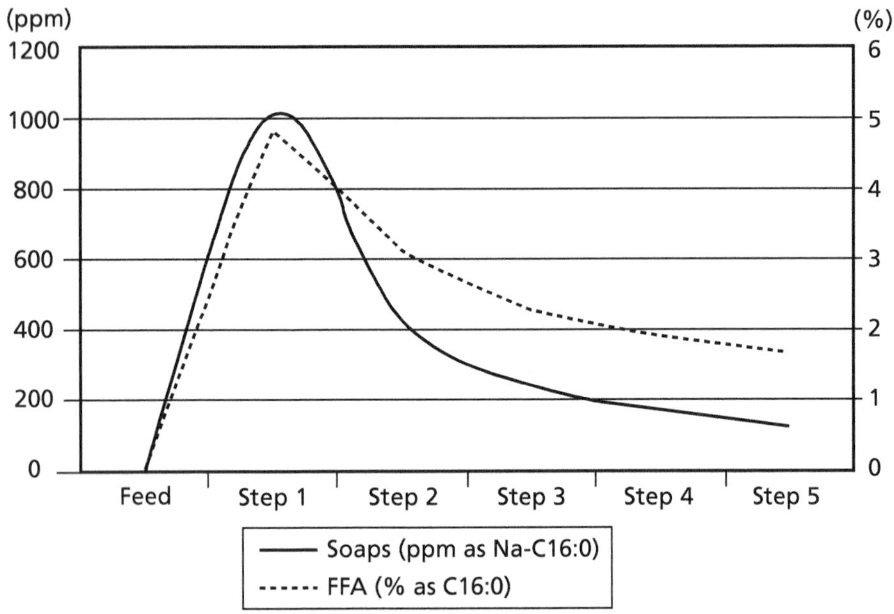

Figure 8.6 Free fatty acid and soap contents in the conditioning oil during a multistep batch enzyme conditioning procedure with TL IM (oil:enzyme ratio 3:1).

(ΔSFC_{sample}) and the degree of interesterification is calculated based on the following equation:

$$DI\ (\%) = 100 \cdot \Delta SFC_{sample}/\Delta SFC_{ref}$$

When the deviation is too big, the reactor is emptied and freshly conditioned enzyme is refilled in this specific reactor, which is placed as the last of the series.

Complementary to SFC, TAG composition determined by reverse-phase high-performance liquid chromatography (HPLC) is another method to calculate the degree of interesterification. Because this requires more sophisticated analytical equipment, it is less frequently used in the frame of an industrial enzymatic interesterification plant. Through this method, the TAG compositions of the native and of the fully interesterified oil are derived and the next formula is applied:

$$DI\ (\%) = 100 \cdot [(A/B)\ \text{native oil} - (A/B)\ \text{EIE oil}]/\ [(A/B)\ \text{native oil} - (A/B)\ \text{random}]$$

A and B are the TAGs that are the most decreased and increased after full conversion, and the term *random* refers to theoretically calculated fully random TAG composition (Costales-Rodriguez et al., 2009). The limit of this method is that formation of positional *sn*-2 saturated isomers cannot be quantified, leading to underestimation of the degree of interesterification (Danthine et al., 2014; De Clercq et al., 2012).

Oil Quality Criteria

Enzymatic interesterification is performed using a biocatalyst that might be sensitive to some impurities present in the native oil. For this reason, quality criteria have been assessed as summarized in Table 8.C for the immobilized TL IM. The native oil must comply with some benchmarks, among which the oxidation parameters (peroxide and anisidine values) and the mineral acidity (pH of the water extract) were shown to be important. The oxidation parameters can easily be controlled by applying good manufacturing practices, that is, by using freshly refined oil or providing adequate storage conditions. On the other hand, this implies that fully refined (NBD or RBD) oils are preferred because the anisidine value of semirefined (NB) oils might still be high. The pH of the water extract of the native oil reflects the sensitivity of the immobilized enzyme with respect to acidic environment; better enzymatic response can be expected at specific pH conditions (pH > 6). This pH, expressed as pH of water extract of the native oil, is easily evaluated by means of a simple laboratory-scale procedure developed by Novozymes (2010). In short, the native oil, is high shear mixed at 70 °C with neutral water at a ratio of about 3:1; after centrifugation, the pH of the water is measured and expressed as pH of the water extract of the oil which should be greater than 6 for the best enzymatic response. The origin of oil acidity (expressed as pH) is not clearly identified, but it is assumed to be related to residual acids

Table 8.C Oil Quality Criteria for Enzymatic Interesterification with Immobilized TL IM (Novozymes)

Quality Criteria	Max.
Free fatty acid (%)	0.1
Peroxide value (meqO_2/kg)	1.0
Anisidine value	5.0
Phosphorus (ppm)	3.0
Moisture + impurities (%)	0.1
Moisture (%)	0.02 (min.)
Iron (ppm)	0.5
Nickel (ppm)	0.2
Copper (ppm)	0.05
pH of water extract	> 6

from refining, such as citric acid or phosphoric acid used during degumming, acids released from the activated bleaching earths during bleaching, or citric acid added as an antioxidant in the refined oil. In practice, a classification was established in terms of "good" oils (typical pH of water extract is 6–7) or in terms of "poor" oils (typical pH of water extract is 4–5) for enzymatic interesterification.

Enzymatic Productivity and Activity

During enzymatic interesterification, the ester–ester exchange takes place at the oil–enzyme interface on the active sites of the enzyme. The interesterification kinetics (expressed as kg of interesterified oil/(kg of enzyme • h)) is determined by the enzymatic activity and also, to a certain extent, by the TAG composition of the oil. It was shown that oils or blends containing substantial amounts of palm kernel or coconut oils (lauric type) usually have slower conversion rates compared to other oils. Therefore, the nominal flow rate can vary between, for example, approximately 2.0 and 1.0 kg of interesterified oil/(kg of enzyme • h) depending on the initial composition of the blend. On the other side, the lifetime of the immobilized enzyme (expressed as kg interesterified oil/kg enzyme, and sometimes referred to *enzymatic productivity*) must be as long as possible in order to keep the cost of the enzymatic interesterification process competitive. The lifetime of the enzyme, which determines when a reactor must be refilled with freshly conditioned enzyme, largely depends on the quality of the native oil (Table 8.C). The expected enzymatic productivity can be 2.5 t of interesterified oil per kilogram of enzyme, which can only be achievable with good quality oils. Similar to the laboratory-scale procedure for the pH of water extract, Novozymes also developed a laboratory-scale procedure to evaluate the impact of the oil quality on the enzymatic productivity and activity (Novozymes, 2008). This procedure is known as MBA (performance tests in multibatch reaction) and, based on solid fat content evaluations, is typically conducted in one incubated shaker over a period of two weeks with daily measurement and replacement with fresh oil. The collected SFC values are introduced in a statistical analysis, which allows derivations of the so-called average production rate and volume-based half-life. Results of MBA tests are usually confronted with the oxidation parameters and the pH of the water extract of the oil. The average production rate reflects the enzymatic activity and the volume-based half-life of the enzymatic productivity. Any increase or decrease in these calculated numbers against a reference means improvement or degradation of the enzymatic performances. Table 8.D shows MBA numbers comparing identical oils having various peroxide and pH of water extract values; combinations of low/high peroxide values and low/high pHs of water extract are presented. The results clearly indicate that low peroxide values, combined with pHs of water extract greater than 6 for the oil, significantly improve the MBA numbers in correlation with better enzymatic performances. A synergic effect of high peroxide values and low pHs of water extract is also observed. Data indicate that the largest effect on the enzyme productivity is due to the peroxide value (instead of the pH of water extract).

Pre- and Post-Treatments of the Oil

Although it is easier to control or to adjust the oxidation parameters by using freshly refined or properly stored oil, or by adding an extra upstream treatment (rebleaching and/or redeodorization), mastery of the pH of water extract can be more problematic. It was recently shown (Desmet Ballestra Engineering, 2012) that creating soaps in the oil with a limited caustic pretreatment was favorable to adjust the pH of the water extract within the expected range, allowing improvement of the MBA numbers. Table 8.E reports two scenarios: RBD palm kernel oil with low pH of water extract and relatively

Table 8.D MBA (Performance Tests in Multi-batch Reaction) Values Calculated for Identical Oil with Various Peroxide and pH of Water Extract

Peroxide Value ($meqO_2/kg$)	pH of Water Extract	Average Production Rate (kg oil/kg Enzyme Jour)	Volume Based Half-time (kg oil/kg enzyme)
0.9	4.2	1.4	909
0.9	6.4	10.4	2214
8.2	4.8	0.4	316
7.9	6.2	1.7	481

Table 8.E MBA (Performance Tests in Multi-batch Reaction) Improvement for RBD Palm and Palm Kernel Oils after Caustic Pre-Treatment

	RBD[a] Palm Kernel Oil	Treated Palm Kernel Oil	RBD Palm Oil	Treated Palm Oil
Free fatty acid (% as C12:0 or C16:0)	0.03	0.03	0.04	0.04
Soaps (ppm as Na-C12:0 or Na-C16:0)	ND[b]	45	N.D.	52
pH of water extract	4.4	7.7	7.0	9.7
Peroxide value (meqO_2/kg)	3.9	4.0	1.1	1.1
Anisidine value	1.2	1.2	1.8	1.5
Average production rate (% improvement)	—	10	—	93
Volume based half-time (% improvement)	—	50	—	25

[a]RBD: Refined, bleached, and deodorized.

[b]ND: Not detected.

high peroxide value, and RBD palm oil with good pH of water extract and low peroxide value. In both cases, the anisidine value was low. The creation of sodium soaps (~50 ppm) by caustic pretreatment enabled an increase of the pH of water extract by about 3 units. MBA tests showed significant increase of the enzymatic productivity in the case of the treated palm kernel oil: 50% improvement of the volume-based half-life, although the enzymatic activity was more weakly modified, and 10% improvement of the average production rate. Surprisingly, the enzymatic activity was strongly boosted in the case of palm oil: 93% improvement of the volume-based half-life when the pH of the water extract was brought above 9. In this case, weaker effect was observed on the enzymatic productivity: 25% improvement of the volume-based half-life. It was shown that, at these levels, the sodium soaps do not accumulate in the enzymatic beds and do not cause any pressure build-up through the columns; the soaps just create an adequate pH environment at the oil–enzyme interface. This pretreatment can easily be implemented on industrial scale: The oil is simply mixed with a caustic soda solution before entering the enzymatic interesterification reactors; the dosage is accurately controlled to ensure a precise adjustment of the pH of water extract. The soaps recovered at the outlet of the enzymatic interesterification plant are converted into free fatty acid with a gentle post-washing with citric acid or removed by post-bleaching with silica.

The use of a specific chromatographic grade silica (SP 535 from Grace) placed in a column upstream of the enzymatic interesterification plant is reported to lead to remarkable improvement of the immobilized enzyme performances during enzymatic interesterification with TL IM (Bunge Oils Inc., 2009); the enzymatic activity is claimed to be prolonged, allowing the process to be conducted at constant flow rate. Pretreatment of the oil with the chromatographic grade silica is capable of producing an oil meeting the predetermined specifications (Table 8.C).

Oil Losses and Byproducts

During enzymatic interesterification, the oil losses are principally due to the amount of oil retained on the wet enzyme: Each kilogram of dry enzyme will retain approximately 1 kg of processed oil, which is negligible in the context of large-capacity continuous plants. However, in case of frequent feed oil changes, cross-contamination can also contribute to oil losses. Cross-contamination can be estimated at about 3.5 times the quantity of immobilized enzyme placed in the packed-bed reactors. Because no chemicals come into play, the side reactions are minimized and, therefore, almost no byproducts are created (Figure 8.7). The increase of free fatty acid content in the enzymatically interesterified oil is very low and usually removed by gentle post-deodorization. Contrary to chemical interesterification, the tocopherols and tocotrienols are well preserved, assuring better oxidative stability to the enzymatically interesterified oils.

Flow Diagram of a Continuous Enzymatic Interesterification Plant

In an enzymatic interesterification plant (Desmet Ballestra Group, 2014) (Figure 8.8), the dry enzyme is automatically conveyed to a high-placed slurry tank where it

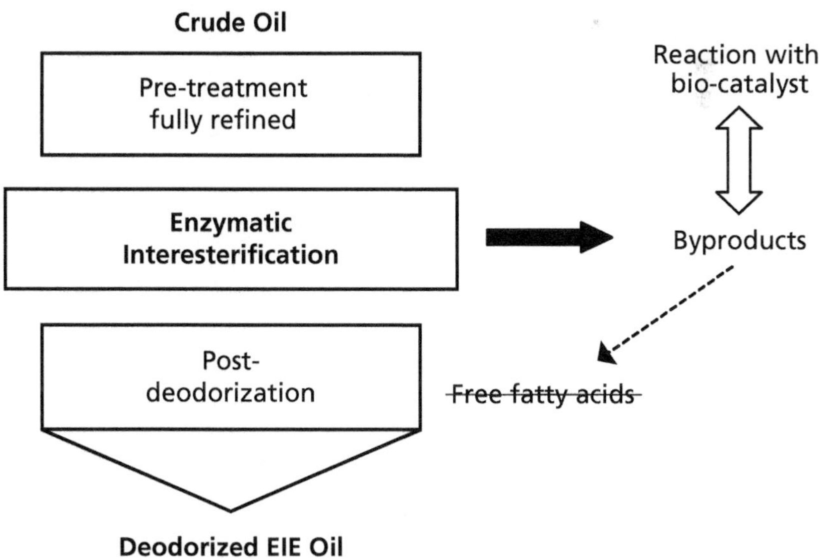

Figure 8.7 Byproducts formed during enzymatic interesterification with TL IM; the crossed out byproducts are removed by post-deodorization.

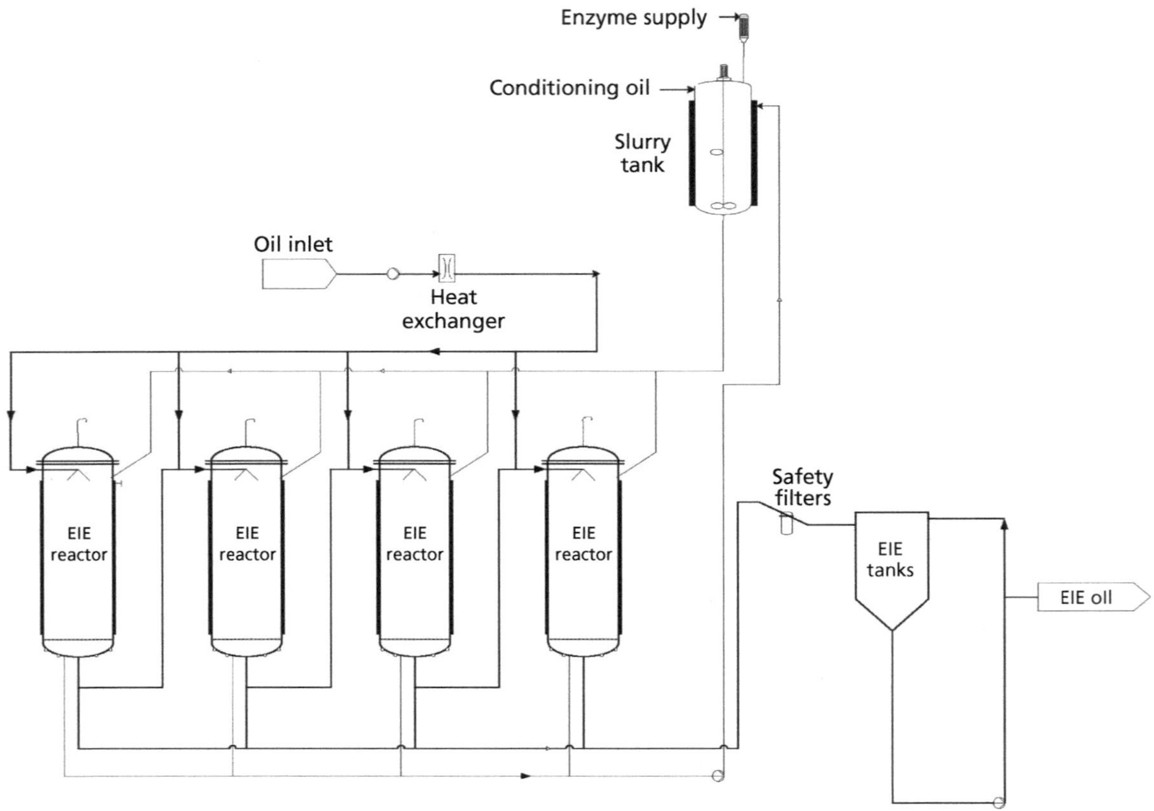

Figure 8.8 Flow diagram of a continuous enzymatic interesterifcation process.

is wetted with a quantity of native or interesterified oil. During the preconditioning step, the wet enzyme is drained by gravity into the enzymatic reactors. The preheated (typically 70 °C) oil is pumped through the packed-bed reactors at an optimal flow rate; when the enzymes in the reactors have lost the expected performance, the enzyme charge is removed after draining the oil content. The first reactor that meets the feed oil generally contains the oldest enzyme (that is, the one with the lowest performance) and a freshly filled reactor is generally attached in the series as the last reactor. The enzymatically interesterified oil leaving the last reactor of the working series enters a safety filter and is transferred to an interesterified oil tank before being pumped to post-deodorization.

Chemical versus Enzymatic Interesterification

Both chemical and enzymatic interesterification processes can be used to randomly modify the compositional properties and, therefore, the melting profile of oils and fats. There are, however, some arguments to select the most appropriate option that will better fit with the industrial requirements.

Pros and Cons for Enzymatic versus Chemical Interesterification

Chemical interesterification is a highly reproducible and cost effective process; it is easily operated as batch and, therefore, very flexible for frequent feed oil changes with relatively low cross-contamination. It uses a chemical catalyst, however, and precautions must be taken to handle it. Side reactions cannot be avoided, and they require proper post-treatments (post-bleaching and post-deodorization) in order to remove byproducts. Unfortunately, the risk of color and flavor reversion cannot be excluded, and molecules like dialkylketones cannot be removed by any of the post-treatments. Dialkylketones can limit the use of chemical interesterification in certain applications (infant formula) due to some toxicity issues (Loders Crokland, 2009). The oxidative stability of the chemically interesterified oils is negatively affected due to degradation of part of the tocopherols and tocotrienols (Table 8.F). Finally, although significantly lower compared to the past, the oil losses are not negligible. Enzymatic interesterification is a cost-effective process principally when it is running continuously on bulk fats; it is a less appropriate solution in the case of frequent feed oil changes due to cross-contamination. It's a simple, clean, and safe process that operates at relatively low temperatures with a biocatalyst. This allows almost no side reactions and less oil loss. Overall, the quality of enzymatically interesterified oils is definitely better due to the fact that tocopherols and tocotrienols are not degraded, improving the oxidative stability compared to chemically interesterified oils (Table 8.F). However, the enzyme might be sensitive to impurities present in the feed oil, which can affect its performance and therefore increase its consumption. Solutions have been recently

Table 8.F Quality Parameters of a Blend of Palm Stearin (70%) and Soybean Oil (30%) Subjected to Chemical and Enzymatic Interesterification

	Initial Blend	Post-Bleached CIE[a] Blend	EIE[b] Blend	Post-Deodorized CIE Blend	Post-Deodorized EIE Blend
Free fatty acid (% as C18:1)	0.03	0.30	0.15	0.02	0.02
α-tocopherol	77	38	78	30	60
α-tocotrienol	37	17	37	16	30
γ-tocopherol	212	163	210	85	151
γ-tocotrienol	65	52	61	31	47
Δ-tocopherol	61	57	59	13	30
Δ-tocotrienol	10	10	9	ND[c]	3
Total tocos	**462**	**337**	**454**	**175**	**321**
Color (Lovibond 5¼")	2.4R/24Y	1.8R/21Y	2.5/26Y	1.7R/20Y	2.2R/23Y
DAG (%)	3.6	5.1	3.6	4.9	3.5

[a]CIE: Chemically interesterified.

[b]EIE: Enzymatically interesterified.

[c]ND: Not detected.

developed, such as caustic pretreatment (Desmet Ballestra Engineering, 2012) or purification with chromatographic grade silica (Bunge Oils Inc., 2009).

Melting and Compositional Properties of Some Interesterified Blends

One of the main objectives of the interesterification process is to modify the melting properties (melting profile and melting point) of an oil or of a blend of oils by allowing random migration of the acyl groups on the glycerol backbone. Figure 8.9 shows the good fit between the solid fat content profiles of a chemically and enzymatically interesterified blend of palm oil, fully hydrogenated palm oil, and palm kernel oil (40/30/30 w/w/w) after post-deodorization. Compared to the native blend, the interesterified blend is harder below 30 °C and softer above 30 °C and the biggest ΔSFC ($\Delta SFC_{ref]}$) is observed at 40 °C. Depending on the desired final applications, a large range of oils and blends of oils are suitable for interesterification: Hard materials such as palm stearin and fully hydrogenated palm oil blended in selected proportions with softer oils such as soybean oil, sunflower oil, palm olein, and palm kernel olein are possible combinations. The final melting profile can be targeted by mixing the inter-

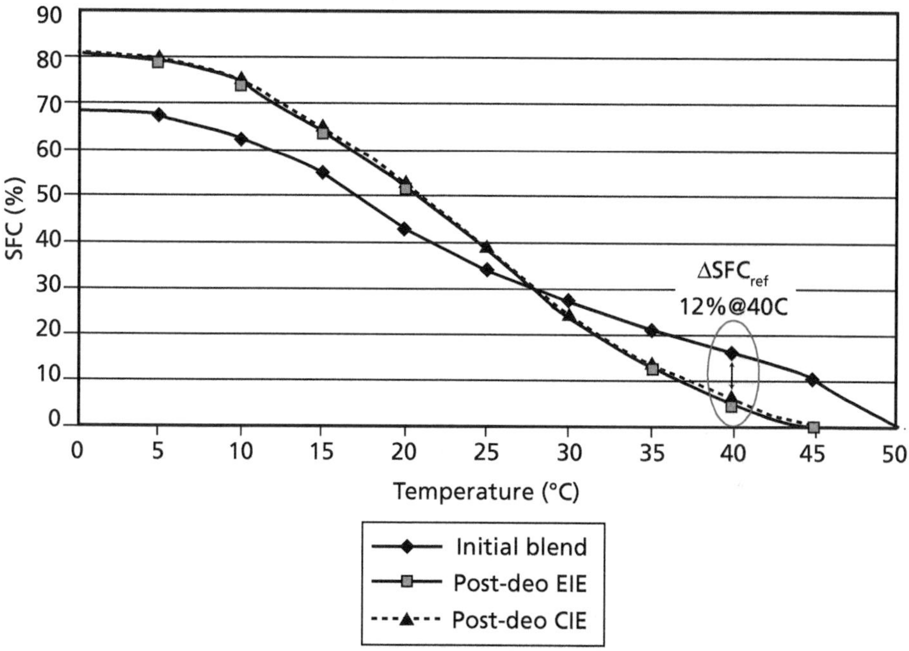

Figure 8.9 Solid fat content profile (IUPAC serial nontempered method) of post-deodorized chemically and enzymatically interesterified blend of palm oil, fully hydrogenated palm oil, and palm kernel oil (40/30/30 w/w/w).

esterified oil with liquid oil. How the fatty acids reorganize on the glycerol depends on the initial triglycerol composition of the oil (Table 8.G). For palm oil and palm olein, the trisaturated and triunsaturated TAG contents are highly increased after interesterification, while the mono- and diunsaturated TAG contents are decreased. In the case of the soft palm mid fraction, all trisaturated, triunsaturated, and diunsaturated TAG contents are increased, while the monounsaturated TAG content is significantly reduced. This results in an increase in the hardness and melting point (Figure 8.10) of the interesterified oils. On the contrary, the monounsaturated and diunsaturated TAG contents are increased when a blend of 70% palm stearin and 30% soybean oil is interesterified; both trisaturated and triunsaturated TAG contents are decreased. This leads to a decrease in the hardness and melting point of the interesterified blend. Compositional modifications are obvious when looking at the melting profile through differential scanning calorimetry (DSC). The DSC melting profiles (recorded at 5 °C/min. heating after full melting and freezing at −60 °C) of palm oil before and after chemical and enzymatic interesterification (Gibon, 2011)

Table 8.G Modification of the Triacylglycerol Composition of Palm Oil, Palm Olein, Soft Palm Mid Fraction, and a Blend of Palm Stearin (30%) and Soybean Oil (70%) during Interesterification

	Palm Oil		Palm Olein		Soft Palm Mid Fraction		Palm Stearin (70%)/ Soybean Oil (30%)	
	Initial	IE	Initial	IE	Initial	IE	Initial	IE
TAG (% by HPLC)[a]								
StStSt	6.9	12.0	1.8	10.5	0.5	15.8	21.5	13.8
StUSt	46.5	38.1	48.0	35.2	72.3	41.1	31.0	39.1
StUU	39.7	37.7	43.0	39.7	23.8	34.0	26.6	36.1
UUU	6.9	12.2	7.2	14.6	3.4	9.1	20.9	11.0

[a]Reported to 100% TAG. St: saturated fatty acids; U: unsaturated fatty acids; IE: interesterified.

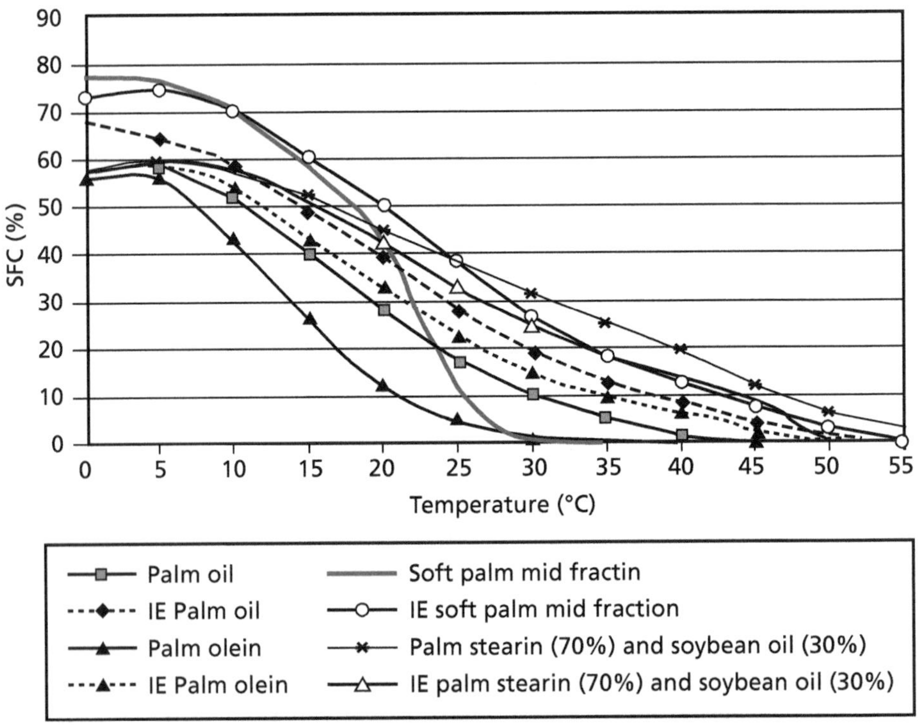

Figure 8.10 Solid fat content profiles (IUPAC serial nontempered method) of palm oil, palm olein, soft palm mid fraction, and a blend of palm stearin (70%) and soybean oil (30%) before and after interesterification.

are presented in Figure 8.11. Palm oil shows two melting endotherms: a low melting endotherm (LME) and a high melting endotherm (HME). As the result of fatty acid re organization on the glycerol backbone and modified intersolubility within the TAGs, the DSC melting profiles of chemically and enzymatically interesterified palm oil are strongly modified. The LME of palm oil is split into a very low (VLME) and medium (MME) melting endotherms and the HME becomes more intense.

Specific Enzymatic Interesterification for Specialty Fat Products

In contrast to random enzymatic interesterification used to formulate commodity oils, regio-selective enzymatic interesterification is principally applied to the manufacture of specialty fat products such as ingredients for cocoa butter equivalents, low calorie fats, easily absorbable MLM-type oils (M: medium chain fatty acid; L: long chain fatty acid), breast milk substitutes, and other functional lipids. The lypozyme RM IM manufactured by Novozymes A/S Denmark is recognized as being *sn*-1,3 specific (positions 1 and 3 on the glycerol backbone); it is produced by immobilization

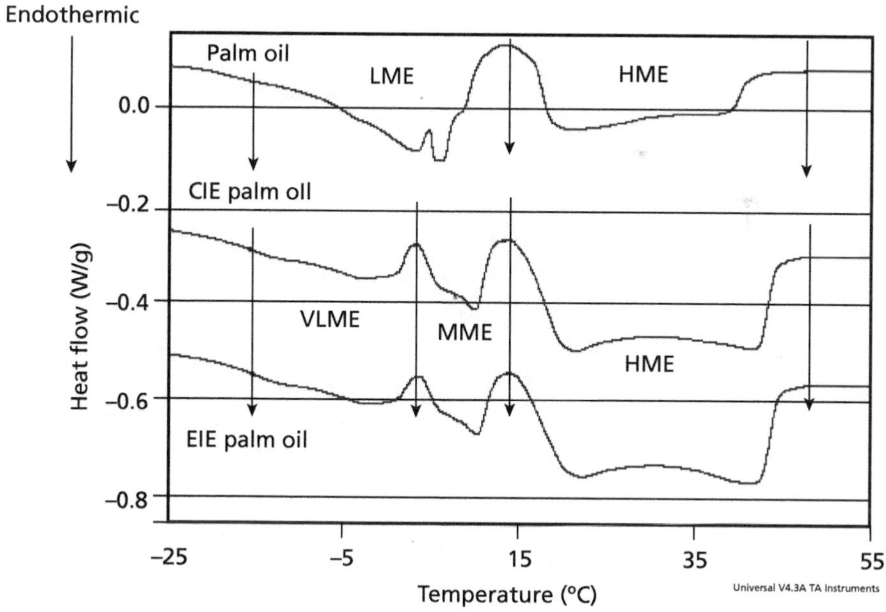

Figure 8.11 Differential scanning calorimetry melting profiles of palm oil and chemically and enzymatically interesterified palm oil (VLME: very low melting endotherm; LME: low melting endotherm; MME: medium melting endotherm; HME: high melting endotherm); the arrows limit each of the melting endotherms.

of a microbial lipase from *Rhizomucor miehei* on a macroporous anion exchange resin (Novozymes A/S, 2012). These kinds of enzymatic modifications can involve ester–ester exchanges or acidolysis reactions.

Cocoa Butter Equivalents

Definition

A true cocoa butter equivalent is a nonhydrogenated product containing almost the same fatty acids and acylglycerols present in a typical cocoa butter (POP, palmitoyl-oleoyl-palmitoylglycerol; POS, palmitoyl-oleoyl-stearoylglycerol; and SOS, stearoyl-oleoyl-stearoylglycerol). As a result of the closely similar chemical composition, the physical properties of cocoa butter equivalents closely match those of cocoa butter. Cocoa butter equivalents are fully compatible with cocoa butter and can be used in any proportion up to 100% for complete replacement. They also require the same tempering procedures as cocoa butter to prevent fat bloom. Cocoa butter substitutes are principally made of palm kernel oil after fractionation and post-hydrogenation. This product is particularly enriched in lauric and myristic fatty acid components and, for this reason, compatibility with cocoa butter is poor. Cocoa butter will not tolerate more than 5% of cocoa butter substitutes in any formulation due to important eutectic effect. Cocoa butter replacers are produced by hydrogenation of liquid oil usually followed by dry fractionation, and they contain amounts of elaidic acids (*trans* type). Compatibility of cocoa butter replacers with cocoa butter is better compared to cocoa butter substitutes; they can tolerate up to 25% of cocoa butter when used in confectionery coatings. However, the high TFA content of cocoa butter replacers makes this alternative less desirable.

Usual Route

Cocoa butter equivalents for confectionery applications are classically made of nonfractionated illipe fat or from solid fractions (stearins) of shea butter, sal fat, and palm oil (the hard palm mid fraction). Unfortunately, compositional properties of these single fats do not fit well enough with the ones of cocoa butter, and for this reason, cocoa butter equivalents are usually formulated by blending. The uncertainty in cocoa butter supply and the volatility in cocoa butter prices have forced confectionary producers to find alternatives. Today, the development of the enzyme technology makes it possible to produce ingredients for cocoa butter equivalents from other vegetable oils that also better fit the compositional and crystallization properties of cocoa butter.

Enzymatic Route

Today, *sn*-1,3 regio-selective enzymatic interesterification is a potential alternative to produce ingredients for cocoa butter equivalents. Some examples are reported below

(Gibon, 2011). The soft palm mid fraction, which is obtained by multistep dry fractionation of palm oil, is characterized by high POP content, whereas the POS and SOS contents are very low. *Sn*-1,3 regio-selective enzymatic intereserification is a way to readjust this POP:POS:SOS ratio in favor of higher amounts of POS and SOS for direct use as cocoa butter equivalent. The original TAG ratio of the soft palm mid fraction can be improved by enzymatic acydolysis with stearic acid or by ester–ester exchange with stearic methyl ester (Danthine et al., 2011). Table 8.H shows how the POP, POS, and SOS contents evolve with time during a laboratory-scale batch acidolysis (32 h, 4% RM IM) of soft palm mid fraction with stearic acid at different dosages: 25% w/w, 50% w/w, and 75% w/w. In each case, the SOS and POS contents were increased and POP was decreased; however, huge amounts of trisaturated TAGs (StStSt) were also formed. Although no substantial difference was observed between 50% and 75% w/w stearic acid dosages, the lowest dosage (25% w/w) was less efficient. Also, a shorter reaction time (15 h vs. 32 h) allowed less StStSt production. With acidolysis, the remaining quantity of fatty acids resulting from the interchange of fatty acids with TAGs must be removed; this is preferentially done by introducing a post-stripping step. Due to the production of substantial amounts of StStSt, multistep post-fractionation is mandatory if the objective is to properly enrich the modified fat into StUSt components. High-oleic sunflower oil is another potential feedstock for cocoa butter equivalents when it is enzymatically acidolysed with stearic acid. The main triacylglycerol component of high-oleic sunflower oil is OOO (~70%) and there is almost no POP, POS, and SOS; after enzymatic reaction with stearic acid,

Table 8.H Triacylglycerol Contents of a Soft Palm Mid Fraction after Laboratory Scale Acidolysis with Stearic Acid (4% w/w RM IM)

TAG (% by HPLC)	StUSt[a]	StStSt	POP	POS	SOS
Cocoa butter	81	2	18	37	26
Soft palm mid fraction	67	<1	47	9	1
After acydolisis					
Soft PMF/stearic acid (75/25% w/w)[b]	54	14	20	22	7
Soft PMF/stearic acid (50/50% w/w)[b]	59	18	13	28	16
Soft PMF/stearic acid (25/75% w/w)[b]	62	16	12	31	17
Soft PMF/stearic acid (50/50% w/w)[c]	64	10	20	30	10

[a]St: Saturated fatty acid; U: unsaturated fatty acid; S: stearic acid; P: palmitic acid; O: oleic acid.

[b]After 32 hours batch enzymatic interesterification.

[c]After 15 hours batch enzymatic interesterification.

quantities of SOS are formed (~20%) (Table 8.I); the POS content is also increased but to a lower extent (~5%). After fatty acid stripping and post-fractionation, this enzymatically produced ingredient for cocoa butter equivalents is generally blended with a POP source (typically the hard palm mid fraction). Alternatively, enzymatically produced cocoa butter equivalents can also result from an ester–ester exchange between high-oleic sunflower oil and high-stearic soybean oil (Table 8.J); in this case, high-stearic soybean oil is the main source of stearic fatty acids. After reaction, the enzymatically interesterified oil may contain high amounts of SOS (~25%) and POS (~10%). Although in this approach post-stripping is not necessary (no fatty acids involved), post-fractionation is usually required to improve the compositional properties of the interesterified blend. In this case, blending with a POP source may be required to better fit with the compositional properties of cocoa butter.

Low Calorie Fats

Attaching long and short chains or long and medium chains on the glycerol backbone gives TAG molecules with low calorie and appropriate melting properties. Typical examples are Salatrim and Caprenin. Salatrim is a TAG molecule consisting of C2:0/C4:0 short-chain and long-chain saturated fatty acids that is industrially produced by chemical interesterification; it was developed by Pfizer and Nabisco and commercialized as Benefat™. Caprenin™, developed by Procter and Gamble, contains behenic and medium-chain C8:0/C10:0 fatty acids; it is industrially produced by

Table 8.I Triacylglycerol Contents of High-Oleic Sunflower Oil after Laboratory-Scale Acidolysis with Stearic Acid (4% w/w RM IM)

TAG (% by HPLC)	High-Oleic Sunflower Oil	After Acidolysis
SSSa	ND	5
POP	1	1
POS	0.5	5
SOS	ND	20
StUSt (POP + POS + SOS)	1.5	26
SOO	7	35
POO	12	2
OOO	68	15
Others	~12	~17

[a]St: Saturated fatty acid; U: unsaturated fatty acid; S: stearic acid; P: palmitic acid; O: oleic acid; ND: not detected.

Table 8.J Triacylglycerol Contents of High-Oleic Sunflower Oil and High-Stearic Soybean Oil after Laboratory-Scale Ester–Ester Exchange (4% w/w RM IM)

TAG (% by HPLC)	High-Oleic Sunflower/High-Stearic Soybean Oils Blend	After Enzymatic Interesterification
POPa	0.5	0.5
POS	0.5	10
SOS	ND	25
StUSt (POP+POS+SOS)	1	35.5

[a]St: saturated fatty acid; U: unsaturated fatty acid; S: stearic acid; P: palmitic acid; O: oleic acid; ND: not detected.

chemical acylation of *sn*-1 monoacylglycerol (MAG) with medium-chain fatty acids. The functionalities of these products come from their fatty acid composition rather than the positions of the fatty acids on the glycerol; they can be functional if long- and medium-chain or long- and short-chain fatty acids are attached within one TAG molecule but do not show any positional specificity.

Easily Absorbable MLM-Type Oils

The production of TAGs with medium-chain fatty acids in *sn*-1 and *sn*-3 positions and functional long-chain fatty acids in the internal *sn*-2 position has increased due to nutritional interest; these are low calorie and dietetic structured lipids for people suffering from fat malabsorption and other metabolism problems. By using *sn*-1,3 regio-specific enzymes, compositional modifications can be made at these selected positions while the fatty acid at *sn*-2 position is not modified. Acidolysis allows selective incorporation of medium-chain C8:0/C10:0 fatty acids into triaglycerols; however, this approach requires post-treatments because the production of desired MLM TAGs is concomitant with the formation of undesired products like fatty acids, partial acylglycerols, and other types of TAGs.

Breast Milk Substitutes

Human milk fat has a specific composition mainly with saturated fatty acids (C16:0) in the *sn*-2 position and unsaturated fatty acids (C18:1) in the *sn*-1 and *sn*-3 positions of the TAGs. In vegetable oils, however, C16:0 is predominantly located in the outer positions and unsaturated fatty acids are located in the central position. This is believed to be why infant formula-fed infants tend to show problems with energy and calcium uptake and increased constipation. Enzymatically produced specialty fats for infant formulation are characterized by selective positioning of C16:0 in *sn*-2 position of the TAG and C18:1 fatty acids at *sn*-1 and *sn*-3 positions (OPO fats). Two routes are possible for designing such products. The first is a two-step process combining *sn*-1,3 specific enzymatic alcoholysis of a high-palmitic substrate, followed by enzymatic re-esterification of the *sn*-2 palmitic monoacylglycerol by high-oleic material. The other route consists of the *sn*-1,3 enzymatic acidolysis of a high-palmitic oil with a high-oleic acid source. Betapol™, initially developed by Unilever and commercialized by IOI-Loders Croklaan, and InFat™, produced by AAK, are two typical examples of such enzymatically produced specialty fats for infant formulation.

Partial Acylglycerols

Sn-*1,3 Monoacylglycerols*

These compounds are common emulsifiers for food, cosmetics, and pharmaceutical industries. As emulsion stabilizers, they are essential ingredients for margarines and low-calorie spreads. They can be obtained by chemical glycerolysis, and purity of the final product after distillation is above 95%. Enzymatic synthesis is an interesting alternative (less energy consumption, less degradation, less toxicity) to the chemical method: Glycerolyisis of TAG, direct esterification of glycerol, and esterification of the protected glycerol are the most practical approaches. Among them, lipase-catalyzed glycerolysis of TAGs is by far the best enzymatic process that can compete with the chemical glycerolysis for the commercial production of *sn*-1,3 monoacylglycerols. The principle of the method is to shift the reaction equilibrium to the *sn*-1,3 monoacylglycerol by significantly lowering the reaction temperature for the precipitation of these molecules.

Sn-*2 Monoacylglycerols*

Because of fast acyl migration creating isomerization, the *sn*-2 monoacylglycerols are not suitable as commercial products; however, they are used as intermediate products for the production of symmetrical structured TAGs (see above). *Sn*-2 monoacylglycerols can be prepared by ethanolysis using an *sn*-1,3 selective lipase. For this reaction, ethanolysis is preferred to hydrolysis because acyl migration is reduced and ethanol can better be removed after reaction. Because the ethanol is in excess and reacts as a substrate and a solvent, the reaction proceeds almost completely.

Sn-*1,3 Diacylglycerols*

Initially appreciated for their emulsifying properties as surface active agents, interest in *sn*-1,3 diacylglycerols progressively moved to specialty oils able to prevent the accumulation of body fat. Such *sn*-1,3 diacylglycerols can be obtained by enzymatic glycerolysis of TAGs in a similar enzymatic way as previously described for the production of *sn*-1 monoacylglycerols (low temperature precipitation and selective crystallization). Alternatively, *sn*-1,3 diacylglycerols can be prepared by direct *sn*-1,3 selective esterification on the glycerol; the reaction is performed under vacuum, allowing the generated water to be evaporated. Econa oil is a functional cooking oil (blend of soybean and canola oils) that was developed by KAO Corporation in Japan; a similar product, known as Enova oil, was available in the United States. Unfortunately, the producer of both products voluntarily suspended sales because the products were said to contain unhealthy fatty acid glycidyl esters as byproducts of the deodorization process.

High Omega-3 Concentrates from Fish Oil

There is considerable evidence of the beneficial role of long-chain polyunsaturated fatty acids in biochemical processes. Marine omega-3 polyunsaturated fatty acids, particularly eicosapentenoic acid (EPA) and docosahexaenoic acid (DHA), can lower plasma lipid concentration, modulate eicosanoid formation, and change cell membrane properties. They are known to reduce incidences of cardiovascular and inflammatory diseases. Because they are better absorbed compared to the corresponding ethyl ester form, omega-3 enriched TAGs are desired. Such products can typically be obtained through a three-step processing route. The first step is conversion to fatty acid ethyl esters of the refined/winterized fish oil; in most cases, the ethyl ester conversion still uses the conventional chemical esterification to convert fish oil into ethyl esters, prior to short path distillation to increase the omega-3 concentration. Enzymatic esterification with ethanol is an alternative that can work at lower temperatures and avoid polymerization, but it still needs some optimization before economical industrial implementation. The Lipozyme 435, developed by Novozymes A/S Denmark, is a suitable immobilized enzyme that allows condensation on the glycerol of the concentrated EPA/DHA ethyl esters on the glycerol. The condensation reaction is conducted under vacuum starting with EPA/DHA as fatty acids or as ethyl esters. Different triacylglycerol purities can be obtained depending on the reaction time and the ethyl ester:glycerol ratio used. Post-distillation allows removal of unreacted partial acylglycerols, increasing the purity of the finished product (at the expense of the yield).

Enzymatic Remediation of Oils

Crude palm oil is characterized by high free fatty acid and high diacylglycerol contents. Its high free fatty acid content makes the physical route the best refining option. Palm oil is also recognized for its potential for dry fractionation in multiple stages, allowing its use in many food-based products. It has long been known that high diacylglycerol content in palm oil negatively affects the crystallization efficiency during

Table 8.K Free Fatty Acid and Diacylglycerol Contents of Crude and Enzymatically Remediated Palm Oils (4% w/w Lipozyme 435)

	Crude Palm Oil	Enzymatically Remediated Crude Palm Oil	Crude Palm Oil	Enzymatically Remediated Crude Palm Oil	Crude Palm Oil	Enzymatically Remediated Crude Palm Oil
Free fatty acid (% as C18:0)	5.3	3.2	5.6	2.8	5.1	3.4
DAG (%)	9.4	5.8	9.4	4.6	7.4	4.4

dry fractionation; the detrimental impact is reflected not only on the quality of the produced fractions, but also on the throughput and yield of the process. More recently, it was shown that palm oil is highly implicated in the problema of toxic 3-MCPD and glycidyl esters (negative health implications); it is increasingly evident that diacylglycerols present in high proportion in crude palm oil play an important role in the synthesis of these unwanted molecules during the physical refining process. In this aspect, a low diacylglycerol crude palm oil is also preferred. Novozymes A/S Denmark has developed an immobilized enzyme (Lipozyme 435) capable of converting diacylglycerols into TAGs by selective condensation with free fatty acids (Table 8.K). This enzymatic condensation route could easily replace the need for high-grade crude palm oils by simply modifying the cheaper and more available standard quality oils.

Conclusions

The majority of oils and fats from natural sources are used directly or after having been refined; some of them need to be modified by physical, chemical, or enzymatic processes. Among these, chemical and enzymatic interesterification allow random migration of the fatty acids on the glycerol backbone; interesterification is principally applied as an alternative to partial hydrogenation for low- and zero-*trans* margarine and shortening formulation. However, chemical modifications usually require drastic operational conditions such as high temperature or pressure, which can degrade the fats and introduce side products. Enzymatic processes using lipases allow processing of the oil under milder conditions, permitting formulation of better quality fat products. While this is not the case for most of the chemical reactions, lipase-catalyzed reactions can show different specificities that enable the modification of oils and fats in more or less sophisticated ways with a number of innovative food, nutraceutical, and pharmaceutical applications.

References

Bunge Oils Inc. (Applicant). Continuous Process and Apparatus for Enzymatic Treatment of Lipids. U.S. Publication Number US2009/03179020283 A1, 2009.

Costales-Rodríguez, R.; Gibon, V.; Verhé, R.; De Greyt, W. Chemical and Enzymatic Interesterification of a Blend of Palm Stearin/Soybean Oil for Low Trans-margarine Formulation. *J. Am. Oil Chem. Soc.* **2009**, *86,* 681–697.

Danthine, S.; Vanden Bossche, S.; Maes, J.; Gibon, V. Regio-selective Enzymatic Acidolysis Combined with Dry Fractionation to Produce Cocoa Butter Equivalent: Optimization of the Enzymatic Reaction. *Récents Progrès en Génie des Procédés* **2011,** *101,* 1–7.

Danthine, S.; De Clercq, N.; Dewettinck, K.; Gibon, V. Monitoring Batch Lipase Catalysed Interesterification of Palm Oil and Fractions by Differential Scanning Calorimetry. *J. Therm. Anal. Calorim.* **2014,** *115,* 2219–2229.

De Clercq, N.; Danthine, S.; Tuyet Nguyen, M.; Gibon, V.; Dewettinck, K. Enzymatic Interesterification of Palm Oil and Fractions: Monitoring the Degree of Interesterification Using Different Methods. *J. Am. Oil Chem. Soc.* **2012,** *89,* 219–229.

De Greyt, W.; Dijkstra, A. Fractionation and Interesterification. In *Trans Fatty Acids;* Dijkstra, A. J.; Hamilton, R. J.; Hamm, W., Eds.; Blackwell Publishing Ltd.: Oxford, UK, 2008; 181–202.

Desmet Ballestra Group. Batch Chemical and Continuous Enzymatic Interesterification Flowcharts, 2014. http://www.desmetballestra.com.

Gibon, V. Enzymatic Interesterification of Oils. *Lipid Technology* **2011,** *23,* 274–277.

Kellens, M.; Gibon, V.; Petrauskaite, V.; Maes J. Enzyme Interesterification Process, Patent Application Publication, Desmet Ballestra Engineering, Belgium. U.S. Publication Number US2012/0270283 A1, 2012.

Novozymes A/S. *Interesterification. Performance Test in Multiple Batch Reactions;* Bagsvaerd, Denmark, 2008.

Novozymes A/S. *pH of Water Extract, Standard Procedure.* Bagsvaerd, Denmark, 2010.

Novozymes A/S. *Lipozyme TL IM Product Data Sheet.* Bagsvaerd, Denmark, 2011.

Novozymes A/S. *Lipozyme RM IM Product Data Sheet;* Bagsvaerd, Denmark, 2012.

Verhe, R.; Van Hoed, V.; De Greyt, W. *Detection of Alkylketones during Chemical Interesterification of Lipids.* AOCS Annual Meeting St. Louis, MO, 2006.

Zand, I. T.; Bouwer, S.; Bhaggan, K.; Schmid, U. Process, Patent Application Publication, Loders Crokland B.V. The Netherlands. International Publication Number WO 2009/012982 A2, 2009.

9

Enzymatic Interesterification

Hong Zhang and Prakash Adhikari ■ *Wilmar Biotechnology Research and Development Center Co., Ltd., Shanghai, China*

Introduction

The term *interesterification* refers to the fats and oils reaction in which fatty acid esters react with other esters or fatty acids or alcohols to produce new esters by an interchange of fatty acid groups. Enzymatic interesterification offers possibilities for the transformation of fats and oils beyond the chemical interesterification because of its positional specificity (region specificity) toward fatty acids in a triacylglycerol (TAG) molecule (Macrae, 1983). Usually, lipase is classified into two categories: random (nonspecificity) and specific (*sn*-1,3 specific). Random interesterification gives a similar product as the chemical interesterification. Region-specific lipases are also widely used to produce symmetric products that could not be achieved by chemical randomization, such as infant formula (OPO) or Econa oil (1,3-DAG) (Jin et al., 2011; Lee et al. 2010).

In this chapter, we will discuss the reaction mechanism of lipase, methods to monitor the interesterification degree, process development of lipase-catalyzed interesterification, and characterization of interesterified fat.

Reaction Mechanism

Enzymatic interesterification (EIE) involves the use of lipase to restructure TAGs, inducing the exchange of fatty acids among and between the TAGs. Unlike hydrogenation, interesterification neither affects the degree of saturation nor causes isomerization of the fatty acid double bond. It maintains the same fatty acid composition of the starting material but rearranges the fatty acid composition on the glycerol backbone. Three types of reactions associated with interesterification are: acidolysis (fatty acid–TAG), glycerolysis (glycerol–TAG), and transesterification (TAG–TAG). The mechanism (chemistry) of lipase-catalyzed interesterification is comparable to that of chemical interesterification in many aspects (Marangoni and Rousseau, 1995).

Lipase-catalyzed interesterification and hydrolysis follow a ping-pong reaction for multisubstrate reaction (Malcata et al., 1992; Reyes and Hill, 1994) in which the initial stage of interesterification hydrolysis of TAGs occurs with the consumption of water to produce diacylglycerols (DAGs), monoacylglycerols MAGs, and free fatty acids (FFAs) in the system. Accumulation of hydrolysis products will continue during interesterification until the equilibrium is reached (Reyes and Hill, 1994). Lipases are activated by oil–water interfaces and must undergo a conformational change before a substrate can diffuse into the active site (Derewenda and Sharp, 1993). For lipase-catalyzed reactions to occur, the lid of the lipase has to be open to make the active site accessible to the substrate. If we accept the premise that lipase functions via acyl-enzyme complex formation, the amino acids, i.e., Asp-His-Ser triad is involved, where serine residue is the nucleophile and the other two amino acids are involved in a charge-relay system designed to improve catalysis (Winkler et al., 1990). The triad is buried under a surface loop referred to as the *flap*. This flap becomes displaced upon binding of the lipase to the interface, exposing the substrate to the active site. At the same time, the hydrophobic environment around the active site becomes exposed and forms a strong binding site for the substrate at the interface. A mechanism for the lipase-catalyzed hydrolysis was proposed by Wong (1995). According to this principle, a proposed mechanism is shown in Figure 9.1 for lipase-catalyzed interesterification (ester–ester exchange). It involves two steps: acylation and deacylation. In the first step, a covalent acyl enzyme is formed by the nucleophilic attack on the carbonyl of the TAG by the essential Ser-OH. The second step occurs with H_2O as the nucleophile, giving the FFA and enzyme, or with DAG as the nucleophile, giving the new TAG and enzyme.

A simplified form, in which E stands for enzyme, is used instead of detailed molecular structure to describe the process of lipase-catalyzed interesterification between TAGs based on the formation of the acyl enzyme complex (Wong, 1995; Zhang, et al., 2001):

$$\mathrm{TAG_1 + E \rightleftharpoons TAG_1 \cdot E \rightleftharpoons DAG_1 + FFA_1 \cdot E} \tag{1}$$

$$\mathrm{TAG_2 + E \rightleftharpoons TAG_2 \cdot E \rightleftharpoons DAG_2 + FFA_2 \cdot E} \tag{2}$$

$$\mathrm{DAG_1 + FFA_2 \cdot E \rightleftharpoons TAG_3 \cdot E \rightleftharpoons TAG_3 + E} \tag{3}$$

$$\mathrm{DAG_2 + FFA_1 \cdot E \rightleftharpoons TAG_4 \cdot E \rightleftharpoons TAG_4 + E} \tag{4}$$

$$\mathrm{TAG_3 \cdot E \rightleftharpoons \ldots} \tag{5}$$

$$\mathrm{TAG_4 \cdot E \rightleftharpoons \ldots} \tag{6}$$

$$\mathrm{FFA_1 \cdot E + H_2O \rightleftharpoons FFA_1 + E} \tag{7}$$

$$\mathrm{FFA_2 \cdot E + H_2O \rightleftharpoons FFA_2 + E} \tag{8}$$

The reactions continue until the equilibrium is reached in the system, involving production of new intermediates and new TAG products (Eqs. 1–6). If the water content increases in the system, the FFA content increases (Eqs. 7 and 8), whereas FFA_1 • E or FFA_2 • E decreases. As a consequence, the content of DAG also increases (Eqs. 3 and 4). The total yield of interesterified new TAG products decreases.

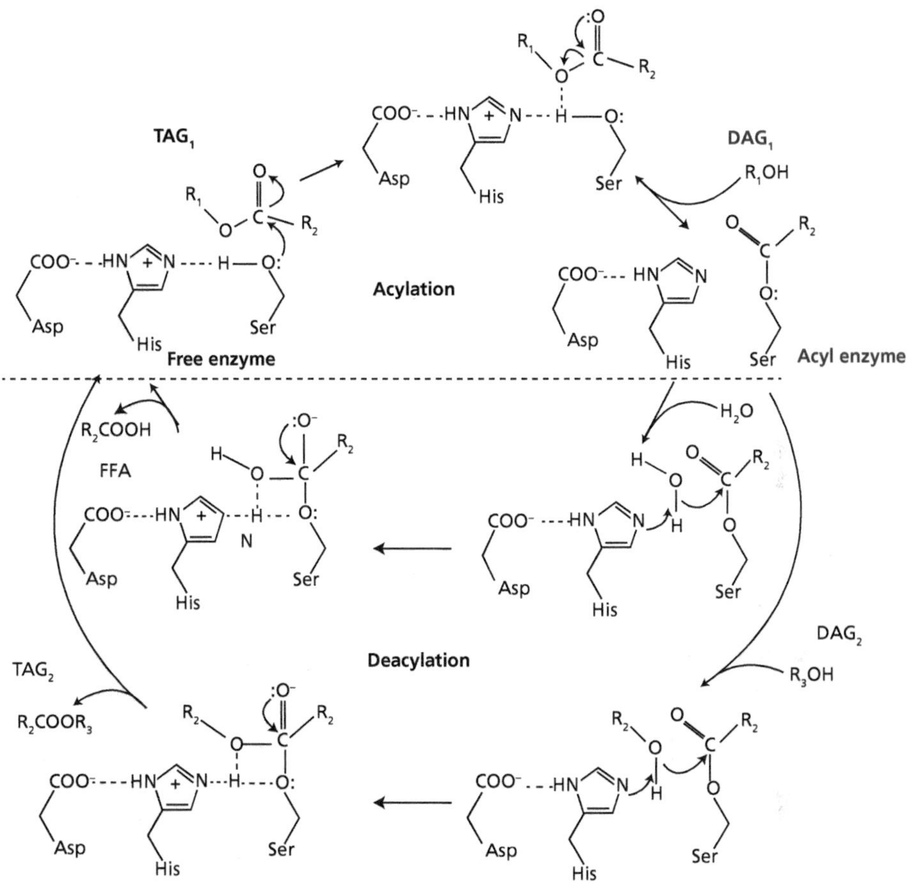

Figure 9.1 Proposed pathway for lipase-catalyzed interesterification.

The free water is the main reason to raise the FFA in the system. One mole of free water in the reaction system generates one mole of FFA (Zhang et al., 2000). Hence, it is very important to control water content in the system in order to reduce the contents of FFA and DAG in the final products.

Monitoring Method for the Process of Lipase-Catalyzed Interesterification Degree

Lipase-catalyzed interesterification is one of the alternative technologies for the replacing the conventional partial hydrogenation process to reduce or eliminate *trans* fatty acids (TFAs). Rearrangement of fatty acids on the glycerol backbone takes place through lipase-catalyzed interesterification. The degree of rearrangement depends on the reaction time. Therefore, it is important to monitor the reaction degree for lipase-catalyzed interesterification in order to get suitable products for a given application.

Enzymatic interesterification has been well-studied for producing modified fats with desired physical and chemical properties (Lee et al., 2007; Xu et al., 1998; Zhang et al., 2004). Different methods can be applied to monitor the interesterification degree. However, widely used methods, such as TAG composition (Paula et al., 2010; Zhang et al., 2004) and solid fat content (SFC) (Zhang et al., 2004), are discussed here.

Triacylglycerol Composition

The change of TAG composition is one of the well-known parameters to monitor the interesterification degree. However, several approaches were used for the calculation. Some of them are discussed below. The interesterification degree can be calculated according to following equation (Paula et al., 2010) based on the blends of milk fat and soybean oil:

$$ID = \left| \left(\frac{[\text{Cc50}]}{[\text{Cc50}]} \right)_t - \left(\frac{[\text{Cc50}]}{[\text{Cc44}]} \right)_0 \right|$$

where Cc50 and Cc44 represent the peaks with carbon numbers equal to 50 and 44, respectively, which represents the highly changed and the most stable group of peaks during the reaction. The index t and 0 represent the concentration of TAG at given reaction time and the initial reaction, respectively.

Zhang et al. (2004) monitored the interesterification conversion degree using peak ratio monitored by HPLC. The conversion degree (X) was defined as follows:

$$X\% = \frac{P_t - P_0}{P_\infty - P_0} \times 100$$

Where P_t is peak ratio at reaction time of t, P_∞ is the peak ratio at equilibrium, and P_0 is the peak ratio at the initial reaction time during the reaction. The peaks with equivalent carbon numbers ECN 44 and ECN 48 were changed most (Figure 9.1). Therefore, the peak ratio of ECN44, ECN 48 was used for monitoring the process.

Figure 9.2 shows that during the enzymatic batch reaction, the ECN 32, 34, 36, 38, 48, and 50 decreased. However, ECN 40, 42, 44, and 46 were increased. This showed that fatty acid compositions on the glycerol backbone were changed during the reaction. The content of TAG from coconut with only shorter chain length (ECN 32, 34, 36, 38) was decreased.

In order to compare different lipase-catalyzed products and to make the comparison clear, the relative degree of interesterification was suggested.

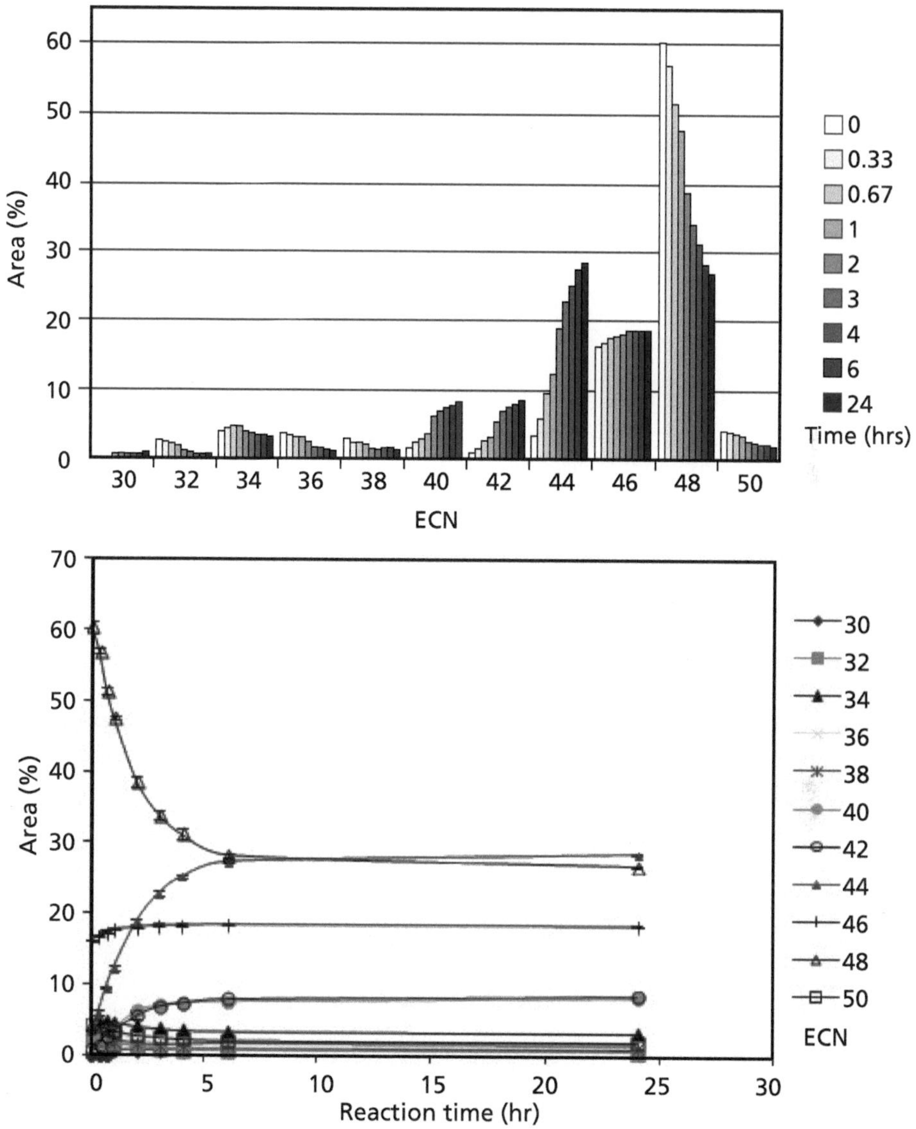

Figure 9.2 Evolution of the relative proportion of TAG as function of the TAG equivalent carbon number (ECN) at different reaction times for lipase-catalyzed interesterification.

$$\text{Relative degree of interesterification} = \frac{\text{Degree of interesterification at specific condition}}{\text{Degree of interesterification at default condition}} \times 100$$

The degree of transesterification is defined as the change of the peak area of the TAG that increased in percentage value at the reaction time t ($TAGI_t$), with respect to the value at the start of the reaction ($TAGI_0$), minus 100%. The rate of transesterification, *X*, was calculated as follows (Ghazali et al., 1995; Lai et al., 1998a, 1998b):

$$X(h^{-1}) = \frac{\text{Initial velocity, \%/h}}{\text{Enzyme activity, \%}}$$

Where initial rate is $(TAGI_t)-(TAGI_0)/t$ in the linear range of reaction, and enzyme activity is total TAG minus remaining TAG. Remaining TAG is the total concentration of TAG after transesterifcation reaction compared to the blend.

The degree of interesterification can be defined as the change of the TAG peak area that showed continuous and constant increases in value during the reaction ($TAGI_t$) with respect to the value at the start of the reaction ($TAGI_0$) (Ghazali et al., 1995):

$$\%\ \text{IE} = \frac{[\text{TAGI}_t]}{[\text{TAGI}_0]}$$

Enzymatic interesterification modified the TAG composition and consequently the consistency properties of fat blends. During the interesterification reaction between coconut oil and palm stearin, only the shorter chain length from coconut oil and the longer chain length of palm stearin were decreased in most cases.

Solid Fat Content

Solid fat content (SFC) is also one of the methods to monitor the interesterification degree of enzymatically interesterified fat (Zhang et al., 2004). The following model is best fitted to monitor the interesterification degree using SFC:

$$\int_{\text{SFC}_0}^{\text{SFC}} \frac{d\text{SFC}}{\text{SFC}-\text{SFC}_\infty} = -\int_0^\tau k \cdot d\tau$$

SFC_0 is the initial SFC value, SFC_∞ is the SFC value when the reaction reaches equilibrium, *k* is the value related to reaction rate of the enzyme on the given blend, and τ is the reaction time.

Figure 9.4 shows the SFC values of the enzymatically interesterified products from two groups of blends. The symbol represents experimental data and lines represent the

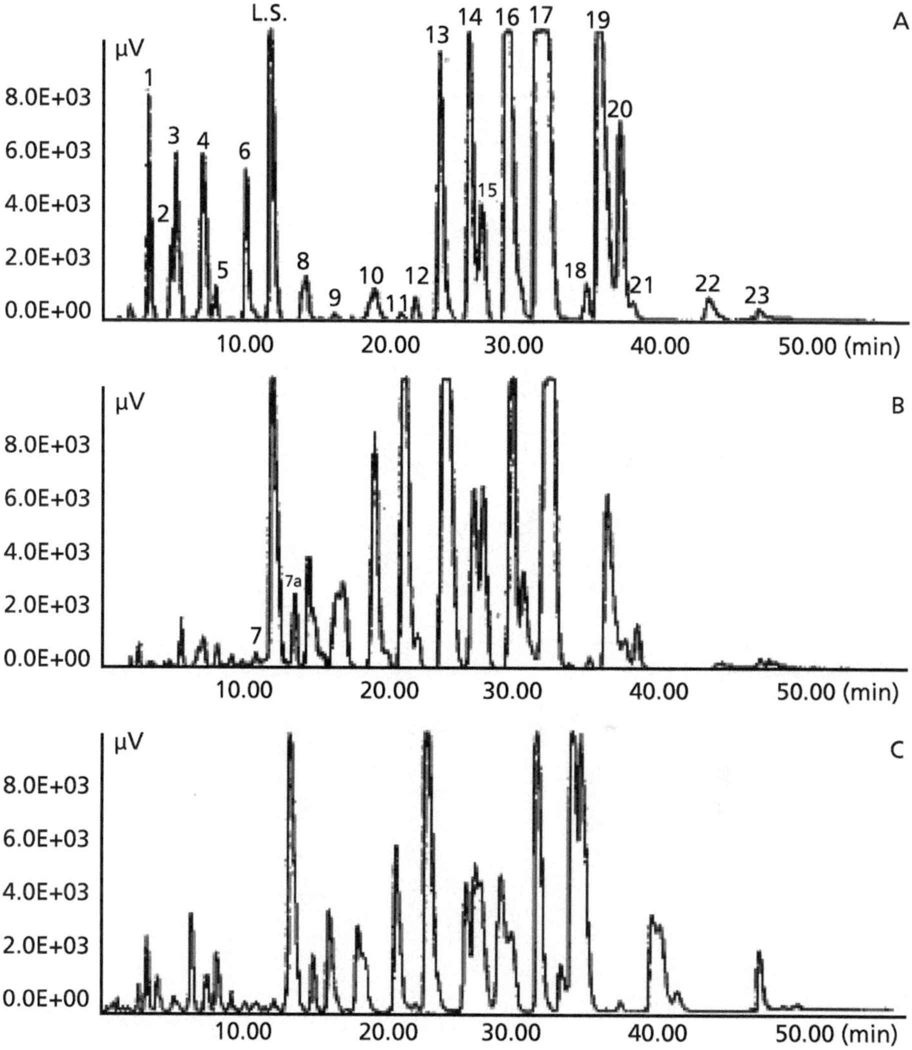

Figure 9.3 (A) High-performance liquid chromatographic TAG chromatogram of the blend (75:25, palm stearin and coconut oil); (B) product from chemical randomization; (C) lipase-catalyzed interesterification. I.S.: internal standard; ECN: equivalent carbon number. Peaks 1–3 (ECN34); Peaks 4–6 (ECN36); peak 7 (ECN 38); peak 7a (ECN 40); peaks 8, 9 (ECN 42); peaks 10–12 (ECN 44); peaks 13–15 (ECN 46); peaks 16–18 (ECN 48); peaks 19–23 (ECN 50).

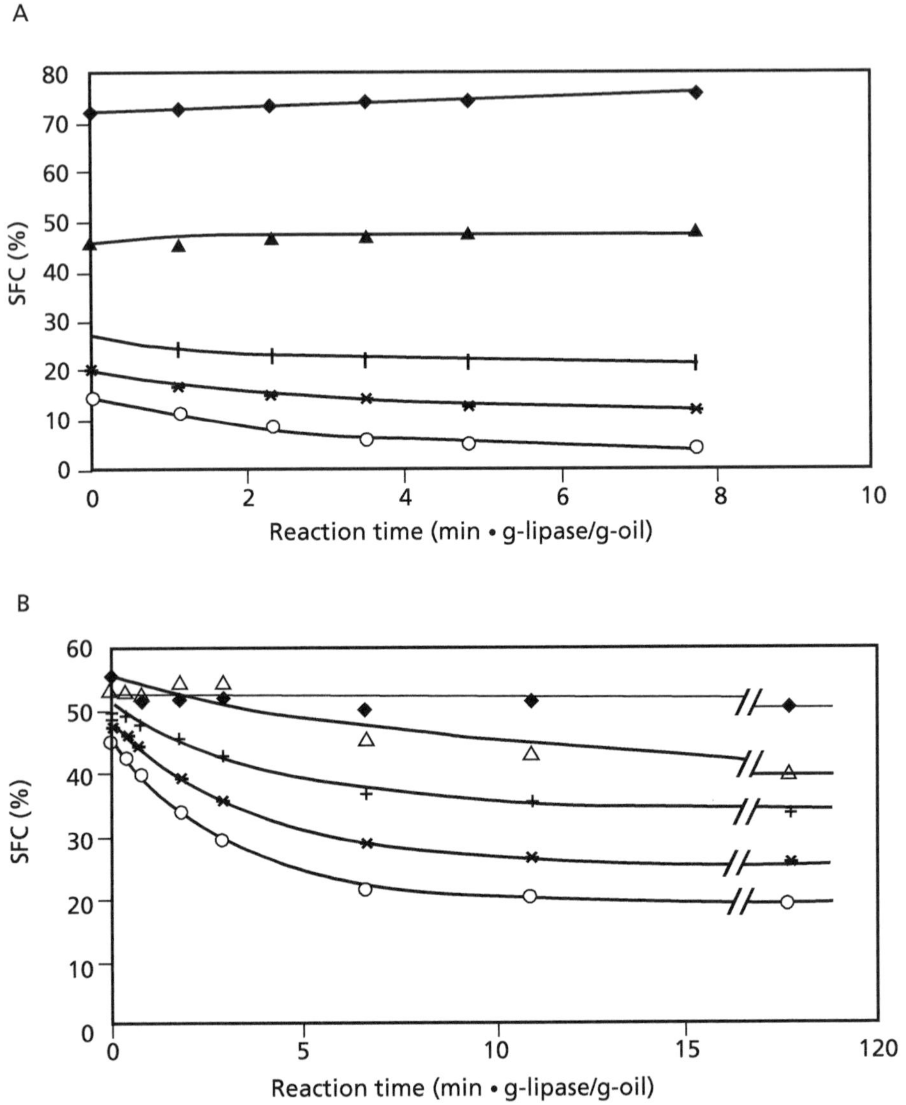

Figure 9.4 Fit of experimental data with the prediction model for blends of (A) PS/CO (70:30) and (B) SBO/FHSBO (50:50). The solid line represents the model, and experimental data are expressed as: ◆ SFC at 10 °C; △ SFC at 20 °C; + SFC at 30 °C; ✱ SFC at 35 °C; ○ SFC at 40 °C.

model. The model had very good fit at the different temperature especially for higher temperature. The derived model is more suitable for SFC at a higher temperature (30 °C, 35 °C, 40 °C) of lipase-catalyzed interesterification for fat modification.

Process Development for Lipase-Catalyzed Interesterification

Lipase-catalyzed interesterification reactions are normally carried out either in a batch or a packed-bed reactor. Therefore, the relationship between the batch and the packed-bed reactor is introduced.

For the industrial-scale production of lipase-catalyzed interesterification, Lipozyme TL IM is currently used as a commercially available lipase and the packed-bed reactor is often chosen for easier operation. When operating a packed-bed reactor, however, several factors have to be considered in order to achieve high efficiency: film diffusion, dispersion, pressure drop, temperature, and productivity. These are discussed and the optimal operation condition is given based on Lipozyme TL IM (Zhang, 2005).

The Relationship between Batch and Packed-Bed Reactors

To design a packed-bed reactor, the relationship between the batch and the packed-bed reactor has to be established. For a packed-bed reactor (Levenspiel, 1999), the relationship between enzyme load, flow rate, reaction rate, and conversion degree is as follows:

$$\frac{w_p}{F_p} = \int_0^{X_a} \frac{dX_a}{-r_a} \tag{1}$$

where w_p is the amount of enzyme in the packed-bed reactor, F_p is the flow rate through the packed-bed reactor, X_a is the substance conversion degree, and r_a is the reaction rate.

For a batch reactor (Levenspiel, 1999) a similar relationship exists, which can be expressed as:

$$\frac{w_p}{V_b} t = \int_0^{X_a} \frac{dX_a}{-r_a} \tag{2}$$

where w_b is the enzyme dosage, V_b is the amount of oil; and t is the reaction time.

Assuming the reaction rate and conversion degree are the same because the same enzyme is used, the right sides of Eqs. 1 and 2 are the same. Therefore, the following equation can be obtained:

$$\frac{w_p}{F_p} = \frac{w_b}{V_b} t \tag{3}$$

If no deactivation is assumed in the packed-bed reactor, Eq. 3 can be written as follows:

$$F_p = w_p \frac{V_b}{w_b \cdot t} \tag{4}$$

On the basis of experimental data from the batch reactor, Eq. 4 can be used to predict the relations between the amount of enzyme (w_p) and the flow rate (F_p) in the packed-bed reactor. Products with a desired conversion degree can be obtained by adjusting the flow rate at a fixed enzyme load.

Film Diffusion

Diffusion resistances, which are diffusions of substrate through a film surrounding an enzyme particle to reach the active surface, can limit the apparent activity of an immobilized enzyme. They may be observed at different levels for different immobilized enzymes. Diffusion resistance varies with the nature of the support material (porous, nonporous), hydrodynamic conditions surrounding the support material, and the distribution of the enzyme inside or on the surface of the support material (Levenspiel, 1999).

For the immobilized lipase, the distribution of the enzyme is both on the surface and inside the porous carrier. It could have both external and internal film diffusion limitations (mass transfer limitations) during the operation. The external film diffusion can be overcome by applying suitable flow rate, whereas the internal film diffusion depends on the particle size of the lipase. The former, however, is related to the process optimization. Therefore, only external film diffusion was considered. Figure 9.5 shows the relationship between linear velocities and conversion degrees monitored by a peak ratio under the same residence time at 70 °C using the "fresh" Lipozyme TL IM. By increasing the linear flow rate, the reaction degree was also increased, indicating that mass transfer limitations did exist. When the linear velocity was above 0.3 m/h in this case, the external film diffusion could be largely overcome. This indicates that an optimal linear velocity for a system is important to ensure an effective operation in a packed-bed reactor for Lipozyme TL IM–catalyzed interesterification. This result was relatively close to a previous observation for Lipozyme RM IM–catalyzed interesterification at 60 °C, in which the critical linear velocity was 0.28 m/h (Luck et al., 1988).

Dispersion

In reality, the ideal plug-flow behavior is never achieved because a certain degree of back mixing or dispersion inevitably occurs. The flow behavior is normally determined by applying an ideal pulse tracer or step tracer in the system. To study the flow behavior, the following equation is used:

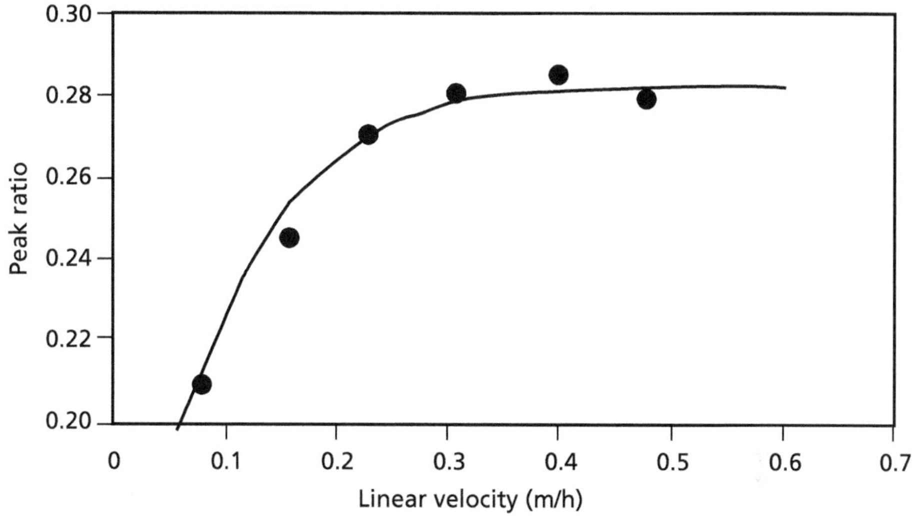

Figure 9.5 Dependence of conversion degree (peak ratio) on critical linear velocity in a packed-bed reactor. A soybean oil/coconut oil (70/30, w/w) blend was used as substrate and the experiments were conducted at 70 °C. Six glass columns (I.D. = 15 mm, L = 24 cm) were set up with enzyme loads of 2, 4, 6, 8, 10, and 13 g, respectively. The experiments were operated at linear velocities of 0.08, 0.16, 0.23, 0.31, 0.40, and 0.48 m/h, respectively, for each column in order to achieve the same retention time.

$$D/uL\left(\sigma_\theta^2 = \frac{\sigma_t^2}{\bar{t}^2} = 2\left(\frac{D}{uL}\right)\right)$$

is a dimensionless group called the *vessel dispersion number* (σ^2 is the variance of a tracer curve, $\theta = \frac{t}{\bar{t}}$) where u is the linear velocity, L is the length of the packed-bed reactor, and D is the dispersion coefficient (m^2/s) that represents the spreading process. It can be used to measure the extent of axial dispersion, which has the following relationship:

- D = 0, meaning no spreading, hence plug flow
- $D/\mu L < 0.01$, small extents of dispersion
- $D/\mu L > 0.01$, large deviations from plug flow

Figure 9.6 shows the results from the laboratory-scale dispersion studies in which soybean oil was used at a flow rate of 2.7 g/h/g-lipase at 70 °C, and red palm oil was used as a tracer. Samples were collected with a time interval of 2 minutes and monitored with a spectrometer. The ratios of reactor inner diameter to the particle

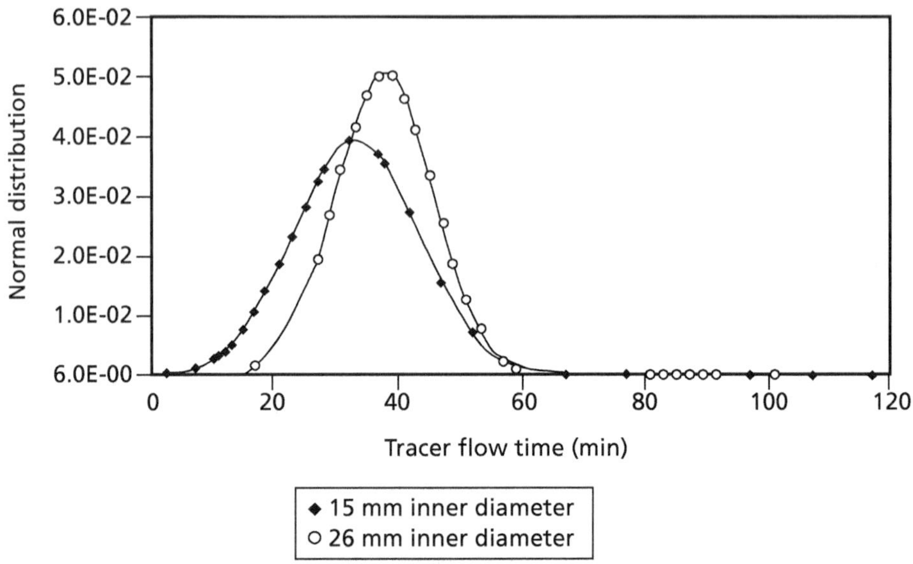

Figure 9.6 Normal distribution of tracer in two packed-bed reactors with inner diameter of 15 (◆) and 26 (○) mm column. Lipozyme TL IM with the load of 13 g in two different inner diameter columns (I.D. = 15 mm, L = 24 cm; I.D. = 26 mm, L = 24 mm).

diameter of lipase were over 20 (15 mm/500 μm and 26 mm/500 μm). Therefore, the effects of the reactor wall on the flow could be neglected (Jung and Bauer, 1992). The dimensionless factors D/μL were 0.010 and 0.023 for the inner diameters of 15 and 26 mm packed-bed columns, respectively. A large dispersion was observed with a large inner diameter packed-bed reactor in this case. This shows that it is important to design a packed-bed reactor with a suitable diameter to avoid dispersions in order to improve the efficiency and to make close to the ideal plug flow.

Pressure Drop

The pressure drop of Lipozyme TL IM across the catalyst bed was determined at 70 °C with a flow rate above the critical linear velocity. The experiments were performed in a thermo-stated glass reactor at 70 °C (I.D. = 10 cm, L = 85 cm). Refined and deodorized rapeseed oil was used as fluid with a downward stream flow. The measurements of pressure drop were carried out by adjusting the flow rate at approximately 8, 12, 16, and 18 kg/h. The pressure drop across the biocatalyst bed

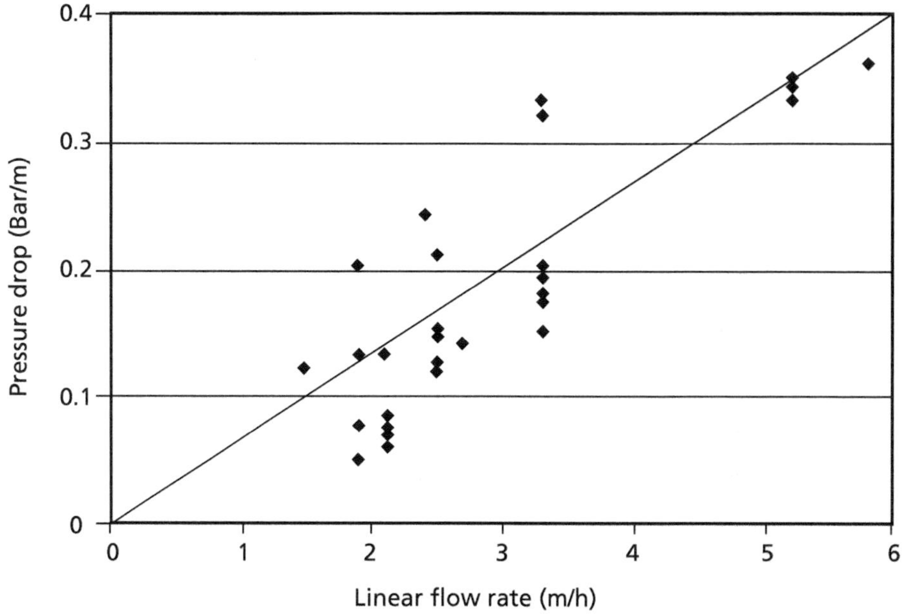

Figure 9.7 Effect of linear flow rate on pressure drop in a packed-bed column.

was measured by a pressure sensor. The data were collected with the same repeated procedure in 10 days.

Figure 9.7 shows that the increase of linear flow rate increased the pressure drop. However, even with 10 times the critical linear flow (3 m/h), the pressure drop was still lower than 0.3 bar/m for Lipozyme TL IM in a pilot-scale operation at the running temperature of 70 °C. This is similar to the observation for Lipozyme RM IM–catalyzed interesterification (Luck et al., 1988). The pressure drop was only 0.5 bar with bed height of 0.7 m when 10 times the critical linear flow rate (2.8 m/h) was used at 60 °C. Thus, these low values allow for the performance of a continuous process with satisfactory operation stability for lipase-catalyzed interesterification processes.

The pressure drop is not only related to the flow rate, but also related to the operation time under the same temperature. A downstream flow is normally used for industrial-scale operation. It allows a packed-bed reactor to be fed by oil gravity. It also ensures that the enzyme bed remains packed and stable during the operation, resulting in a maximum contact between the enzyme and fluids. However, the bed might be compressed in a long term operation, which might lead to a higher pressure drop. Therefore, a further study is needed for the measurement of pressure drop in a long-term operation.

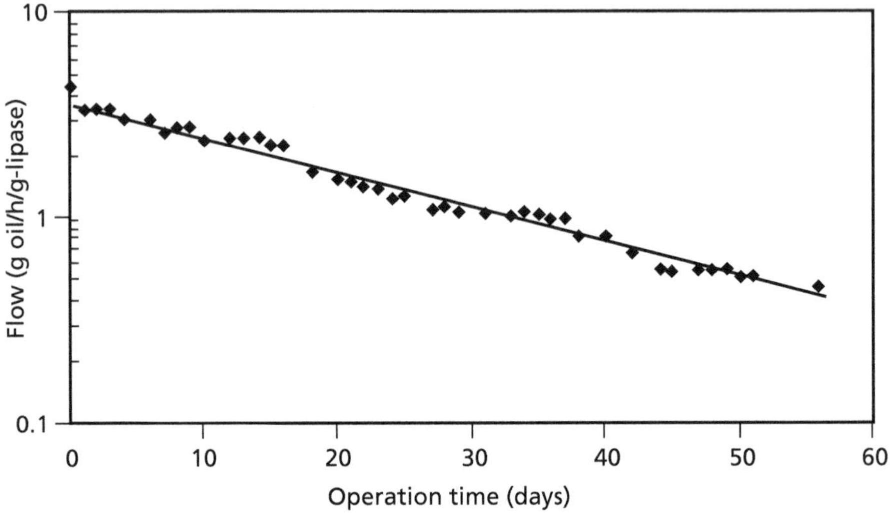

Figure 9.8 Isoconversion flow rate as function of operation time in a packed-bed reactor. Reaction conditions: soybean oil/coconut oil (70/30, w/w) blend; temperature 70 °C; column I.D. = 16 mm, L = 60 cm; upward flow; enzyme loading 64 g.

Productivity

Productivity is an important issue to describe the performance of a process or a catalyst. It is important to know the capability of the lipase in terms of the output of the product per unit enzyme. To measure this, the product quality (reaction degree) should be maintained throughout the operation. This way, it can be determined how much product is produced from the given amount of catalyst.

Figure 9.8 shows the change of flow in a packed-bed reactor with the operation time based on the amount of oils treated per hour per gram of lipase. This reflects the change of enzyme activity during the operation.

As can be seen, the enzyme decay followed the first order, which can be described by $\ln A = kt + \ln A_0$ or $A = A_0e^{-kt}$. A linear relationship existed between the logarithmic form of activity and running time. The area under the curve represents the total amount of product that was produced when the actual scale of flow rate versus the operation time was plotted. Therefore, the productivity of Lipozyme TL IM–catalyzed interesterification was roughly calculated as about 2 t product/kg of Lipozyme TL IM for 50 days operation at 70 °C (Figure 9.8). In a previous study for Lipozyme RM IM–catalyzed interesterification, about 2.4 t of fat/kg of lipase were obtained (Hansen and Eigtved, 1986), indicating a similar productivity of these two lipases. The latter lipase required a particular control of water activity in the system, so a pre-column was installed in the system to saturate the oil fluid with water in order to maintain the lipase activity. This led to a higher DAG content (6.4%) in the products. From this point, it is more advantageous to use Lipozyme TL IM for the process since water is not necessary to be adjusted during the operation.

Characterization of Lipase-Catalyzed Interesterified Fat

Fat modification has long been practiced in the oils and fats industry because vegetable fats, particularly, do not have the desirable melting/crystallization properties in their original state that make them suitable for various food product applications. To widen their application, oils and fats need to be modified either physically, chemically, or enzymatically (Anderson, 1996). The new developing method to improve the nutritional and functional properties of fats and oils is of great interest for the food industry (Marangoni, 2002).

Interesterification has been widely used for the modification of fats and oils, in which molecular weight, unsaturation, and positional distribution of fatty acid residues on the glycerol backbone of triacylglycerol are the main factors determining the physical properties of fats and oils. There are several ways to characterize the modified fats. Among them, widely used methods were solid fat content (Adhikari et al., 2009; Lee et al., 2007), TAG composition (Chu et al., 2002), melting and crystallization (Jeyarani and Reddy, 2010), crystal microstructure (Zhang et al., 2004), and polymorphic forms (Shin et al., 2009).

Solid Fat Content

SFC is the percentage of the solid part in the lipid at various temperatures. The SFC profile is responsible for many characteristics of fats, such as physical appearance, ease of packing, organoleptic properties, oil exudation, and spreadability (Farmani et al., 2006; Khatoon and Reddy, 2005; Norizzah et al., 2004). Therefore, SFC is becoming an important parameter to characterize physical properties of solid fats such as margarines, shortenings, cocoa butter (CB), cocoa butter substitute (CBS), cocoa butter equivalent (CBE), and so forth.

The effect of interesterification can be clearly observed in the SFC profile where interesterified fat shows lower SFC than the noninteresterified blends and chemically interesterified fat (Alpaslan and Karali, 1998; Lee et al., 2007). Dramatic reduction of PPP (tripalmitin) and SSS (tristearin) could be responsible for the reduction of SFC after interesterification. Drastic reduction in slipping melting point (SMP) and SFC would be obtained if the palm stearin or fully hydrogenated soybean oil was used for the interesterification with liquid oil (sunflower oil, palm kernel oil, rice bran oil, etc.) (Adhikari et al., 2009; Lai et al., 1998a, 1998b).

Adhikari et al. (2009, 2010) reported a dramatic lowering of SFC after enzymatic interesterification from the mixtures of fractionated rice bran oil/fully hydrogenated soybean oil, and pine nut oil/palm stearin. Li et al. (2010) reported lower SFC values in the interesterified fat from high-oleic sunflower oil and fully hydrogenated soybean oil compared to physical mixture. Slightly increased SFC below 20°C and significantly decreased SFC at higher temperatures (30°C, 35°C, and 40°C) after interesterification are common phenomena for the interesterified fat from palm stearin/coconut oil and palm stearin/rice bran oil (Reshma et al., 2008; Zhang et al., 2004). Long chain TAGs such as 1,3-palmitic-2 oleic-triacylglygcerol/1,2-palmitic-3 oleic–triacylglygcerol (POP/PPO), tripalmitin (PPP), tristearin (SSS), and 1,3-stearic-2 oleic–triacylglygcerol/1,2-stearic-3 oleic-triacylglygcerol (SOS/SSO) decreased in overall size because of the interesterification; therefore, there is a decrease in solids content at higher temperatures, especially in samples that contain palm stearin and fully hydrogenated soybean oil.

The plasticity of shortening helps air incorporation to increase the volume during the creaming stage in cake batter and cookie dough formation (Litwinenko et al., 2002). Lipase-catalyzed interesterification is one of the alternative technologies for replacing the conventional hydrogenation process to reduce or eliminate *trans* fatty acids. Therefore, lipase-catalyzed interesterification could be one of the alternative choices to get desirable products. Normally, a wide range of plasticity is required for bakery shortenings; therefore, the SFC is one of the important characteristics for shortenings and is used to assess their performance in the bakery products. After interesterification, a wide range of plasticity can be achieved compared to non-esterified blends (Litwinenko et al., 2002).

The SFC profiles of lipase-catalyzed interesterified Mahua oil/Kokum fat (1:1) blends and commercial fats are shown in Figure 9.9. Before interesterification, a narrow melting range was observed. However, after 30 minutes and 1 hour of interesterification, the drastic reduction in the SFC at a lower temperature was observed. After 3 hours, gradual increases in the SFC at all the temperatures was shown. Wider plastic range was obtained, which is desired for plastic fats, and the melting profile was similar to that of hydrogenated at 6 hours. After 24 hours, very high solids at higher temperature were observed. (Jeyarani and Reddy, 2010).

The drastic reduction of SFC at certain temperatures could be related to the melting point of TAG. For example, if the TAG of 1,3-palmitic-2-oleic-triacylglygcerol (POP) and 1,2-stearic-3 linoleic–triacylglygcerol (SSL) contain above 40% in the blend, the dramatic reduction of SFC within 30–38°C at interesterification can be expected because the melting points of POP and SSL are about 31–36°C.

Overall, after interesterification between two oils (hard fat and liquid oil), there is a drastic change in the SFC profile, and SFC was significantly decreased in the lower

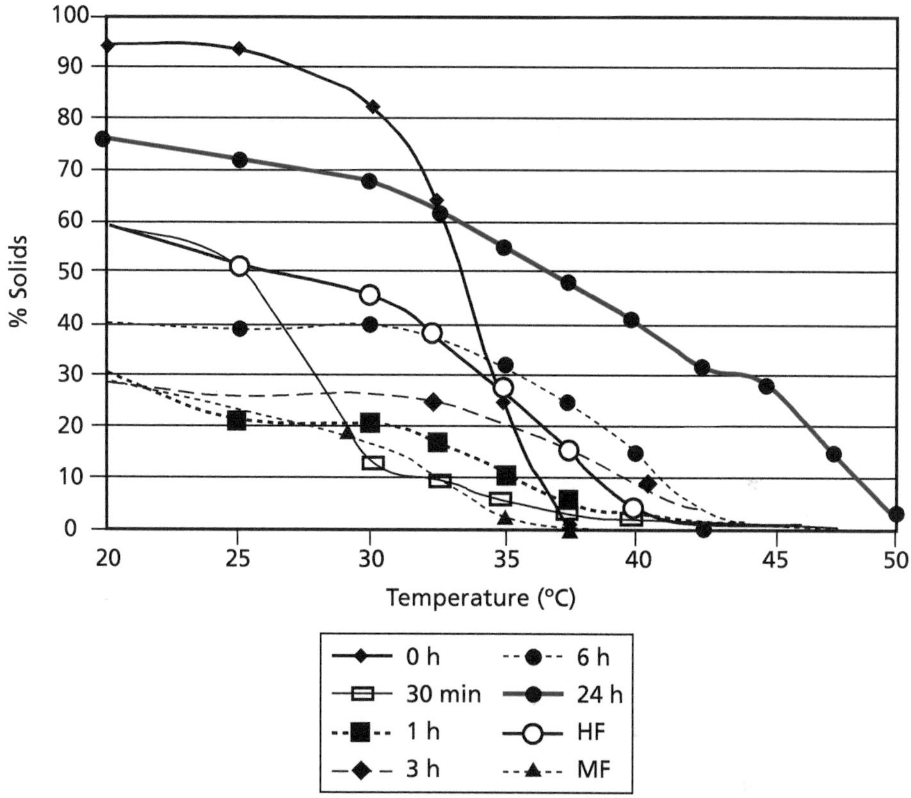

Figure 9.9 Melting profile of lipase-interesterified Mahua oil/Kokum fat (1:1) blends and commercial hydrogenated fat (HF) and milk fat (MF). Based on Jeyarani and Reddy (2010).

temperature region. However, this phenomenon may not be applied in the single oil interesterification.

Triacylglycerols

Every fat shows a direct relationship between its TAG composition and its physical properties. During the interesterification, rearrangement of fatty acids within TAG occurs, which changes the physical properties of the interesterified fat, such as solid fat content, polymorphic form, crystal micro structure, melting point, hardness, and so forth.

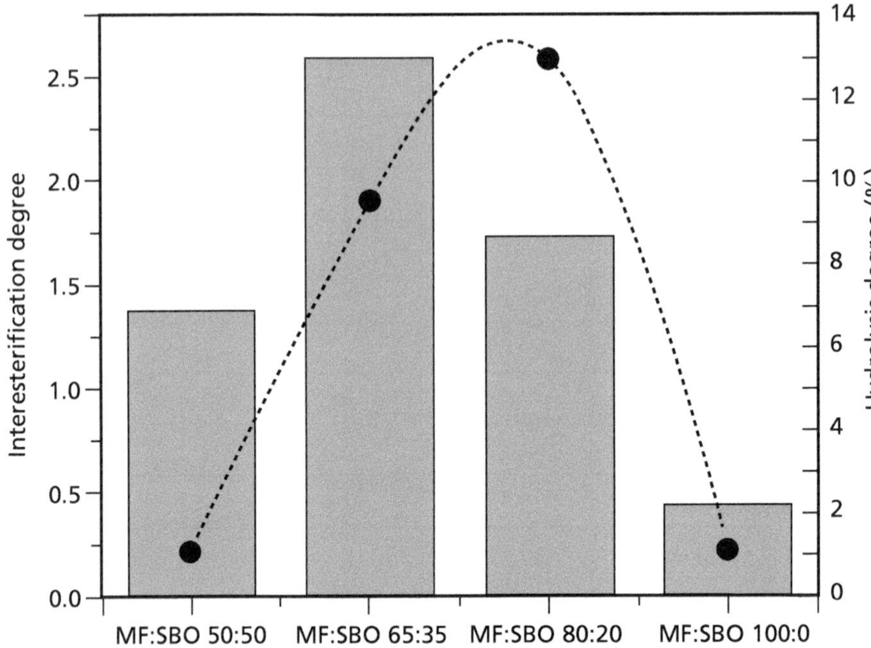

Figure 9.10 Interesterification degree (gray bars) and hydrolysis degree (dotted black line) at 48 hours for milk fat (MF) and soybean oil (SBO). Based on Paula et al. (2010).

Changes in textural properties can also be explained by distinct TAG compositions between interesterified and noninteresterified products. Increasing and decreasing the concentration of several TAG species indicate interesterification taken place which is compared to blends (non-esterified fat). Previous literature reported that the concentration of the medium-chain TAGs (1,2-lauric-3 oleic-triacylglygcerol [LaLaO], 1,2-lauric-3 myristic-triacylglygcerol [LaLaM], 1-lauric-2 oleic-3 palmitic-triacylglygcerol [LaOP], 1-lauric-2,3 palmitic-triacylglygcerol [LaPP], and 1,3-myristic-2 oleic-triacylglygcerol [MOM]) showed substantial increases after the reaction and a substantial decrease of high melting TAGs (POP and PPP) after interesterification from palm stearin and palm kernel olein (Chu et al., 2002).

Interesterification using milk fat, linseed, and rapeseed oils was reported by Augedo et al. (2008), and interesterification occurred quickly during the first hour of the reaction and reached a quasi-equilibrium state after 4–6 hours with no further significant change until 24 hours.

Figure 9.10 displays values attained for interesterification and hydrolysis for each reaction. The highest interesterification degree (2.60) was observed using MF:SBO (65:35). When the ratio of milk fat was increased in the mixture, a fall in the interesterification degree was observed. The fall of the interesterification degree could be because of reaction limitation imposed by the loss of TAG containing unsaturated 18-carbon fatty acids in soybean oil.

TAG composition of interesterified and noninteresterified fat is presented in Table 9.A, in which several TAG species were increased and decreased during interesterification. The increased and decreased amounts of TAG species were dependent on the oil type and their ratios (liquid oil and hard fat). Some new TAGs were also formed during interesterification (Table 9.A 1. SSL was not observed in the blends. However,

Table 9.A Triacylglycerol Composition of Interesterified and Noninteresterified Fat

1			2		
TAG[a] Species	Before IE	After IE	TAG[a] Species	Before IE	After IE
LLL	—	1.2	LLLn	1.3	—
LLO/OLL	2.5	11.1	LLL	5.2	1.1
PLL/LPL	1.5	1.3	MLO	0.2	3.2
OLO/OOL	1.0	11.9	PLL	5.1	12.0
PLO	5.1	12.7	OLL	5.1	3.3
PLP	2.1	0.5	PLP	4.8	13.4
OOO	—	—	PLO	6.1	14.2
POO	—	—	OLO	3.1	3.9
POP	—	—	PPP	21.5	8.8
PPP	—	—	POP	19.7	14.9
SSL	—	28.7	POO	8.7	7.7
PPS/PSP	—	2.7	PLS	1.4	3.0
SOS/SSO	—	9.2	OOO	2.1	1.4
SPS/PSS	18	11.3	SLO	1.4	1.6
SSS	69	8.3	PPS	4.0	2.8
			POS	3.3	3.1

[a]Ln: Linolenic acid; L: Linoleic acid; M: Myristic acid; P: Palmitic acid; S: Stearic acid; O: Oleic acid.

Sources: Adhikari et al. (2009).

the high concentration (28.7%) of SSL was observed in the interesterified fat due to the rearrangement of fatty acids during interesterification (Adhikari et al., 2009).

Several factors can influence interesterification, such as enzyme type and doses, reaction temperature, reaction time, chain length of fatty acids, and so forth. Any of these parameters can influence some of the interesterification degree. For example, lipase *Rhizopus oryzae* prefers C18 fatty acids and C2–C4 alcohols. Therefore, a blend containing a higher proportion of C18 may favor the reaction. Similarly, *Pseudomonas* lipase caused a drastic drop (15.6%) in the slip melting point for the palm stearin and anhydrous milk fat (PS:AMF, 40:60) blends as compared to a *R. Miehei* lipase (12.5%). It showed that *Pseudomonas* lipase is a better biocatalyst in randomizing the fatty acids in the TAG molecule than *R. Miehei* (Lai et al., 2000).

In conclusion, rearrangement of TAG composition after interesterification plays a vital role in changing the physical properties of oils and fats.

Polymorphic Form

The main polymorphic forms of fat crystals are: alpha, beta prime, beta. Each polymorphic form has different characteristics. The alpha form is characterized as an unstable crystal form with a low melting point and can be characterized with a single short spacing at 4.15 Å in X-ray analysis. The beta prime form is known as metastable, having an intermediate melting point with two major short spacings at

Table 9.B Polymorphic Form and Short Spacings (Å) of Noninteresterified and Enzymatic Interesterified Modified Butterfats

	Substrate Ratios	Short Spacing (Å)			Relative Content (β/β')	Polymorphic Form
		4.6	4.2	3.8		
Non-interesterified	8:6:6	4.630m[a]	4.232s	3.826w	56.44	β>β'
	6:6:8	4.602s	4.229m	3.827w	44.56	β<β'
	6:6:9	4.603s	4.232m	3.823w	48.52	β<β'
	4:6:10	4.625s	4.232m	3.827w	45.55	β<β'
Interesterified	8:6:6	4.605m	4.229m	3.827w	56.44	β>β'
	6:6:8	4.601m	4.232s	3.824w	54.46	β>β'
	6:6:9	4.607m	4.232s	3.827w	95.50	β>>β'
	4:6:10	nd	4.365s	3.828w	100.0	β

w: weak; m: medium; s: strong.

Source: Shin et al. (2009).

3.80 and 4.20 Å or three minor short spacings at 4.27 Å, 3.97 Å, and 3.71 Å. The beta form is the most stable, having the highest melting point with a strong short spacing at 4.60 Å.

Table 9.B presents the polymorphic forms of interesterified and noninteresterified fats, in which noninteresterified fat blends showed predominately β-polymorphic forms except one blend, which contained high amounts of anhydrous milk fat. After interesterification, β'-polymorphic forms of all blends were predominantly presented and the β-polymorphic forms became weaker.

In Figure 9.11, interesterified fat showed stronger intensities at 3.86, 4.22, or 4.37 Å than 4.66 Å. Similar intensities were observed in the case of physical blends.

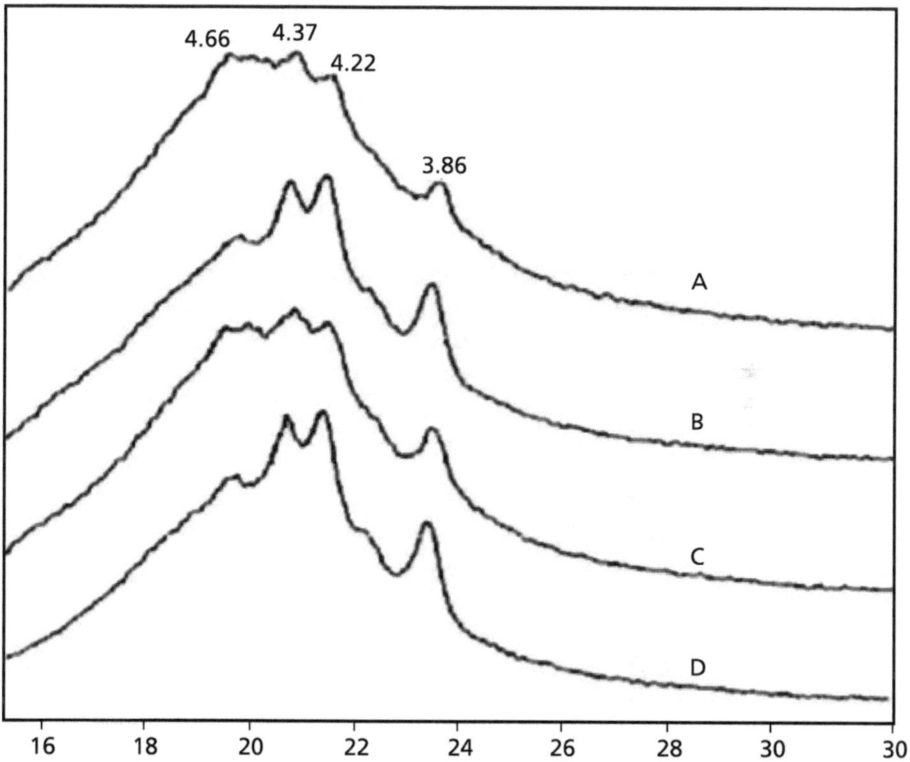

Figure 9.11 X-ray diffraction spectroscopy of interesterified product (A) and physical blend (B) of pine nut oil/palm stearin in a ratio of 40:60, and interesterified product (C) and physical blend (D) of pine nut oil/palm stearin in a ratio of 30:70, respectively. Based on Adhikari et al. (2010).

The interesterified product (pine nut oil/palm stearin, 30/70) contained 72.1% β' polymorphic forms, which was higher than the other product (pine nut oil/palm stearin, 40/60) (57.7%). The β' form (at 3.86 and 4.22 Å) was increased and the β form (4.66 Å) was decreased as the amount of palm stearin was increased, in the case of the intererterified product. Reshma et al. (2008) did not observe increasing effect on the β'-polymorphic form after interesterification. The reason could be the resultant enzyme interesterified product has not been subjected to the crystallization process using the scraped surface heat exchanger, which modifies the crystal polymorphism.

Crystal Microstructure

The intereserification process also affects the crystal microstructure. The β polymorphic form is more stable, has a larger crystal size (40–100 μm), and is harder in texture compared to β' form. Before interesterification, fat crystals appeared much coarser and larger with a more complex crystalline structure, which represents a sandy mouth feel. However, those larger crystals from the initial source became small crystals and agglomerated into the spherical crystal that has a higher density of β' form (Adhikari et al., 2011; Shin et al., 2009). The blend formed very coarse, condensed, branched, and leaf-like bigger crystals, whereas absolutely different crystals can be observed in interesterified fat. The interesterified fat with a 31% conversion degree had a mixture of leaf-, ball-, and needle ball–like spherulites; the longest was about 50 μm. When the conversion degree was over 70%, only needle-like or needle ball–like crystals appeared, having a higher concentration of β'-polymorphic form (Figure 9.12) (Zhang et al., 2004). Therefore, the interesterification degree has great effect on the crystal microstructure.

Melting and Crystallization Behavior

Enzymatic interesterification is a process in which a lipase (enzyme) is used to catalyze the exchange of fatty acids attached to the glycerol backbone of a fat. The purpose of the interesterification is to change the physical (melting and crystallization) properties of the resulting fats.

The thermal behavior of edible fats and oils is commonly characterized by two physical events, melting and crystallization, which are determined using differential scanning calorimetry (DSC). The features of melting peaks that are not readily interpretable, such as shoulder peaks and the recrystallization step, represent a transition of the polymorphs from their less stable form to a more stable form (Yap et al., 1989). Physicochemical property changes during interesterification can be explained by the rearrangement of fatty acids within the TAG molecule. First, the changes in the TAG composition are observed, followed by melting and crystallization thermograms. Lit-

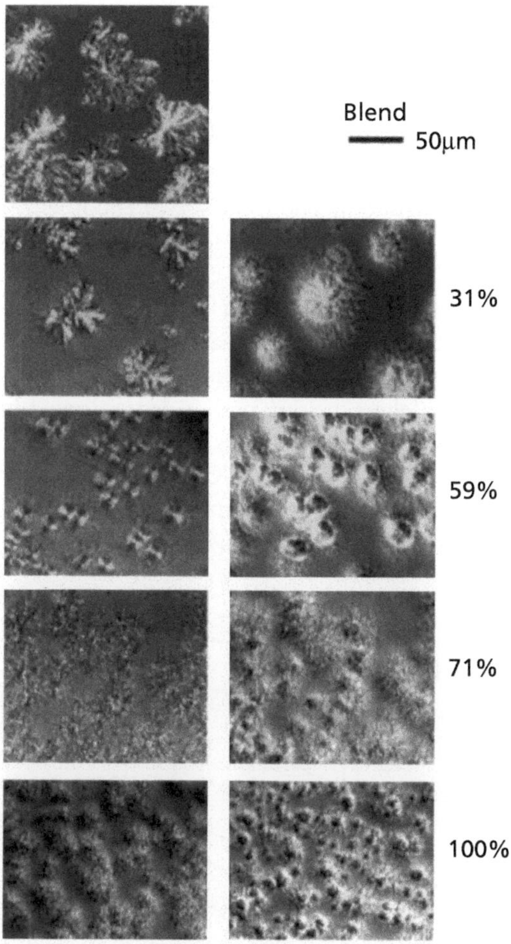

Figure 9.12 Morphology of the blends (palm stearin:coconut oil, 70:30) and interesterified products with addition of 50% liquid rapeseed oil (Zhang et al., 2004).

erature references report a decrease of melting and crystallization thermograms after interesterification compared to their physical blends (Jeyarani and Reddy, 2010; Zhang et al., 2004). The decrease of melting and the crystallization thermograms could be explained by the reduction of high-melting TAGs and the increase in low-melting TAGs after interesterification. However, the TAG composition created by interesterification of a single oil could be different. For example, after interesterification of palm oil, it becomes more solid-like (more easily solidified at room temperature) as the reaction time increases. That could be because of the increased formation of PPP in palm oil after interesterification that results in a substantially harder product. On the other hand, intermediates, such as MAG and DAG, also formed when the reaction time was increased (De and Patel, 2010).

Melting and crystallization thermograms of interesterified and noninteresterified fats from Mahua and Kokum (1:1) are presented in Figure 9.13. Before interesterification, a single, sharp endothermic peak was observed. However, a prominent lower melting peak (peak I) was observed after a 30 minute reaction time using 10% enzyme. With the increase in the time of interesterification, the size of endothermic peak in the lower temperature region (peak I) was reduced, while in the higher temperature region (Peak II) it was broadened (Figure 9.13A). The cooling curves of the noninteresterified fat showed a single, sharp exothermic peak at 12 °C. All the interesterified samples showed two distinct exothermic peaks: a broad peak in the lower temperature region and sharp peak in the high temperature region (Figure 9.13B).

The effect of interesterification on the highest melting peak is demonstrated in Table 9.C. Increasing the amount of palm stearin in the blends from 40% to 70%, the highest melt peak temperature (Tp) increased from 44.42 °C to 47.63 °C. Tp is decreased, however, if the reaction time is increased. For example, in 40:60 blends, Tp at 0 hours is 44.42 °C, after 2 hours Tp was decreased to 35.44 °C, and after that

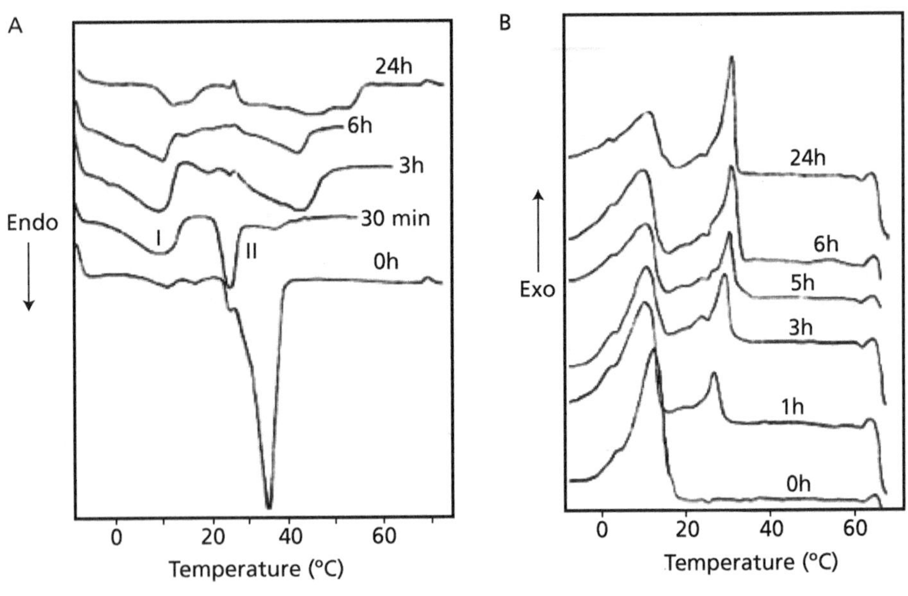

Figure 9.13 DSC melting (A) and crystallization (B) curves of Mahua/Kokum fat (Jeyarani and Reddy, 2010).

Table 9.C Effect of Enzymatic Interesterification[a] on Tp[b]

Palm Stearin: Rice Barn Oil PS:RBO (ratios)	Tp (°C) at Different Time (h) Durations						
	0	1	2	3	4	5	6
40:60	44.42	44.18	35.44	35.26	34.42	32.93	32.67
50:50	45.72	45.28	45.28	44.95	35.18	34.69	34.18
60:40	46.99	46.48	46.24	45.52	45.03	36.26	36.25
70:30	47.63	46.89	46.75	46.60	46.27	46.02	45.69

[a]Reaction conditions: temperature 60°C; reaction time 6 h; 3% lipase dosages, stirring 400 rpm.

[b]Tp: Highest melt peak temperature.

Source: Reshma et al. (2008).

there was a minor change until 6 hours. In the blends 50:50 and 60:40 there were minor changes until 3 hours and a major reduction was observed in 4 hours. A different pattern was observed in 70:30 blends, in which there were no major changes in the Tp until 6 hours. Increasing the concentration of hard fat, such as palm stearin, may not have much more effect on the reaction or it may take long time to complete the reaction.

In conclusion, interesterification has a great effect on the physicochemical properties of fats and oils, such as TAG composition, solid fat content, microstructure, polymorphic forms, melting and crystallization behavior, and others. In most of cases, melting point, SFC, and crystal microstructure (up to 5 μm) were decreased and polymorphic forms were changed after interesterification.

References

Adhikari, P.; Shin, J.-A.; Lee, J.-H.; Hu, J.-N.; Hwang, K.-T.; Lee, K.-T. Enzymatic Production of *Trans* Free Hard Fat Stock from Fractionated Rice Bran Oil, Fully Hydrogenated Soybean Oil and Conjugated Linoleic Acid. *J. Food Sci.* **2009,** *74,* 87–96.

Adhikari, P.; Zhu, X.-M.; Gautam, A.; Shin, J.-A.; Hu, J.-N.; Lee, J.-H.; Akoh, C.C.; Lee K.-T. Scaled-up Production of Zero *Trans* Margarine Fat Using Pine Nut Oil and Palm Stearin. *Food Chem.* **2010,** *119,* 1332–1338.

Adhikari, P.; Shin, J.-A.; Lee, J.-H.; Kim, H.-R.; Kim, I.-H.; Hong, S.-T.; Lee, K.-T. Crystallization, Physicochemical Properties and Oxidative Stability of the Interesterified Hard Fat from Rice Bran Oil, Fully Hydrogenated Soybean Oil and Coconut Oil through Lipase-catalyzed Reaction. *Food Bioprocess Technol.* **2011,** 6, 2474–2487.

Adhikari, P.; Peng, H.; Yafei, Z. Oxidative Stability of Enzymatically Interesterified Fat Containing Conjugated Linoleic Acid. *J. Am. Oil Chem. Soc.* **2012,** 89, 1961–1970.

Aguedo, M.; Giet, J. M.; Hanon, E.; Lognay, G.; Wathelet, B.; Destain, J.; Brasseur, R.; Vandenbol, M.; Danthine, S.; Blecker, C.; Wathelet, J. P.; Calorimetric Study of Milk Fat/Rapeseed Oil Blends and Their Interesterification Products. *Eur. J. Lipid Sci. Technol.* **2009**, 111, 376–385.

Alpaslan, M.; Karaali, A. The Interesterification-induced Changes in Olive and Palmoil Blends. *Food Chem.* **1998,** *61,* 301–305.

Anderson, D. A. Primer on Oils Processing Technology. In *Bailey's Industrial Oil and Fat Products,* 5th ed.; Huy, Y. H., Ed.; Wiley-Interscience: New York, 1996; pp 1–60.

Chu, B. S.; Ghazali, H. M.; Lai, O. M.; Man, Y. B. C.; Yusof, S. Physical and Chemical Properties of a Lipase-transesterified Palm Stearin/Palm Kernel Olein Blend and its Isopropanol-solid and High Melting Triacylglycerol Fractions. *Food Chem.* **2002,** *76,* 155–164.

De, B. K.; Patel, J. D. Modification of Palm Oil by Chemical and Enzymatic Catalyzed Interesterification. *J. Oleo. Sci.* **2010,** *59,* 293–298.

Derewanda, Z. S.; Sharp, A. M. News from Interface: The Molecular Structures of Triacylglyceride Lipase. *Trends Biochem. Sci.* **1993,** *18,* 20–25.

Farmani, J.; Safari, M.; Hamedi, M. Application of Palm Olein in the Production of Zero *Trans* Iranian Vanaspathi through Enzymatic Transesterification. *Eur. J. Lipid. Sci. Technol.* **2006,** *108,* 636–643.

Ghazali, H. M.; Hamidah, S.; Che Man, Y. B. Enzymatic Transesterification of Palm Olein with Nonspecific and 1,3-Specific Lipases. *J. Am. Oil Chem. Soc.* **1995,** *72,* 633–639.

Hansen, T. T.; Eigtved, P. New Immobilized Lipase for Interesterification and Ester Synthesis. *J. Am. Oil Chem. Soc.* **1986,** *63,* 365–369.

Jeyarani, T.; Reddy, Y. Effect of Enzymatic Interesterification on Physicochemical Properties Muhua Oil and Kokum Fat Blend. *Food Chem.* **2010,** *133,* 49–53.

Jin, J.; Li, D.; Zhu, X. M.; Adhikari, P.; Lee, K.-T.; Lee, J.-H. Production of Diacylglycerols from Glycerol Monooleate and Ethyl Oleate through Free and Immobilized Lipase-catalyzed Consecutive Reaction. *New Bio. Technol.* **2011,** *28,* 190–195.

Jung, H. J.; Bauer, W. Determination of Process Parameters and Modeling of Lipase-catalyzed Transesterification in a Fixed Bed Reactor. *Chem. Eng. Technol.* **1992,** *15,* 341–348.

Khatoon, S.; Reddy, S. R. Y. Plastic Fats with Zero *Trans* Fatty Acids by Interesterification of Mango, Mahua and Palm Oils. *Eur. J. Lipid. Sci. Technol.* **2005,** *108,* 636–643.

Lai, O. M.; Ghazali, H. M.; Cho, F.; Chong, C. L. Properties of Lipase-catalyzed Transesterified Blends of Palm Stearin and Anhydrous Milk Fat. *Food Chem.* **2000,** *70,* 215–219.

Lai, O. M.; Ghazali, H. M.; Chong, C. L. Effect of Enzymatic Transesterification on the Melting Points of Palm Stearin:Sunflower Oil Mixtures. *J. Am. Oil Chem. Soc.* **1998a,** *75,* 881–886.

Lai, O. M.; Ghazali, H. M.; Chong, C. L. Physical Properties of *Pseudomonas and Rhizomucor miehei* Lipase-catalyzed Transesterified Blends of Palm Stearin:Palm Kernel Olein. *J. Am. Oil Chem. Soc.* **1998b,** *75,* 953–959.

Lee, J.-H.; Akoh, C. C.; Lee, K.-T. Physical Properties of *Trans*-free Bakery Shortenings Produced by Lipase-catalyzed Interesterification. *J. Am. Oil Chem. Soc.* **2007,** *85,* 1–11.

Lee J.-H.; Son, J.-M.; Akoh, C. C.; Kim, M. R.; Lee, K. T. Optimized Synthesis of 1,3-Dioleoyl-2-palmitoylglycerol-rich Triacylglycerol via Interesterification Catalyzed by a Lipase from *Thermomyces lanugianosus. New Bio. Tech.* **2010,** *27,* 38–45.

Levenspiel, O. *Chemical Reaction Engineering*, 3rd ed. John Wiley & Sons: New York, 1999; pp 38–60, 427–446.

Li, D.; Adhikari, P.; Shin, J.-A.; Lee, J.-H.; Kim, Y.-J.; Zhu, X.-M.; Hu, J.-N.; Jin., J.; Akoh, C. C.; Lee K.-T. Lipase-catalyzed Interesterification of High Oleic Sunflower Oil and Fully Hydrogenated Soybean Oil Comparision of Batch and Continuous Reactor for Production of Zero *Trans* Shortenings Fats. *Food Sci. Technol.* **2010,** *43,* 458–464.

Litwinenko, J. W.; Rojas, A. M.; Gerschenson, L. N.; Marangoni, A. G. Relationship between Crystallization Behavior, Microstructure and Mechanical Properties in a Palm Oil-based Shortening. *J. Am. Oil Chem. Soc.* **2002,** *79,* 647–654.

Luck, T.; Klesser, T.; Bauer, W. Engineering Parameters for the Application of Immobilized Lipases in a Solvent-free System. In *Proceedings of World Conference on Biotechnology Fats and Oils Industry*; Applewhite, T. H., Ed.; AOCS Press: Champaign, IL, 1988; pp 343–345.

Macrae, A. R. Lipase-catalyzed Interesterification of Oils and Fats. *J. Am. Oil Chem. Soc.* **1983,** *60,* 291–294.

Malcata, F. X.; Reyes, H. R.; Garcia, H. S.; Hill, C. G.; Amundson, C. H. Kinetics and Mechanisms Catalyzed by Immobilized Lipases. *Enzyme Microb. Technol.* **1992,** *14,* 426–446.

Marangoni, A. G.; Rousseau, D. Engineering Triacylglycerol: The Role of Interesterification. *Trends Food Sci. Technol.* **1995,** *6,* 329–335.

Marangoni, A. G. Food Lipids. In *Chemistry, Nutrition, and Biotechnology,* 2nd ed.; Akoh, C. C., Min, D. B., Eds.; CRC Press: New York, 2002.

Norizzah, A. R.; Chong, C. L.; Cheow, C. S.; Zaliha, O. Effect of Chemical Interesterification on Physicochemical Properties of Palm Stearin and Palm Kernel Olein Blends. *Food Chem.* **2004,** *86,* 229–235.

Paula, A. V.; Nunes, G. F. M.; Freitas, L.; de Castro, H. F.; Santos, J. C. Interesterification of Milk Fat and Soybean Oil Blends Catalyzed by Immobilized *Rhizopus Oryzae* Lipase. *J. Molec. Catal. B: Enzymatic* **2010,** *65,* 117–121.

Reshma, M. V.; Saritha, S. S.; Balachandran, C.; Arumughan, C. Lipase-catalyzed Interesterification of Palm Stearin and Rice Bran Oil Blends for Preparation of Zero *Trans* Shortening with Bioactive Phytochemicals. *Bioresource Technol.* **2008,** *99,* 5011–5019.

Reyes, H. R.; Hill, C. G., Jr. Kinetic Modeling of Interesterification Reaction Catalyzed by Immobilized Lipase. *Biotechnol. Bioeng.* **1994,** *43,* 171–182.

Shin, J.-H.; Akoh, C. C.; Lee, K.-T. Production and Physicochemical Properties of Functional-butterfat through Enzymatic Interesterification in a Continuous Reactor. *J. Agric. Food Chem.* **2009,** *57,* 888–900.

Winkler, F. K.; D'Arcy, A.; Hunziker, W. Structure of Human Pancreatic Lipase. *Nature* **1990,** *343,* 771–774.

Wong, D. W. S. *Food Enzymes Structure and Mechanism.* Chapman & Hall: New York, 1995; pp 37–84.

Xu, X.; Balchen S.; Høy, C.-E.; Adler-Nissen, J. Pilot Batch Production of Specific-structure Lipids by Lipase-catalyzed Interesterification: Preliminary Study on Incorporation and Acyl Migration. *J. Am. Oil Chem. Soc.* **1998,** *75,* 301–308.

Yap, P. H.; de Man, J. M.; de Man, L. Polymorphic Stability of Hydrogenated Canola Oil as Affected by Addition of Palm Oil. *J. Am. Oil Chem. Soc.* **1989,** *66,* 1784–1791.

Zhang H., Lipase Catalyzed Interesterification for Margarine Fat Production, PhD Thesis, BioCentrum-DTU, Technical University of Denmark, 2005.

Zhang, H.; Xu, X.; Mu, H.; Nilsson, J.; Adler-Nissen, J.; Høy, C.-E. Lipozyme IM-catalyzed Interesterification for the Production of Margarine Fats in a 1kg Scale Stirred Tank Reactor. *Eur. J. Lipid Sci. Technol.* **2000,** *102,* 411–418.

Zhang, H.; Xu, X.; Nilsson, J.; Mu, H.; Adler-Nissen, J.; Høy, C.-E.; Production of Margarine Fats by Enzymatic Interesterification with Silica-granulated *Thermomyces lanuginosus* Lipase in a Large-scale Study. *J. Am. Oil Chem. Soc.* **2001,** *78,* 57–64.

Zhang, H.; Smith, P.; Adler-Nissen, J. Effects of Degree of Enzymatic Interesterification on the Physical Properties of Margarine Fats: Solid Fat Content, Crystallization Behavior, Crystal Morphology and Crystal Network. *J. Agric. Food Chem.* **2004,** *52,* 4423–4431.

10

Structured Emulsions and Edible Oleogels as Solutions to *Trans* Fat

Alexander K. Zetzl and Alejandro G. Marangoni ■ *Department of Food Science, University of Guelph, Guelph, Canada*

Introduction and Recent Progress in Regard to *Trans* Fat Reduction

Trans fatty acids (TFAs) were created and used by industry to fill a demand for functional fats that were solid at room temperature and could withstand the oxidation stresses provided by temperatures in excess of 160 °C when frying (Kodali, 2005). By simply changing the configuration of an unsaturation from *cis* to *trans*, a greater ease of packing can be achieved, due to more symmetrical molecules. This creates a corresponding increase in the melting points of these fatty acids and increases their stability when subjected to high temperatures (Kodali, 2005). When greater functionality was combined with what were believed to be health improvements over saturated fat, the widespread use of *trans* fats seemed to be ensured. Many years later, the shocking truth about *trans* fat and its deleterious effects on cardiovascular disease were reported (Judd et al., 1994; Mensink and Katan, 1990; Willet et al., 1993). In 2006, mandatory labeling of TFAs became a requirement in the United States, in an attempt to force producers to reformulate products and reduce our consumption of these harmful fatty acids (U.S. Food and Drug Administration, 2012).

In December 2009, Health Canada released its final monitoring report that reported the level of TFAs in certain Canadian foods, including french fries, desserts, cookies, frozen appetizers, popcorn and snacks, and chicken products (Health Canada, 2012). The results were rather shocking, with only 4 of the 21 different product types tested meeting the required *trans* fat level. Only 40% of cookies from small- and medium-sized family and quick service restaurants met the requirements, and only 25% of margarines from cafeterias located in institutions met the *trans* requirements. Although 18 of the 21 categories had 50% or more of the tested products meet the necessary requirements, *trans* fats clearly remain a problem (Health Canada, 2012). It is possible that for many of these products the producers were unable to effectively replace *trans* fats with a substitute, either due to lack of availability, poor functionality on the substitute's part, or cost.

The small change in unsaturated fatty acid bond configuration from *cis* to *trans* has represented a large problem to the food industry with regard to its replacement. This created a great challenge for both academic and industrial scientists: Provide a solid-like structure similar to highly saturated or *trans*-containing triacylglycerols, keeping functionality, yet without having negative impacts on human health. Other additional factors such as cost, availability, versatility, efficiency, and food-grade status should also be considered when trying to find a replacement for *trans* fats (Co and Marangoni, 2012). A distinction can be made here: Replacements that fulfill only some of these requirements should be considered as "substitutes," while those that fulfill all of these requirements, and potentially provide additional benefits, can be deemed "solutions" to *trans* fats. Many previously proposed substitutes for TFAs have found their way into our diets. Their effectiveness as a solution to the issue can now be seen, well over five years after January 1, 2006, which was when the new labeling requirements were put into place (U.S. Food and Drug Administration, 2012). This chapter focuses on structured emulsions and edible oleogels, two potential solutions to the *trans* fat dilemma. However, to understand why these are potential solutions, background information in regard to how specific fatty acids affect our cardiovascular health is required.

Effects of Specific Fatty Acids on Our Cardiovascular Health

Cardiovascular disease (CVD) continues to be the leading cause of death and disability in the world, resulting in an estimated 17.3 million deaths in 2008, and a predicted 23.6 million deaths in 2030 (WHO, 2012). Blood serum cholesterol levels have been used for many years as an indicator for cardiovascular health, as a strong correlation was seen between high total serum cholesterol levels and CVD (Klag et al., 1993; LaRosa et al., 1990). Today, many different types of serum cholesterol have been identified, including the following: high-density lipoprotein (HDL), low-density lipoprotein (LDL), intermediate-density lipoprotein, very-low-density lipoprotein, and chylomicrons (LaRosa et al., 1990; Nordestgaard and Tybjærg-Hansen, 1992). Of these different types of lipoprotein, LDL and HDL are by far the most utilized to report effects on cardiovascular health, with increased LDL levels having a negative effect and increased HDL levels having a positive effect on cardiovascular health compared to baseline levels (LaRosa et al., 1990). Typically, serum cholesterol levels are measured after the consumption of meals or diets containing a specific amount and type of fat or fatty acid. These levels are then compared to a control meal or diet, which is often carbohydrates or one specific fatty acid, such as oleic acid. The work of Mensink and Katan (1990) was one such study that used oleic acid in their control diet, providing 10% of the subject's daily energy.

Although many studies in the 1990s looked only at total changes in serum cholesterol levels, or change in LDL, it has since been shown that it is much more advantageous to report both the change in LDL and HDL, or more specifically, as a cholesterol ratio, ΔTotal:HDL (Mensink et al., 2003). The ratio is determined by adding the change for both LDL and HDL cholesterol, and comparing this to the change in HDL only. If the reported ratio is positive or close to 0, this means that there was primarily an increase in LDL levels, while a negative ratio indicates a larger increase in HDL relative to LDL. With this ratio, it is very clear what specifically increased, and whether this indicates a negative, neutral, or positive effect on CVD. The work of Mensink et al. in 2003 showed *cis*-polyunsaturated fatty acids had the greatest positive effect on CVD, with a ΔTotal:HDL ratio of approximately –0.032, while TFAs showed the worst effect, resulting in a ratio of just over 0.02 (Mensink et al., 2003). Saturated fatty acids showed a fairly neutral effect on the ΔTotal:HDL cholesterol ratio, while *cis*-monounsaturated fatty acids showed a ratio of –0.026, also indicating a positive effect on cardiovascular health (Mensink et al., 2003).

TFAs are considered to be the most deleterious type of fatty acids, predominately due to their effect on this cholesterol ratio. While TFAs caused the greatest increase in LDL levels, it was also the only type of fatty acid to decrease HDL levels (Mensink et al., 2003). This has been confirmed by many other groups, including Mozaffarian and Clarke (2009). This group also showed impact on the ΔTotal:HDL ratio if TFAs replaced poly, mono, or saturated fatty acids, on a basis of percentage of calories replaced by *trans* fat. At the level of 1% replacement of calories, the values are very similar to the 0.02 reported by Mensink et al. (2003). However, when *trans* fat replaces 5% of calories formerly provided by polyunsaturated fatty acids, this value jumps to above 0.3, more than a tenfold increase (Mozaffarian and Clarke, 2009). When *trans* fat replaced 5% of calories from monounsaturated and saturated fat, the ratios were approximately 0.27 and 0.17, respectively (Mozaffarian and Clarke, 2009).

As with cholesterol, the general term "saturated fat" can be broken down into specific fatty acids, with two of the most heavily studied and prevalent in edible fats and oils being palmitic acid (C16) and stearic acid (C18). The effects of these fatty acids on serum cholesterol have been shown to be significantly different, and they should not be grouped together (Mensink et al., 2003). Stearic acid, which has been estimated to make up 3% of daily energy in the average American diet, has a slightly beneficial effect on serum cholesterol levels, with a ratio of –0.013 in the Mensink et al. (2003) study (Hunter et al., 2010). Palmitic acid shows a more negative effect on cardiovascular health, with a ΔTotal:HDL ratio of 0.005, and was the most atherogenic saturated fatty acid studied (ΔTotal:HDL). This is troubling because palmitic acid is the most heavily consumed saturated fatty acid in the United States, making up 56.3% of total saturated fat intake and resulting in 1.8–4.4% of daily energy for 14 European countries (Hunter et al., 2010).

Recently, the true effect of saturated fatty acids on human health has come under debate (Siri-Tarino et al., 2010a, 2010b). Contrary to what serum cholesterol values may indicate, a meta-analysis study covering close to 350,000 subjects found no relationship between saturated fat consumption and increased risk of stroke or CVD (Siri-Tarino et al., 2010a). Although saturated fat may not be as damaging to health as once previously believed, it can still be concluded that saturated fats, individually or as a whole, do not have the same positive benefits that mono- and especially polyunsaturated fatty acids possess. When replacing 1% of energy formerly held by stearic acid with mono- or polyunsaturated fatty acids, ΔTotal:HDL cholesterol can be lowered by 0.043 and 0.055, respectively (Hunter et al., 2010). An overwhelming amount of evidence has shown that polyunsaturated fatty acids possess the greatest cholesterol lowering effects of all other types of fatty acids (Hunter et al., 2010; Kris-Etherton et al., 2004; Mensink et al., 2003). Many oils from vegetable sources contain a high percentage of polyunsaturates, as shown in Table 10.A. For the development of any solutions to *trans* fat, the inclusion of a high level of polyunsaturates should be a priority, while minimizing the level of saturated fat. Both edible oleogels and structured emulsions have the potential to take advantage of polyunsaturated fatty acids, while possessing highly reduced levels of saturates and zero TFAs. Although either of these fairly new approaches for creating a solid-like fat can achieve a goal of zero *trans* fat, each has its own set of advantages and specific applications.

Structured Emulsions Using Monoglycerides

Emulsions consist of at least two immiscible phases, with one phase being dispersed in the other as tiny droplets (McClements, 2010). The most common type of emulsion is oil in water (O/W), with some examples including milk, cream, and mayonnaise (McClements, 2010). It can be a challenge trying to differentiate between a structured emulsion and a simple O/W or water-in-oil emulsion, as often they involve many of the same ingredients and production procedures. For example, both commonly rely on a mixing or homogenization step to disperse one phase into the other, and they both commonly use a minute amount of emulsifier to help stabilize the

Table 10.A Fatty Acid Composition (wt%) of Common Fats and Oils from Vegetable Sources

	Lauric	Myristic	Palmitic	Stearic	Oleic	Linoleic	Linolenic
Oil Type	C12	C14	C16	C18	C18:1	C18:2	C18:3
Palm	—	2	44	4	39	11	—
Olive	—	—	13	3	75	8	1
Canola	—	—	5	2	62	21	10
Soybean	—	—	12	4	23	54	7
Corn	—	—	11	2	26	60	1
Flaxseed	—	—	6	4	15	16	59

Gunstone and Harwood (2007).

emulsion (McClements, 2010). Traditional emulsions are prone to physical instability (coalescence and phase separation) and are not able to provide a solid-like texture that is similar to hard-stock triacylglycerol molecules (McClements, 2010). Although mayonnaise certainly has structure, it is unlikely that it would ever be described as looking "shortening-like." With structured emulsions, products with a wide variety of textures can be created, including something that is similar to a traditional partially hydrogenated shortening (Batte et al., 2007a; Zetzl and Marangoni, 2011). Several varieties of structured emulsions have been listed in a review by McClements (2010) and include the following: multiple emulsions, solid lipid particles, filled hydrogel particles, and multilayer emulsions. Here the focus will be on one variety of multilayer emulsions, as described by Marangoni (2007), which use monoglycerides to entrap multiple layers of water around oil droplets (Marangoni, 2007; Marangoni et al., 2007).

To understand more about this system, it is first important to describe how this type of emulsion is produced. The system can be created by first heating a cosurfactant-saturated monoglyceride–oil mixture above the Krafft temperature of the monoglycerides until they have become fully dissolved in the oil. This mixture is then added to water while briefly exposing the system to a gentle external shear field. This leads to the formation of a multilayer lamellar monoglyceride structure in the liquid crystalline state, which surrounds the oil droplets. Upon cooling below the Kraft temperature, the monoglycerides undergo a liquid-crystalline to crystalline phase transition and adopt a solid-like structure (Batte et al., 2007a, 2007b). The final product contains vegetable oil "droplets" surrounded by the hydrated, saturated, monoglyceride multilayers (Batte et al., 2007a; Marangoni et al., 2008; Zetzl and Marangoni, 2011). These droplets can be easily observed when using freeze fracture cryo-scanning electron microscopy, as shown in Figure 10.1 (A and B). By making adjustments regarding the charged cosurfactant ratio and/or pH, a semisolid material of high viscosity, similar to a shortening in appearance, can be formed (Batte et al., 2007a). Structured emulsions such as those mentioned here are already commercially available. One such product has been trademarked under the name Coasun™. This shortening-like material contains no TFAs, limited saturated fatty acids, and is 30–40% structured water (Figure 10.1C) (Zetzl and Marangoni, 2011).

The structure from the term *structured emulsion* comes from the monoglycerides, which are only incorporated at a level of a few percent, yet are able to stabilize the emulsion, greatly reducing phase separation and providing structure. In fact, the monoglycerides could potentially be the only actual solid component in these structured emulsions at room temperature. This structure can be seen when analyzing X-ray diffraction spectra in the small angle region, where the structured emulsion (4.5% monoglyceride and 35% water) will show diffraction peaks (001, 003, 005, 007), yet mayonnaise will not (Figure 10.2). These peaks, which signify sizes of

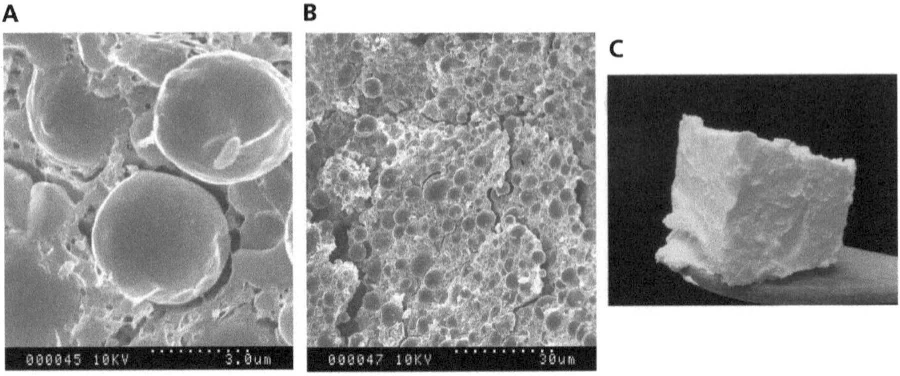

Figure 10.1 (A, B) Cryo-scanning electron micrographs of a structured oil-in-water emulsion, similar to the commercial product Coasun™. (C) Structured emulsion Coasun™, which can possess a shortening-like texture through the use of a surfactant and careful control of pH. Coasun™ can successfully be used for a variety of baking applications by replacing traditional fats high in saturated and TFAs.

approximately 61 Å, 18 Å, 13 Å, and 8 Å for 001, 003, 005, and 007, respectively, indicate that there is a lamellar crystalline structure in the long spacing that is not shown by a traditional O/W emulsion, such as mayonnaise. Three definitive peaks were also noted in the wide angle region for the structured emulsion sample, whereas the mayonnaise emulsion showed no definitive peaks. Peaks in this region signify that there is subcell packing; specifically, the peaks indicate that the sample had converted from the metastable α-form to the more stable β-form.

Rheology can also be used to show the difference between an O/W emulsion (mayonnaise) and a structured emulsion (Coasun™), as shown in Figure 10.3. When analyzing the storage modulus (G') for the two different types of emulsions, at 10 Pa the structured emulsion has a G' of 3022 Pa, which is more than six times that of mayonnaise (461 Pa). This indicates a material that is stiffer and more solid-like, which might be unexpected considering that the Coasun™ product contains an additional 15% water compared to the mayonnaise. The differences in the loss modulus (G") is also quite substantial, with the structured emulsion showing a loss modulus over seven times that of mayonnaise (424 vs. 59 Pa).

Work was completed by Huschka et al. (2011) in an attempt to determine how similar this type of structured emulsion would behave to an actual interesterified vegetable shortening. The doughs containing structured emulsion showed a lower amount of water absorption compared to all other samples, including the interesterified

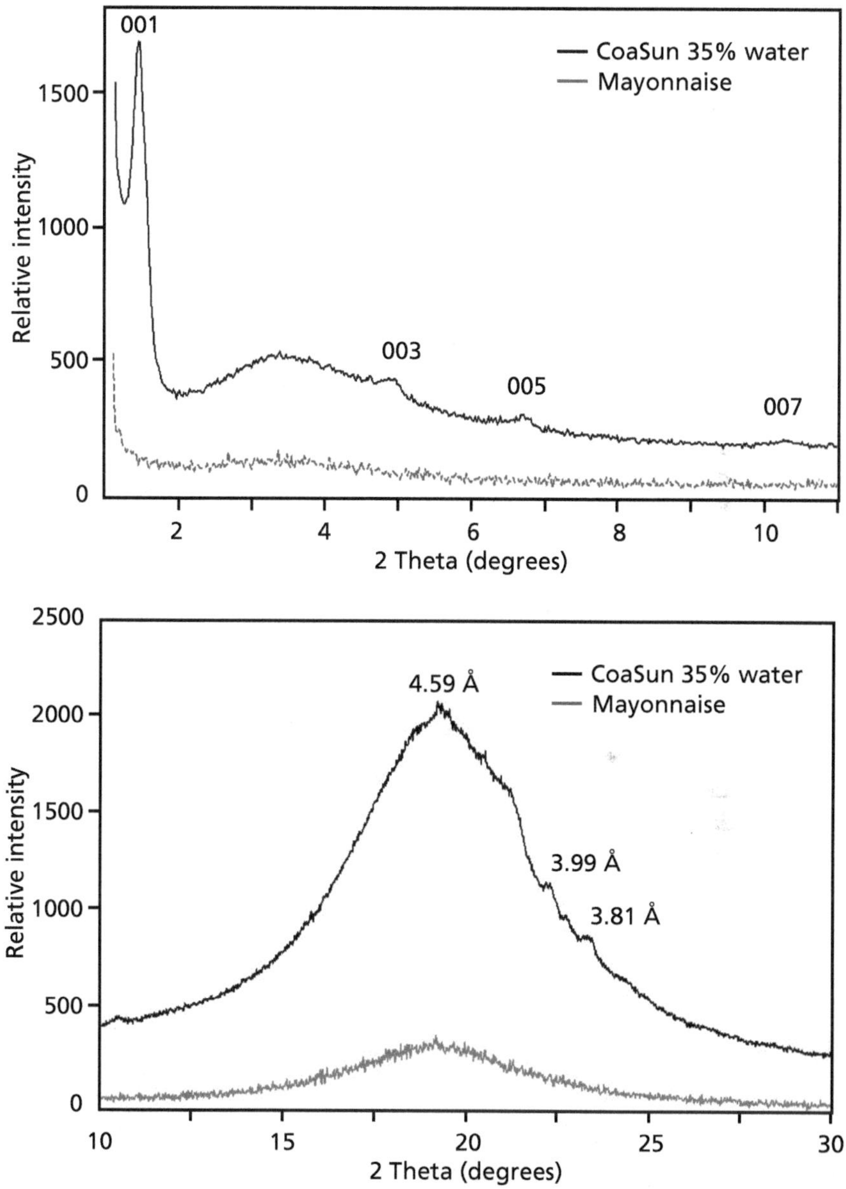

Figure 10.2 Small and wide angle X-ray diffraction spectra for Coasun™ and mayonnaise.

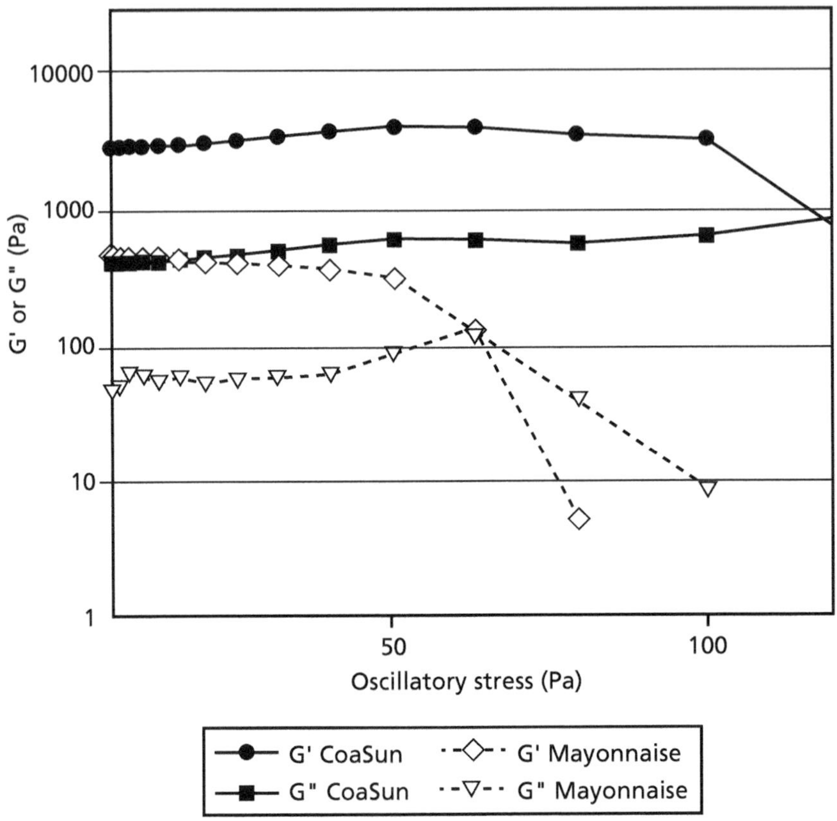

Figure 10.3 Storage modulus (G') and loss modulus (G") for the structured emulsion Coasun™ and a typical oil-in-water emulsion, mayonnaise, over a range of oscillatory stresses.

soy oil, at lipid contents above 6%. This suggests the formation of a softer dough that had been "shortened." This prevention of cross-linkages between gluten molecules was especially noticeable in the dough samples using hard wheat flower, which contains a higher protein (gluten) content compared to soft wheat flower. Preventing gluten aggregation through the use of shortenings is beneficial for baked products that are not reliant on gluten for structure, such as cakes and tarts (Huschka et al., 2011). Based on these results, it is likely that a structured emulsion (Coasun™) could pose as a viable substitute for highly saturated and TFA-rich shortenings in these types of products. The same ingredients used in Coasun™, although not heated and mixed together, were used as a control and did not demonstrate these same shortening properties, signifying the importance of the specific structure of these emulsions rather than simply the presence of the ingredients (Huschka et al., 2011).

Other than a low saturated, and zero *trans* fat content, additional physiological benefits have been discovered after consuming these multilayer structured emulsions. The unique structure of Coasun™ also has shown the ability to help regulate blood lipid and insulin responses in humans and to lower postprandial triacylglycerol levels (Marangoni et al., 2007; Rush et al., 2009). Once again, these lowering effects were not demonstrated when the raw ingredients alone were consumed, or when the structure was destroyed by cooking (Rush et al., 2008). Furthermore, there is potential for nutraceuticals such as phytosterols, omega-3 fatty acids, fat soluble antioxidants, and other compounds (which will be discussed further later in this chapter) to be incorporated into the water or oil component of these structured emulsions as an added nutritional benefit (Zetzl and Marangoni, 2011).

Due to the increased incorporation level of water, the final product is fairly inexpensive, especially when its multitude of potential health benefits are taken into consideration. Although continued research is required as to how these structured emulsions behave in food systems, they may be one of the best solutions to the *trans* fat dilemma, especially in the bakery industry where its shortening-like structure would be ideally suited (Lin and Appleby, 2012).

Organogels

Organogels, also known as *oleogels,* can be defined as an organic liquid entrapped within a thermo-reversible, three-dimensional gel network (Zetzl and Marangoni, 2011). The process of forming an organogel is called *organogelation.* Molecules capable of forming nonpolar aggregated molecular or crystal networks, with the ability of entrapping or structuring oil, were certainly not unheard of in the scientific community and industry prior to the 1990s. However, it was not until the late 1990s that the potential for these molecules to be used as a vegetable oil structurant and food ingredient began to be realized (Co and Marangoni, 2012). As of 2012, there have been several reviews published regarding the many known organogelators, their properties, advantages, and disadvantages (Bot et al., 2009; Co and Marangoni, 2012; Pernetti et al., 2007a; Rogers, 2009).

The following are general categories of network-forming edible oil structurants that have been identified: monoacylglycerols (MAGs), fatty acids, fatty alcohols, waxes, wax esters, sorbitan monostearate, lecithin and sorbitan tri-stearate, and phytosterols and oryzanol (Pernetti et al., 2007a). In addition, the following organogelators or mixtures thereof are well known for having an ability to structure edible oils: 12-hydroxystearic acid (Rogers and Marangoni, 2008; Rogers et al., 2007, 2008; Terech and Weiss, 1997), ricinelaidic acid (Wright and Marangoni, 2006), candelilla wax (Toro-Vazquez et al., 2007), rice bran wax (Dassanayake et al., 2009), sunflower wax (and other waxes) in soybean oil (Hwang et al., 2012), several waxes in canola oil (Blake and Marangoni, 2013), mixtures of β-sitosterol and γ-oryzanol (Bot and Agterof, 2006), mixtures of stearic acid and stearyl alcohol (Gandolfo et al., 2003), mixtures of lecithin and sorbitan tri-stearate (Pernetti et al., 2007b), and more recently, mixed ceramides and ethylcellulose (Rogers, 2011; Zetzl et al., 2012).

Waxes and Wax Organogels

For decades waxes have played an important part outside of the food industry. A wax can be defined as a fatty substance that contains long hydrocarbon chains with or without a functional group (Dassanayake et al., 2011). It is unknown as to how far back their uses go, but the oil structuring ability and texture they provide to products such as lipstick, lip balms, and lotion bars are necessities (Toro-Vazquez et al., 2007). Previously, to structure oil effectively, waxes had to be used at levels close to or in excess of 5%, making them impractical for most food uses because they would impart a waxy mouthfeel. Carnauba wax, for example, is only able to structure oil at levels in excess of 4% (Dassanayake et al., 2009). More recent studies have shown the superior oil-binding ability of certain waxes that are able to gel oil at levels as low as 1% (Blake and Marangoni, 2013; Dassanayake et al., 2011; Toro-Vazquez et al., 2007, 2011). With wax incorporation levels of only a few percent of the fat phase, this may provide a texture and mouthfeel that is more acceptable to consumers.

Candelilla wax is one such wax that shows great potential as an organogelator. Obtained from the leaves of a small shrub native to the southern United States and northern Mexico, candelilla wax consists of 49–50% n-alkanes with 29 to 33 carbons, and 20–29% esters of acids and alcohols with 28 to 34 carbons (Toro-Vazquez et al., 2007, 2011). Candelilla wax has been shown to structure safflower oil at levels as low as 1%, while actual gelation was not found to occur until concentrations were raised to 2% (Toro-Vazquez et al., 2007, 2011). This wax appears to be limited by the type of crystals it forms, which are usually less than 10 μm in size and spherulitic in shape (Toro-Vazquez et al., 2011). To effectively entrap oil, much longer and thinner crystals, such as those formed when using rice bran wax, are usually needed (Co and Marangoni, 2012). Wax derived from rice (*Oryza sativa*) bran possesses long needle-like crystals in oil, ranging from 20 to 50 μm, that are very effective in entrapping oil within a crystalline matrix (Co and Marangoni, 2012; Dassanayake et al., 2011). These crystalline strands are so effective, in fact, that they have been shown to gel oil as low as 1% w/w (Blake and Marangoni, 2013).

With the large production levels of rice in eastern Asia, rice bran wax is very inexpensive, and was traditionally considered a waste product of the rice milling process (Dassanayake et al., 2011). This means that it is largely available and cost effective, with the possibility to greatly reduce the amount of saturated fatty acids while eliminating any TFAs. Unfortunately, gels containing only 1% wax are very soft and have an oily appearance. It is probable that much higher levels would have to be used to produce a fat that is similar to lard or shortening in texture. At such a high incorporation level, it is unknown as to how noticeable and waxy the mouthfeel of the fat would be, which would have a negative effect in regard to consumer perception.

In Figure 10.4, the structure of the aforementioned wax oleogels can be seen at a wax incorporation level of 10% (w/w) in canola oil. These images give a better understanding as to why rice bran wax is able to gel oil at the lowest concentration compared to the other two waxes. Carnauba wax, the wax with the highest critical gelator concentration, formed large, open, dendritic clusters or aggregates, which are not very effective in entrapping oil. Although the structure of candelilla wax is better

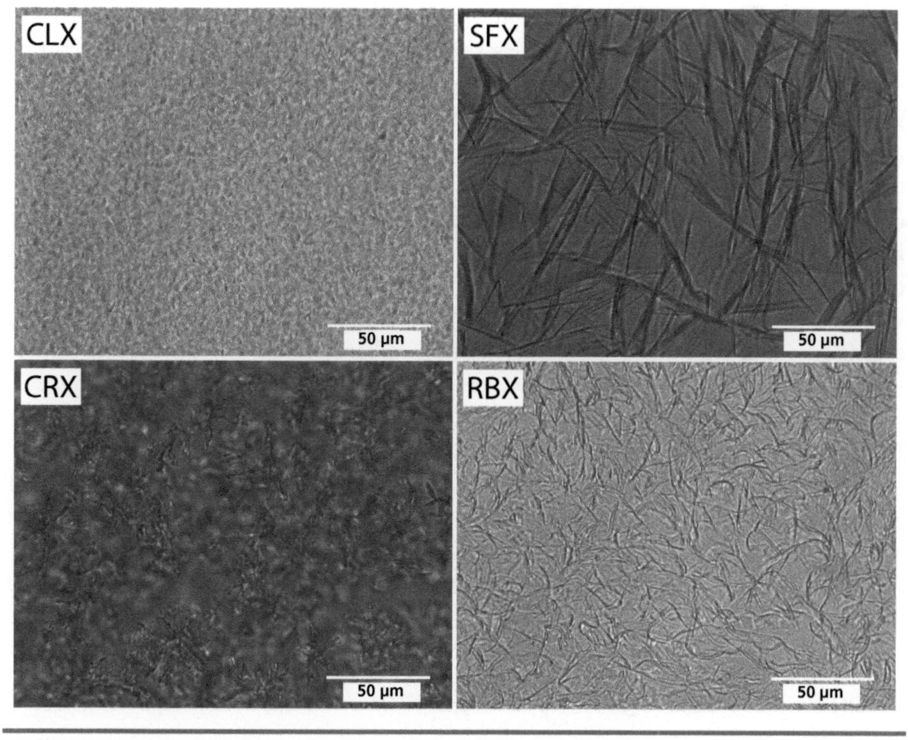

Figure 10.4 Brightfield light micrographs of wax–oil gels consisting of 10% wax (w/w) in canola oil at a temperature of 25 °C. The different waxes are labeled as follows: candelilla wax (CLX), carnauba wax (CRX), sunflower wax (SFX), and rice bran wax (RBX).

for gelling oil compared to carnauba wax, it is only rice bran wax out of the three that forms very long, needle-like crystals that are very effective in forming gels (Blake and Marangoni, 2013; Co and Marangoni, 2012).

Sunflower wax, derived from sunflower seeds, has barely been mentioned in literature compared to these three other waxes, yet it may provide oil-binding properties that are similar or even superior to rice bran wax (Blake and Marangoni, 2013; Hwang et al., 2012). As can be seen in Figure 10.4, sunflower wax has formed crystals that are in excess of 100 μm, which allows for more junction zones to be formed along each crystal strand and increases the strength of the gel network (Blake and Marangoni, 2013; Hwang et al., 2012). Compositional purity has also been shown to have an effect on wax gelation. Minor components in the waxes have the potential to act as impurities, impairing gelation and changing morphology in regard to crystal size and potentially shape (Blake and Marangoni, 2013). While rice bran wax consists of over 90% esters, sunflower wax contains 97–100% esters and contains the fewest minor components out of the four aforementioned waxes (Blake and Marangoni, 2013). This high level of compositional purity also aids in the understanding as to why rice bran and sunflower wax are such good organogelators in comparison to other waxes. Although low critical gelator concentrations can be achieved when using these two waxes, it seems that their ability to hold the oil in its gel state is fairly low, with the percentage oil loss exceeding 50% when gels were made with 1% wax (w/w). Oil loss was measured by placing gel samples inside a glass funnel lined with Whatman #5 filter paper and measuring the amount of oil collected in a beaker below the funnel for 24 hours. In comparison, candelilla wax showed only a 25.8% oil loss at the 1% (w/w) incorporation level, and only 11.1% oil loss at the 2% (w/w) incorporation level (Blake and Marangoni, 2013). Although oil loss values are dependent on the test conditions, these differences show that there are a variety of factors that should be taken into consideration when choosing a wax for organogelation purposes, not just the critical gelation concentration.

Clearly there is great potential in the field of waxes to structure oils, although many questions still remain, especially in regard to how these gels will behave in food systems. Although they have the possibility to become a substitute or solution to TFAs in the future, a significant amount of research and development must still take place in this field.

Oleogels Made Using 12-Hydroxystearic Acid

Similar to waxes, the low molecular weight organogelator 12-hydroxystearic acid (12-HSA) also has the ability to gel vegetable oil at levels below 2% (w/w) (Hughes et al., 2011). This molecule is derived from castor oil, and has been used for decades by industry in the production of lithium grease (Co and Marangoni, 2012). Structurally,

12-HSA is 18 carbons long and possesses a hydroxyl group at position 12 (Rogers and Marangoni, 2011). Oleogels are formed by heating the 12-HSA-in-oil mixture to above the melting point of the 12-HSA, which occurs at approximately 76 °C (Co and Marangoni, 2012). Upon cooling, 12-HSA fibers form throughout the oil, growing one dimensionally to hundreds of micrometers in length. In Figure 10.5, a bright to dark striation pattern can be seen on each of these fibrillar crystals. This is the result of a helical twist of the 12-HSA fibers, causing them to pass in and out of birefringence under polarized light (Co and Marangoni, 2012; Rogers and Marangoni, 2011). An extensive characterization of these oleogels has been previously described by Rogers and Marangoni (2011) and Co and Marangoni (2012), though it is perhaps the health implications of consuming such an oleogel that are of greatest interest to the food industry.

A review chapter by Hughes et al. (2011) reported the results of a clinical trial reported in which subjects were fed standardized test meals that differed only by the fat source they contained, which were butter, margarine, canola oil, or gelled canola oil (using 12-HSA) (Hughes et al., 2011). After consumption of the test meals, blood samples were taken every hour for six hours and were analyzed for triacylglycerols, free fatty acids, glucose, and insulin levels. No significant differences were found between the treatments in regard to glucose or insulin levels; however, the oleogel and canola oil meals significantly reduced the serum triacylglycerol response curves, compared to those from the margarine and butter meals, for the

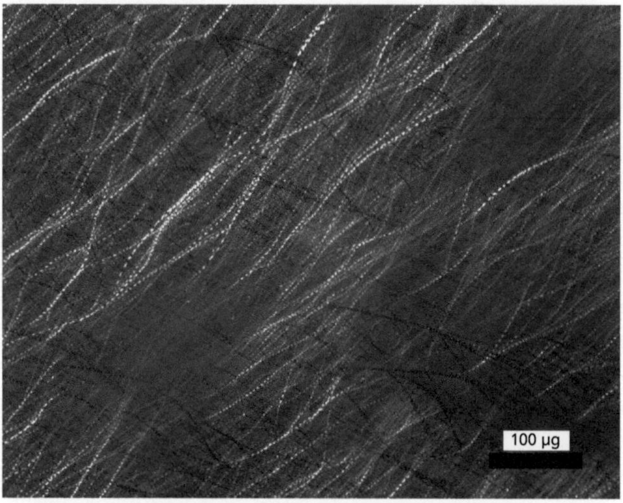

Figure 10.5 A polarized light micrograph showing the fibrillar crystals of 12-hydroxystearic acid in canola oil at a concentration of 2.5% (w/w).

majority of the measurements (Hughes et al., 2011). The oil gelled with 2% w/w 12-HSA also showed the lowest maximum serum free fatty acid levels compared to all other meals (though it was not significantly less than the meal containing canola oil) (Hughes et al., 2011). These effects are added benefits that go beyond the fatty acid compositional benefits provided by all oleogels made with a high percentage of vegetable oil. Although this study utilized 12-HSA, it is possible that, if consumed in a similar manner, oleogels made using other oraganogelators could show similar beneficial physiological effects.

While 12-HSA is an exceptional organogelator, it unfortunately does not currently have full food-grade status (Co and Marangoni, 2012). In addition, for any food systems in which the shearing or mixing of these oleogels would be required, the use of 12-HSA as the organogelator would not be possible because the long fibrillar crystals are very delicate and essentially shatter under these conditions. This damage to the fibrillar network is nonrecoverable and results in a high percentage of oil loss. It is therefore likely that while oleogels show a great deal of potential in food systems, it is probable that other organogelators, such as polymers, will be used in place of the fibrillar network forming 12-HSA.

Ethylcellulose (Polymer) Oleogels

For the purposes of creating a food-grade oleogel, the use of a polymer such as ethylcellulose (EC) is highly novel, although this is rather surprising considering that its solubility properties were reported as early as 1937. The work of W. Koch stated that "solubility in both polar and nonpolar organic solvents is best with ethylcellulose of substitutions between 2.4 and 2.5 ethoxy groups" (Koch, 1937). At the time, this must have seemed like a trivial detail; however, this means that EC can be used as an organogelator of food-grade oils, as a common vegetable oil would classify as a nonpolar solvent. It is likely that this detail was originally simply overlooked, as there was no need to create a substitute for *trans* or saturated fats. Not until the past decade has the potential of oleogels, and in particular polymer oleogels, become fully realized. Figure 10.6A shows an example of a firm and stable oleogel made using only soybean oil and ethylcellulose, while 10.6B shows a laminate-type pastry where an oleogel replaced 50% of the traditionally used fat (discussed further in the "Production Considerations and Food Applications of Ethylcellulose Oleogels" section).

Ethylcellulose is a chemically modified version of the plant cell wall–based polymer cellulose. Ethylcellulose differs from cellulose only by the substitution of hydroxyl groups for ethoxyl groups, with a maximum of three substitutions possible. Solubility in water is achieved when the average substitution is between 1 and 1.5, while only in the narrow range of 2.4–2.5 substitutions, 47–48% ethoxy content, is solubility in oil possible (Zetzl and Marangoni, 2011; Zetzl et al., 2012). Though solubility in

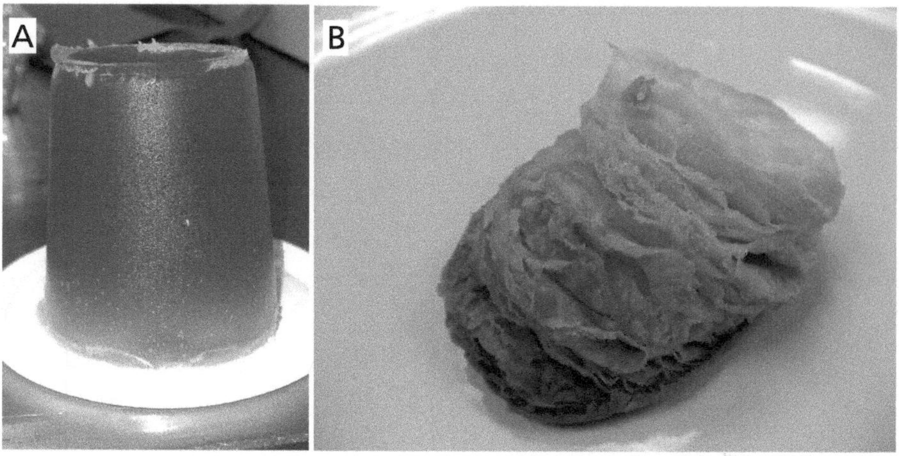

Figure 10.6 (A) Ethylcellulose oleogel consisting of 10% 45 cP ethylcellulose (w/w) and 90% soybean oil. The oleogel remains stable and is very solid at room temperature. (B) A laminate type pastry made with a 50% substitution of butter with an ethylcellulose oleogel.

oil was not a requirement of the commercial product, the 2.4–2.5 substitution level has been the standard substitution level used by industry since the 1930s. Compared to organogelators used in the past, ethylcellulose is rather inexpensive and can be produced (and purchased) in large volumes. This makes the large-scale use of EC for organogelation both possible and feasible.

For solubility in oil to occur, the ethylcellulose must be heated above the glass transition temperature (T_g), which occurs at approximately 130 °C. A variety of molecular weights are available, expressed as a cP value, with 10–100 cP being the range that is most practical for organogelation purposes. Molecular weights can be calculated, but they are not provided by ethylcellulose suppliers (Zetzl et al., 2012). Table 10.B shows the melting point, as well as the onset, midpoint, and final temperature for the glass transition of three varieties of ethylcellulose, in addition to the matching cP values and calculated molecular weights. Figure 10.7 shows a sample differential scanning thermograph of 10, 45, and 100 cP ethylcellulose powder, which can be used to determine the T_g and melting point of the polymer. Though it is only the T_g that is needed to create a gel, the melting point for these varieties is useful information because at temperatures above this point it is highly likely that the polymer will begin to break down or degrade. By remaining within the functional range between the T_g and the melting temperature, the quality of the EC can be preserved while retaining its ability to make oleogels.

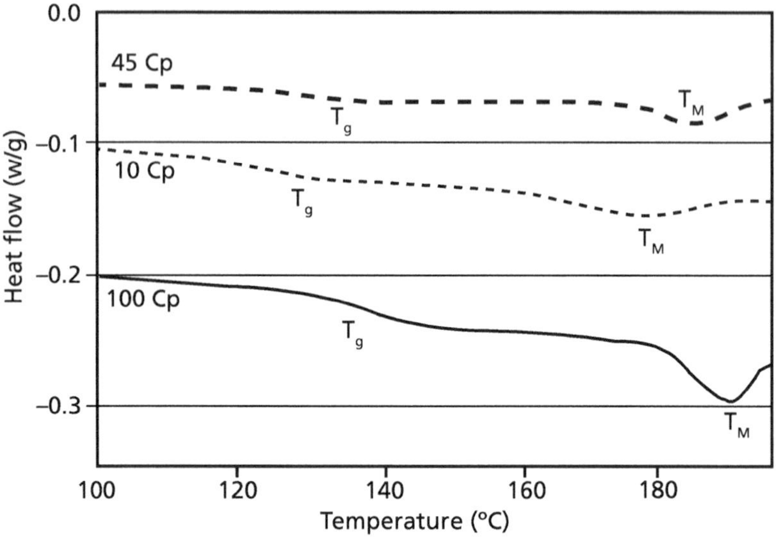

Figure 10.7 Sample differential scanning calorimetry thermogram showing the glass transition and melting for 10, 45, and 100 cP ethylcellulose powder.

A great deal is already known about the mechanical properties of EC oleogels. Recent studies have shown that the mechanical strength of these gels is highly dependant on the fatty acid composition of the vegetable oils used in making the gels (Figure 10.8) (Laredo et al., 2011; Zetzl et al., 2012). Oils such as canola, which contain a fairly low comparative degree of unsaturation (approximately 60% oleic acid, 18:1), produce fairly soft gels. Flaxseed oil, which contains close to 60% linolenic acid (18:3), produces substantially harder gels (Laredo et al., 2011; Zetzl et al., 2012). This increase in gel hardness corresponds to a statistically similar change in the elastic modulus of gel samples made with different vegetable oils. It is believed that these differences are caused by a change in the molar density of the oils within the gels. Essentially, oils with a higher degree of unsaturation are able to pack more tightly within the gel network, causing a firmer gel (Laredo et al., 2011; Zetzl et al., 2012). Even prior to gelation, a relationship can be seen regarding level of unsaturation and molar density. At 25 °C, canola oil has a density of 0.9134 g/cm^{-3}; soybean oil, 0.9167 g/cm^{-3}; and flaxseed oil, 0.9250 g/cm^{-3} (Laredo et al., 2011). Attenuated total internal reflection infrared spectroscopy has been used to look at the differences between these oils in their gelled state. As the level of unsaturation increased, so did the intensity ratio between the band at 3007 cm^{-1} (=C-H stretching) and 2870 cm^{-1} (CH_3 symmetric stretching). This signifies an increasing difference in the level of =C-H stretching between the gels and the pure oils as unsaturation increases (Laredo

Table 10.B Glass transition and melting temperatures for ethylcellulose powder of different molecular weights, determined using a TA Instruments Q1000 differential scanning colorimeter with a temperature ramp of 5 °C / min. Letters indicate significance at a confidence level of 95% for three replicates using a Tukey post-test, while standard error is indicated after the ± symbol.

Ethylcellulose viscosity[a]	10 cP	45 cP	100 cP
Ethylcellulose molecular weight[b]	24 kDa	57 kDa	74 kDa
T_g onset temperature	$125.0^{a} \pm 0.57$	$130.6^{ab} \pm 0.13$	$131.1^{b} \pm 2.02$
T_g mid-point temperature (°C)	$131.0^{bde} \pm 0.15$	$137.8^{c} \pm 0.33$	$136.1^{cd} \pm 2.79$
T_g final temperature (°C)	$136.1^{ce} \pm 0.53$	$141.1^{cf} \pm 0.67$	$146.0^{f} \pm 0.05$
Melting point (°C)	$178.8^{g} \pm 0.35$	$185.8^{h} \pm 0.36$	$188.2^{h} \pm 0.91$

[a]Determined by making a 5% solution of ethylcellulose in a solvent (80% toluene and 20% ethanol), and measuring at 25 °C in a rotational viscometer.

[b]As calculated in Zetzl et al. (2012).

et al., 2011). In addition, Raman spectroscopy revealed a higher number of *gauche* conformers in the gels compared to the pure oils, with the fatty acid chains becoming more disordered or bent when they were in their gelled state (Laredo et al., 2011). This supports the hypothesis that the linolenic acid molecules in flaxseed oil are more tightly packed within the gel network compared to the oleic acid molecules in canola oil. It is possible that analysis of scanning electron and atomic force micrographs could provide additional evidence regarding the density of the gel network when using vegetable oils containing different unsaturation levels.

The effect of polymer molecular weight has also been shown to have a significant impact on the mechanical properties of these polymer oleogels. As previously mentioned, molecular weight is expressed as a cP value, with ethylcellulose of 10 cP possessing a lower molecular weight, on average, than 20, 45, or 100 cP. Increases in molecular weight have been shown to produce gels that were significantly harder than low molecular weight varieties (Figure 10.8). Compared to 10 cP, oleogels made with 45 cP are nearly 10 times harder, while gels made using 100 cP ethylcellulose are more than 20 times harder when using soybean oil (Zetzl et al., 2012). As higher molecular weight varieties of ethylcellulose would contain longer polymer chains, it is hypothesized that these longer chains would be able to form a higher number of junction zones, improving network strength.

Polymer concentration is one additional factor that has a very significant effect on gel strength. When using 45 cP ethylcellulose, critical gelator concentrations of 4% and 6% were determined when using soybean and canola oil, respectively (Zetzl et al., 2012). In addition, when the hardness values at different polymer concentrations were plotted, both canola oil and soybean oil followed a power-law function with a

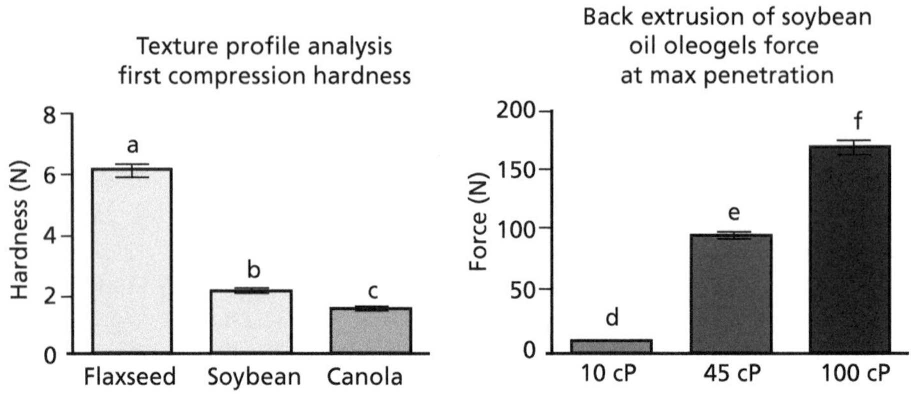

Figure 10.8 Texture profile analysis and back extrusion results for testing the mechanical properties of oleogels made with 10% ethylcellulose (w/w) in vegetable oil. The texture profile analysis results show the effect of oil type on hardness, while the back extrusion results illustrate the differences in hardness due to ethylcellulose molecular weight.

scaling factor of approximately 6, with an r^2 value of 0.99 (Zetzl et al., 2012). Using this data, it might be possible to predict the approximate hardness of gels made with a certain polymer concentration.

Imaging the Polymer Network Structure of Ethylcellulose Oleogels

Attempting to image the polymer network structure of a polymer oleogel such as this has posed a great challenge. Many organogelators display birefringence under polarized light, allowing networks or dispersions to be easily viewed using a polarized light microscope, as previously shown in Figure 10.5. When EC in water or oil is viewed under polarized light prior to heating, some birefringence can be observed, as shown in Figure 10.9A. Typically, a glass should not show any birefringence under polarized light; however, it appears that after the production process to the glassy state, crystallinity of some sort is still present in the ethylcellulose powder. This crystallinity can also be seen when using small angle X-ray scattering (SAXS), where 10 cP ethylcellulose powder produces a diffraction peak corresponding to a lattice parameter of 57.97 Å. Although a diffraction peak is seen in the SAXS region, there are no identifiable peaks in the wide angle region.

These results indicate that no crystalline packing of the ethylcellulose chains is occurring, yet it is possible that crystalline arrangements or bundles of ethylcellulose are forming, resulting in the diffraction peak in the small angle region. In cellulose,

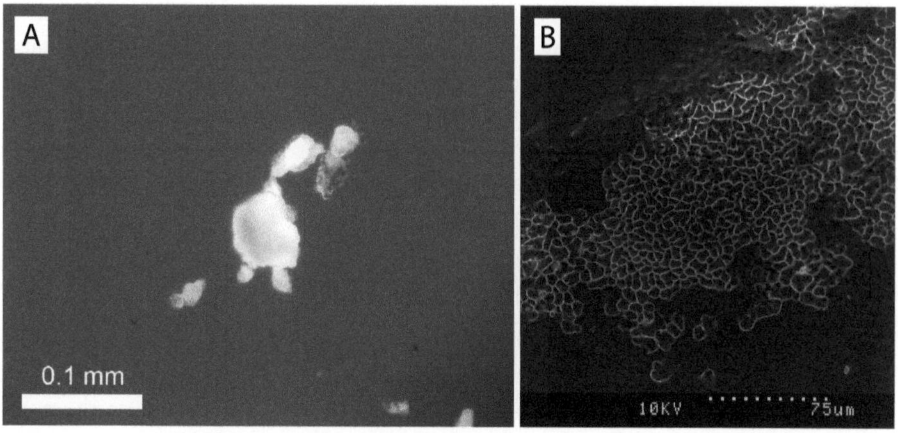

Figure 10.9 (A) Polarized light micrograph of 10 cP ethylcellulose powder in water. (B) A cryo-scanning electron micrograph of a canola oil organogel using 45 cP ethylcellulose, treated with 3.4 mL of isobutanol to remove surface oil.

individual cellulose chains interact via van der Waals and hydrogen bonding, forming microfibrils, which can be identified by a diffraction peak in the SAXS region (Müller et al., 1998). The exact position of the peak is highly variable, depending on the size and arrangement of the microfibrils, which is organism specific (Müller et al., 1998). The mean diameter of microfibrils has been shown to range from 25 to 200 Å, depending on the source of the cellulose (Müller et al., 1998). The 57.97 Å peak noted for ethylcellulose falls within this range and may indicate a similar grouping or bundling of ethylcellulose chains, which show birefringence under polarized light. After oleogels are made through heating of the ethylcellulose, any noted crystallinity disappears completely because birefringence is no longer seen under polarized light and no peaks are visible in the SAXS region. This means that techniques other than polarized light microscopy or powder XRD have to be utilized to try to view the microstructure of these polymer oleogels.

Preliminary images taken using cryo-scanning electron microscopy using a freeze-fracture technique also did not uncover many details in regard to the polymer network structure (Laredo et al., 2011). The work of Dey et al. (2011) also shows cryo-scanning electron micrographs of ethylcellulose oleogels. These researchers submerged 0.2 g gel samples into 40 mL of solvent in an attempt to expose a polymer network structure; however, yet again, few clear structures were discernible (Dey et al., 2011). Finally, in 2012, by using only a small amount of solvent in an attempt to wash away only oil at the surface of the oleogel, it was possible to uncover a view of the polymer network structure below, as shown in Figure 10.9B (Zetzl et al.,

2012). This image shows what is believed to be a continuous polymer network of ethylcellulose strands surrounding pores that would normally be filled with vegetable oil. Without the use of a solvent, the sample surface is completely smooth, as can be seen on the top and bottom portion of Figure 10.9B. Through the analysis of cryo-scanning electron micrographs, it is possible that these images may reveal further details regarding ethylcellulose oleogels, including a possible connection between gel microstructure and mechanical properties.

Production Considerations and Food Applications of Ethylcellulose Oleogels

On a slightly negative note, it appears that the preparation method used to produce ethylcellulose oleogels has a significant effect on gel properties, in particular, the number of oxidation products found in the sample (Gravelle et al., 2012). An increase in the thiobarbituric acid (TBA) value can be seen with extended holding time above the glass transition temperature (Gravelle et al., 2012). This value, along with the peroxide value, can give a good indication as to the level of oxidation in a vegetable oil. For canola oil oleogels, the TBA value increased from just over 0.08 to close to 0.13 after 90 minutes holding time above the T_g (Gravelle et al., 2012). The peroxide value of these gels also increased from approximately 2.5 meq/kg to approximately 14 meq/kg after 60 minutes (Gravelle et al., 2012). It was suggested that a holding time of 20 minutes should be used, as any longer and the oil quality would no longer be acceptable based on the peroxide values (Gravelle et al., 2012). In addition, an increase in the percent of total polar components was also noted as a function of holding time, increasing from 2.5% at 0 minutes to 4.0% and 6.5% after 60 and 120 minutes, respectively (Gravelle et al., 2012). The higher prevalence of these oxidation components caused a significant increase in the mechanical strength of the oleogels. It is believed that as the polarity of the oil increases, it is able to form hydrogen bonds to the ethylcellulose, helping to increase the strength of the gel network (Gravelle et al., 2012).

When heating a vegetable oil to temperatures in excess of 100 °C, oxidation will always be a factor. As previously mentioned, to produce these gels, a temperature in excess of 140 °C is required, which is above the glass transition temperature of the ethylcellulose powder (~135 °C). This causes not only oxidation of the oil, but also has the potential to degrade any surfactants used, in addition to degrading of the polymer itself. It was, therefore, necessary to develop a standard procedure for the production of these gels, as described by Gravelle et al. (2012), to improve reproducibility and reduce oxidation. By combining this improved production method with an antioxidant such as butylated hydroxytoluene (BHT), it is likely that the overall acceptance of the produced oleogels in regard to palatability would be greatly improved.

Something unique about ethylcellulose oleogels compared to most other oleogels is that they have actually been used in real food systems as a replacement for more highly saturated animal fats. A number of recent studies have discussed potential applications of these gels, including their use in cookies, comminuted meat products, creams for various fillings (predominately baked goods), and chocolate (Stortz and Marangoni, 2011; Stortz et al., 2012; Zetzl et al., 2012). Figure 10.10 shows cooked ground and comminuted meat products that were made using 100% replacement of added animal fat with ethylcellulose oleogels. This replacement significantly reduced the amount of saturated fat in these products. While nongelled oil tends to leak out of the ground products, or make comminuted meat products significantly harder and chewier, gelling the oil prevents both of these problems. Oil is immobilized, and is not lost from breakfast sausages upon cutting, while cooked comminuted meat products made with gelled canola oil showed no significant differences in regard to chewiness and hardness when compared to a beef fat control product (Zetzl et al., 2012). This textural improvement compared to products made with nongelled oil appears to be caused by an increase in the size of the fat/oil globules in the cooked meat batter. As can be seen in Figure 10.11, the average fat globule size is greatly increased once the oil is in its gel form. Although these globules are still smaller than those found in the beef fat products, this increase in size still has a great impact on product texture. It is believed that the smaller globules in the canola oil product allow for a larger surface area to be coated by proteins, increasing the strength of the protein network (Zetzl et al., 2012).

Outside of meat systems, ethylcellulose oleogels have also very recently been used in the production of pastries, in particular, laminate type products that are notorious for being difficult to produce with any fat other than butter. The product shown in

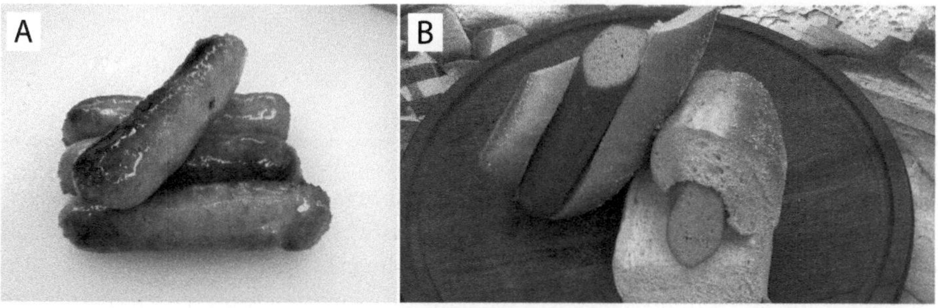

Figure 10.10 (A) Breakfast sausages (a ground meat product) and (B) frankfurters (a comminuted meat product) containing a 100% replacement of the traditionally added animal fat with an ethylcellulose oleogel.

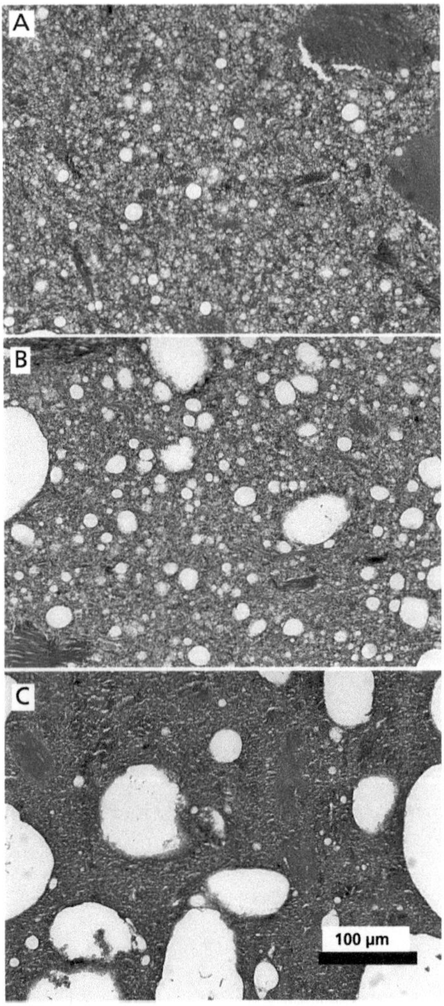

Figure 10.11 Cooked comminuted meat batter micrographs with various fat sources: (A) canola oil, (B) canola oil oleogel, and (C) beef fat. The white circular globules are fat globules (removed during the paraffin embedding process), while the dark surrounding area is the protein network in which some small intact muscle fibers still exist. The scale bar is the same for all three images, and is 100 μm.

Figure 10.6B contains a 50% replacement of butter with an ethylcellulose oleogel, significantly reducing the amount of saturated fat while still allowing the formation of lamination layers. Creams for the purpose of fillings in the baking industry can also be made using ethylcellulose oleogels, reducing oil migration from the filling into the surrounding product and also improving the fatty acid profile of the cream. Creams consisting of 60% gelled vegetable oil and 40% interesterified palm oil showed almost 0% oil leakage after 12 days, while creams made with nongelled oil showed close to 25% oil leakage (wt%/g sample) after 12 days (Stortz et al., 2012).

Although the primary focus of these replacement experiments was to reduce the amount of saturated fat while retaining functionality, it may be very possible to use ethylcellulose oleogels as a method to reduce *trans* fat in similar products. The baking industry in particular still has many items, including donuts, muffins, and cookies, that are high in saturated fat and still contain *trans* fat. If these gels are able to replace saturated fat in such a wide variety of products, while at the same time retaining product texture and palatability, it is possible they can be used in similar products to finally eliminate any *trans* fat they still contain.

In North America, ethylcellulose is currently approved for indirect food uses, such as use in inks to mark fruits and vegetables, and as a component of paper and paperboard that is in contact with fatty or water-based foods (Zetzl and Marangoni, 2011). In Europe, ethylcellulose has been approved for food uses since late 2006 (Zetzl and Marangoni, 2011). Internationally, the Food and Agriculture Organization of the United Nations, in collaboration with the World Health Organization, has listed ethylcellulose as a food additive that may be used in a variety of foods under the conditions of good manufacturing practices as outlined in the Preamble of the Codex GSFA (FAO and WHO, 2012). Some of the foods listed include processed comminuted meat, poultry and game products, fat spreads, fat emulsions, cheeses, bakery wares, and confectionery products (FAO and WHO, 2012). Although EC may not yet have full food-grade status worldwide, it is highly likely that such a development will occur in the near future.

Using Oleogels for Nutraceutical Delivery or Encapsulation

There have been recent discussions into how to make an oleogel, usually consisting of at least 90% vegetable oil, even healthier. One of the easiest ways to do so would be to use the oleogel to deliver lipid-soluble nutraceuticals. Nutraceuticals can be defined as "a food (or part of a food) that provides medical or health benefits, including the prevention and/or treatment of a disease" (Brower, 1998). For incorporation into an oleogel, it would be most advantageous to use a fairly purified compound because it would not be hindered or restricted by the food matrix where it was originally contained. Oil-soluble compounds such as omega-3 fatty acids, the carotenoids β-carotene and lycopene, phytosterols, coenzyme Q, and vitamin E have all been identified as potential compounds of interest for incorporation into oleogel systems (Zetzl and Marangoni, 2012). These compounds are discussed in detail elsewhere; however, some of their benefits include decreased platelet aggregation, blood viscosity, and fibrinogen; antioxidant properties; and lower incidences of chronic disease, including cardiovascular disease and certain cancers, in particular, prostate, breast, and lung cancer (Zetzl and Marangoni, 2012). Clearly, the addition of any one of these compounds to an oleogel would have a significant impact on its healthfulness.

The availability/presence of dietary fat also has a significant impact on the absorption of most of the aforementioned molecules, as they are all at least partly fat soluble.

The difficulty in incorporating any one of these nutraceutical compounds lies in trying to minimize degradation. Many of these compounds contain a large number of double bonds, and they would degrade very quickly if exposed to the high heat required to create an ethylcellulose oleogel, for example. By adding these compounds during the cooling process, just before gelation occurs, this could maximize the quality and effectiveness of any added nutraceuticals.

Phytosterol–Oryzanol Mixtures for Organogelation Purposes

Phytosterols are compounds of particular interest, as they not only possess cholesterol-reducing properties, but also certain varieties can be used as organogelators (Bot and Flöter, 2011). Mixtures of β-sitosterol and γ-oryzanol in vegetable oil can be used to form optically transparent (when a 1:1 molar ratio of structurant is used) or hazy/semi-opaque gels at incorporation levels as low as 2–4% total sterols at 5 °C (Bot and Flöter, 2011; Bot et al., 2009). It is proposed that these components are able to structure the vegetable oil by forming tubules with a diameter of approximately 7.2 nm and a wall thickness of 0.8 nm (Bot and Flöter, 2011). These tubules are able to aggregate and interact, effectively forming a network and entrapping the liquid oil (Co and Marangoni, 2012). The small size of these tubules—smaller than the wavelength of visible light—gives an explanation as to why they are able to form optically transparent gels (Bot and Flöter, 2011). Although these phytosterol–oryzanol mixtures are very effective at gelling oil when used together, this gelation does not take place when one of the components is excluded. Instead, sterol or sterol ester crystals are formed and simply settle to the bottom of the container without gelling or structuring the liquid oil (Co and Marangoni, 2012).

The β-sitosterol and γ-oryzanol mixture in vegetable oil is one of the first oleogel systems that consists entirely of food-grade or near-food-grade materials (Bot and Flöter, 2011). This is a major step forward in the field of organogelation, as most organogelators to date have not been even given GRAS (generally recognized as safe) status or letters of no objection from governing bodies (Co and Marangoni, 2012). An extensive summary of the β-sitosterol and γ-oryzanol system was completed by Bot and Flöter (2011), providing a concise review of the work completed on these components as organogelators thus far.

Although the prospect of phytosterol-based oleogels appears very promising, they unfortunately suffer from significant limitation in regard to food applications. In the presence of water, the surfactant-like organogelators have a reduced ability to structure oil (Bot and Flöter, 2011). In a system such as a baked good or meat emulsion, compatibility with water is a critical property. Because the gelling capabilities of β-sitosterol and γ-oryzanol are so greatly affected by water, it has been suggested that they will most likely only be effective gelators in an anhydrous system (Bot and Flöter, 2011). Moreover, most low-molecular weight gelators that form self-assembled fibrillar networks are extremely shear sensitive. This is unfortunate since most food manufacturing processes as well as the actual food consumption involve high levels of shear. In addition, the high cost of sterols and sterolesters further renders these organogelators applicable for only more specific applications, where a greater cost can be justified. Therefore, even with the promising health benefits of such a nutraceutical organogelator, it is unlikely that we will be seeing a phytosterol-based oleogel on supermarket shelves in the near future.

Even though clearly many technical challenges still exist, there have been great advancements in recent replacements for TFAs, in particular, the development of structured emulsions using monoglycerides and edible oleogels. The promise of incorporating additional nutraceuticals into these substitutes further increases their value, as they would become essentially free of unhealthy fatty acids and would contain highly beneficial nutraceuticals. Due to these factors, both structured emulsions and certain edible oleogels could be considered "solutions" to the *trans* fat problem.

Conclusion

Although many promising solutions to TFAs have been proposed and are currently in use, development is still required to ensure that we are not just simply substituting *trans* fats with something that is equally, or similarly, harmful. We should attempt to develop solutions that not only provide all the requirements of a viable substitute, but also ideally contain components or ingredients that actually improve our cardiovascular health, such as phytosterols or polyunsaturated fatty acids. With the development of many functional and comparatively healthy replacements over the past five years, such as oleogels and structured emulsions using monoglycerides, it is possible that we may be able to overcome the *trans* fat problem in the near future.

Funding

We acknowledge funding from the Natural Sciences and Engineering Research Council of Canada and the Ontario Ministry of Agriculture and Food. We would also like to thank Fernanda Svaikauskas for technical assistance with rheology and X-ray diffraction.

References

Batte, H. D.; Wright, A. J.; Rush, J. W.; Idziak, S. H. J.; Marangoni, A. G. Phase Behavior, Stability, and Mesomorphism of Monostearin-oil-water Gels. *Food Biophys.* **2007a,** *2,* 29–37. DOI: 10.1007/s11483–007–9026–7.

Batte, H.; Wright, A. J.; Idziak, S. H. J.; Marangoni, A. G. Effect of Processing Conditions on the Structure of Monostearin-oil Water Gels. *Food Res. Int.* **2007b,** *40,* 982–988.

Blake, A. I.; Marangoni, A. G. Structure and Physical Properties of Wax Crystal Networks and Their Relationship to Oil Binding Capacity. *J. Am. Oil Chem. Soc.,* submitted for publication, 2013.

Bot, A.; Agterof, W. G. M. Structuring of Edible Oils by Mixtures of γ-Oryzanol with β-Sitosterol or Related Phytosterols. *J. Am. Oil Chem. Soc.* **2006,** *83,* 513–521.

Bot, A.; Flöter, E. Edible Oil Oleogels Based on Self-assembled β-Sitosterol and γ-Oryzanol Tubules. In *Edible Oleogels;* Marangoni, A. G., Garti, N., Eds.; AOCS Press: Urbana, IL, 2011; pp 49–80.

Bot, A.; Veldhuizen, Y. S. J.; den Adel, R.; Roijers, E. C. Non-TAG Structuring of Edible Oils and Emulsions. *Food Hydrocoll.* **2009,** *23,* 1184–1189.

Brower, V. Nutraceuticals: Poised for a Healthy Slice of the Healthcare Market? *Nat. Biotechnol.* **1998,** *16,* 728–731.

Co, E. D.; Marangoni, A. G. Organogels: An Alternative Edible Oil-Structuring Method. *J. Am. Oil Chem. Soc.* **2012,** *89,* 749–780. DOI: 10.1007/s11746-012-2049-3.

Dassanayake, L. S. K.; Kodali, D. R.; Ueno, S.; Sato, K. Physical Properties of Rice Bran Wax in Bulk and Organogels. *J. Am. Oil Chem. Soc.* **2009,** 86, 1163–1173.

Dassanayake, L. S. K., Kodali, D. R.; Ueno, S.; Sato, K. Physical Properties of Organogels Made of Rice Bran Wax and Vegetable Oils. In *Edible Oleogels;* Marangoni, A. G., Garti, N., Eds.; AOCS Press: Urbana, IL, 2011; pp 149–172.

Dey, T.; Kim, D. A.; Marangoni, A. G. Ethylcellulose Oleogels. In *Edible Oleogels;* Marangoni, A. G., Garti, N., Eds.; AOCS Press: Urbana, IL, 2011, pp 295–312.

Food and Agriculture Organization of the United Nations (FAO) in collaboration with the World Health Organization (WHO). Food additive details—Ethylcellulose (462). http://www.codexalimentarius.net/gsfaonline/additives/details.html?id=356 (accessed October 2012).

Gandolfo, F. G.; Bot, A.; Flöter, E. Phase Diagram of Mixtures of Stearic Acid and Stearyl Alcohol. *Thermochim Acta* **2003,** *404,* 9–17.

Gravelle, A. J.; Barbut, S.; Marangoni, A. G. Ethylcellulose Oleogels: Manufacturing Considerations and Effects of Oil Oxidation. *Food Res. Int.* **2012,** *48* (2), 578–583.

Gunstone, F. D.; Harwood, J. L. Occurrence and Characterisation of Oils and Fats. In *The Lipid Handbook,* 3rd ed.; Gunstone, F. D., Harwood, J. L., Dijkstra, A. J., Eds.; CRC Press: Boca Raton, FL, 2007; pp 37–142.

Health Canada. Trans fat Monitoring program—fourth set of monitoring data. http://www.hc-sc.gc.ca/fn-an/nutrition/gras-trans-fats/tfa-age_four-data_quatr-donn-eng.php (accessed June 2012).

Hughes, N.; Rush, J. W.; Marangoni, A. G. Clinical Study on 12-Hydroxystearic Acid on Organogel Ingestion. In *Edible Oleogels;* Marangoni, A. G., Garti, N., Eds.; AOCS Press: Urbana, IL, 2011; pp 313–330.

Hunter, J. E.; Zhang J.; Kris-Etherton, P. M. Cardiovascular Disease Risk of Dietary Stearic Acid Compared with *Trans*, Other Saturated, and Unsaturated Fatty Acids: A Systematic Review. *Am. J. Clin. Nutr.* **2010,** *91,* 46–63.

Huschka, B.; Challacombe, C.; Marangoni, A. G.; Seetharaman, K. Comparison of Oil, Shortening, and a Structured Shortening on Wheat Dough Rheology and Starch Pasting Properties. *Cereal Chem.* **2011,** *88* (3), 253–259.

Hwang, H.; Kim, S.; Singh, M.; Winkler-Moser, J. K.; Liu, S. X. Organogel Formation of Soybean Oil with Waxes. *J. Am. Oil. Chem. Soc.* **2012,** *89* (4), 639–647.

Judd, J. T.; Clevidence, B. A.; Muesing, R. A.; Wittes, J.; Sunkin, M. E.; Podczasy, J. J. Dietary *Trans* Fatty Acids: Effects on Plasma Lipids and Lipoproteins of Healthy Men and Women. *Am. J. Clin. Nutr.* **1994,** *59,* 861–868.

Klag, M. J.; Ford, D. E.; Mead, L. A.; He, J.; Whelton, P. K.; Liang, K. Y.; Levine, D. M. Serum Cholesterol in Young Men and Subsequent Cardiovascular Disease. *New Eng. J. Med.* **1993,** *328* (5), 313–318.

Koch, W. Properties and Uses of Ethylcellulose. *Ind. Eng. Chem.* **1937,** *29* (6), 687–690.

Kodali, D. R. *Trans* Fats—Chemistry, Occurrence, Functional Need in Foods and Potential Solutions. In Trans *Fats Alternatives;* Kodali, D. R., List, G. R., Eds.; AOCS Press: Urbana, IL, 2005; pp 1–25.

Kris-Ehterton, P. M.; Hecker, K. D.; Binkoski, A. E. Polyunsaturated Fatty Acids and Cardiovascular Health. *Nutr. Rev.* **2004,** *62* (11), 414–426.

Laredo, T.; Barbut, S.; Marangoni, A. G. Molecular Interactions of Polymer Oleogelation. *Soft Matter* **2011,** *7,* 2734–2743.

LaRosa, J. C.; Hunninghake, D.; Bush, D.; Criqui, M. H.; Getz, G. S.; Gotto, A. M.; Grundy, S. M.; Rakita, L.; Robertson, R. M.; Weisfeldt, M. L. The Cholesterol Facts. A Summary of the Evidence Relating Dietary Fats, Serum Cholesterol, and Coronary Heart Disease. A Joint Statement by the American Heart Association and the National Heart, Lung, and Blood Institute. The Task Force on Cholesterol Issues, American Heart Association. *Circulation* **1990,** *81* (5), 1721–1733.

Lin, P.; Appleby, D. Challenges for the Food Industry in the Post-trans Era. *Inform* **2012,** *23* (8), 527–529.

Marangoni, A. G. A *Trans* Fat Free Future—A Commentary. *Inform* **2007,** *18* (4), 281–283.

Marangoni, A. G.; Idziak, S. H. J.; Vega, C.; Batte, H.; Ollivon, M.; Jantzi, P. S.; Rush, J. W. Oil Microencapsulation Attenuates Acute Elevation of Blood Lipids and Insulin in Humans. *Soft Matter* **2007,** *3,* 183–187.

Marangoni, A. G.; Idziak, S. H. J.; Rush, J. W. E. Controlled Release of Food Lipids Using Monoglyceride Gel Phases Regulates Lipid and Insulin Metabolism in Humans. *Food Biophys.* **2008,** *3,* 241–245. DOI: 10.1007/s11483-008-9054-y.

McClements, D. J. Emulsion Design to Improve the Delivery of Functional Lipophilic Components. *Annu. Rev. Food Sci. Technol.* **2010,** *1,* 241–269.

Mensink, R. P.; Katan, M. B. Effect of Dietary *Trans* Fatty Acids on High-Density and Low-Density Lipoprotein Cholesterol Levels in Healthy Subjects. *New Eng. J. Med.* **1990,** *323* (7), 439–445.

Mensink, R. P.; Zock, P. L.; Kester, A. D. M.; Katan, M. B. Effects of Dietary Fatty Acids and Carbohydrates on the Ratio of Serum Total to HDL Cholesterol and on Serum Lipids and Apolipoproteins: A Meta-analysis of 60 Controlled Trials. *Am. J. Clin. Nutr.* **2003,** *77,* 1146–1155.

Mozaffarian, D.; Clarke, R. Quantitative Effects on Cardiovascular Risk Factors and Coronary Heart Disease Risk of Replacing Partially Hydrogenated Vegetable Oils with Other Fats and Oils. *Eur. J. Clin. Nutr.* **2009,** *63* (Suppl. 2), S22–S33.

Müller, M.; Czihak, C.; Vogl, G.; Fratzl, P.; Schober, H.; Riekel, C. Direct Observation of Microfibril Arrangement in a Single Native Cellulose Fiber by Microbeam Small-Angle X-ray Scattering. *Macromolecules* **1998,** *31* (12), 3953–3957.

Nordestgaard, B. G.; Tybjærg-Hansen, A. IDL, VLDL, Chylomicrons and Atherosclerosis. *Eur. J. Epidimiol.* **1992,** *8,* 92–98.

Pernetti, M.; van Malssen, K. F.; Flöter, E.; Bot, A. Structuring of Edible Oils by Alternatives to Crystalline Fat. *Curr. Opin. Colloid In.* **2007a,** *12,* 221–231.

Pernetti, M.; van Malssen, K. F.; Kalnin, D.; Flöter, E. Structuring Edible Oil with Lecithin and Sorbitan Tri-stearate. *Food Hydrocolloids* **2007b,** *21,* 855–861.

Rogers, M. A. Novel Structuring Strategies for Unsaturated Fats—Meeting the Zero-*trans,* Zero-saturated Fat Challenge: A Review. *Food Res. Int.* **2009,** *42,* 747–753.

Rogers, M. A. Ceramide Oleogels. In *Edible Oleogels: Structure and Health Implications;* Marangoni, A. G., Garti, N., Eds.; AOCS Press: Urbana, IL, 2011; pp 221–234.

Rogers, M. A.; Marangoni, A. G. Non-isothermal Nucleation and Crystallization of 12-Hydroxystearic Acid in Vegetable Oils. *Cryst. Growth Des.* **2008,** *8,* 4596–4601.

Rogers, M. A.; Marangoni, A. G. Hydroxystearic Acid Oleogels. In *Edible Oleogels;* Marangoni, A. G., Garti, N., Eds.; AOCS Press: Urbana, IL, 2011; pp 101–118.

Rogers, M. A.; Smith, A. K.; Wright, A. J.; Marangoni, A. G. A Novel Cryo-SEM Technique for Imaging Vegetable Oil Based Organogels. *J. Am. Oil Chem. Soc.* **2007,** *84* (10), 899–906.

Rogers, M. A.; Wright, A. J.; Marangoni, A. G. Engineering the Oil Binding Capacity and Crystallinity of Self-assembled Fibrillar Networks of 12-Hydroxystearic Acid in Edible Oils. *Soft Matter* **2008,** *4,* 1483–1490.

Rush, J. W. E.; Jantzi, P. S.; Dupak, K.; Idziak, S. H. J.; Marangoni, A. G. Effect of Food Preparation on the Structure and Metabolic Responses to a Monostearin-oil-water Gel-based Spread. *Food Res. Int.* **2008,** *41,* 1065–1071.

Rush, J. W. E.; Jantzi, P. S.; Dupak, K.; Idziak, S. H. J.; Marangoni, A. G. Acute Metabolic Responses to Butter, Margarine, and a Monoglyceride Gel-structured Spread. *Food Res. Int.* **2009,** *42,* 1034–1039.

Siri-Tarino, P. W.; Sun Q.; Hu, F. B.; Krauss, R. M. Meta-analysis of Prospective Cohort Studies Evaluating the Association of Saturated Fat with Cardiovascular Disease. *Am. J. Clin. Nutr.* **2010a,** *91,* 535–546.

Siri-Tarino, P. W.; Sun, Q.; Hu, F. B.; Krauss, R. M. Saturated Fatty Acids and Risk of Coronary Heart Disease: Modulation by Replacements Nutrients. *Curr. Atheroscler. Rep.* **2010b,** *12,* 384–390.

Stortz, T. A.; Marangoni, A. G. Heat Resistant Chocolate. *Trends Food Sci. Tech.* **2011,** *22* (5), 201–214.

Stortz, T. A.; Zetzl, A. K.; Barbut, S.; Cattaruzza, A.; Marangoni, A. G. Edible Oleogels in Food Products to Help Maximize Health Benefits and Improve Nutritional Profiles. *Lipid Technology* **2012,** *24* (7), 151–154.

Terech, P.; Weiss, R. G. Low Molecular Mass Gelators of Organic Liquids and the Properties of Their Gels. *Chem. Rev.* **1997,** *97,* 3133–3159.

Toro-Vazquez, J. F.; Morales-Rueda, J. A.; Dibildox-Alvarado, E.; Charó-Alonso, M.; Alonzo-Macias, M.; González-Chávez, M. M. Thermal and Textural Properties of Organogels Developed by Candelilla Wax in Safflower Oil. *J. Am. Oil Chem. Soc.* **2007,** *84,* 989–1000.

Toro-Vasquez, J. F.; Charó-Alonso, M. A.; Pérez-Martínez, J. D.; Morales-Rueda, J. A. Candelilla Wax as an Organogelator for Vegetable Oils—An Alternative to Develop *Trans*-free Products for the Food Industry. In *Edible Oleogels;* Marangoni, A. G., Garti, N., Eds.; AOCS Press: Urbana, IL, 2011; pp 119–148.

U.S. Food and Drug Administration. Federal Register—68 FR 41433: Food Labeling; *Trans* Fatty Acids in Nutrition Labeling; Consumer Research to Consider Nutrient Content and Health Claims and Possible Footnote or Disclosure Statements; Final Rule and Proposed Rule. http://www.fda.gov/food/labelingnutrition/labelclaims/nutrientcontent claims/ucm110179.htm (accessed October 2012).

Willet, W. C.; Stampfer, M. J.; Manson, J. E.; Colditz, G. A.; Speizer, F. E.; Rosner, B. A.; Sampson, L. A.; Hennekens, C. H. Intake of *Trans* Fatty Acids and Risk of Coronary Heart Disease among Women. *The Lancet* **1993,** *341* (8845), 581–585.

World Health Organization (WHO). Cardiovascular disease. http://www.who.int/cardiovas cular_diseases/en/ (accessed November 2012).

Wright, A. J.; Marangoni, A. G. Formation, Structure, and Rheological Properties of Ricinelaidic Acid–Vegetable Oil Organogels. *J. Am. Oil Chem. Soc.* **2006,** *83,* 497–503.

Zetzl, A. K.; Marangoni, A. G. Novel Strategies for Nanostructuring Liquid Oils into Functional Fats. In *Edible Oleogels;* Marangoni, A. G., Garti, N., Eds.; AOCS Press: Urbana, IL, 2011; pp 19–47.

Zetzl, A. K.; Marangoni, A. G. Structured Oils as Food Ingredients and Nutraceutical Delivery Systems. In *Encapsulation Technologies and Delivery Systems for Food Ingredients and Nutraceuticals;* Garti, N., McClements, D. J., Eds.; Woodhead Publishing Limited: Cambridge, 2012; pp 392–411.

Zetzl, A. K.; Marangoni, A. G.; Barbut, S. Mechanical Properties of Ethylcellulose Oleogels and Their Potential for Saturated Fat Reduction in Frankfurters. *Food Funct.* **2012,** *3,* 327–337. DOI: 10.1039/c2fo10202a.

11

Trans Fats Replacement Solutions for Frying and Baking Applications, Shortenings, Margarines, and Spreads

G.R. List ■ *U.S. Department of Agriculture, Peoria, Illinois, USA (Retired)*

Introduction

On July 11, 2003, *trans* fat labeling became law of the land, with key provisions that *trans* fat is to be listed as a separate line on nutrition labels and foods containing less than 0.5 g *trans* fat per serving could be declared zero (Anon, 2003). The law became effective January 1, 2006. Many companies began reformulating foods to meet *trans* fat labeling well in advance of the 2006 compliance date. In 1999, the zero-*trans* foods were essentially nonexistent. The period of 2003–2007 saw the number of zero/low *trans* fat foods increase from about 200 to over 1900. A recent report indicates that over the period 2005–2010, the *trans* fat content of baked goods has decreased from 0.49% to less than 0.2% (Rahovsky et al., 2012). Prior to labeling, baked goods were a major source of *trans* fats in the diet (Satchithanandam et al., 2004). Government dietary guidelines published in 1980 and 1985 recommended that consumption of saturated fat be avoided. Thus, the food industry sought replacements for coconut, palm, and animal fats in vegetables/dairy, confections, baked goods, margarines, snacks, and cereals. Partially hydrogenated oils (soy, cottonseed, canola), liquid oils, and high stability oils served in many food applications, but saturates were replaced with *trans* fats (Norris and Gingras, 1990).

A review of new and existing fats and oils used in reduced-*trans* food applications was published in the *Journal of the American Dietetic Association* (Tarrago-Trani et al., 2006).

Snack food manufacturers took the lead in reformulation by switching from heavily hydrogenated frying shortenings to naturally stable liquid vegetable oils including corn, cottonseed, and sunflower oils. Since these oils are free of linolenic acid and very low in *trans* fats, they proved to be satisfactory alternatives to conventional cube or fluid products. In some cases, reformulation proved to be both expensive and time consuming. For example, the reformulation of 187 products made in 46 plants (requiring 7200 man hours) required over 240 analytical tests and 24 consumer studies at a cost of $25 million (Eckel et al., 2007). At the time, only three oil suppliers were used and supply issues had to be overcome. Eventually, a blend of naturally stable oils was chosen as the *trans* fat replacement.

Soft margarines and spreads proved to be relatively easy to reformulate to zero *trans* by using both hydrogenated and liquid oil components. However, stick products have proven more difficult to reformulate because more solid fat is required for functionality in baking applications and storage considerations at ambient temperatures. Without question, the most difficult applications for *trans* fat replacements are baking shortenings. For many years, baking shortenings have been formulated from hydrogenated stocks high in *trans* fats or, to a lesser extent, from animal fat–based components. Hydrogenated oils are popular for food formulation (Podmore, 2008) because they are versatile, oxidatively stable, and they crystallize well in the desired beta-prime form (Floeter and Dujin, 2006). Animal fats, while essentially *trans* free, are higher in saturated acids and contain cholesterol, qualities that detract from a health/nutrition perspective. However, from a functional point of view, hydrogenated vegetable and animal fat–based shortenings are equivalent with regard to aeration/creaming and icing volume in all-purpose baking applications (Woerfel, 1960). Zero *trans* baking shortenings formulated from beef tallow and liquid cottonseed oil were introduced in the mid 1890s and were popular in retail/baking products well into the 1930s. In 1893, Cottolene was marketed by NK Fairbank and Co. and, shortly thereafter, Cottosuet was marketed by Swift and Co. Both were very popular among bakers because they performed well in both cake and pie applications.

Processing Methods to Reduce *Trans* Fats

A review of oil processing methods to reduce *trans* fats is beyond the scope of this chapter. The reader is referred to a number of excellent reviews on chemical/enzymatic interesterification (Binder et al., 2006; Going, 1967; Holman and Going, 1959; Rozendaal and McRae, 1997; Screenivasan, 1978; Xu et. al 2006). The fractionation of tropical oils has been reviewed by Timms (1997). The patent literature on fractionation has been covered by Dijkstra (2012). Gibon (2006) has reviewed food uses of fractionation products. Technologies to control the physical properties of blended fats by triacylglycerol (TAG) compositions have been reviewed by Dijkstra (2008).

Interesterification

Interesterification is an old processing tool dating back to the 1920s. The process does not change the overall fatty acid composition or the degree of unsaturation, but it modifies TAG structure affecting the melting profile and the crystal habit (Karabulit et al., 2004; Norris and Mattil, 1947). In the 1950s, interesterified lard was produced by a number of companies (Hawley and Holman, 1956; Mattil and Nelson, 1953; Mattil and Norris, 1953; Van der Wal and Van Akkeren, 1951) in order to overcome the poor performance of natural lard in cake baking applications (Slater, 1953). Although it was highly prized for pie crusts, natural lard gave poor results in cakes. The TAG structure of natural lard contains palmitic acid in the 2 position, whereas after randomization the fat is changed from a beta to a beta-prime crystal structure that allows better incorporation of air into cake batters, yielding increased cake volume. In addition, beta-prime fats crystallize in finer crystal structures and, upon passage through scraped surface heat exchangers, the fat has a white creamy smooth texture.

Historically, both random (van Loon, 1927) and directed intresterification (Eckey, 1948) have been used as fat modification tools. In random methods (Minal 2003a, 2003b), the reaction is usually carried out with a chemical catalyst (sodium methoxide or sodium metal) at relatively high temperatures (70–100 °C) while the directed interesterification is conducted at lower temperatures, allowing the higher-melting triglycerides to crystallize out of the reaction medium (Hawley and Holman 1956; Holman and Going, 1959).

Fractionation of Tropical Oils

Palm oil has been used in food products for 5000 years. However, many of the existing technologies for incorporation into frying fats, baking shortenings, and spreads have been developed over the past 30 years or so. Unmodified palm oil performs well in most bakery products. It is rated highly suitable or suitable for shortenings, margarines, frying fats, cookies, crackers, cake mixes, icings, and biscuits. Palm oil is unsuitable as a coating fat. Fractionation of palm oil yields palm olein, soft stearins, and hard stearins. Palm olein is highly suitable in shortenings, margarines, and frying fats. The soft stearins are suitable in most applications, with the exception of icings. Hard stearins find use in shortenings. Hydrogenation of palm oil is useful in shortenings, margarines, frying fats, biscuits, and cookies. Double fractionated palm oil is highly suitable in frying applications. Palm mid fractions are suitable in icings. Palm kernel oil is highly suitable in margarines, coating fats, crackers, and biscuits (Ranhotra, 1993). A detailed description of the chemical and physical properties of palm oil and its fractions is given by Kheiri (1987), and a number of excellent reviews on the food uses of palm oil have appeared recently (Berger, 2005, 2007, 2010) and summarize many of the formulations used for low-/zero-*trans* frying, baking shortenings, and spreads.

The highly saturated fatty acid composition of palm oil/palm kernel combined with fractionation, hydrogenation, interesterification, and blending provide a number of options for *trans* fat free foods. The patent literature contains a wealth of information on formulations employing these processing techniques (Ainger and Coverly, 1980; Babayan, 1966; Berlin, 1974; Delfosse, 1971; Dijkshoorn et al., 1982; Dijkstra, 2012; Fondu and Willems, 1971, 1972; Gillies, 1974; Graffelman,1966; Huizinga et al., 1999; Lansbergen and Schijf, 1996; Lindsay, 1961; List and Pelloso, 2007; Mat Sahri and Dian, 2011; Poot et al., 1978; Pronk et al., 1986; Read, 1975; Sassen and Westdorp, 2001; Schmidt, 1986a, 1986b; Seiden,1971; Tafuri and Tao, 1984; van Heteren et al., 1983; Ward, 1982; Weiske, 1977; Weiske et al., 1976).

Much of the research conducted on food uses of palm, palm kernel oils, and their fractions has been done by the Malaysian Palm Oil Board, and a list of their publications is available online (www.mpob.gov.my)

Modified Hydrogenation for *Trans* Fat Reduction

A considerable amount of research has been done to reduce isomerization during catalytic hydrogenation of edible oils (Beers, 2004; Beers et al., 2008; Hasman, 1995; List et al., 2007). By changing temperatures, pressure, agitation, catalyst loading, use of noble metal catalysts (platinum, palladium), and modification of traditional nickel catalysts, significant reduction in *trans* acids can be achieved. Traditionally high temperatures, low pressures, moderate agitation, and low nickel catalyst loadings have been employed to reduce polyunsaturates in commercial practice. However, these conditions promote *trans* isomerization at a rate of about 0.73% *trans*/IV drop (List and King, 2006). Conversely, at lower temperatures (140–170 °C) and pressures of 200 lbs psi, over 55% reduction in *trans* can be achieved (Eller et al., 2005) However, the higher pressures would require refitting converters that normally operate at 50 psi or less. Other approaches to *trans* reduction include hydrogenation in supercritical fluids (King et al., 2001), use of low IV oils for spreads/shortenings (List et al., 2007a), electrochemical hardening (List et al., 2007b), and hydrogenation by use of nickel/platinum catalysts (Jackson et al., 2008). The use of modified nickel catalysts has shown industrial applications. Treatment of nickel supported catalysts with phosphoric acid allows a significant lowering of *trans* isomers during catalytic hydrogenation. At least two lines of baking shortenings are commercially available employing this technology (Higgens, 2007; Van Toor et al., 2009a, 2009b, 2010).

Blending as Zero *Trans* Options

Many suppliers are offering custom blends for food applications in which oxidative stability and sensory properties are primary considerations. Commodity soybean oil performs well in most applications with the exception of heavy duty frying, in which high temperatures promote breakdown of the 7–8% linolenic acid with loss of fry life. Naturally stable oils (free of linolenic acid), when blended with soybean oil to 3% or less linolenic acid, provide increased stability for frying. Blending of commodity or trait-modified oils with lightly hydrogenated soybean oil can also be used as a *trans* fat replacement in lower fat containing foods. Such products are custom made and available commercially (Matlock, 2005).

Studies have shown that frying oils should contain about 60% oleic, 20% linoleic, and 3% or less of linolenic acid for better performance and flavor. Linoleic acid and its breakdown products contribute to the desirable fried food flavors (Warner et al., 2001). The high-oleic canola, soybean, and sunflower oils (75–80% oleic acid) provide a wide range of custom fatty acid profiles for specific applications. Thus, by blending the high-oleic oils with oils containing higher amounts of linoleic acid (cottonseed, soybean, canola, corn, sunflower), a balance between the oxidatively stable oleic and the increased linoleic needed for flavor is achieved. Lui and Iassonova (2012) have reported on food uses of canola oils having varying amounts of oleic acid. Debonte et al. (2012) reported that cereals formulated with high-oleic canola oils and packaged with both high and low oxygen barriers show little deterioration after 12 days of storage at 60 °C, which corresponds to 1 year of shelf life at room temperature.

Trait Modified Oils as *Trans* Fat Replacements

Trait-modified oils were commercialized in the early 1990s. Low-linolenic soybean oil (Hammond, 1984), mid-oleic sunflower (Gupta, 1998; Miller et al., 1987) and low-linolenic canola oil (Debonte et al., 1999) were not very successful because of higher costs associated with grower premiums and identity preservation (Krawczyk, 1999). However, *trans* fat labeling has generated new interest in the trait-modified oil industry. Mid- and high-oleic and low-linolenic soybean and mid- and high-oleic sunflower, along with high-oleic canola, now command about 20% of domestic consumption. A low saturate, high-oleic soybean oil is expected to be commercialized very shortly (Wilkes, 2010). In addition, an omega-3 enriched soy is nearing completion (Wilkes, 2008). A number of factors have driven the development of trait-modified oils, including health/nutrition issues such as the removal of *trans* and saturated acids from the food supply. Because trait-modified oils are essentially free of *trans* acids, food labels do not carry hydrogenation on them. Trait-modified oils are considered heart healthy and do not contain cholesterol like other vegetable oils. Because trait-modified oils are liquids, they are easily pumped and handled in bakeries and food service kitchens. Food applications include deep-fat frying, pan/griddle frying, spray oils, sautéing, pan release agents, nutritional bars, sauces and dressings, and some baking applications. These applications will be covered in separate sections.

Frying

A number of reference books covering all aspects of deep-fat frying are available and should be consulted for further information (Della Porta, 2008; Erickson, 2007; Gupta et al., 2004). Wainwright et al. (2006) reviewed options for reducing/eliminating *trans* acids in deep-fat frying and labeling implications.

Frying fats have evolved from heavily hydrogenated soybean oil (40% *trans*) in the form of 50-lb plasticized cubes wrapped in cellophane/plastic and packaged in cardboard boxes. The next generation was beta-stable hard fats suspended in a lightly hydrogenated base. They were very popular in the food service sector because they were stable and easily handled because of their fluid nature. Although they contained less *trans* than cube shortenings, they did not provide a *trans*-free solution. Although popular in other parts of the world, palm-based frying fats have not entered into U.S. markets to any great extent. Trait-modified soybean, canola, and sunflower oils have been adopted by the food service industry as *trans* fat replacements. Trait-modified oils are characterized by increased amounts of oleic acid, decreased polyunsaturated acid levels, and, in some cases, reduced saturates compared to commodity oils. As a result, trait-modified oils have increased oxidative stability toward high temperatures used in frying. Examples now in commercial production include low-linolenic, and mid- and high-oleic soybean oils, low-linolenic and high-oleic canola, mid- and high-oleic sunflower oils. Several other trait-modified oils are nearing commercialization, including a low-saturate/high-oleic soybean oil and a stearidonic acid–enriched omega-3 soybean oil (Wilkes, 2008).

An early study (Erickson and Frey, 1994) compared several trait-modified soy and sunflower oils in frying tests against hydrogenated frying shortenings. Parameters investigated included foam height in the fryer, color, free fatty acids, and organoleptic tests. The results showed that the trait-modified oils performed better than fluid opaque and liquid frying fats, but were slightly inferior to solid cube frying fats. Other work carried out at Texas A&M University supports these findings (www.frytest.com).

Pan and Grill Shortenings

It has been estimated that 75–80% of fast food breakfast items are prepared on grills or frying pans. The source oils are soybean, coconut, palm kernel, and cottonseed. Both unsalted and salted pourable products are available and have low solid contents. Unsalted shortenings are all purpose, suitable for pan frying, grilling, soups, gravies, basting, and brush-on dressings. Salted shortenings are seasoned but serve in many of the same applications. The solid shortenings are used for pan frying, griddle oils, and in-bun toasting. Common additives include lecithin (anti-sticking/spattering function), artificial coloring, butter flavor, silicones (reduce oxidation/oxygen barrier), and antioxidants to prolong storage life. The pourable shortenings are low in *trans* fat. Solid pan/griddle products may be low in *trans* fat, but they are higher in saturates because they are formulated from coconut, palm kernel, and cottonseed oils (O'Brien, 2009).

Case Studies on *Trans* Reformulation in Fast Food Chains and Laboratory Frying (Trait-Modified Oils)

Numerous laboratory frying studies have been reported and the reader is referred to them for further information (Gerde et al., 2007; Kiatscrichart et al., 2003; Lui and

White, 1992; Matthius et al., 2009; Miller and White, 1988; Normand et al., 2006; Prevot et al., 1990; Soheli et al., 2002; Su et al., 2003; Warner and Gupta, 2003; Warner and Knowlton, 1997, Warner and Moser, 2009; Warner and Mounts, 1993; Warner et al., 1997). Several frying studies from the fast food industry have been reported (Miller, 2007; Nagy-Nero, 2006; Reid, 2007). Many factors influence the choice of frying oils, including cost, availability, fry life, and consumer acceptance (Tiffany, 2007).

Other factors include: no transfer of unwanted flavors added to the food, oil resistance to polymerization and oil should not form films or residues in equipment. Frying fats tend to darken upon continued use and should remain clear for the entire fry life. Because frying oils tend to foam after extended use, resistance to foaming is highly desirable. From a health/nutrition standpoint, frying oils should be low in TFAs and saturated acids.

A major national chain, Kentucky Fried Chicken, using 160 million pounds of oil per year, began the task of replacing a hydrogenated fluid shortening with a *trans*-free alternative. Some 26 different oils and blends were evaluated for fry life and consumer acceptance. By 2004, the search was narrowed to two oils. Although both performed equally well in testing, a trait-modified soybean oil was selected for test marketing in eight restaurants in New York City. Consumers were asked for their reaction to the new frying oil. The results were overwhelmingly positive and the decision was made to supply some 5500 stores with the *trans*-free oil. A major concern was oil stability. The company uses an active filtration to polish the oil with magnesol, which extends fry life and retains seasonings added to the food. The company concluded that fry life of the replacement was equal to the hydrogenated shortening it replaced. By April 2007, all stores were serving zero-*trans* food (Miller, 2007).

A regional chain having 1800 employees operating 40 restaurants prides itself in offering nutritional, good tasting foods made with local ingredients. A TFA-free solution was sought because it was the right thing to do for their customers. They began with a TFA-free soybean oil packaged in 35 pound jugs. Employees were educated about TFA fats and a testing was conducted in one of the chain restaurants by comparing french fries fried in *trans* replacement against the existing shortening. The tests showed satisfactory performance, and the chain made the decision to switch despite increased price (an additional $2/35 lbs) and some decrease in fry life from 16 to 14 days and some as short as 7–12 days. It was estimated that the additional cost amounted to 6 plus cents per pound of oil with an additional loss of fry life (Debe-Nero, 2006; Eckel et al., 2007). The fatty acid composition of low-linolenic soybean oil lends itself well to deep-fat frying because of the increased amount of the oxidatively stable oleic acid and reductions in the polyunsaturated linoleic and linolenic acid content. The same is true for low-linolenic canola and mid-oleic soybean oils (Warner and Gupta, 2003, 2005).

Ruby Tuesday is a national chain with about 850 restaurants (Reid, 2007). In late 2003, a corporate decision was made to switch from partially hydrogenated soybean oil to canola oil. Two challenges were encountered: increased cost and shorter fry life. However, by switching, the number of foods with *trans* acids decreased from 30 to about 10. French fries contained *trans* because they are purchased par fried in partially hydrogenated oil. At the time, it was estimated that french fries par fried in canola would add an additional $1 million per year. However, in the meantime, zero-*trans* frying shortenings have been marketed specifically for par/deep-fat frying.

Baking

Bakery Shortenings and Applications of Liquid Oils in Baking

An extensive review of baking shortenings can be found in Ghotra et al. (2002), Hartnett (1977), and Weiss (1983). Troubleshooting problems in bakery/deep-fat frying applications is covered by Stauffer (1996) and should be consulted for further information. The role of fats, oils, and emulsifiers in bakery applications has also been covered in other reviews (Orthoefer, 2008; Stauffer, 2005).

Many baking applications require solid fat for functional needs, including aeration, plasticity for dough products, lubricity, texture, tenderness, mouth feel, and richness. Liquid oils have been used for bread baking for many years, and the use of emulsifiers and surfactants has played a major role in the switch from lard to liquid oils. Hartnett and Thalheimer (1979) reported studies on the baking of sweet doughs, bread, and cakes formulated from liquid soybean oil containing emulsifiers and surfactants. In bread baking, 3% soybean oil containing 0.5% monoglycerides/polysorbate performed as well as a commercial fluid shortening with respect to dough handling, grain, and softness. Similar results were obtained in baking cakes. However, the emulsifier polyglycerol monostearate (PGMS) at concentrations of 8–12% was required. This system was equal to or better than a commercial fluid shortening. Sweet doughs made from liquid soybean oil handled poorly; the dough was sticky, had low specific volume, and had an open irregular grain. Soybean oil with 2% added monoglycerides only slightly improved dough handling. However, soybean oil containing 1.5% monoglycerides and polysorbate 60 performed well in sweet doughs. Kamel (1992) studied the characteristics of bread and buns made with lard and liquid vegetable oils with different iodine values. When emulsifiers are incorporated into soybean and canola oils, baking performance was equal to lard/palm oils with a reduction of 30% total fat. Baldwin et al. (1972) reviewed the uses of liquid oils in bread and cakes. Cakes baked with soybean oil with added surfactants showed excellent crumb softness and moisture retention equal to a standard hydrogenated shortening. These authors point out that solid fat profiles of the two fat systems are markedly different, but at the temperature at which leavening power (100–110 °F) occurs the soy/surfactant system is equal to the hydrogenated product.

Liquid Oil/Monoglyceride/Diglycerides and Oleogels in Baking Shortening: Applications for *Trans* Reduction

The use of liquid oil/partial glyceride mixtures for *trans* reduction in baking is the subject of several patents (Doucet, 1999; Skogerson and Boute, 2010). The use of these systems allows a zero-*trans* and a reduced-saturate composition. Applications include cakes, cookies, Danishes, icings, puff pastry, and laminated products. They are powders containing 8% monoglycerides with a Mettler dropping point of 131–140 °F. The products are Generally Recognized as Safe (GRAS).

The use of oleogels/structured emulsions to provide structure and functionality in baking applications is recent technology (Marangoni and Garti, 2011). They are produced by shearing monoglycerides, water, and common liquid vegetable oils. Oleogels are reduced-saturate, zero-TFA fat replacements in a variety of food products including cookies, cakes, biscuits, pie shells, muffins, pizza, and frozen dough (Marangoni and Idziak, 2008).

Liquid Oil Applications in Cookies, Baked Snack Crackers, Spray Oils, Liquid Shortenings, Pan Release Agents, Pretzels, Muffins, and Tortillas

Cookies

Soft cookies require creaming. Traditionally, all-purpose shortenings, either hydrogenated or animal-based with added emulsifiers, have been the industry standard with a short plastic range and high stability desirable. Palm and animal-based soft cookie shortenings offer a *trans*-free solution at the possible expense of increased saturates. Idris et al. (1991) evaluated "biscuits" (short dough cookies) baked with 100% palm oil, blends of palm oil and butter (3:1, 1:1), and 100% butter against a commercial cookie. Sensory evaluations of texture, flavor, and force to break were performed on freshly baked products and after 3 months of storage. Although few significant differences in sensory tests were found among the experimental cookies, the all-butter products were liked the best. Force to break tests indicated the four experimental cookies were softer in texture than the commercial products.

Hard cookies require fat for lubrication. Thus, any recipe calling for vegetable oil can include any commodity or trait-modified soy, canola, or sunflower oil. In commercial cookie baking, spread is a crucial factor affecting packaging. Too much or too little spread affects the number of cookies per stock keeping unit. Several studies made with hydrogenated and TFA-free shortenings indicate that the latter does not increase or decrease spread in sugar cookie baking (McNeil, 2005; Tiffany, 2008).

Baked Snack Crackers

Several well-known snack crackers have been successfully reformulated to zero *trans* with liquid unhydrogented soybean oil (Klemann, 2005). Trait-modified soy, canola, and sunflower oils should also serve well because they are more oxidatively stable than commodity unhydrogenated soy containing 7–8% linolenic acid.

Spray Oils

In addition to extensive food service and home uses, spray oils are used in the cracker baking industry. Crackers, croutons, and crisps are often sprayed with a thin layer of oil to serve as a moisture barrier, which protects the product from flavor and textural deterioration. Traditionally, hydrogenated soybean oil (IV 70–80) or coconut oil has been used for the spraying of crackers. The former is high in *trans,* while the latter is very high in saturates. Thus, trait-modified soy, canola, and sunflower should perform well in spray applications. Limited published data confirm that low-linolenic soy and mid-oleic sunflower oils were equal to hydrogenated controls in cracker spray tests (Erickson and Frey, 1994).

Pan Release Agents: Zero Trans *Options*

Bread is baked in loaf pans arranged on racks that are inverted on exiting the oven. Thus, it is imperative that loaves release readily from the pans (Weiss, 1983). A number of pan release agents have been described in the patent literature (Carey, 1974; Gawrilow, 1975; Hanson, 1980). Because they must be easily applied by spraying, they are usually in liquid form. However, solid-stick pan lubricants have also been described in the patent literature (Mahler and Doummani, 1977).

Stick pan lubricants can be formulated from liquid (unhydrogenated) vegetable oil, lecithin, hydrogenated fatty acid glycerides, or wax in the following proportions: 30–45 parts oil, 5–20 parts lecithin, 40–60 parts wax/fatty acid TAG. A typical formulation consists of 50% hydrogenated tallow, 15% double-bleached lecithin, and 35% liquid soybean oil. Other base vegetable oils include those liquid at room temperature or petrolatum approved for food use. Since they are applied by hand pressure, an effective layer of lecithin is deposited on the pan such that food does not stick. In addition to zero-*trans* oils as bases, other common ingredients include aluminum stearate, lecithin, partial glycerides, animal and vegetable waxes, polysorbate esters, and flours. Trait-modified oils should perform well in pan release products. Although more costly than commodity oils, they provide added oxidative stability.

Pretzels, Muffins, Tortillas

Traditionally, pretzel dough has been formulated with hydrogenated soybean oil. Reformulation to zero *trans* can be achieved by switching to liquid unhydrogenated oil (Manirath et al., 2006). Pretzels normally contain about 2% fat needed for tenderness, mouth feel, and structure/strength. Many home recipes for muffins call for vegetable oil, for which either commodity or trait-modified soybean, corn, canola, or cottonseed oils can furnish a TFA-free solution. Flour tortillas also contain hydrogenated oils or animal fats because of improved machineability and reduction of dough stickiness. However, TFA fat labeling has stimulated interest in 100% liquid oil in tortillas despite the possibility of them sticking together when stacked in packages. Liquid oils provide not only a TFA-free solution, but also eliminate the heating of the fat before usage. The reader is referred to a recent patent describing use of liquid oil in tortilla manufacture (Gerardus et al., 2009).

Trait-Modified Oils in Fluid Shortenings

Fluid shortenings have been used for many years in the baking and food service industries (Norris, 1975, 1976). However, fluid shortenings have never been well received in the retail market place despite a large amount of research and development by the oil processing/food industries (Andre and Going, 1957; Brock, 1959; Cross and Griffin, 1956; Houser, 1961; Howard and Koren, 1965; Linteris, 1959). Proctor and Gamble marketed such a product (SWIRL) but it was discontinued after a short time (Weiss, 1983). Typically, fluid shortenings have been formulated from either an unhydrogenated soybean oil with a completely hardened soybean oil (IV +5 or less) or a hydrogenated oil (IV 90–100). The hard fat is in a beta stable form suspended in the liquid portion (Widlak, 2001). The solid portion contains 2–6% hard fat. Applications for these products include frying, grilling, toppings, and popping. Silicone and antioxidants are normally added to frying oils to stabilize them against foaming and oxidation. Grilling, toppings, and popping oils may contain antioxidants, lecithin and colors, salt, and flavor components. Bread and cake fluid shortenings are formulated from liquid oils (IV 90–130) with the solid portion furnished by partial glycerides and their esters, lecithin, and polysorbates. Antioxidants are added for oxidative stability.

Shortenings prepared in this manner can be used for yeast-raised bakery products (Norris, 1976). Because trait-modified oils show increased oxidative stability, hydrogenation may not be required and would serve well in *trans*-free fluid shortenings for the baking/food service industry market (Orthoefer, 2005).

Palm-Based Baking Shortenings

As mentioned previously, palm-based shortenings have been increasingly popular as a *trans* fat solutions for many foods and baking shortenings because they furnish the solid fat needed for functionality and are strong beta-prime crystal formers, which is desirable in shortenings and spreads. Fully refined, bleached, and deodorized palm serves as an all-purpose baking shortening after plasticization. However, while very low in *trans,* such shortenings contain about 50% saturated acids. Palm kernel oil and its fractions have uses in baking shortenings, confections, and spreads, but also are very high in saturates. Palm and palm kernel oils are particularly well-suited to formulate products low in *trans* and saturates when combinations of fractionation, interesterification, hydrogenation, and blending are combined. Fractionation of palm/palm kernel oils yields liquid oleins (lower in saturates) and a stearin fraction higher in saturates. These can be further fractionated to yield super oleins and stearin. Further fractionation yields even harder fractions. Very hard stearins form structuring fats capable of holding large amounts of liquid oil in emulsified systems and are particularly useful for the manufacture of margarines and spreads (Ullanoormadam, 2004). Blending of structural fats (5–15%) with liquid oils (85–95%) such as canola and high-oleic canola and soybean oils yields melting points and solid fat matching those of soft spread oils. The hard structuring fats (20%) can be interesterified with soybean oil (80%) to produce a product with physical properties matching an all-purpose baking shortening. Thus, the use of palm stearins in conjunction with liquid oils allows a *trans*-free solution with minimal increases in saturated fatty acids.

Both unemulsified and emulsified palm-based shortenings are commercially available. Nonemulsified shortenings are used primarily for frying and are offered in plasticized cubes, in bulk, and in specialty fats for doughnut frying. Doughnut frying oils are formulated to reduce oiliness and assure adhesion of frosting and glazes. Palm-based emulsified shortenings are formulated with mono-/diglycerides, polysorbate 60 esters, polyglycerol monostearate (PGMS), and lecithin, depending on the application. Cake icing, creamy icings, and scoopable icings normally contain mono-/diglycerides and polysorbate esters as emulsifiers. Cake shortenings designed to give enhanced aeration are emulsified with mono-/diglycerides. Palm-based shortening specially designed for packaged cake mixes contains mono-/diglycerides, PGMS, and lecithin. Other palm-based shortenings are formulated with the foregoing emulsifier system and are designed for low-fat cakes.

Palm-based coating fats are available for a wide variety of baking applications including cookies, doughnuts, and cakes. Firmer coating fats for baked goods and snack bars, as well as rapidly crystallizing shortenings for baked goods and bars, are available commercially. Palm kernel–based fats for hard coatings (e.g., confections, snack bars) are likewise available. These products are lower in saturated fat and are designed to be bloom free for the shelf life of products and are compatible with both palm and hydrogenated shortenings.

Performance Testing of Palm-Based Baking Shortenings

In 2006, the American Institute of Baking presented a study of the performance of zero-*trans* baking shortenings at the American Heart Association *Trans* Fat (AHA

TFA) Conference held in Washington, DC, and it is available online (Strouts, 2006). A summary of the entire meeting was published in the *AHA Journal* (Eckel et al., 2007).

Although many of the problems encountered in early baking applications with TFA fat replacements have probably been solved, the fact remains that TFA-free fats do not always behave like their replacements (Loh, 2006). Differences in functionality, including loss of aeration, volume, appearance, and greasy/oily handling, may occur. Processing issues may include achieving specific gravity of batters and cream fillings leading to package fill issues, curdling of batter emulsions, loss of sheet forming capabilities, and disruption of dough film formation. Flavor and finished product quality issues include off flavors in high fat products like cookies and doughnuts. Mouth feel may be affected when the shortening leaves a coating effect in the mouth from higher-melting triglycerides. Flavor development may also occur during the frying process.

Hydrogenated bakery shortenings (*trans*-containing fats) are/were produced with specific melting points and solid fat index/solid fat content depending on their final end uses (Johnson, 1999). As a result, drop-in solutions for baking were not always successful (Loh, 2006). Both palm-based and interesterified baking fats may contain higher amounts of saturated TAGs that crystallize differently than hydrogenated fats. Palm oil has a tendency to crystallize slowly, with the net effect that products may have a smooth creamy texture after passing through a scraped surface heat exchanger (votator), but after storage they become harder. This phenomenon is known as post-hardening and has been attributed to diacylglycerols (DAGs) or the presence of POP (where P is palmitic acid, O is oleic acid) (Sudin et al., 1991). Because interesterification greatly alleviates the post-hardening problem, the latter seems more likely. Processing conditions during the chilling and crystallization of emulsions in scraped surface heat exchangers and pin workers may also contribute to post hardening of palm-based margarines. In pilot plant studies, emulsion temperatures of 10 °C above the fat's melting point, flow rates of 45kg/hour through the A unit, a super cooling temperature of 20 °C, and pin worker (B unit) speeds of 200 rpm are optimal for controlling post-hardening and delays of transformation from the beta-prime to the higher-melting beta crystal habit (Sahri and Idris, 2006). Kirkeby (2008) reported full scale (1000 kg) data for residence times in scraped heat exchangers, pin workers, and resting tubes, which in turn determines product throughput and properties of finished margarines and spreads.

Other studies on formulation of zero-*trans* soft soybean margarines from interesterified oils indicate that solid fat index is not reliable to predict spreadibility (List et al., 1995, 2001). Less solid fat is needed for interesterified margarines compared to hydrogenated oils. Typical SFC values at 10, 21.1, and 33.3 °C are about half that of similar products formulated from hydrogenated oils.

Performance of Palm-Based Baking Shortenings (Zero *Trans*)

The majority of baking studies with palm oil shortenings have been done in the laboratory (Idris et al., 1987, 1988, 1989, 1991). Zero-*trans* shortenings prepared from hydrogenated palm oil, palm stearin, and blended with cottonseed, low-erucic rapeseed, cottonseed, and soybean oils in various proportions were evaluated in the baking of maderia cakes (chosen because they are low in fat and are most sensitive to the properties of the shortening). A hydrogenated shortening was used as a control. The results showed that all of the 10 formulations yielded excellent specific cake volumes, and creaming performance exceeded that of the control. However, they concluded that good creaming performance does not necessarily ensure good baking performance. Interesterified palm olein (100%) was judged to be superior for cream fillings and baking.

Dogan et al. (2007) studied the effects of interesterified and simple blends of palm/cottonseed oil shortenings on cake quality. Batter density, creaming, crust color, crumb color, and sensory properties were evaluated against a hydrogenated emulsified baking shortening. They concluded that levels of 25–50% palm oil in the interesterified blends gave good aeration and creaming properties and cakes with excellent crumb grain, moistness, and sensory properties, and would be a suitable replacement for hydrogenated shortenings. Ranhotra (1993) reported cake volume data on six palm oil formulations compared to standard shortening. All gave cake volumes ranging from 95–99% of the hydrogenated control.

Waheed et al. (2010) reported a baking study in which sugar cookies were evaluated with interesterified palm/cottonseed blends against a hydrogenated baking shortening. The cookies were evaluated for width, height, color, taste texture, and overall acceptability both as fresh products and after storage at ambient temperatures up to 45 days. Few differences in spread factors were noted after 45 days of storage. Control shortening showed the best overall acceptability, closely followed by the 50:50 interesterified blend of palm/cottonseed oil. All cookies showed a gradual deterioration in storage with respect to overall acceptability.

The American Institute of Baking presented performance tests in which commercially produced palm oil–based shortenings were compared against a hydrogenated shortening in cookies, crackers, puff pastry, doughnuts, and pie crusts (Strouts, 2006). The results showed that compared to a standard hydrogenated shortening, palm-based fats performed as well or better in these applications. In 2003, a major oil supplier marketed a line of zero-*trans* baking/spread fats based on enzymatic interesterification of liquid and completely hydrogenated stearins (Anon, 2004; Lee et al., 2008). The process involves blending liquid soybean oil with soybean or cottonseed stearins and passing the mixture through a series of four reactors containing a 1-3 specific enzyme where rearrangement occurs. The technology is versatile because the physical properties (melting point, solid fat content) of the rearranged fat can be controlled by the amount of hardstock in the simple blend. For example, an 85%/15% blend yields margarine/spread oils, while increasing the hardstock to about 30% results in an all-purpose baking shortening and about 40% yields fats suitable for puff pastry.

Enzymatically interesterified shortenings (soybean, soy plus cottonseed) were compared to an all-purpose baking shortening prepared from hydrogenated soybean oil, a palm-based shortening, and a hydrogenated soybean/cottonseed blend in baking tests including sugar cookies, high ratio cakes, and pie shells (Tiffany, 2008).

Parameters tested for sugar cookies included texture analysis (force to break), stack height, width, and wicking. High ratio cake testing involved texture, specific gravity, and height. Pie dough tests included texture analysis and wicking.

The sugar cookies prepared from the five shortenings all showed comparable stack heights with minimal differences. However, the all-purpose shortening showed the smallest spread and force to break after three days. Wicking or the seepage of fat showed little difference between the five shortenings, but the interesterified soy shortening showed the least amount of wicking. The spread factors (width/height) were very similar for all shortenings tested.

High ratio cakes were tested for texture (grain), force to break, height, and batter-specific gravity. The all-purpose shortening produced cake with the coarsest open grain, while the interesterified soy and the soy with added cottonseed oil (post-interesterification) had a closed fine grain. Although the differences were small, the hydrogenated shortening showed the highest batter-specific gravity, but the interesterified soy oil shortening had the best cake volume height. Texture or peak force measurements after one and three days indicated that the interesterified soy oil shortening was equal to the hydrogenated control, which indicates equal cake softness. The pie dough evaluations showed that the interesterified soy shortening has the lowest amount of wicking and the lowest peak force required for breakage, both of which are highly desirable. In summary, limited data suggest that interesterified zero-TFA baking shortenings perform in a wide variety of applications as well or better than the hydrogenated fats they replaced.

Troubleshooting *Trans*-Free Frying and Baking

Standard baking tests employed by the baking industry are outlined in Official Methods of the American Association of Cereal Chemists. Many of these methods are designed to evaluate flours rather than fats and oils. Typically, cakes are formulated from "bakers" hydrogenated emulsified shortening, while cookies and pies require non-emulsified all-vegetable hydrogenated shortenings for evaluation of finished baked goods. Thus, substituting *trans*-free shortenings for hydrogenated fats posed problems for bakers, many of whom were overcome by making adjustments to the baking process and the handling/storage of TFA replacements.

Common complaints included: shortenings that were too hard or too soft, margarines with off-flavors, and loss of quality with time. Cookie doughs were too hard when chilled, cookies were too crisp, there was excessive spreading, and macaroons were too dense. Icing/buttercreams had off-flavors and colors, breakup of stored icing, and icing was too soft or too stiff. Doughnuts were oily and "off-tasting."

Problems encountered included poor creaming, off-flavors, storage life, stiff doughs, and cookie texture and spread, icing performance, and poor performance in doughnut frying fats.

The following describes performance problems with zero-*trans* shortenings in commercial baking operations.

- Palm oil shortenings tend to be harder in winter and softer in summer, leading to difficult creaming properties. Palm-based shortenings tend to be sensitive to temperature changes. During the winter months, storage in warmer conditions is advised. On the other hand, storage in summer requires a cooler spot to get the desired firmness.
- Palm-based baking margarines can, on occasion (rarely), develop slight off-flavors (typical of tropical fats) in sweet rolls and pound cakes. A solution might be found in a different brand or in the addition of butter flavor to the recipe.
- Complaints that *trans* fat replacements do not last as long as the hydrogenated products have been expressed. The latter can often be stored for a year, compared to 6–9 months for the new margarine or shortening. Oftentimes the supplier gives storage instructions to ensure preservation of keeping qualities. Other options include the purchase of smaller quantities more frequently.
- Some bakeries pre-make dough in advance of the next day's needs, followed by resting in a cooler. As a result, the dough becomes too stiff to roll out. Palm-based margarines are temperature sensitive, allowing the chilled dough to sit at room temperature long enough to become soft enough to work. However, doughs should not be allowed to sit at ambient temperatures for more than 2 hours.
- Sugar cookies become too crisp with *trans* fat replacements. Adjustments to baking time and temperatures, such as a slight reduction in baking time or a reduction in baking temperature, may solve the problem. Other options include replacement of part (up to 25%) of the granulated sugar with liquid sweeteners. However, liquid sweeteners may cause increased browning. Thus, by varying bake time, temperature, and liquid sweeteners, the problem of crispy texture may be resolved.
- Chocolate chip cookies may spread too much with the new shortening. This can be solved by baking at 25 degrees higher than usual to "set" the cookies

earlier in the baking cycle and reduce baking time. Another solution involves substituting some of the flour with high-gluten bread flour (up to 20%).

- Icings made with alternative shortenings turn brown in color and have an off flavor. This problem is common to some palm-based icing shortenings. Different products may be different in flavor and whiter in color.
- Freshly prepared buttercreams are excellent, but overnight loss of volume and "oil off" occurs. This can be traced to improper emulsification of the shortening. All-purpose shortening may not be emulsified at all. All icing shortenings are emulsified, but not all perform the same way. Options include use of different brands, adding extra emulsifier (as directed by supplier), or making smaller batches and using them the same day.
- Soft/stiff icing problems can be solved by either refrigeration of soft icing before use or by adding up to 10% of extra powdered sugar. Stiff icings result from cool temperatures. Tempering at room temperature for not more than 2 hours, or the addition of up to 5% water, are helpful.
- Over-mixing may cause breakdown of icings. Softer *trans*-free sandwich cookie fillings may need a longer set time before crowning.
- Doughnut frying oils may lead to greasy, bitter-tasting doughnuts. Use of fresh oil at the proper frying temperature may solve the problem. Switching to a different brand of palm-based or palm-free reduced-*trans* shortening may be an option.

Zero-*Trans* Margarines and Spreads

Health and nutrition issues over *trans* and saturated acids have greatly impacted the spread market. Consumption in the United States is down about 50% from the peak years of the mid 1990s. A number of factors are responsible, including government dietary guidelines that have become increasingly critical of dietary fat. This, coupled with the "poisoning of America" campaign in the mid 1980s, prompted the low-fat food craze that followed. The spread industry began a concerted effort to reduce both *trans* and saturated acids from products, and by 1999, a survey showed a marked decrease (about 55%) in *trans* fatty acids in a short period of time (List et al., 2000). Social issues have also brought decline to the domestic spread industry. Eating habits have changed from the traditional breakfast of toast and so forth to a trip through the drive through, which may be convenient but is just as unhealthy as a touch of margarine on a piece of toast, a muffin, or a bagel. In addition, numerous press releases on the potentially harmful effects of *trans* and saturated fats has educated consumers to read food nutrition labels, avoid *trans* and saturated fats, and choose heart-healthy products. In addition, hydrogenated, interesterified, and tropical oils are portrayed as unhealthy, as well as products advertised as having less saturated fat than butter.

Technologies to prepare improved margarine and spreads have been available for many years (Gooding, 1963; Melnick and Gooding, 1960; Seiden, 1971). An excellent summary of the patent literature has been published up until 1974 (Gillies, 1974). However, early focus was not on removal of *trans* and saturated acids, but to increase the amounts of essential fatty acids. Zero-*trans* margarines were first commercialized in Europe during the 1960s under the acronym BECEL (blood and cholesterol lowering); these are still popular in Europe and Canada but are marketed under different brand names (Nieuwenhuis, 2000). The original formulation consisted of interesterified palm fats and low-IV hardstocks as the solid portion and liquid sunflower oil to furnish high levels of linoleic acid. Since only 8–10% hardstock was needed, BECEL contained low *trans,* low saturates, and increased essential fatty acids (Graffelman, 1967).

The first U.S. generation of zero-*trans* soft margarines and spreads was formulated from lightly hydrogenated oils blended with liquid soybean, canola, corn, and, to a lesser extent, olive and palm oil and its fractions (List and Peloso, 2007). Consumers were educated that hydrogenation on labels was not healthy despite meeting zero-*trans* requirements under the 2003 and 2006 federal mandates. Today, most soft tub spreads are reformulated with the same liquid oils, but solids are now furnished by tropical oils including palm and palm kernel and their fractions.

Stick products (80% fat) have proven to be difficult to reformulate because they must have sufficient solid fat for storage under ambient conditions. Typically, stick products contain 1.5–2.5 g *trans* fat per serving. However, retail stick fat products (with < 0.5g *trans*/serving) are marketed as zero *trans* but require refrigeration.

A recent study reported that palm stearin (PS) (IV 20–40), as well palm kernel olein, can be used to formulate *trans*-free block/stick margarines. By blending the hardstocks with varying amounts of liquid sunflower oil, margarines with sufficient solid fat content to ensure spreadability at low temperatures, structure (resistance to oil off) at ambient temperatures, and complete melting at body temperature are obtained. Pastry margarines can also be produced with the long plastic range needed for rolling dough and folding needed for the flaky texture of the final baked goods (Mat Sahri and Idris, 2010).

Kirkeby (2008) reviewed formulation of low-/zero-*trans* food products in the European industrial and retail sectors. Industrial products, including soft table/table margarines, contain 4–8% and 10–13% *trans,* respectively. Cake, puff pastry, and pumpable liquid shortenings contain 8–26% *trans* because partially hydrogenated palm (mp 42 °C) and vegetable oils (mp 34 °C) (25–75%) are included for solid fat in the formulations. Liquid oils and/or palm and coconut account for the remainder. The *trans* contents of these formulations is similar to products produced in the United States by blending hydrogenated base stocks with liquid oils and/or hardstocks (fully hydrogenated, low IV [5–10] from soybean and cottonseed oils). The *trans* content of these products can be reduced to about 3% by substituting palm stearin interesterified with coconut oil (25–80%) for solid fat. Both types of products are designed for usage temperatures of 5 °C, ambient, 25 °C, or 30 °C. It should be pointed out that small amounts (1–2%) of *trans* isomers are formed during bleaching and deodorization of fats and oils. These isomers are formed from thermal isomerization of polyunsaturates rather than industrial hydrogenation where C18 *trans* monoenes are the major *trans* isomers. Labeling requires that all *trans* isomers be included, that is, *trans* monoenes and all *trans* with conjugated or non conjugated diene/triene configurations.

The European spread/margarine market amounts to about 2.5 million t or 5.6 billion lbs per year, with Germany, the UK, Poland, the Netherlands, and Belgium accounting for about 65% of production in EU 27 countries. Total consumption in the EU countries has remained static over the 2003–2010 timeframe. However, in 2010, Germany, Austria, France, and Belgium imported about 65% of the spreads consumed. The export market for 2010 shows that Belgium, the Netherlands, and Germany furnished about 75% of spreads consumed in the EU. The consumption in the 27 EU countries amounts to about 5.6 billion lbs per year. With a population of 502 million, per capita consumption amounts to about 10 lbs per year. On the other hand, the U.S. (population 311 million) consumption of spreads in 2010 was about 1.2 billion lbs, or a per capita of 3.4 lbs. According to Korver and Katan (2006), the European spread market has prospered because of an early awareness of the possible adverse effects of dietary fatty acids and their removal from spreads, coupled with modification of technology developed in the 1960s in which hardstocks were blended with liquid sunflower oil (Graffelman, 1967). The old technology involved hardstock with 16.5% saturates and 10.5% *trans*, yielding 27% saturates plus *trans*. *Trans*-free hardstocks in the reformulated products contained less than 1% *trans* and 21–22% saturates, and oil-binding properties were similar. Further information can be found in a 2005 review (Upritchard et al., 2005). Thus, modern technology has provided removal of *trans* fats from spreads and decreased saturates, and they are heart healthy as well.

Spread and margarine oils are formulated for functionality, including spreadability, resistance to oil off, and mouth feel. Typically, solid fat contents at 50, 70, and 92 °F, along with melting point, define spread functionality. An early report of the physical properties of *trans*-free retail spreads indicated that oil off was a potential problem because of their lower melting points (25–28 °C) compared to hydrogenated counterparts (31–32 °C) (List and Pelloso, 2007). Despite having a *trans*-free claim and being fortified with cholesterol-lowering sterols, these products are expensive and command a minor share of the U.S. spread market.

Trans-Free Bakery Margarines

Unlike all-purpose shortenings, bakery margarines are emulsified and serve in a number of bakery applications. Generally, they fall into five categories: table grade, baker's margarine, roll-in margarines, puff pastry, and specialty roll-in (Johnson, 1999). Prior to *trans* fat labeling, these products were formulated from hydrogenated oils with specific solid fat indexes and melting points according to the specific application. However, bakery margarines can be substituted for butter and all-purpose shortening in most applications, with the exception of doughnut frying. An excellent review of bakery margarines and applications has been published by Johnson (1999), and Wainwright (1999) has reviewed oils and fats for the baking industry.

Both low-*trans* and *trans*-free free baking margarines are commercially available and are formulated with either hydrogenated (from a proprietary process) (Higgens, 2007) or tropical oils. Both lines of products show reduced *trans* and minimal increases in saturates, and the tropical fats do not carry hydrogenation on the label nor do the hydrogenated fats carry a tropical oil label. Both lines of bakery margarines are reported to offer an 80% reduction in *trans* and a 33% reduction in *trans* plus saturates, compared to standard bakers-grade products. The hydrogenated products reportedly can be used as a drop-in solution for icings, fillings, cookies, and Danishes. A beta-prime stable, low-saturate/low-*trans,* all-purpose shortening has been patented (Scavone, 1995).

The tropical-based fats are specifically designed for croissants, roll-in applications, biscuits, and emulsified doughs. Palm-based fats for frozen bread bakery doughs have been tested in the laboratory and found to be equivalent in height (before thawing and baking), bread volume, and sensory evaluation compared to a commercial product designed for baking bread (Ruihong et al., 2006).

The performance and formulation of *trans*-free roll-in margarine has been reported (Kanagaratnam, 2009). Palm, palm stearin (IV 14–44), palm kernel oil, palm kernel stearin, and interesterified palm/kernel blends were processed into margarine emulsions (82% fat) and processed in the pilot plant consisting of three A units and a single resting tube. The margarines were tempered at 20 °C for 4 days. The melting point of the experimental margarine was 43 °C, compared to 42–45 °C for commercial (hydrogenated) products. Optimum blends matching the hydrogenated margarines consist of palm stearin IV 20 or less at levels of 15–25% (promotes fast crystallization at temperature below 30 °C and provides structure above 30 °C). Medium melting fats [palm oil, palm stearin (IV 35), and palm kernel stearin interesterified] at levels of 30–50% ensure good mouth melt properties. Liquid oils and palm olein, palm kernel oil, and olein are used at levels of 25–40% to obtain solid fat profiles according to customer needs. Texture analysis showed that the roll-in margarine is similar to that of Play-Doh, having the unique ability to be formed and reformed according to stress applied. Thus, in roll-in pastries, the fat forms even, continuous layers during sheeting and lamination. Flexibility is crucial to the performance of roll-in fats through the formation of even layers of continuous fat needed for even puffing up during baking. If roll-in fats are too hard or soft, the sheeting and lamination steps preclude their use because hard fats resist sheeting by lumping or tearing the dough. Similarly, soft fats cannot stand stress during sheeting and may form pools of oil that may seep out of the dough during sheeting.

Retail Zero-*Trans* Shortenings

Crisco all-purpose baking shortenings have been popular for over 100 years (List and Jackson, 2007, 2009). Crisco was originally formulated from hydrogenated and liquid cottonseed oil, followed by hydrogenated and liquid soybean oil. In 2003, a portion of the Crisco brand was reformulated to zero *trans*, but by 2006 the entire Crisco brand became *trans* free. The formulation consists of fully hydrogenated hard stocks and liquid sunflower oil. Orthoefer (2005) described the formulation of zero-*trans* shortenings by blending soybean, cottonseed, or palm stearins with high-oleic canola oil either as simple mixtures or after interesterification. These shortenings have a wide plastic range and should perform well in most baking and/or frying applications.

Animal fat–based all-purpose shortenings are popular retail items and perform well in commercial baking/deep-fat frying (Kincs, 1985; Woerfel, 1960) and are low in *trans* acid content. In 2010, the food use of animal fats (lard, tallow) amounted to 1530 million lbs, with a per capita consumption of 4.9 lbs. In the same year, butter consumption was 1510 million lbs with a per capita of 4.9 lbs. Per capita consumption of all food products in 2010 was about 82 lbs. Thus, the 9.8 lbs of animal fats account for nearly 12% of U.S. per capita consumption of fats.

Conclusion

In summary, the food, oil processing, and agribusiness sectors have overcome many technical issues in order to bring healthier products to the market place in spite of working with just a few fats and oils (i.e., palm, soybean, canola, sunflower, corn, cottonseed, and animal fats). The reemergence of the trait-modified oils industry will continue to grow and provide TFA-free oils.

The aforementioned technologies of oleogels for structuring baking fats and improved emulsifier/surfactant blends with liquid oils are very promising as TFA replacements. The time-honored fat modifications, including hydrogenation, interesterification, and fractionation are still valuable, and further research may extend their usefulness as food formulation methods. Only time will tell if the expense and time required to meet labeling regulations are merited.

References

Ainger, G.; Coverly, B. Fat Compositions. U.S. Patent 4,214,012, 1980.

Andre, J. R.; Going, L. H. Liquid Shortening. U.S. Patent 2,815,286, 1957.

Anon. ADM Chooses Trouble Free Process for *Trans* Free Fats. *Oil Mill Gazeteer* **2004,** *109,* 2–5.

Babayan, V.; Lehman, H. Interesterified Mixture of Lauric and Non Lauric Oils. U.S. Patent 3,268,340, 1966.

Baldwin, R. R.; Baldry, R. P.; Johansen, R. G. Fat Systems for Bakery Products. *J. Am. Oil Chem. Soc.* **1972,** *49,* 473–477.

Beers, A. M.; Mangus, G. (2004) Hydrogenation of Edible Oils for Reduced *Trans* Fatty Acid Content. *Inform* **2004,** *15,* 404–405.

Beers, A. M.; Aariaansz, R.; Okonek, D. *Trans* Isomer Control in Hydrogenation of Edible Oils. In Trans *Fatty Acids;* Dijkstra, A. J., Hamilton, R. J., Hamm, W., Eds.; Blackwell Publishing: Oxford, UK, 2008; pp 147–180.

Berger, K.; Idris, N. A. Formulation of Zero Trans Shortenings, Margarines and Other Food Fats with Products from the Oil Palm. *J. Am. Oil Chem. Soc.* **2005,** *82,* 775–782.

Berger, K. *Trans* Free Fats with the Products of the Oil Palm: A Selective Review. *Czech. J. Food Sci.* **2007,** *25,* 174–181.

Berger, K. *Quality and Functions of Palm Oil in Food Applications: A Layman's Guide;* Malaysian Palm Oil Council, Kelana Jaya, Selangor, Malaysia, 2010.

Berlin, K. Margarine Fats Containing Interesterified Constituents. U.S. Patent 3,796,581, 1974.

Binder, T. P.; Bloomer, S.; Lee, I.; Solheim, L.; Wickland, L. Method for Producing Fats or Oils. U.S. Patent Application 0257982, 2006.

Brock, F. Liquid Shortening and Method of Making Same. U.S. Patent 2,868,652, 1959.

Carey, W. C. Spray Type Pan Release and Method for Making Same. U.S. Patent 3,821,007, 1974.

Cross, S. T.; Griffin, W. C. Fluid Shortening Composition. U.S. Patent 2,746,868, 1956.

Debonte, L. R.; Fan, Z.; Loh, W. Oil from Canola Seed with Altered Fatty Profiles and a Method of Producing Oil. U.S. Patent 5,861,187 (also U.S. Patent 6,270,828), 1999.

Delfosse, J. Margarine Fat Composition. British Patent 1,244,868, 1971.

Della Porta, R., Ed. *Edible Oils Manual,* 2nd ed.; AOCS Press: Urbana, IL, 2008.

Dijkshoorn, W.; Huizinga, H.; Pronk, J. Fat Blend Substantially Free of Hydrogenated and Interesterified Fats. U.S. Patent 4,366,181, 1982.

Dijkstra, A. J. Controlling the Physical and Chemical Properties of Fat Blends through Their Triglyceride Composition. In Trans *Fatty Acids,* Dijkstra, A. J., Hamilton, R. J., Hamm, W., Eds.; Blackwell Publishing, Oxford, UK, 2008; pp 132–146.

Dijkstra, A. J. *Edible Oil Processing from a Patent Perspective.* Springer Publishing: New York, 2012.

Dogan, I.; Javidpour, I.; Akin, T. Effects of Intereseterified Palm and Cottonseed Oil Blends on Cake Quality. *Intl. J. Food Science and Technol.* **2007,** *42,* 157–164.

Doucet, J. Shortening System Products There with and Methods for Making the Same. U.S. Patent 5,908,655, 1999.

Eckel, R. H.; Borra, S.; Lichtenstein, A.; Piazza, S. Understanding the Complexity of *Trans* Fatty Reduction in the American Diet. *Circulation* **2007,** *115,* 2231–2246.

Eckey, E. W. Directed Interesterification of Glycerides. *Ind. Eng. Chem.* **1948,** *40,* 1183–1190 (also U.S. Patents 2,442,532; 2,442,537; 2,442,536; 2,442,538).

Eller, F.; List, G. R.; Teel, J. A.; Steidley, K. R.; Adlof, R. O. Preparation of Spread oils meeting FDA Labeling Requirements for *Trans* Fatty Acids. *J. Ag. Food. Chem.* **2005,** *53,* pp 5982–5984.

Erickson, M. D., Ed. *Deep Frying: Chemistry, Nutrition and Practical Applications,* 2nd ed.; AOCS Press: Urbana, IL, 2007.

Erickson, M. D.; Frey, N. Property Enhanced Oils in Food Applications. *Food Tech.* **1994,** *50,* 63–68.

Floeter, Z. E.; van Duijn, G. *Trans* Free Fats for Use in Food. In *Modifying Lipids for Use in Food;* Gunstone, F. D., Ed.; Woodhead Publishing: Cambridge, UK, 2006; pp 429–443.

Fondu, M.; Willems, M. Margarine Fat Formulation. British Patent 1,245,531,1971.

Fondu, M.; Willems, M. Margarine Fat Containing Randomized Fat Components. U.S. Patent 3,634,100, 1972.

Gawrilow, I. Hydrated Pan Release Agent. U.S. Patent 3,906,117, 1975a.

Gawrilow, I. Process for Preparing Bakery Products. U.S. Patent 3,914,453, 1975b.

Gerde, J.; Fehr, W.; White, P. J. Frying Performance of No *Trans* Low Linolenic Soybean Oils. *J. Am. Oil Chem. Soc.,* **2007,** *84,* 557–563.

Gerardus, M.; Lee, M.; Gerardus van Oort, M.; Bright, M. U.S. Patent Application 0142465, 2009.

Ghotra, B. S.; Dyal, S.; Narine, S. S. Lipid Shortening: A Review. *Food Res. Intl.* **2002,** *35,* 1015–1048.

Gibon, V. Fractionation of Lipids for Use in Foods. In *Modifying Lipids for Food;* Gunstone, F. D., Ed.; Woodhead Publishers: Cambridge, UK, 2006; pp 201–233.

Gillies, M. T. *Shortenings, Margarines and Food Oils.* Noyes Data Corporation: Park Ridge, NJ, 1974.

Going, L. H. Interesterifcation Products and Processes. *J. Am. Oil Chem. Soc.* **1967,** *44,* 414A.

Gooding, C. M. Highly Nutritious Fat Composition. U.S. Patent 3,099,564, 1963.

Graffelman, H. Margarine Fat and Process for Preparing a Spread. U.S. Patent 3,617,308, 1967.

Gupta, M. NuSun the Next Generation of Oils. *Inform* **1998,** *9,* 150–154.

Gupta, M.; Warner, K.; White, P. J., Eds.; *Frying Technology and Practices.* AOCS Press: Urbana, IL, 2004.

Hammond, E. G. Improving the Fatty Acid Composition of Soybean Oil. *J. Am.Oil Chem. Soc.* **1984,** *61,* 1713–1716.

Hanson, H. W. Food Release Agent. U.S. Patent 4,192,898, 1980.

Hartnett, D. I. Cake Shortenings. *J. Am. Oil Chem. Soc.* **1977,** *54,* 557–560.

Hartnett, D. I.; Thalheimer, W. G. Part 1: Use of Oil in Baked Products, Background and Bread. Part 2: Sweet Goods and Cakes. *J. Am. Oil Chem. Soc.* **1979,** *56,* 944–952.

Hasman, J. (1995) *Trans* Suppression in Hydrogenated Oils. *Inform,* **1995,** *6,* 1206–1213.

Hawley, H. K.; Holman, G. W. Directed Interesterification as a New Processing Tool for Lard. *J. Am. Oil Chem. Soc.* **1956,** *33,* 29–35.
Higgens, N. Low Trans Stereoisomer Shortening Systems. U.S. Patent 7,149,430, 2007.
Holman, G. W.; Going, L. H. Rapid Directed Interesterification of Glycerides. U.S. Patent 2,875,066, 1959.
Houser, C. J. Shortening. U.S. Patent 2,968,562, 1961.
Howard, N. B.; Koren, P. Fluid Shortening for Cream Icings. U.S. Patent 3,208,857, 1965.
Huizinga, H. C.; Sassen, C.; Verimas, I.; Schur, P. Process for Making a Margarine Hardstock. U.S. Patent 5,858,445, 1999.
Idrus, N. A. Palm Oil Products for Cake Shortenings. *Palm Oil Developments PORIM,* 1987, 1–4.
Idrus, N. A. (1988) Characteristics and Performance of Palm Based Shortenings, *Sains Malaysiana,* 17. pp 269–281
Idrus, N. A.; Berger, k.; Ong, A. S. Evaluation of Shortenings Based on Various Palm Oil Products. *J. Sci. Food Agric.* **1989,** *46,* 481–493.
Idrus, N. A.; Abdullah, A.; Embong, M.; Hassan, H. Use of Palm Oil and Butterfat as Shortenings for Short Dough Biscuits: Sensory and Instrumental Analysis, *Elaeis* **1991,** *3,* 8.
Idris, N.; Dian, N. Interesterified Palm Products as Alternatives to Hydrogenation. *Asia Pacific J. Clin. Nutr.* **2005,** 14, 396–401.
Jackson, M. A.; List, G. R.; Palmquist, D. Low *Trans* Spreads and Shortening Oils via a Catalyst Switching Strategy. *J. Am. Oil Chem. Soc.* **2008,** *8,* 481–486.
Johnson, R. Bakery Margarines (Special Report). *Cereal Foods World* **1999,** *44,* 9–12.
Kamel, B. Characteristics of Bread and Buns Made with Lard and Vegetable Oils of Different Iodine Values. *J. Am. Oil Chem. Soc.* **1992,** *69,* 794–796.
Kanagaratnam, S.; Mat Sahri, M.; Idrus, N. A.; Tangavelu, T.; Ahmad, M. J. Palm Based *Trans* Free Roll in Margarine. *Palm Oil Developments,* **2009,** *48,* 7–12.
Kheiri, S. A. End Use of Palm Oil: Human Food. In *Palm Oil;* Gunstone, F. D., Ed.; John Wiley and Son: New York, 1987; pp 71–83.
Kiatsrichart, S.; Brewer, M. S.; Cadwallader, K. R.; Artz, W. Pan Frying of Nusun: A Mid Oleic Sunflower Oil. *J. Am. Oil Chem. Soc.* **2003,** *80,* 792–795.
Kincs, F. Meat Fat Formulation. *J. Am. Oil Chem. Soc.* **1985,** *62,* 815–818.
King, J. W.; Holliday, R. L.; List, G. R.; Snyder, J. M. Hydrogenation of Soybean Oil in Supercritical Carbon Dioxide and Hydrogen. *J. Am. Oil Chem. Soc.* **2001,** *78,* 815–818.
Kirkeby, P. G. Food Products without *Trans* Acids. In Trans *Fatty Acids;* Dijkstra, A.J., Hamilton, R. J., Hamm, W., Eds.; Blackwell Publishing: Oxford, UK, 2008; pp 219–234.
Klemann, L. Oils and Fats: Role in Baking Applications. In *Proceedings, IFT Short Course,* Orlando, FL, 2005.
Korver, O.; Katan, M. B. The Elimination of *Trans* Fats from Spreads: How Science Helped to Turn an Industry Around. *Nut. Rev.* ***2006,*** *64,* 275–279.
Krawczyk, T. Edible Specialty Oils: An Unfulfilled Promise. *Inform* **1999,** *10,* 555–561.
Lansbergen, A. J.; Shijf, R. *Edible Fats.* U.S. Patent 5,547,698, 1996.
Lee, I. Methods for Producing Fats and Oils. U.S. Patent 7,452,702, 2008.
Lindsay, D. Margarine Oil Manufacture. U.S. Patent 2,996,388, 1961.

List, G. R.; Jackson, M. A. Battle over Hydrogenation (1903–1920) Part 1. *Inform* **2007,** *18,* 403–405.

List, G. R.; Jackson, M. A. Battle over Hydrogenation (1903–1920) Part 2. *Inform* **2007,** *20,* 395–397.

List, G. R.; King, J. W. Hydrogenation of Lipids for Use in Foods. In *Modifying Lipids for Use in Foods;* Gunstone, F. D., Ed.; Woodhead Publishing: Cambridge, UK, 2006; pp 173–200.

List, G. R.; Pelloso, T. Zero/low *Trans* Margarines, Spreads and Shortenings. In Trans *Fats in Foods;* List, G. R., Kritchevsky, D., Ratnayake, N., Eds.; AOCS Press: Urbana, IL, 2007; pp 155–176.

List, G. R.; Mounts, T. L.; Orthoefer, F.; Neff, W. E. Margarine and Shortening Oils by Interesterification of Liquid and Trisaturated Triglycerides. *J. Am. Oil Chem. Soc.,* **1996,** *73,* 379–382.

List, G. R.; Steidley, K.; Neff, W. E. Commercial Spreads, Formulation, Structure and Properties. *Inform* **2000,** *11,* 980–986.

List, G. R.; Pelloso, T.; Warner, K.; Neff, W. E. Soft Margarines from High Stearic Acid Soybean Oil. *J. Am. Oil Chem. Soc.* **2001,** *78,* 103–104.

List, G. R.; Jackson, M. A.; Eller, F.; Neff, W. E. Low *Trans* Spread and Shortening Oils via Hydrogenation of Soybean Oil. *J. Am. Oil Chem. Soc.* **2007a,** *84,* 609–612.

List, G. R.; Warner, K.; Pintauro, P.; Gil, M. Low *Trans* Spreads and Shortening Fats by Electrochemical Hardening. *J. Am. Oil Chem. Soc.* **2007b,** *84,* 497–501.

Linteris, L. L. Fluid Shortening. U.S. Patent 2,909,432, 1959.

Loh, W. *Trans* Fat Labeling: A Quiet Revolution in the Food Industry. *Inform* **2006,** *17,* 283–285.

Lui, H. R.; White, P. J. High Temperature Stability of Soybean Oils with Altered Fatty Acid Compositions. *J. Am. Oil Chem. Soc.* **1992,** *69,* 533–537.

Lui, L.; Iaasonova, D. High Oleic Canola Oils and Their Food Applications. *Inform* **2012,** *23,* 491–494.

Mahler, D.; Doummani, C. Solid Stick Pan Lubricant. U.S. Patent 4,023,912, 1977.

Manirath, K.; Karleskind, D.; Lowery, C. Dough Compositions and Pretzels. U.S. Patent Application 0198936, 2006.

Marangoni, A.; Garti, N., Eds. *Edible Oleogels: Structure and Health Implications;* AOCS Press: Urbana, IL, 2011.

Marangoni, A.; Idziak, S. Spreadable Food Product. U.S. Patent 7,357,957, 2008.

Mat Dian, N.; Ibraham, N.; Idris, N. A. Interesterified Palm Oil Products for Solid Fat Applications. *Palm Oil Developments* **2006,** *45,* 12–19.

Matlock, M. In Trans *Fats Alternatives;* Khodali, D., List, G. R., Eds.; AOCS Press: Urbana, IL, 2005; pp 110–113.

Mat Sahri, M.; Dian, N. Formulation of *Trans* Free and Low Saturate Margarine. *J. Oil Palm Res.* **2011,** *23,* 958–967.

Mat Sahri, M. M.; Idris, N. A. Properties of Palm Oil Margarines during Storage: Effects of Processing Conditions. *Palm Oil Developments* **2006,** *46,* 20–26.

Mat Sahri, M.; Idris, N. A. Palm Stearin as Low *Trans* Hard Stock for Margarine. *Sans Malaysiana* **2010,** *39,* 821–827.

Mat Sahri, M.; Che Man, Y.; Yusoff, M.; Rahman, R. Effect of Scraped Surface Cooler Temperatures on the Physical Properties of Palm Oil Margarine. *J. Am. Oil Chem. Soc.* **2002,** *79,* 931–936.

Mat Sahri, M.; Che Man, Y.; Yusoff, M.; Rahman, R. A. Quality of Margarine: Fats Selection and Processing Parameters. *Asia Pacific Clin. Nutr.* **2005,** *14,* 387–395.

Matthius, B.; Haase, N.; Ubenend, G. Chemical and Sensory Characteristics of Products Fried in High Oleic Low Linolenic Rapeseed Oil. *J. Am. Oil Chem. Soc.* **2009,** *85,* 799–808.

Mattil, K. F.; Nelson, D. Process for Producing Modified Lard. U.S. Patent 2,625,483, 1953.

Mattil, K. F.; Norris, F. A. Modified Lard and Process for Making Same. U.S. Patent 2,625,478, 1953 (also U.S. Patents 2,625,479; 2,625,480; 2,465,481; 2,465,482).

McNeil, G. P. Loders Croklan Commercial Solutions. In Trans *Fat Alternatives;* Kodali, D., List, G. R., Eds., AOCS Press: Urbana, IL, 2005; 119–123.

Melnick, D.; Gooding, C. M. Highly Nutritional Oil Blends. U.S. Patent 2,921,855, 1960 (also U.S. Patent 2,955,039).

Miller, H. R.; White, P. J. High Temperature Stabilities of Low Linolenate, High Stearic and Common Soybean Oils. *J. Am. Oil Chem. Soc.* **1988,** *65,* 1324–1327.

Miller, J. W.; Zimmerman, D. C.; Vick, B. Genetic Control of High Oleic Acid Content in Sunflower Oil. *Crop Science* **1987,** *27,* 923–926.

Miller, M. *Alternative Oils: KFC's Journey to Low Lin Soybean Oil.* AOCS Meeting, Quebec City, QC, 2007.

Minal, J. Applications of Palm Based Interesterified Fats. *Palm Oil Developments* **2003a,** *39,* 11–21.

Minal, J. An Introduction to Random Interesterfication of Palm Oil. *Palm Oil Developments* **2003b,** *39,* 1–6.

Nagy-Nero, D. *Proceedings of AHA Trans Fat Conference,* Washington, DC, October 2006.

Nieuwenhuis, H. Putting Science on the Supermarket Shelf. In *Scientia Gras, A Select History of Fat Science and Technology,* Gunstone, F. D., Firestone, D., Eds.; AOCS Press: Urbana, IL, 2000; pp 141–148.

Normand, L. N.; Eskin, A. M.; Przbylski, R. Comparison of the Frying Stability of Regular and High Oleic Sunflower Oils. *J. Am. Oil Chem. Soc.* **2006,** *83,* 331–334.

Norris, F. A.; Mattil, K. F. A New Approach to the Glyceride Structure of Natural Fats. *J. Am. Oil Chem. Soc.* **1947,** *24,* 274–275.

Norris, M.; Gingras, L. Oil Substitution in Food Formulations. *Inform* **1990,** *1,* 388–392.

Norris, M. E. Fluid Shortening. U.S. Patent 3,941,452, 1975.

Norris, M. E. Preparing Fluid Shortening for Use in Yeast Raised Bakery Products. U.S. Patent 3,943,259, 1976.

O'Brien, R. D. Food Service Pan and Grill Shortenings. In *Fats and Oils: Formulating and Processing for Applications,* 3rd ed.; CRC Press: Boca Raton, FL, 2009; pp 414–415.

Orthoefer, F. Performance of *Trans* Free Vegetable Oils in Shortenings and Deep Fat Frying. *Lipid Technol.* **2005,** *17,* 101–106.

Orthoefer, F. Applications of Emulsifiers in Baked Goods. In *Food Emulsifiers and Their Applications,* 2nd ed.; Hasenhuettl, G. L., Hartel, R. W., Eds.; Springer: New York, 2008; 263–284.

Podmore, J. Food Applications of *Trans* Fatty Acids. In Trans *Fatty Acids,* Dijkstra, A. J., Hamilton, R. J., Hamm, W., Eds.; Blackwell Publishing: Oxford, UK, 2008; pp 203–218.

Poot C.; Verburg, C.; Kirton, D.; McNeil, A. Fractionated Co-randomized Fat Blend and Use. U.S. Patent 4,087,564, 1978.

Prevot, A.; Perrin, J.L.; Auge, P. H.; Coustelle, J. I. A New Variety of Low Linolenic Rapeseed Oil: Characteristics and Room Odor Tests. *J. Am. Oil. Chem. Soc.* **1990,** *67,* 161–164.

Pronk, J.; Saltau, M.; Weiske, M. Fat Having Butter like Properties and a Reduced Tendency to Develop Graininess and Process for Producing Such. U.S. Patent 4,590,087, 1986.

Rahovsky, I.; Martinez, C.; Kuchler, F. *New Food Choices Free of Trans Fats Better Align with Health Recommendations.* ERS/USDA Info Bulletin 95, 2012.

Ranhotra, G. S. Nutritional and Functional Considerations of Tropical Oils. *Cereal Foods World* **1993,** *38,* 486–489.

Read, C. Fat Products. U.S. Patent 3,889,011, 1975.

Reid, J. *Trans* Reformulation: Ruby Tuesday. *Circulation* **2007,** *115,* 2231–2246.

Roberio, A.; Grimaldi, R.; Gioielli, L.; Gonclaves, L. Zero *Trans* Fats from Soybean Oil and Fully Hydrogenated Soybean Oil: Physico-chemical Properties and Food Applications. *Food Res. Intl.* **2009,** *42,* 401–410.

Robinson, H. E.; Mattil, K. F. Fifty Years of Progress in the Technology of Fats and Oils. *J. Am. Oil Chem. Soc.* **1959,** *36,* 434–446.

Rousseau, D.; Marangoni, A. Chemical Interesterification of Food Lipids: Theory and Practice. In *Food Lipids;* Akoh, C. C., Min, D., Eds.; Marcel Dekker: New York, 2002; pp 301–334.

Rozendaal, A.; McRae, A. R. Interesterification of Fats and Oils. In *Lipid Technologies;* Gunstone, F. G., Padley, F. B., Eds.; Marcel Dekker: New York, 1997; pp 223–263.

Ruihong, G.; Meng, C. E.; Cali, L.; Chuanguo, M.; Dezhi, W. Special Palm based Fat Spread, for Bakery Frozen Dough. *Palm Oil Developments* **2008,** *48,* 7–13.

Sassen, C.; Westdorp, L. Edible Fat Spread. U.S. Patent 6,238,723, 2001.

Satchithanandam, S. C.; Oles, J.; Spease, C. J.; Brandt, M.; Yurawecz, M.; Rader, J. *Trans,* Saturated and Unsaturated Fat in Foods in the United States Prior to Mandatory *Trans* Fat Labeling. *Lipids* **2004,** *39,* 11–18.

Scavone, T. A. Beta Prime Stable Low Saturate Low *Trans* All Purpose Shortening. U.S. Patent 5,470,598, 1995.

Schmidt, W. Edible Fat and a Process for Producing Such Fat. U.S. Patent 4,567,056, 1986 (also U.S. Patent 4,610,889).

Screenivasan, B. Interesterification of Fats. *J. Am. Oil Chem. Soc.* **1978,** *55,* 796.

Seiden, P. Interesterified Triglycerides Containing Long and Short Chain Fatty Acids. U.S. Patent 3,253,964, 1967.

Seiden, P. Margarine Oils Containing Intermediate Melting Randomly Esterfied Triglycerids of High Content. U.S. Patent 3,592,661, 1971.

Skogerson, L.; Boute, T. Non-hydrogenated Vegetable Based Shortening Containing an Elevated Diglyceride Emulsifier Composition. U.S. Patent 7,691,428, 2010.

Slater, L. Lard Scores Again. *Food Eng.* **1953,** *100,* 72–73.

Soheli, K. C.; Artz, W. E.; Tippaywat, P. Pan Heating of Low Linolenic and Partially Hydrogenated Soybean Oils Using Pan Fried Hash Browns. *J. Am. Oil Chem. Soc.* **2002,** *79,* 1197–1200.

Stauffer, C. *Fats and Oils. Bakery Product Applications;* Eagan Press: St. Paul, MN, 1996; pp 61–79.

Stauffer, C. Fats and Oils in Bakery Products. In *Bailey's Industrial Oil and Fat Products,* 6th edition, Vol. 4; Shahidi, F., Ed.; John Wiley and Sons: Hoboken, NJ, 2005; pp 207–227.

Strouts, B. *Challenges in Commercial Baking Applications.* AHA *Trans* Fat Conference, Washington, DC, 2006.

Su, C.; Gupta, M.; White, P. J. Oxidative and Flavor Stabilities of Soybean Oils with Low and Ultra Low Linolenic Acid Composition. *J. Am. Oil Chem. Soc.* **2003,** *80,* 171–176.

Sudin, N. A.; Mat Sahri, M.; Kun, Y.; Oh, F. Modification of Palm and Palm Kernel Oil and Their Fractions for Margarine. *Palm Oil Developments (PORIM)* **1991,** *18,* 1–3.

Tafuri, M. B.; Tao, B. Structural Fat and Methods for Making Same. U.S. Patent 4,447,462, 1984.

Tarrago-Trani, K.; Phillips, L.; Lemar, L. E.; Holden, J. New and Existing Oils Used in Products with Reduced *Trans* Fatty Acid Content. *J. Am. Dietetic Assoc.* **2006,** *106,* 867–870.

Tiffany, T. Oil Options for Deep Fat Frying. *Food Technol.* **2007,** *61* (7), 46–56.

Tiffany, T. *Enzymatic Interesterified Soybean based Shortening and Margarine: Functional 0 Grams/serving Alternatives for the Food Industry.* IFT Annual Meeting, New Orleans, LA, 2008.

Timms, R. Fractionation. In *Lipid Technologies;* Gunstone, F. D., Padley, F. B., Eds.; Marcel Dekker: New York, 1997; pp. 199–222.

Ullanoormadam, S. R. Trans Free Hard Structural Fat for Margarine Blends and Spreads. U.S. Patent 6,808,737,2004 (also U.S. Patent 7,807,208, 2010).

Upritchard, J.; Zeelenberg, M. J.; Huizinga, H.; Verschuren, P. M.; Trautwein, E. Modern Fat Technology: What Is the Potential for Heart Health? *Proc. Nutr. Soc.* **2005,** *64,* 379–386.

Van der Wal, R. J.; Van Akkeren, L. A. Modified Lard and Process for Producing Same. U.S. Patent 2,571,315, 1951.

van Heteren, J.; Pronk, J.; Vermass, L. Fat Blend. U.S. Patent 4,386,111, 1983.

van Loon, C. Process for the Conversion of Triglycerides with Other Esters. U.S. Patent 1,744,596, 1927 (also U.S. Patent 1,873,513).

Van Toor, H.; van Rossum, G.; Kruidenberg, M. Low *Trans* Fat Compositions/Low Temperature Hydrogenation of Edible Oils. U.S. Patents 7,585,990; 7,498,453; 7,820,841, 2009.

Van Toor, H.; van Rossum, G.; Kruidenberg, M. Low *Trans* Fat Compositions/Low Temperature Hydrogenation of Edible Oils. U.S. Patent 7,820,841, 2010.

Waheed, A.; Rasool, G.; Asghar, A. Effect of Interesterified Palm and Cottonseed Blends on Cookie Quality. *Agric. Biol. N. America* **2010,** *33,* 402–406.

Wainwright, R. Oils and Fats for the Baking Industry. *Cereal Foods World* **1999,** *44SR,* 16–19.

Wainwright, R.; Fallow, D.; Morehart, L.; Womack, J. Options for Reducing/eliminating *Trans* Acids in Deep Fat Frying and Labeling Implications. In *Deep Frying;* Erickson, M. D., Ed.; 2006; pp 397–414.

Ward, J. Edible Fat Products. U.S. Patents 4,341,812 and 4,341,813, 1982.

Warner, K. A.; Fehr, W. Mid Oleic Low Linolenic Acid Soybean Oil: A Healthful, New Alternative to Hydrogenated Oil for Frying. *J. Am. Oil Chem. Soc.* **2008,** *85,* 945–951.

Warner, K. A.; Gupta, M. Frying Quality of Ultra Low and Low Linolenic Acid Soybean Oil. *J. Am. Oil Chem. Soc.* **2003,** *80,* 275–280.

Warner, K. A.; Gupta, M. Potato Chip Quality and Frying Oil Stability of High Oleic Soybean Oil. *J. Food Sci.* **2009,** *70,* 395–400.

Warner, K. A.; Knowlton, S. Frying Oils and Oxidative Stability of High-oleic Corn Oil. *J. Am. Oil Chem. Soc.* **1997,** *74,* 1317–1322.

Warner, K. A.; Moser, J. Frying Stability of Purified Mid Oleic Sunflower Triacylglycerols with Added Pure Tocopherols and Tocopherol Mixtures. *J. Am. Oil Chem. Soc.* **2009,** *85,* 1461–1469.

Warner, K. A.; Mounts, T. L. Frying Stability of Soybean and Canola Oil with Modified Compositions. *J. Am. Oil Chem. Soc.* **1993,** *70,* 983–988.

Warner, K. A.; Parrot, L.; Glynn, M. P. Effect of Frying Oil Composition on Potato Chip Stability. *J. Am. Oil Chem. Soc.,* **1994,** *71,* 1117–1121.

Warner, K. A.; Orr, P.; Glynn, M. P. Effect of Fatty Acid Composition of Oils on Flavor and Stability of Fried Foods. *J. Am. Oil Chem. Soc.* **1997,** *74,* 347–356.

Warner, K. A.; Neff, W. E.; Byrdwell, W. C.; Gardner, H. W. Effect of Oleic and Linoleic Acids on the Production of Deep Fried Odor in Heated Triolein and Trilinolein. *J. Agric. Food Chem.* **2001,** *49,* 899–905.

Weiske, T.; Hannewijk, J.; Willems, M. Margarine Fat. U.S. Patent 3,949,105, 1976.

Weiske, T. Margarine Fat. U.S. Patent 4,045,588, 1977.

Weiss, T. *Food Oils and Their Uses,* 2nd ed.; AVI Publishing: Westport, CT, 1983; pp. 157–186.

Widlak, N. Formulation of Fluid Shortenings. In *Proceedings of World Conference on Oilseed Utilization;* Wilson, R. F., Ed.; AOCS Press: Urbana, IL, 2001; pp 39–43.

Wilkes, R. Low Linolenic Soybeans and Beyond. *Lipid Tech* **2008,** *20,* 277–279.

Wilkes, R. *Fry Studies Utilizing a Novel Low Saturate High Oleic Soybean Oil.* AOCS Meeting, Phoenix, AZ, 2010.

Woerfel, J. B. Shortenings. In *Bakery Technology and Engineering;* Matz, S., Ed.; Avi Publishing: Westport, CT, 1960; pp 134–169.

Xu, X.; Guo, Z.; Zhang, H.; Vikbjerg, A. F.; Damstrup, M. L. Chemical and Enzymatic Interesterifiation of Lipids for Food Use. In *Modifying Lipids for Use in Food;* Gunstone, F. D., Ed.; Woodhead Publishers: Cambridge, UK, 2006; pp 234–272.

12

Trans Fats Replacement Solutions in North America

G.R. List ■ *U.S. Department of Agriculture, Peoria, Illinois, USA (Retired)*

Introduction

Trans fat replacements in North America have focused on the food service industry, the baking industry, and myriad fat-containing foods. Replacement of the traditional hydrogenated fats in order to meet nutritional labeling requirements has evolved over the past decade in the form of new processing technologies, improved oilseeds with trait-enhanced or modified oils, a switch to commodity oils, and the resurgence of tropical oils and animal-based fats in the marketplace. The U.S. food processing industry consists of about 60 plants producing nearly 300 brand names. Many of these products have been reformulated to 0 g *trans* fat per serving, and often contain reduced saturated fatty acid content as well. Major suppliers have taken different approaches to provide customers with *trans* fat replacements. One supplier includes both chemically and enzymatically interesterified margarine/shortening oils along with a line of naturally stable oils, lauric fats for confections, and palm-based shortening products in their portfolio. Other commercial approaches include baking shortenings made by modified hydrogenation technologies. High stability trait-modified oils serve as *trans* fat replacements. Several suppliers offer exclusively palm-based products. A summary of commercial offerings as of 2006 has been reported (Tarrago-Trani, 2006). Federal dietary guidelines have increasingly emphasized the need for consumption of less saturated fat and for foods that contain low/no *trans* fatty acids (TFAs). This chapter will review steps taken by North American companies to replace TFAs and saturated fats in food oils.

Consumption Patterns: Effect of *Trans* Fat Labeling

The global production of oils amounts to nearly 152 million t, of which palm, soybean, canola, and sunflower oils account for over 85%. Palm and soy account for 61% of the world's output. Thus, reduction of *trans* fats must focus on soybean and palm oils. For many applications for which solid fat is needed (spreads, baking, heavy duty frying), hydrogenation is required for needed functionality and oxidative stability. Over the past decade, statistics show that in the United States, the amount of oil going into baking/frying fats has decreased markedly since *trans* fat labeling requirements were announced in 2003 with an effective date of January 1, 2006 (see Table 12.A). The consumption of salad/cooking oils over this period, however, has increased dramatically. This category includes liquid (unhydrogenated) and/or lightly (brush) hydrogenated oils (10% *trans*). In 2000, soybean oil commanded over 80% of the U.S. edible oil market, whereas today soybean oil accounts for about 65% of U.S. consumption. The trend toward increased usage of liquid oils began in about 2004, corresponding to the beginning of zero-TFA reformulation. Another factor promoting the increased usage of liquid oils is reduction of saturated fatty acids. Liquid oils also provide omega-3 acids and can be labeled as heart healthy. Although the spread market has declined markedly over the past 20 years, omega-3 and heart healthy oils are of value in this food category, especially when fortified with plant sterols.

A major factor in edible oil consumption patterns is the development and expansion of the canola industry in Canada and increased U.S. demand. The United States has doubled canola production from about 640 million lbs to 1228 million lbs between 2003 and 2011. Domestic usage, however, has tripled over this timeframe, and imports amount to over 3500 million lbs.

Sunflower, cottonseed, and corn oils are considered naturally stable oils because they are free of linolenic acid. During the 2003–2011 timeframe, domestic usage of these oils has remained fairly static and it would appear that TFA labeling has had little effect. In 2004, combined usage of these three oils amounted to 2908 million lbs compared to 2585 million lbs in 2011.

Animal fats, including edible tallow and lard, offer a *trans* fat replacement. However, only slight increases in food use have occurred. Over the period of 2003–2011, lard in food products amounted to a low of 220 million lbs to a high of about 500 million lbs. On the other hand, edible tallow consumption has been largely static,

Table 12.A U.S. Per Capita Consumption of Edible Fats and Oil (pounds)

Year	Butter	Lard	Tallow	Margarine	Baking/ Frying	Salad/ Cooking	Other Edible	All Food Products (Total)	Total Consumption (Million pounds)
2000	4.5	0.8	4.0	8.3	23.0	33.7	1.5	73.2	20674
2001	4.4	1.1	3.0	7.1	32.6	35.6	1.4	83.0	23682
2002	4.4	1.3	3.4	6.6	33.3	39.7	1.4	87.9	25311
2003	4.4	1.3	3.8	5.3	32.8	40.2	1.3	87.3	25375
2004	4.5	0.8	3.8	5.3	32.6	40.0	1.5	86.8	25421
2005	4.5	1.6	3.8	4.1	29.2	42.7	1.6	85.8	25404
2006	4.7	1.7	3.9	4.6	24.9	44.6	2.1	84.6	25295
2007	4.7	1.6	2.9	4.6	21.0	50.2	1.7	84.9	25636
2008	5.0	1.0	2.9	4.3	18.1	54.0	1.6	85.2	25959
2009	5.0	1.5	0.7	3.7	16.0	51.0	1.7	77.8	23908
2010	4.9	1.5	3.4	3.6	15.3	53.5	1.6	82.1	25466

Table 12.B Food Use U.S. Tropical Oils/Animal Fats

	Palm Kernel		Palm oil		Total Palm Oils		Coconut	Lard	Tallow	Butter
Year	MT 1000	Lbs.[a]	MT 1000	Lbs.	MT 1000	Lbs.	Lbs.	Lbs.	Lbs.	Lbs.
2000	36	80.6	152	340	421	188	999	221	1125	1311
2001	69	154.6	196	439	594	265	1137	325	869	1332
2002	82	183.7	154	345	499	236	874	370	974	1444
2003	98	219.5	212	474	694	310	885	369	1108	1431
2004	83	186	301	674	860	384	815	220	1163	1392
2005	90	202	531	1189	1391	621	1134	460	1116	1431
2006	110	246	600	1344	1590	710	1017	499	1160	1540
2007	67	150	878	1967	2117	945	1138	487	889	1677
2008	173	388	870	1949	2337	1043	959	317	896	1831
2009	136	305	858	1922	2227	994	1340	448	212	1726
2010	117	262	852	1922	2184	969	1089	480	1050	1510
2011	138	309	937	2010	2319	1075	1154	N/A	N/A	1911
2012	152	340	1056	2365	2705	1396	1122	N/A	N/A	N/A

[a]All lbs in millions.

ranging from 815–1163 million lbs, except in 2009, when unusually low amounts were consumed (see Table 12.B).

Palm, palm kernel, and their fractions are very popular TFA replacements and are major players in the edible oil marketplace worldwide. In 2003, the United States imported 693 million lbs of palm/palm kernel oil, compared to 2705 million lbs in 2012. Coconut oil usage has increased from 885 million lbs in 2003 to 1154 million lbs in 2011. Thus, the tropical oil market has rebounded from the poor image it had in the 1980s (see Table 12.B).

Food Service Applications and Products

Although the food service industry is exempt from federal labeling requirements, local and municipal laws have banned *trans* fats. Fast food and other restaurants and school lunch programs are affected. Most notably, New York City took the lead and provided assistance to comply. In other locations, compliance was voluntary.

The food service industry uses a variety of fats and oils for deep-fat frying, pan/griddle use, par frying, sauteing, and spray oils. These products have evolved over the years from heavily hydrogenated cube shortenings to fluid products containing hydrogenated oil with beta stable hardstocks incorporated for increased stability and ease of handling. Heavy duty frying oils can also be produced by hydrogenation followed by fractionation. However, these products may contain 20–40% *trans*. To offer a *trans*-free solution, the industry has introduced blends of commodity/trait-modified and palm-based products for heavy duty frying. Studies conducted by Texas A&M University, in which a number of frying fats were used to prepare french fries and a standard soybean (hydrogenated, 32% *trans*) oil was used as a control, showed that the *trans*-free fats were equal to or superior to the control (findings at www.frytest.com). Factors evaluated included fry life by total polar materials (TPM) and sensory properties. Although Europe has set a limit for TPM of 24% for discarding frying oil, the United States does not have a TPM requirement and all of the oils were well below 24% after 14 days of frying.

Doughnut frying does not lend itself well to *trans*-free liquid oils. Although they function as a heat transfer medium, the doughnuts absorb oil and tend to be soggy and as they cool. Solid fat is required so that icings and glazes will adhere to the doughnut. On the other hand, it is claimed that frying doughnuts in canola oil does not present these problems (www.frytest.com).

Several TFA-free frying oils have been introduced especially for doughnut frying, and they are formulated from blends of palm and high-stability trait-modified canola oil.

A study published in 1994 compared the frying performance of low-linolenic soybean and mid-oleic sunflower oils against a standard high-TFA hydrogenated frying shortening (Erickson and Frey, 1994). These oils performed well in both frying and as spray oils for crackers.

In food service, french fries are often par fried followed by deep-fat frying prior to serving. A low-saturate TFA-free oil formulated from high-oleic canola oil was introduced in 2008. This par frying system is claimed to alleviate problems of increased crumbs in the fryer and a reduced grease line. The fry life is comparable to a partially hydrogenated shortening, and french fries have excellent flavor and color (USDA, 2013).

Traditionally, high stability oils were produced by hydrogenation followed by fractionation (Lampert, 2000). These oils are typically used when long shelf life is needed. Examples include the roasting of nuts, spray oils, moisture barriers, pan release agents, and foods for military use. High-stability oils are characterized by high *trans* fat content and very high stability as measured by the active oxygen method (AOM).

Trans Fat Regulation in Canada

In 2004, the Canadian government appointed a task force to develop *trans* fat labeling regulations. Unlike U.S. regulations, which require less than 0.5 g *trans* fat per serving to be declared zero, Canada has declared that for a food to be declared zero *trans* it must contain less than 0.2 g per serving, less than 2 g of saturates plus *trans*, and less than 15% of energy from saturates plus TFA. To be labeled 0.0 g TFA, a food must contain less than 0.1 g per serving of the food (for fats and oils, serving size is

12–14 g). The TFA level is not dependent on the saturates level. The food industry claimed that these requirements were too stringent and difficult to achieve. In 2006, the Canadian government appointed another taskforce which recommended that foods should not contain more than 5% *trans* in the total fat. In 2007, the government announced that it would regulate *trans* to the 2006 recommendation unless the industry voluntarily complied within 2 years. The city of Calgary and the province of British Columbia complied in 2008 and 2009, respectively.

As a result of labeling regulations, the volume of hydrogenated fats has decreased, imports of palm and lauric oils have increased, and, as a result, the *trans* levels in Canadian foods have been decreasing. However, TFA replacements have significantly different characteristics than hydrogenated products. These include shelf life and packaging, textural changes in fried foods, loss of functionality, and decreased fat levels in some baked goods (Forster, 2006).

Commercial *Trans* Fat Replacements

The commercially available products as of 2005 are presented in Trans *Fat Alternatives* (Kodali and List, 2005). Although not a complete compilation, the products are typical of U.S. technology. More recent products are covered in the food service section that follows.

Palm Based: Company A (Fractionation/Blending)

- Three families of margarine and shortening oils; nonhydrogenated, zero *trans*, low saturates, wide range of melting points
- Baking applications, pastries, frying, filling fats for cream cookies and icings
- Cocoa butter replacements, palm/palm kernel based

Palm Based: Company B (Fractionation/Blending)

- Seven baking shortenings; wide range of applications: icing stabilizer, structuring fat, cookies/crackers, all purpose, cakes, cookies, fillers, dairy substitutes, liquid oil applications
- Nonemulsified and emulsified offerings
- Frying shortenings (plastic/liquid) for doughnut frying
- Coating fats

Palm Based: Company C

- *Trans*-free structural fats
- Blending with liquid oils allows formulation of margarines, shortenings with low saturates, zero *trans*

Diverse Approach: Company D (Interesterification, Blending Tropical and Liquid Oils, Blends Partially Hydrogenated)

- Interesterified (chemical, enzymatic), baking fats, margarine/spread bases
- Naturally stable oils (corn, cottonseed, Nusun, sunflower), blends with partially hydrogenated soybean oil and liquid oils
- Palm oil/soybean oil blends
- Palm kernel oil, partially hydrogenated palm kernel, coconut, partially hydrogenated coconut; used in spray oil coatings

Company E (Baking, Frying, Trait Modified Canola, Soybean Oils)

- Baking shortenings (interesterified canola/fully hydrogenated soybean oil; modified hydrogenation)
- All-purpose baking shortening with reduced-TFA saturates as drop-in solutions for cookies, biscuits, pie crusts, tortillas, mixes; formulated from a proprietary hydrogenation process from commodity oils
- Palm/palm kernel based
- All purpose, cake and icing, specialty icing, specialty cake shortening, baker's margarine, croissant margarine, pastry margarine, roll-in shortening, emulsified dough shortening, biscuit flakes
- Trait-modified canola, soybean oils for spray oils, frying, blending, salad dressings, crackers, and snack spray
- Par/deep-fat frying shortenings (low *trans*/saturates)
- Doughnut frying oils (low *trans*/saturates)

*Company F (Low-*Trans *Shortenings, High-Stability Oils; High-Oleic Canola Based)*

- Low-*trans* shortenings produced by interesterification or modified hydrogenation
- Three offerings: soft (for cookies, crackers, bread, pizza dough, scones, cake mixes); medium (soft cookies, biscuits, dough mix, doughnuts); relatively hard (pastry biscuits, pie crusts)
- All have a maximum of 2% *trans*, 10–22% saturates, lowered melting points of 109–122 °F, AOM 70–85 hours

Innovations in *Trans* Fat Replacements in the Food Service Sector

Although exempt from federal labeling requirements, many local and municipal governments have proposed or enacted bans on *trans* fats in the food service industry. Schools, hospitals, fast foods restaurants, and small bakeries are affected. As a result, myriad *trans*-free products are available through local suppliers. These include fully refined, bleached, and deodorized (RBD) liquid oils (no hydrogenation), as well as trait-modified oils, which may be considered suitable for heavy duty frying. RBD commodity oils include soybean, cottonseed, corn, peanut, and olive. Trait-modified oils include low linolenic, mid-/high-oleic soybean, high-/mid-oleic sunflower, and low-linolenic/high-oleic canola. Although the RBD and trait-modified oils contain no industrial *trans* fats, small amounts (1–2%) of *trans* are produced primarily by deodorization. The polyunsaturated *trans* fat is not included in federal labeling regulations.

In addition to liquid frying oils, a number of palm-based frying shortenings have been introduced by major oil processors and marketed under private labels. Palm and hydrogenated soy/cottonseed oils are blended to meet a zero-*trans* claim. Because oils act as both a heat *trans*fer media and a solid fat in doughnut frying, palm-based shortenings have proven to be *trans*-free replacements for heavily hydrogenated doughnut frying shortenings. As the doughnuts cool, solid fat forms and allows glazes and icings to adhere to the doughnuts without collapse or loss of sugar.

Many foods are par fried, frozen, and then deep-fat fried prior to serving. In 2008, a product was introduced to function as both a par and a deep-fat frying medium. The frying fat is formulated from fully hydrogenated cottonseed and soybean oils and trait-modified vegetable oils. The blended oil has 0 g TFA and contains less saturated fat than heavily hydrogenated frying shortenings. Because the trait-modified oil is rich in oleic acid, extended fry life is to be expected.

Traditionally, pan and grill oils have been formulated from soybean, coconut, palm, palm kernel, and cottonseed oils. Both pourable and salted/pourable products serve in a variety of applications, including pan/grill frying, soups, gravies, seasonings, sauces, basting, and dips. These products are generally low in TFAs.

Applications for solid products include bun/bread toasting for sandwiches, dressing for corn on the cob, and grilling. Although they may be lower in *trans* fat, palm kernel and coconut oils contribute to increased saturated fat. Butter and margarine are popular among chefs for these applications because of the flavors and color imparted to the food. However, the moisture and milk solids may scorch and/or spatter.

Within the past few years, a number of low-TFA, reduced-saturates pan/grill shortenings have been introduced to the food service industry, and they are marketed as liquid butter alternatives. Typically they are unsalted, pourable, butter-flavored oils that contain lecithin as an antistick spattering agent. Other ingredients may include artificial color, antioxidants, and methyl silicones. Additional features include a microencapsulated flavor system which ensures that flavors carry through to foods. The products are shelf stable and refrigeration is not required.

Since 2006, much research and development has brought a greatly expanded portfolio of low-/zero-*trans* and reduced-saturate baking shortenings to the food service sector. The first generation of products was produced by random interesterification of liquid oils and hardstocks or proprietary hydrogenation technologies. At least two major suppliers are now offering products using enzymes as rearrangement catalysts. This technology is versatile because the physical properties of the rearranged fat can be controlled by the amount of hardstock in the simple blend. Typically, soybean oil and fully hydrogenated soy hardstocks are blended before rearrangement. Both soft and firm all-purpose baking shortenings are offered commercially. Other all-purpose shortenings made with domestic oils (hydrogenated cottonseed/soybean oils) contain reduced TFAs without increased saturates. Nonhydrogenated, all-purpose shortenings are available for customers wishing to eliminate "hydrogenation" from labels and to maintain a zero-*trans* claim. Palm, palm kernel, and canola oils are used in formulating these products. Thus, the solid fat content can be adjusted to yield products ranging from very soft to very firm, which allows flexibility in each bakery requirement.

Specialty shortenings for use in pies, very cold pie doughs, industrial pie manufacture, and refrigerated and frozen doughs are commercially available. They are nonhydrogenated and formulated from soybean, high-oleic canola, palm, and palm kernel oils. Although they are TFA free, the saturated fatty acid content of these products ranges from 36–61%.

Nonhydrogenated, zero-TFA plastic bakery margarines for all-purpose and roll-in applications are formulated from palm and soybean oils. The all-purpose shortenings are recommended for cookies, Danishes, croissants, and general baking, including cakes and icings. Roll-in margarines perform well in puff pastry and other laminated doughs. This product was designed for use in automated dough lines structure, and lamination. Both emulsified and unemulsified products are available. Other specialty shortening applications include tortillas, cake mixes, bread and yeast-raised doughs, icings and cream fillers, and biscuits.

Trait-modified oils (soybean, canola, sunflower) are becoming important food oils, making up about 18% of U.S. consumption. Major applications include deep-fat frying, spray oils, and applications for which long shelf life is needed. They offer a TFA-free solution and, in the case of canola and mid-oleic sunflower, reduced saturates. The high-oleic oils are ideal for blending with other oils when specific flavor profiles are needed. For example, the desirable fried food flavors originate from the breakdown of linoleic acid hydroperoxides. A linoleic acid content of 20% is considered optimum (Warner et al., 1997). A linolenic acid content of 3% or less is recommended for frying oils.

Other *Trans* Fat Alternatives

The use of unhydrogenated liquid oils in combination with emulsifiers and surfactants for baking bread has been an industry practice for many years. Hartnett and Thalheimer (1979) have shown that unhydrogenated soybean oil containing monogylcerides and polysorbate 60/ssl can be used in white and devils food cakes with even regular grain as well as being rich and tender. Sweet doughs made with soybean oil containing monogylcerides and polysorbate 60 handled well, with good structure and softness. Sweet doughs made with liquid soybean oil without emulsifiers, however, were sticky, had open grain, and poor softness (Hartnett and Thalheimer, 1979).

Zero-*trans* oils can be formulated from liquid vegetable oils and high amounts of digylcerides; these oils are *trans* free and are lower in saturated fats than commercial baking shortenings (Skogerson and Boutte, 2010). Other approaches to zero-*trans* and low-saturate baking shortenings use a liquid-base oil (74–90%) and a hardstock (10–26%) consisting of PSP and PSS (where P = palmitic, S = stearic) TAG. Plastic shortenings prepared in this manner are beta-prime stable, low in *trans* and saturated fatty acids, and are reported to be useful in confections, frying, and baking applications (Scavone, 1995). Doucet (1999) describes a shortening system based on liquid oil (86–95%) and interesterified stearines (5–14%) from coconut, palm, and palm kernel oils. Because the gylcerolysis is carried out in the presence of excess glycerol, mono- and diacylglycerols (MAG and DAG) are formed. Sugar cookies prepared from 86% oil and 14% emulsifier had good texture and flavor release and left negligible oil prints when placed on paper towels overnight. A shortening prepared with 93% soybean oil and 7% emulsifier was evaluated as a spray oil for buttery snack crackers. The crackers had a uniform appearance, were semidry to the touch, and had a good mouth feel and flavor release.

The use of oleogels for *trans* reduction in food uses is a recent phenomenon. Liquid vegetable oil, when sheared in the presence of water and monogylcerides, forms a gel that gives structure to baked goods (Marangoni and Idziak, 2008). Common vegetable oils, including canola, soybean, and sunflower, and trait-modified oils can serve as the liquid portion. The gels are white, tasteless, and creamy in texture. Oleogels can be substituted for vegetable shortening, butter, or lard in baking applications and perform well in cookies, cakes, biscuits, pie shells, brownies, waffles, pizza dough, frozen dough, and muffins.

New Low-Saturate/No-*Trans,* Omega-3-Enriched Oils in the Commercial Pipeline

In response to the need for reducing saturated fatty acids and the need for increased omega-3 acids in dietary fats, new oils are nearing commercial completion. Vistive gold is a low-saturate, high-oleic acid soybean oil produced by a combination of traditional plant breeding and transgenic gene insertion. Compared to commodity oil, which has about 15% saturates, vistive gold contains about 6% saturates. The oleic acid content is around 75%, which is very attractive for deep-fat frying and high stability applications. Its use for frying potatoes and chicken resulted in a reduction of

TFA plus saturates amounting to 66% and 31%, respectively, compared to a hydrogenated frying shortening. The low-saturate soybean oil had a fry life (chicken frying) identical to the standard shortening and high-oleic canola oil (4.5 h to a total polar content of 24%) (Wilkes, 2010).

Commodity soybean oil (unhydrogenated) contains 7–8% omega-3 acids (linolenic acid). A stearidonic acid (SDA)-enriched soy oil is nearing commercialization and contains 36% omega-3 acids. Despite the high unsaturated fatty acid composition, SDA oil has a clean neutral taste and is more stable than other omega-3 oils, offers a broad range of food applications, and maintains traditional flavor and shelf life. Potential applications include beverages, dairy products, oil-based foods, baking, snack foods, and prepared foods (Wilkes, 2010). Unlike other omega-3 fatty acids, SDA readily converts to EPA in the human body (Wilkes, 2010).

Margarines and Spreads

Virtually all U.S. soft tub margarines and spreads have been reformulated to 0 g of TFA per serving. This has been accomplished by blending liquid oils with lightly hydrogenated base stocks and/or tropical oils and their fractions. Stick products, on the other hand, have proven more difficult to reformulate and typically contain 1.5–2.5 g TFA fat/serving. A few stick margarine brands have reformulated to zero *trans*, but owing to less solid fat in the formulation, they require refrigeration whereas traditional products can be stored at ambient temperatures. The U.S. consumption of margarines and spreads has decreased by over 50% from peak years in the mid 1990s. In order to reverse a shrinking market, the spreads industry has introduced products advertised as "heart healthy" that are low in saturated and TFA fats and fortified with plant sterols to lower cholesterol in blood lipids. While popular in Europe, these products command a small market share in the United States. Higher costs are no doubt a factor contributing to a lack of success. In Canada, BECEL (blood and cholesterol lowering) margarine, first introduced in 1960 by Unilever, is popular and has been reformulated to zero TFA per serving (Korver and Katan, 2006).

References

Doucet, J. Shortening Systems Therewith and Methods for Making the Same U.S. Patent 5,908,655, 1999.

Erickson, M.; Frey, N. Property Enhanced Oils in Food Applications. *Food Technol.* **1994,** *50,* 63–68.

Forster, D. Emerging Technologies to Partially Hydrogenated Vegetable Shortenings and Margarines in Canada. *Abstracts AOCS Meeting,* St. Louis, MO, 2006.

Hartnett, D. I.; Thalheimer, W. G. Part 1. Use of Oil in Baked Products, Background and Bread. Part 2. Sweet Goods and Cakes *J. Am. Oil Chem. Soc.* **1979,** *56,* 944–952.

Kodali, D.; List, G. R., Eds., Trans *Fat Alternatives.* AOCS Press: Urbana, IL, 2005.

Korver, O.; Katan, M. B. The Elimination of *Trans* Fats from Spreads: How Science Helped Turn an Industry Around. *Nutr. Rev.* **2006,** *64,* 275–279.

Lampert, D. High Stability Oils: What, How and Why. In *Physical Properties of Fats, Oils, and Emulsifiers;* Widlak, N. Ed.; AOCS Press: Urbana, IL; 1999, pp 238–246.

Scavone, T. A. Beta Prime Stable Low Saturate Low *Trans* All Purpose Shortening U.S. Patent 5,470,598, 1995.

Skogerson, L.; Boute, T. Non-hydrogenated Vegetable Based Shortening Containing an Elevated Digylceride Emulsifier Composition. U.S. Patent 7,691,428, 2010.

Marangoni, A.; Idziak, S. Spreadable Food Product. U.S. Patent 7,357,597, 2008.

Tarrago-Trani, M. T.; Phillips, K.; Lemar, L.; Holden, J. New and Existing Oils Used in Prod ucts with Reduced *Trans* Fat Content. *J. Am. Dietetic Assoc.* **2006,** *106,* 867–880.

Texas A&M University, www.frytest.com (accessed February 2014).

Warner, K. A.; Orr, P.; Glynn, M. Effect of Fatty Acid Composition of Oils on Flavor and Stability of Fried Foods. *J. Am. Oil Chem. Soc,* **1997,** *74,* 347–356.

Wilkes, R. Fry Studies Utilizing a Novel Low Saturate High Oleic Soybean Oil. *Abstracts AOCS Meeting,* Phoenix, AZ, 2010; p. 50.

United States Department of Agriculture (USDA). *Oil Crop Yearbook,* No 89002, ERS.

13

Trans Fats Replacement Solutions in Europe

Leendert H. Wesdorp, Sergey M. Melnikov, and Estelle A. Gaudier ■ *Unilever Foods R&D Vlaardingen, The Netherlands*

Introduction

Trans fatty acids (TFAs) are formed by natural biohydrogenation of fats in the rumen of cattle and sheep, as well as by partial hydrogenation of vegetable oils in industrial processing. The negative health impact of TFAs was first discovered in the mid 1990s (Zock, 1997), and there is now consistent evidence that industrial and ruminant TFAs adversely affect the blood cholesterol profile (Brouwer et al., 2010). The impact of different dietary sources of TFAs on coronary heart disease is still subject to controversy; most of the scientific evidence relates to industrial TFAs and strongly shows a negative impact on coronary heart disease (CHD) risk. Dietary intake of ruminant TFAs is generally not seen as a large health problem because intake is relatively low. However, the available data on ruminant TFAs indicate that the potential impact on CHD risk of equal intakes of ruminant and industrial TFAs can be considered similar (Brouwer et al., 2010, 2013). Public health authorities recommend limiting dietary intakes of TFA to below 1% of total dietary energy, because of their established adverse effects on heart health (EFSA, 2004; WHO, 2008).

The major source of TFAs in processed food products in Europe used to be partially hydrogenated vegetable oils. Partially hydrogenated vegetable oils were used because of their properties to structure fat-continuous margarines and spreads, to increase the stability and shelf life of frying oils, or used as affordable and functional alternatives to cocoa butter in confectionary.

This chapter first describes the decrease in TFA intake in Europe, which occurred since the discovery of their adverse effects; the corresponding evolution in TFA content in foods products; and the voluntary and regulatory measures that have enabled such a drastic change. Such decrease in TFA intake was made possible by the various technological strategies developed to replace partially hydrogenated vegetable oils.

In many countries in Europe, intakes of ruminant TFAs are now higher than those of industrial TFAs due to significant industrial reformulation. Public health measures and programs to further reduce TFA intake should focus both on further elimination of partial hydrogenation of vegetable fats and industrial TFAs, as well as reducing the intakes of saturated fats, which will also limit the intake of ruminant TFAs.

TFA Intake in Europe

After the discovery of their adverse effects on the blood cholesterol risk profile for CHD, TFA intakes have considerably reduced in Europe. The comprehensive pan European TRANSFAIR study assessed the intake of TFAs and other fatty acids in 14 Western European countries, based on a combination of data from food consumption databases and actual analysis of TFA levels in up to 100 foods per country (Hulshof et al., 1999). Overall, the TRANSFAIR study found that the TFA intake in Western Europe was lower than previously assumed: 1.2–6.7 g/day, corresponding to 0.5–3.0% of energy, assuming 2000 calories daily. In populations with the highest average TFA intake (2.1% energy), the 90th percentile was 2.8% energy. Intake was lowest in the Mediterranean countries, but also below 1% energy in Finland and Germany. Moderate intakes were seen in Belgium, the Netherlands, Norway, and the U.K., and the highest intake was in Iceland. Major sources of TFA were edible fats and ruminant fat, with bakery products and french fries as additional contributing foods in some countries. The contribution of TFA from ruminant fat ranged from about 30% to 80%, corresponding to 0.3–0.8% energy. These results were based on consumption surveys from 1989 up to 1996, depending on the country, and food samples that were analyzed were purchased in 1995–1996; therefore, they probably already took into account some reformulation of industrial products that occurred in the mid 1990s.

Evidence from a number of countries indicates that the intake of TFA in the EU has continued to decrease below the recommendation of less than 1% energy over recent years (Figure 13.1), owing to further reformulation of food products such as fat spreads, sweet bakery products, and fast food (EFSA, 2010).

In the Netherlands, the Zutphen Elderly study data confirmed that average TFA intake steadily declined markedly in Dutch men between 1985, 1990, and 1995, from 4.3% energy to 2.9% energy and 1.9% energy, respectively, corresponding to daily amounts of 10.9 g/d to 6.9 g/d and 4.4 g/d (Oomen et al., 2001). Decreases in TFA intake have continued over the years. According to the most recent national consumption survey in the Netherlands, performed in 2007–2010 (van Rossum et al., 2011), the median habitual TFA intake ranged from 1.1–1.5 g/d for men and 1.2–1.3 g/d for women. Over 95% of the Dutch population was found not to exceed the recommended upper bound for TFA intake at 1% energy.

Similarly, TFA intake in the French population has decreased during the last two decades (AFSSA, 2009). The INCA-1 study, performed in 1998–1999, found TFA intake of 3.4 g/d for men and 2.8 g/d for women (1.2–1.4% energy). The 95th percentile intake was estimated at 5.8 g/d for men and 4.9 g/d for women (for both 2% energy). The dietary sources of TFA were primarily dairy products (53% of TFA intake in adults). Total animal products represented 67% of TFA intake, whereas industrial bakery products represented 18% of TFA intake. The most conservative estimate of

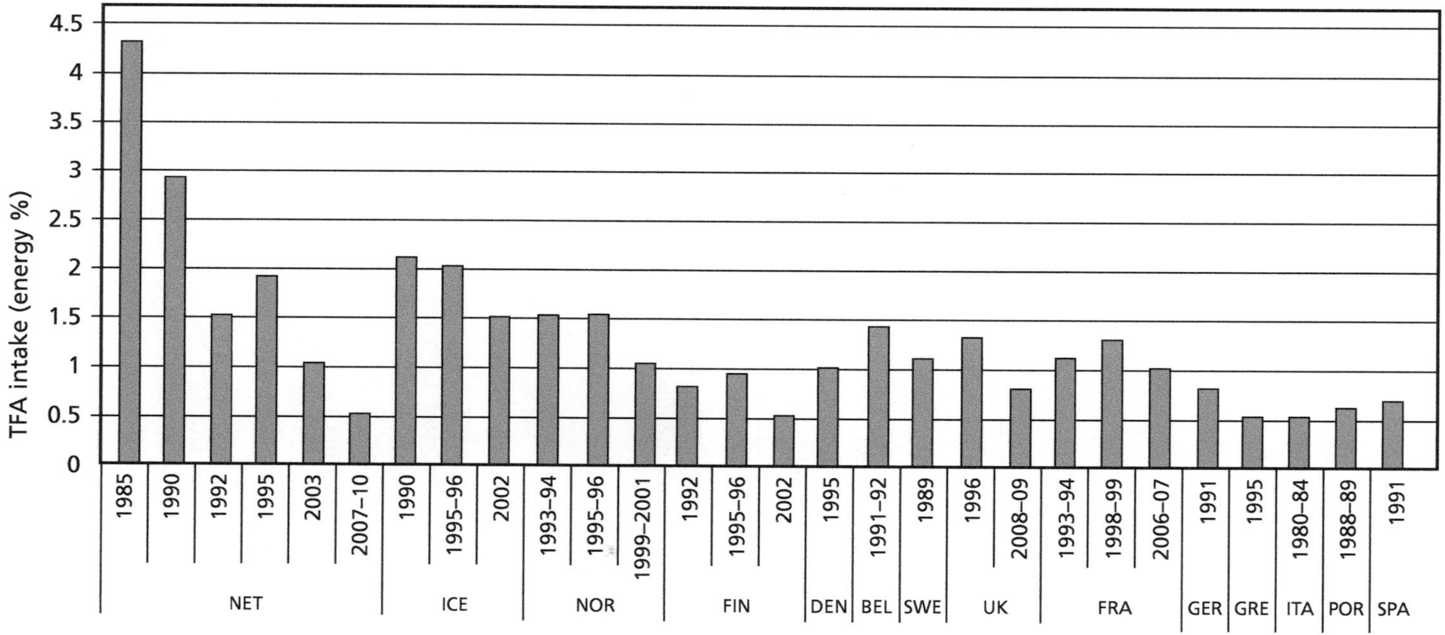

Figure 13.1 Evolution of TFA intake as energy percent at different time intervals in several European countries.

TFA intake in the INCA-2 study performed in 2006–2007 found a reduction compared to the INCA-1 study: an average of 2.3 g/d in adults (corresponding to 1% energy, including 0.6% energy for TFA from ruminant sources and 0.4% energy for TFA from other sources), with the 95th percentile reaching 3.9 g/d (1.5% energy). Only 5% of adults are estimated to have a TFA intake higher than 1.2% energy.

In 2008–2009 in the U.K., TFA intake averaged 0.8% energy. Similar to France, the major contributors to TFA intake in the U.K. were meat and meat products, milk and milk products, and cereal and cereal products (Pot et al., 2012). In Nordic countries, further decrease in TFA intake has also been observed. In Finland, average intakes in 2002 were 0.5% energy compared with 0.9% energy in 1995–1996; in Iceland, 1.5% energy in 2002 compared with 2% energy in 1995–1996; in Norway, 1% energy in 1999–2001 compared with 1.5% energy in 1995–1996 (Anon, 2003; Henderson et al., 2003; Männistö et al., 2003; Steingrimsdottir et al., 2003).

As a result of the steady decrease in TFA intake in Western Europe to reach the recommended levels, TFAs no longer represent a primary health concern. The impact on health of high saturated fats intake above recommendation is now a stronger concern for Western European public health authorities. Intake data of TFA are less abundant for Eastern European countries and there are indications that progress has not been made as rapidly as in Western Europe, as the decline of TFAs in foods has occurred more recently, and some dietary patterns rich in snacks that are high in TFAs can still lead to higher-than-recommended TFA intake (Stender et al., 2012).

TFA in Foods in Europe

The margarine industry was one of the first food sectors to start reformulating their products after the discovery of the deleterious effects of TFAs on cardiovascular risk factors (Korver and Katan, 2006). For example, in Denmark, comparisons of TFA levels in margarines between 1992 and 1995 revealed a noteworthy decrease in the content of *trans*-18:1 for the semisoft margarines, from 9.8 + 6.1% of total fat in 1992 to 1.2 +/− 2.2% of total fat in 1995. At that time, significant amounts of *trans*-18:1 were found only in hard margarines (mean: 4.2 + 2.8%) and shortenings (mean: 6.8+ 3.1%) (Ovesen et al., 1996). In Germany, the total TFA content in sunflower margarines decreased from 21.77% to 5.37% between 1994 and 1999 (Precht and Molentin, 2000). The total TFA content in cooking fats and oils strongly decreased on average from 11.77% in 1994 and 12.52% in 1996 down to 5.91% in 1999. A subsequent study analyzed 45 different retail margarines collected in several European countries during 2004–2005. Out of these 45 samples, TFA in amounts of 4–6% of total fatty acids were detected in only 3 margarines. Only trace amounts (<1%) were detected in the other 42 samples (Pedersen and Kirkhus, 2008). The very recent food analysis data from the U.K. show that spreads and margarines nowadays contain very low levels of TFA: 0.5–0.15 g/100 g product (United Kingdom Department of Health, 2013). Such progress has been made in all Western European countries and can also now be observed in Eastern European countries. In a survey of 26 edible fat brands available in the Estonian retail market in 2011, the total TFA for blended spreads varied from 1.18% to 9.08%, from 0.04% to 34.96% for margarines, and from 0.14% to 39.50% for shortenings. Compared to 2008–2009, the industrially produced TFA content in several of the dietary fat brands was much reduced in 2011 (Meremäe, 2012).

Beyond the margarine industry, levels of TFA have considerably decreased across the total food basket in Europe. The recent U.K. survey concluded that levels of artificial *trans* fats in processed foods have reduced considerably compared with previous analyses of similar foods carried out over the last 20–30 years, where available. Where samples contain higher levels of *trans* fats, this is generally due to the presence of natural sources of *trans* fat in the product (e.g., dairy sources) (United Kingdom Department of Health, 2013). In Denmark, food samples were collected in 2002–2003, 2004–2005, and 2006–2007. In 2002–2003, 65 out of 253 (26%) samples contained more than 2 g TFA/100 g product, mostly among sweets, cookies, french fries, frozen potatoes, and ice cream. In 2006–2007, only 4 samples out of 45 collected contained more than 2 g TFA/100 g. The surveys showed that the industrially produced TFA content has been reduced or removed from most products with originally high industrially produced TFA content, like french fries, microwave popcorn, and various bakery products; therefore, industrially produced TFA are now insignificant for the intake of TFA in Denmark (Bysed et al., 2009). A recent study compared TFA content is foods in 16 EU countries in 2005 and 2009. TFA levels in various food baskets decreased markedly all over Europe and have reached low levels in Western Europe, but progress still needs to be made in some Eastern European countries (Figure 13.2) (Stender, 2012).

Trans Fat Regulations in Europe

The vast majority of the decrease in TFA content in foods, and hence reduction in TFA intake in Europe, has been achieved through industry self-regulation. For example, the margarine industry in Europe has made consistent commitments and progress in reducing TFA content in its products. Launched already in 1995 and now updated for the third time, the IMACE code of practice is the cornerstone of the sector's reformulation objectives (IMACE, 2013). It states that retail margarines and vegetable fat spreads should contain no more than 2% TFA. Retail margarines, vegetable fat spreads, and business to business margarines used as ingredients in food products have never been lower in TFAs than they are today. The removal of TFAs from retail margarines and fat spreads has been accompanied by other beneficial changes: The level of mono- and polyunsaturated fatty acids has consistently increased, while the

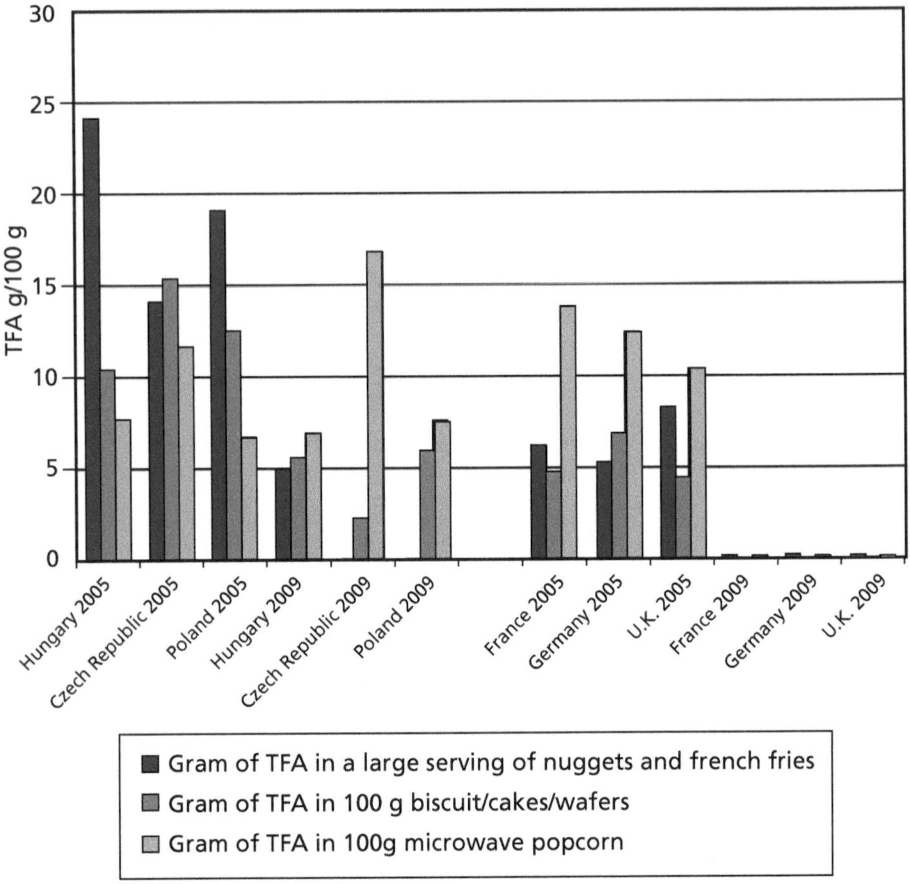

Figure 13.2 Amounts of industrial TFAs in various foods bought in three Eastern European countries in 2005 and 2009 and in three Western European countries in 2005 and 2009. Adapted from Stender et al. (2012).

level of saturated fatty acids has decreased. Business to business margarines, which have to face additional technical challenges, reduced their average TFA level on fat basis by 76% from 2004 to 2012, from 7.1% to 1.7% (IMACE website). This decreasing trend was already acknowledged by EFSA in 2004, which stated that "the intakes of *trans* fatty acids have decreased in a number of EU countries, mainly due to reformulation of food products, e.g., fat spreads, to reduce the *trans* fatty acids content" (EFSA, 2004). and in the latest FAO report of the expert consultation on fats and fatty acids: "*trans* fatty acids have been reduced or eliminated from retail fats and spreads in many parts of the world" (FAO, 2008). In 2010, Unilever committed, as part of their Unilever Sustainable Living Plan, to remove from all their products any TFA originating from partially hydrogenated vegetable oils (Unilever Sustainable Living Plan). In September 2012, 100% of the Unilever portfolio by volume did not contain TFA originating from partially hydrogenated vegetable oils (Unilever Sustainable Living Plan, 2012). This is true both in high income countries but also in middle and low income countries.

To date, the content of TFA in food stuffs is not regulated at the EU level. However, a few individual countries in Europe have taken the approach of setting legal limits of industrial TFA content in foods (Downs et al., 2013). In 2003, Denmark decided to impose a maximum level of 2 g/100 g fat on industrially produced TFA (executive order Denmark), which contributed to the reduction of TFA levels in foods (Leth et al., 2006). Other countries have followed, such as Switzerland in 2007, Austria in 2009, and Iceland in 2011. Hungary is also currently considering legislation on TFA levels. In Switzerland, 100 g of vegetable cooking oil and vegetable cooking fat are only permitted to contain a maximum of 2 g of TFAs (Switzerland, 2007). Austria also introduced legislation similar to Denmark, with a general maximum limit of industrial TFAs set at 2 g/100 g of total fat, with specific conditions for products of lower fat content (Austria, 2009). In Iceland, legislation prohibits companies from putting food on the market that has more than 2 g of TFA per 100 g of total fat content (Iceland, 2011). Finally, Hungary intends to introduce a similar regulation to the Danish and Austrian legislations in 2013 (Hungary, 2013). In terms of providing additional voluntary information to the consumer about the content of TFA, the list of permitted nutrition claims in the nutrition and health claims legislation does not include nutrition claims that refer to TFA.

The specific labeling of TFA in food by means of nutrition declaration was not regulated until the official publication of the Food Information to Consumers (FIC) regulation in October 2011. Before the FIC implementation date (December 2014), TFA can still be declared in the nutrition table. FIC legislation introduced a limited list of mandatory and voluntary nutritional compounds that can be declared in the nutrition table from October 2014 onward that does not include TFA.

In the Netherlands, the self-regulation approach has been adopted and has enabled a reduction in TFA in food without an increase in saturated fats (Temme et al., 2011). In Germany and the U.K., voluntary agreements between governments and the food industry have been put in place, also leading to marked reduction in TFA in foods (U.K. Department of Health, 2013).

Thus, since the discovery of the deleterious effect of TFAs on risks of coronary heart disease in the 1990s, Europe has been the theater of considerable reformulation by the food industry, led by the margarine and spreads sector, to remove TFAs originating from partially hydrogenated vegetable oil. Such efforts have occurred mostly in the context of voluntary reformulation programs, but a few European countries have taken the approach to set legal limits to TFA levels in food products. In most of those cases, the majority of products already complied with national limits before they were introduced. Nowadays, TFA intake in Europe is mostly below recommendations of 1% energy and not a health concern anymore, but efforts need to continue to completely remove TFA in the last pockets of products or populations (mostly in Eastern European countries) where progress has not been as fast. Such a decrease in the industrial TFA content in foods has been made possible by the development of various technological strategies.

Why Industrial TFAs Were Used in Food Products in Europe

The key source of TFAs in processed food products in Europe used to be partially hydrogenated vegetable oil. The main reasons for that are:

1. Partial hydrogenation of liquid oils and soft fats increases their melting point and makes them suitable as oil structurants in the process of manufacturing of fat-continuous margarines and spreads. These food products are water-in-oil emulsions, and their appearance, stability and oral behavior are directly linked to the crystallization and melting behavior of corresponding fat blends (Chrysan, 2005).
2. Partial hydrogenation of polyunsaturated liquid oils increases their stability to oxidation and, therefore, increases the shelf life of these oils in high temperature applications (e.g., shallow frying of foods) (Gupta, 2005).
3. Partially hydrogenated vegetable oils were extensively used in the confectionary industry as affordable and functional alternatives to cocoa butter (Shukla, 2005).
4. Partial hydrogenation enabled practically infinite flexibility of starting materials in the process for each of the applications previously mentioned. Implementation of partially hydrogenated vegetable oil allowed formulating superior consumer products at the lowest possible cost, depending on the current market prices of various oils and fats.

When the industry in Europe came to the insight that TFA had to be reduced, various strategies were developed to do so, not all of which were successful.

Low *Trans* Partial Hydrogenation

Naturally, researchers looked at the adjustment of the process of partial hydrogenation of oils and fats and attempted to modify it in order to control the amount of TFAs formed during the process. It is known from the literature that the degree of TFA formation during partial hydrogenation strongly depends on the processing parameters, such as the type/amount of catalyst, process temperature, hydrogen pressure, and agitation. In general, TFA content in partially hydrogenated vegetable oil is varying in the interval between 25 and 45 wt% (Ackman and Mag, 1998). Maximum formation of TFA isomers happens at low hydrogen pressures (100–200 kPa), temperatures above 200 °C, and relatively low (ca 50 ppm) concentrations of nickel catalyst. Increase of hydrogen pressures to ca 300 kPa, lowering temperatures to 160–180 °C, and enhancement of nickel catalyst concentrations to above 80 ppm leads to a significant decrease in TFA formation upon partial hydrogenation (Ackman and Mag, 1998).

Several studies were devoted to the optimization of hydrogenation catalysts for the reduction of TFA levels during partial hydrogenation. Hsu et al. (1986, 1988) reported that the use of palladium on alumina support instead of nickel catalysts, in combination with high hydrogen pressure (5 MPa) and moderate hydrogenation temperatures (ca 70 °C), enabled the formation of partially hydrogenated oils with reduced TFA content (ca 10–15%). Wright et al. (2003) found that the addition of Ni to a *cis*-selective Pd catalyst did not result in significant advantage for *cis*-selective hydrogenation compared to application of only Pd catalysts.

Carbon-supported platinum catalysts (Pt/C) were used by the Unilever research team to hydrogenate regular soybean oil (Kemps et al., 1977–1979, unpublished results). The process was accomplished at 25–40 °C in a solvent (acetone) medium and at atmospheric pressure, in the presence of 3–5% Pt/C. It was also noticed that the addition of tetraethyl ammonium hydroxide decreases the activity of the catalyst, improves selectivity, and suppresses *trans* isomerization of oils and fats. Application of Pt/C catalysts enabled partial hydrogenation of liquid oils with the formation of very low *trans* levels; for example, soybean oil with iodine value (IV) of 112 (compared to IV 133 for the original soybean oil) with less than 1% of TFAs was obtained (Kemps et al., 1977–1979, unpublished results).

Alternative processing aimed at TFA reduction in partially hydrogenated vegetable oil was also the subject of several investigations. King et al. (2001) demonstrated that the use of mixtures of hydrogen and supercritical carbon dioxide at reaction pressures up to 14 MPa and temperatures in the range of 120–140 °C is a promising technology to deliver partially hydrogenated vegetable oil with reduced TFA levels. Lalvani and Mondal (2004) reported a low temperature (25–75 °C) electrochemical process for the hydrogenation of vegetable oil, which is accomplished by the reduction of unsaturated fatty acids via a chemical pathway using formate ion as a mediator in combination with Ni and Pd catalysts. This method, based on a model described in an earlier work by Mondal and Lalvani (2000), helped to significantly limit the formation of TFA during the partial hydrogenation process.

Therefore, we can conclude that although the process of partial hydrogenation of oils and fats could be optimized to control the amount of generated TFAs, it still results in the formation of significant amounts of TFA (often above 10%). Also, fairly high processing costs are associated with all alternative methods for partial hydrogenation of oils and fats. In addition to that, the use of partially hydrogenated oils/fats requires their labeling on retail consumer products and reduces attractiveness of these foods to the consumers. Modified hydrogenation processes were therefore not implemented; instead, the industry developed alternatives to partially hydrogenated vegetable oil for each of the three applications, as described below.

Elimination of Partially Hydrogenated Vegetable Oils as Structurants from Fat-Continuous Margarines and Spreads

The main challenge in the process of partially hydrogenated vegetable oil elimination from fat-continuous margarines and spreads was to eliminate TFA without increasing the total amount of saturated and *trans* fatty acids, in order not to decrease the nutritional quality of the fat in the product.

Theoretically, traditional hardstocks of dairy/animal origin, such as milk fat, tallow, and lard, can be used as an alternative for structuring of fat-continuous margarines and spreads. Milk fat fractionation has been described in detail elsewhere (Kaylegian and Lindsay, 1995; Kontkanen et al., 2011), and it leads to the isolation of butter stearin. Butter stearin can be used as such, but also after blending and interesterification (Kontkanen et al., 2011; Majumdar and Bhattacharyya, 1986; Pal et al., 2001; Petrauskaite et al., 1998) it is a functional hardstock for making butter melanges and other fat-continuous spreads. Although hardstocks of dairy/animal origin are low in industrial TFA, they are high in ruminant TFA and cholesterol. Dairy fat is not very effective as hardstock as it contains short chain (saturated) fatty acids that hardly contribute to structure. The best hardstocks give maximal structure at minimal content of saturated fat. In addition, more functional hardstocks of dairy origin, such as butter stearin, are quite costly, their supply is fairly limited, and their environmental footprint is also high compared to the hardstocks of plant origin (Nilsson et al., 2010). Combination of all these factors virtually excludes dairy and animal fats from consideration for industrial-scale implementation as partially hydrogenated vegetable oil alternatives.

It is known that in-use properties of fat blends in spreads are adequately described by their solid fat content (SFC) curves, which depict the amount of solid fat at a given temperature. An example of such a curve (also called an SFC profile) is given in Figure 13.3. In the case of margarine and spread formulations, product developers are usually interested in SFC profile values of fat blends in three regions of SFC curves: at 5–10 °C (corresponding to product appearance in use), 20–30 °C (linked to the ambient stability of a spread/margarine), and 35 °C (corresponding to the oral melting of product and release of tastants and flavors). Fat blends with low

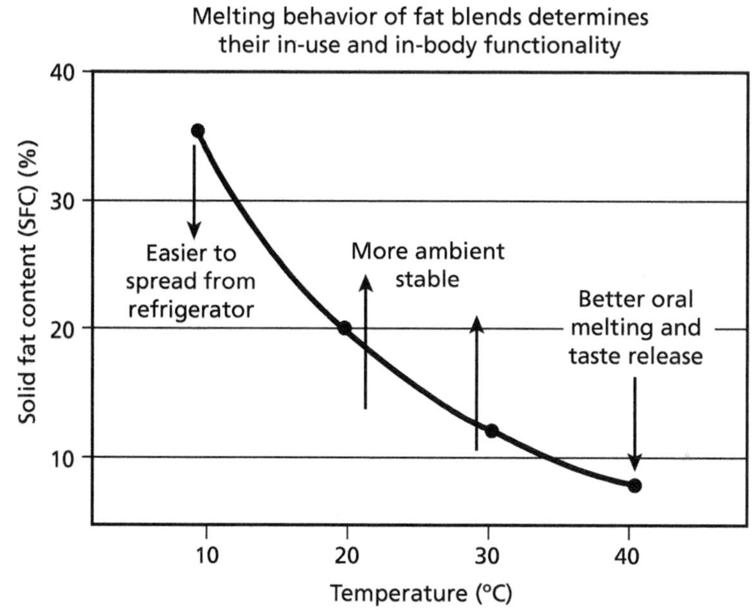

Figure 13.3 Effect of solid fat content in a fat blend of a fat-continuous spread on the functional properties of the product at various temperatures.

N35 values (preferably around 1%) are required for spreads to deliver their buttery melting behavior, whereas cooking/baking margarines may have much higher N35 values in the interval of 5–10%. Looking at oils and fats available in nature, in the amounts sufficient for the industrial scale applications in margarines and spreads, we can conclude that natural oils and fats (i.e., seed/bean oils and tropical fats such as palm, palm kernel, and coconut) could not deliver appropriate SFC profile shapes similar to the partially hydrogenated oils and fats (Figure 13.4a). The SFC profiles of these natural ingredients do not meet the prerequisites of optimal SFC profiles in the whole range of temperatures between 5 and 35 °C (Figure 13.4b). Therefore, these abundant natural oils and fats need to be subjected to physical and/or chemical modification prior to their use in consumer products.

Key tools for oil and fat modification include: (1) fractionation, (2) full hydrogenation, and (3) chemical or enzymatic rearrangement of triacylglycerols, in combination with (4) blending. Next we will briefly review these methods in relation to their applicability for the reduction of TFA content in margarines and spreads.

The fractionation process is well known and described elsewhere (Bockisch, 1998a). In brief, solvent-assisted (wet) and solvent-free (dry) fractionation processes are used in manufacturing of various oil and fat fractions. Dry fractionation is one

A

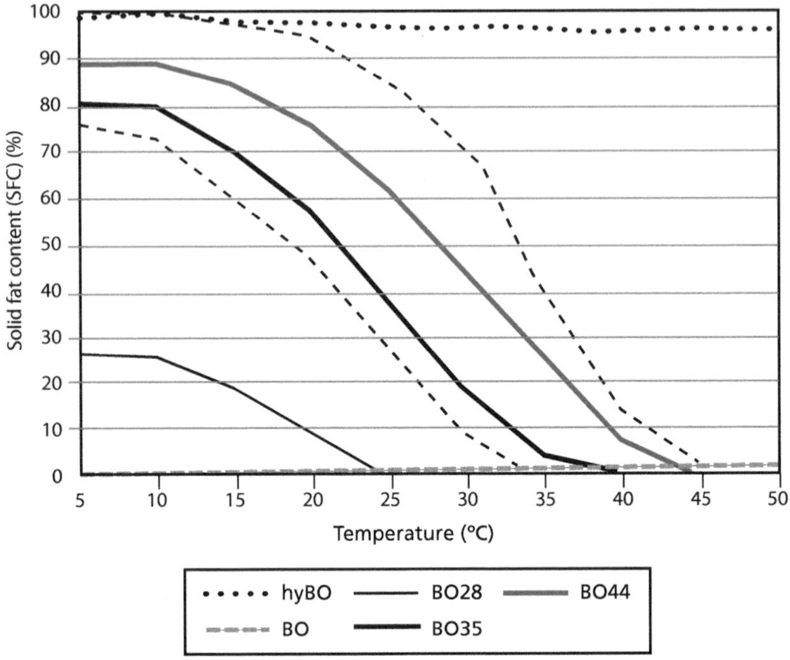

Figure 13.4 (A) Solid fat content profiles of straight soybean oil (BO), fully hydrogenated soybean oil (hyBO), and various partially hydrogenated soybean oils (BO28, BO35, and BO44). Dotted lines define the interval of solid fat content profile values for the hardstocks that are of key importance for applications in fat-continuous spreads. (B) Solid fat content profiles of straight sunflower oil (SF), fully hydrogenated soybean oil (hyBO), straight palm oil (PO), straight palm kernel oil (PK), straight coconut oil (CN), dry fractionated palm olein (dfPOf), and palm stearin (dfPOs). Dotted lines define the interval of solid fat content profile values for the hardstocks that are of key importance for applications in fat-continuous spreads. (C) Solid fat content profiles of various rearranged hardstocks (HS1–HS5) that are commonly used as partially hydrogenated vegetable oil replacers in modern fat-continuous spreads. Dotted lines define the interval of solid fat content profile values for the hardstocks that are of key importance for applications in fat-continuous spreads.

B

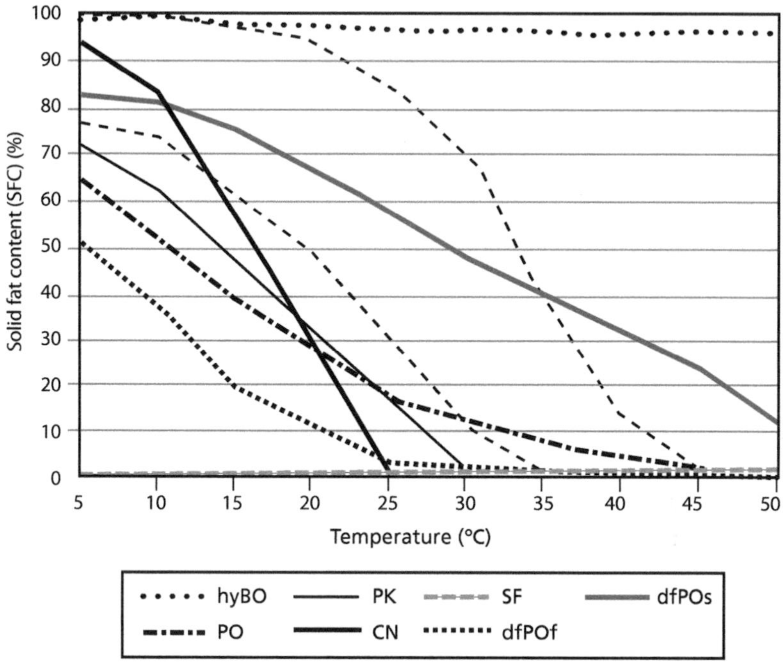

100
90
80
70
60
50
40
30
20
10
0
Solid fat content (SFC) (%)
5
10
15
20
25
30
35
40
45
50
Temperature (°C)
hyBO
PK
SF
dfPOs
PO
CN
dfPOf

C

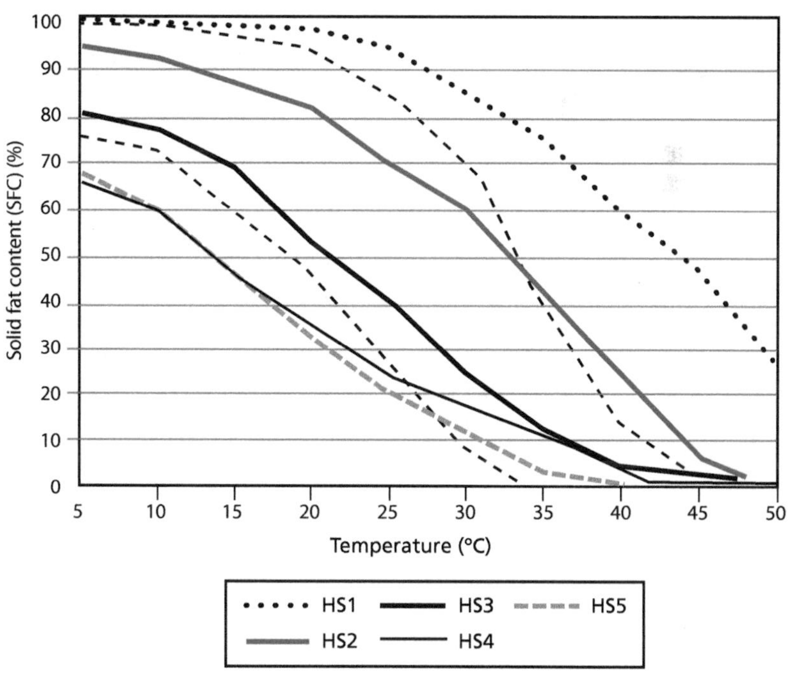

100
90
80
70
60
50
40
30
20
10
0
Solid fat content (SFC) (%)
5
10
15
20
25
30
35
40
45
50
Temperature (°C)
HS1
HS3
HS5
HS2
HS4

stage of a multistage process. It enables separation of triacylglycerols in natural oils and fats according to their slip melting point temperature in a rapid and cost-efficient manner. For example, single-stage fractionation of palm oil results in separation of palm stearin and palm olein; a consequent fractionation of these two intermediates leads to the isolation of palm superstearin, soft stearin, palm mid-fractions, and palm superolein. All these materials can potentially be used as such for making fat blends of margarines and spreads, but still a very limited range of product properties can be delivered. Both SFC profiles and triacylglycerol compositions of palm (and palm kernel) oil fractions could not make them equal substitutes for partially hydrogenated oils and fats from technical perspective (Figure 13.4b). In general, a wider variety of hardstocks with various SFC profile shapes and triacylglycerol compositions is required.

Full hydrogenation of oils and fats is long known as a method of delivering structuring hardstocks from liquid and soft oils and fats (Farr, 2005). Because it leads to the formation of triacylglycerols with three saturated fatty acid chains, hardstocks obtained via full hydrogenation have only a limited scope for application as such, without further modification. SFC profiles of fully saturated hardstocks are flat in the whole interval of relevant temperatures (i.e., from 5 °C to 40 °C and above) and are not capable of delivering desired melting curves for spread applications, as exemplified in Figure 13.4b.

Various triacylglycerols in a fat blend have different functionalities that determine processing conditions for margarines and spreads (e.g., crystallization behavior, tendency to form separate or mixed crystals) and their consumer-relevant properties (e.g., appearance, physical/chemical stability, spreadability, and oral behavior). Rearrangement of fatty acids in oils and fats helps to modify triacylglycerol composition of a fat blend in the desired direction. Excellent reviews on the details of the process are available elsewhere (Bockisch, 1998b) but, in brief, rearrangement implies either random or selective exchange of fatty acid chains between triacylglycerol molecules of a selected blend of starting oils, resulting in formation of new triacylglycerol molecules without changing the overall fatty acid composition.

This process can be done using immobilized lipases at temperatures between 30 and 60 °C, or at elevated temperatures (ca 90 °C) using sodium methylate as a catalyst. Depending on the composition of the initial blend, tailored triacylglycerol compositions can be delivered using rearrangement of oils and fats.

An important starting oil in making rearranged blends is palm oil (Basiron, 2005), as it is less costly than all liquid seed oils. Taking into account that palm fractions are usually used in limited amounts during the process of hardstock manufacturing, the move from partially hydrogenated vegetable oil toward non–partially hydrogenated vegetable oil (i.e., rearranged and/or fractionated and/or fully hydrogenated) hardstocks has minimal impact on the cost of fat blends and, therefore, on the retail prices of consumer products. Application of enzymatically rearranged hardstocks is gaining increased popularity among major manufacturers of margarines and spreads. Compared to chemical rearrangement, the more natural enzymatic treatment occurs under milder conditions, ensuring fewer side reactions, less post-treatment, and, as a result, fewer oil losses. Several studies concentrated on comparative analysis of properties of chemically and enzymatically rearranged hardstocks made from identical fat blends (Costales-Rodrıguez et al., 2009; Zhang et al., 2000, and references therein). The results of these studies demonstrated that enzymatic rearrangement is a suitable alternative to chemical rearrangement, as key functional parameters of these hardstocks (e.g., SFC profiles, diglyceride amounts, crystallization behavior, and organoleptic properties) can be made comparable. In general, however, there are differences in composition and properties of products prepared by chemical and enzymatic interesterification.

Major oil and fat suppliers now deliver the whole range of rearranged oils and fats with different functionalities. Figure 13.4c summarizes the area of SFC profiles covered by a set of selected rearranged margarine hardstocks. It can be easily seen by comparing Figures 13.4a–13.4c that rearrangement applied to a combination of straight and/or fractionated and/or fully hydrogenated oils and fats enable production of hardstocks with functional properties that make them suitable replacers of partially hydrogenated vegetable oils. Most rearranged hardstocks are blends of palm oil, palm stearin, and a lauric oil, such as coconut or palm kernel oil.

We should mention that processing of fat-continuous margarines and spreads needs some modification as a result of replacement of partially hydrogenated vegetable oils by hardstocks originating from tropical oils and fats. Regular margarine and spread processing involves fat crystallization and simultaneous emulsification in a scraped-surface heat exchanger (SSHE), where α-crystals of fat are formed. At a later stage of the process, α-crystals are transformed into β'-crystals upon agitation using crystallizer units supplied with pin stirrers (this approach is usually used in spreads manufacturing, when plasticity of the consumer product is required), or upon static conditions in static residence units (e.g., during manufacturing of wrappers/bricks). Upon substitution of partially hydrogenated vegetable oil hardstocks with TFA-free hardstocks from the oils and fats modification toolbox, processing parameters often need to be tailored, although the overall design of processing facilities for margarines and spreads remains unchanged.

We can conclude that the expansion of oils and fats modification toolbox toward the area of enzymatic rearrangement allows delivering even more blends for making products with desired consumer properties. We can also conclude that consumer needs can be met using existing oils and fats modifications such as fractionation, full hydrogenation, rearrangement, and blending of various natural oils and fats low in TFAs. It is important to underline that partially hydrogenated vegetable oil–free margarines and spreads are, in most cases, nutritionally superior compared to historical partially hydrogenated vegetable oil–based products. Table 13.A summarizes nutritional properties (saturated fatty acid and TFA content) of typical soft and firm spreadable tubs,

Table 13.A Total saturated fatty acid (SFA) and TFA content, and TFA-only content of representative spreads and margarines with identical SFC profiles made using partially hydrogenated vegetable oil–based and partially hydrogenated vegetable oil–free oil and fat blends (Unilever, unpublished data).

	PHVO-based		PHVO-free	
	SFA + TFA (%)	TFA (%)	SFA + TFA (%)	TFA (%)
Soft tub	22	6	21	<1
Firm tub	33	13	33	<1
Wrapper	45	20	43	<1

as well as cooking/baking wrappers, made using partially hydrogenated vegetable oil–based and partially hydrogenated vegetable oil–free oil and fat blends (Unilever, unpublished data). It is clear that in the reformulated products the sum of saturated fatty acids (SAFA) and TFA is reduced to that in the historical high-*trans* recipes.

Recently, consumers began associating the use of palm oil with sustainability aspects of its production. In this connection, we should underline that a number of major food companies in Europe, including Unilever and Nestle, have together formed a roundtable on sustainable palm oil (RSPO). The main goals of the RSPO could be summarized as follows (RSPO, 2013):

1. To advance the production, procurement, finance, and use of sustainable palm oil products
2. To develop, implement, verify, assure, and periodically review credible global standards for the entire supply chain of sustainable palm oil
3. To monitor and evaluate the economic, environmental, and social impacts of the uptake of sustainable palm oil in the market
4. To engage and commit all stakeholders throughout the supply chain, including governments and consumers

In addition, companies commit to the use of sustainable palm oil in their products; for example, the Unilever Sustainable Living Plan (USLP) sets clear measurable targets for the palm oil used in Unilever products, as follows (USLP, 2013):

1. We will purchase all palm oil from certified sustainable sources by 2015.
2. We will purchase all palm oil sustainably from certified, traceable sources by 2020.
3. All palm oil was coming from sustainable sources by the end of 2012: 97% via RSPO GreenPalm certificates and 3% of palm oil purchased from certified, traceable sources (through a segregated supply).

These initiatives clearly help to improve the image of palm oil in the eyes of consumers, even further enhancing its acceptability as partially hydrogenated vegetable oil replacement in margarines and spreads.

Replacement of Partially Hydrogenated Vegetable Oil as a Cocoa Butter Alternative

Another significant industrial application of partially hydrogenated vegetable oil in consumer products was in manufacturing of confectionary fats, as alternatives to cocoa butter. Cocoa butter, and the tropical butters used as cocoa butter alternatives, are all fats primarily containing symmetric triacylglycerols composed of two long saturated fatty acid chains (H = C16:0 palmitic and C18:0 stearic) in sn-1,3 positions and one monounsaturated (U = C18:1 n-9 oleic) in sn-2 position. These fats give the excellent steep melting profile of chocolate, and such triacylglycerols are nearly ideal structurants of liquid oil-in-fat blends of margarines and spreads (Shukla, 2005). Because the price of cocoa butter and tropical butters is very high, very steeply hardened partially hydrogenated vegetable oils with high TFA content were used for manufacture of cheap cocoa/fantasy products in Western and Eastern Europe. Nowadays, they tend to be substituted by blends with palm oil mid fractions and/or rearranged blends of palm stearin and lauric oils.

Cocoa butter is sometimes rearranged with lauric oils to substitute palm oil in the rearranged margarine hardstocks, in order to create palm oil–free products. It is clear that such hardstocks remain too costly to find wide-scale application. Therefore, researchers looked at other plant fats that could be potential alternatives for cocoa butter. Next we present a summary of these alternatives.

Sal butter is produced from the seed kernel of sal trees grown in India and Southeast Asia. It is recommended to fractionate sal butter and isolate sal stearin for applications in cocoa butter equivalents (Jahurul et al., 2013; Kochhar, 2011; Reddy and Prabhakar, 1989), but this treatment increases the in-use cost of sal butter. While fractionation seems necessary for applications of sal butter in the chocolate industry, it may not be necessary for use in spreads.

Shea butter is an edible fat manufactured by solvent extraction from the kernels of shea trees grown in Western and Sub-Saharan Africa. Similar to sal butter, shea butter can be used in structuring of margarines and spreads as such, but fractionation and rearrangement of shea butter help to further enhance its structuring functionality. In this connection, blending of fractionated palm stearin and shea stearin has been reported (Kang et al., 2013).

Illipe butter is recommended (Kochhar, 2011) for the use as cocoa butter equivalent without further processing (i.e., fractionation and/or interesterification). It should also be suitable as a hardstock in the manufacturing of margarines and spreads. However, there is a fairly limited supply of Illipe butter available on the market, and the effect of agricultural factors (i.e., growing geographies and climate) on fatty acid and triacylglycerol composition of Illipe butter still needs to be established.

Allanblackia seed oil is obtained from the seeds of *Allanblackia floribunda,* a typical tropical rain forest belt tree, commonly found in the Western, Central, and Eastern Africa. Allanblackia trees bear large fruits up to 12 inches long, which may contain up to 40–50 seeds. The seed kernels amount to 60–80% of the whole seed weight. Allanblackia seed oil is used in Africa as a substitute for palm oil to produce commercial products. Similar to Illipe butter, Allanblackia seed oil is suitable for use as cocoa butter equivalent without further processing (i.e., fractionation and/or interesterification), and it is also perfectly suitable as a hardstock in manufacturing of confectionary products, margarines, spreads, and nondairy creams (Avramis et al., 2006; Floter, 2003).

Mango, one of the most abundant tropical fruits in the world (Ramteke et al., 1999), could also be considered as a source of tropical fats capable of replacing partially hydrogenated vegetable oils (Gunstone, 2006; Kochhar, 2011). Using tailored extraction and fractionation approaches, mango kernel fat suitable for the replacement of cocoa butter can be isolated (Dhinigra and Kapoor, 1985; Lakshminarayana et al., 1983; Narashima-Char et al., 1977). However, despite the fact that there is significant knowledge on the compositional properties of mango kernel fat, only lab-scale experiments with this fat are reported as of now, and building a supply chain for large-scale industrial applications of mango kernel fat is another technical challenge.

Kokum butter is isolated from the seeds of the kokum tree, which mainly grows in the coastal regions of India. This material is not only suitable as a structuring hardstock for margarines and spreads, but also as a cocoa butter replacer in the chocolate industry (Baliga et al., 2011; Jahurul et al., 2013). Similar to other tropical sources of stearic-oleic-stearic triacyglycerol-rich hardstocks, additional efforts need to be invested into the development of a supply chain of kokum butter to enable cost-efficient industrial scale applications of this hardstock in fat-continuous margarines and spreads.

It should also be mentioned that various factors influence composition and properties of the above-mentioned tropical oils. Because they come from rainforest area trees, their availability, as well as triacylglycerol composition, can change significantly from year to year and between different geographies (Di Vincenzo et al., 2005; Sanou et al., 2006).

Attempts have been made to produce seed/bean oils that can be used as hardstocks for structuring of fat-continuous products (Bootello et al., 2012; Garces et al, 2012). When only a breeding approach was used, the content of stearic acid in plant oils was moderate; for example, a sunflower oil containing 21% of stearic acid and 62% oleic acid was reported by Pleite et al. (2006). At the same time, combination of breeding and mutagenesis techniques makes it possible to isolate high-stearic rapeseed oil containing up to 27–35% of stearic acid (Fernandez-Moya et al., 2005; Karim Zarhloul et al., 2006; Kodali, 2003; Serrano-Vega et al., 2005), which was comparable with best transgenic genotypes of cottonseed (40% stearic acid) (Liu et al., 2002) and rapeseed (40% stearic acid) (Knutzon et al., 1992). Genetically modified high palmitic and stearic soybean oils (stearic acid content of 30–40%) were also described by Hammond and Fehr (1983), Graef et al. (1985), and Wilson and Bulton (1992). In addition to that, List et al. (1997) demonstrated that properties of high-stearic soybean oils can be further improved by interesterification, making them suitable as hardstocks for spreads manufacturing. The applicability of tailored seed/bean oils with high stearic content for structuring of fat-continuous food emulsions, such as high-fat (70–80%) stick and tub margarines, as well as light (40%) spreads, has been confirmed (DiRienzo et al., 2008).

In summary, we can conclude that all hardstocks described in this chapter are rich in HUH triacylglycerols; therefore, various natural stearic-rich fats could be used as cocoa butter alternatives but also have a potential as structuring hardstocks in the manufacturing of fat-continuous margarines and spreads. Supply chain aspects for the majority of mentioned hardstocks still need to be addressed to make them suitable for the replacement of partially hydrogenated vegetable oil in industrial food applications.

Replacement of Partially Hydrogenated Vegetable Oil in Stable Frying Oils

Finally, elimination of partially hydrogenated vegetable oils from food applications implied the need for the replacement of partially hydrogenated liquid oils used for shallow frying purposes. The main benefit that is achieved by applying partial hydrogenation to liquid oils used in high-temperature applications is the increase of oil stability against oxidation and prolongation of its usage interval. Partial hydrogenation of liquid oils leads to the dramatic reduction of polyunsaturated fatty acid content, which enables enhanced stability of oils at elevated temperatures.

Logically, liquid oils with reduced polyunsaturated fatty acid content could be suitable replacements for partially hydrogenated vegetable oils in frying applications, but the availability of such oils in nature is limited. Therefore, various agricultural research programs were aimed at the manipulation of fatty acid compositions of liquid seed/bean oils using genetic engineering and conventional plant breeding. These programs resulted in identification of sunflower, rapeseed, and soybean plants as containing mid- and high-oleic oils for high-temperature food applications (Tarrago-Trani et al., 2006, and references therein). Newer seed variants are tailored to deliver a high content of oleic acid in combination with exceptionally low saturated fatty acid levels. For example, omega-9 oils manufactured from tailored breeds of canola and sunflower seeds by Dow AgroSciences have exceptionally high levels of oleic (>70%)

and very low levels of linolenic (<3%) fatty acids (Ohr, 2009). According to information provided by Dow AgroSciences (www.dowagro.com), such oils are virtually free of *trans* fat, and they also help in lowering saturated fat claims on menus or labels because there is only 3% of saturated fatty acid in omega-9 sunflower oil (http://www.dowseeds.eu/products/healthier_oil.htm).

Therefore, we can conclude that mid- and high-oleic seed oils have found application in Europe as alternatives to partially hydrogenated vegetable oil–based frying oils. They deliver excellent in-use properties in frying applications and are superior from the nutritional perspective. These oils are still distributed at a price premium compared to regular seed/bean oils, but impressive developments in the establishment of a supply chain for these innovative high-oleic oils imply that their availability for frying food applications should further improve in the coming years.

Although other types of partially hydrogenated vegetable oil alternatives, such as organogels and synthetic hardstock substitutes, are reported in literature, we leave them out of the scope for this review. These alternatives are often not natural, are costly, have notably different physical properties and functionality compared to oil- and fat-based hardstocks, and require significant rebuilding of manufacturing facilities. Also, labeling, regulatory, and legal aspects associated with the use of these ingredients in foods do not make them feasible alternatives for partially hydrogenated vegetable oil replacement.

Conclusion

In summary, Europe was at the front of the discovery of TFA negative health effects, and has taken rapid actions to remove them from most products, to a large extent through voluntary removal. The margarine industry has been a frontrunner. Nowadays, TFA intake in Europe is mostly below recommendations of 1% energy and is no longer a health concern at the population level; however, efforts need to continue to completely remove TFAs in the last pockets of products or populations (mostly in Eastern European countries), where progress has not been as fast. TFA intake reduction has been achieved thanks to several alternative ingredients or technologies. Primary partially hydrogenated vegetable oil applications were in frying oils and in the structuring of margarines/spreads. In the case of frying oils, successful implementation of breeding methods resulted in high-oleic seed oils that deliver superior stability in use. In the case of margarine hardstocks, application of tropical oils (mainly palm and coconut, as well as their fractions), in combination with fully hydrogenated oils, helped to populate the list of potential hardstocks. Their functionality was further improved and tailored for particular applications using chemical and enzymatic rearrangement in combination with blending, and allowed to perfectly match current industrial needs at an acceptable cost in use. Other hardstocks, such as stearic fractions of seed and tropical oils, could be potentially in scope, but for several reasons (mainly cost, availability, and natural variation in triacylglycerol composition) are not yet widely used; however, this situation might change in time. In many countries in Europe, intakes of ruminant TFA are now higher than those of industrial TFA due to these significant industrial reformulations. Therefore, public health measures and programs to further reduce TFA intake should focus both on further elimination of partial hydrogenation of vegetable fats and even more on reducing the intake of saturated fats, which will also limit the intake of ruminant TFA.

References

Ackman, R. G.; Mag, T. K. *Trans* Fatty Acids and the Potential for Less in Technical Products. In Trans *Fatty Acids in Human Nutrition;* Sebedio, J. L; Christie, W. W., Eds.; The Oily Press: Dundee UK, 1998; pp 35–58.

Agence Française de Sécurité Sanitaire des Aliments (AFSSA). Avis de l'Agence française de sécurité sanitaire des aliments sur l'estimation des apports en acides gras *trans* de la population française. Request 2007-SA-220. 2009.

Anon. (2003). Utviklingen i norsk kosthold (Developments of the Norwegian diet). Directorate for Health and Social affairs. IS:1143. Oslo 2003.

Austria. Verordnung des Bundesministers für Gesundheit über den Gehalt an *trans*- Fettsäuren in Lebensmitteln (*Trans*-Fettsäuren-Verordnung). Jahrgang 2009 Ausgegeben am 20. August 2009

Avramis, C. A.; Floeter, E.; Persson, H. K.; Stellema, C. S. Patent WO2006002739A1, 2006.

Baliga, M. S.; Bhat, H. P.; Pai, R. J.; Boloor, R.; Palatty, P. L. The Chemistry and Medicinal Uses of the Underutilized Indian Fruit Tree *Garcinia indica* Choisy (Kokum)—A Review. *Food Research International* **2011,** *44,* 1790–1799.

Basiron, Y. Palm Oil. In *Bailey's Industrial Oil and Fat Products,* 6th ed.; Shahidi, F., Ed.; Wiley, 2005; Vol. 2.

Bockisch, M. Fractionation. In *Fats and Oils Handbook.* AOCS Press: Urbana, IL, 1998a; pp 449–507.

Bockisch, M. Interesterification. In *Fats and Oils Handbook.* AOCS Press: Urbana, IL, 1998b; pp 516–545.

Bootello, M. A.; Hartel, R. W.; Garces, R.; Martinez-Force, E.; Salas, J. J. Evaluation of High Oleic-High Stearic Sunflower Hard Stearins for Cocoa Butter Equivalent Formulation. *Food Chem.* **2012,** *134,* 1409–1417.

Brouwer, I. A.; Wanders, A. J.; Katan, M.B. Effect of Animal and Industrial *Trans* Fatty Acids on HDL and LDL Cholesterol Levels in Humans—A Quantitative Review. PLoS ONE 2010, 5.

Brouwer, I. A.; Wanders, A. J.; Katan, M. B. *Trans* Fatty Acids and Cardiovascular Health: Research Completed? *Eur. J. Clin. Nutr.* **2013,** 67, 541–547.

Bysted, A.; Mikkelsen, A.; Leth, T. Substitution of *Trans* Fatty Acids in Foods on the Danish Market. *Eur. J. Lipid Sci. Technol.* **2009,** *111.*

Chrysan, M. M. Margarines and Spreads. In *Bailey's Industrial Oil and Fat Products,* 6th ed.; Shahidi, F., Ed.; Wiley, 2005; Vol. 4.

Costales-Rodrıguez, R.; Gibon, V.; Verhe, R.; De Greyt, W. Chemical and Enzymatic Interesterification of a Blend of Palm Stearin: Soybean Oil for Low *Trans*-Margarine Formulation. *J. Am. Oil Chem. Soc.* **2009,** *86,* 681–697.

Denmark: Executive Order No. 160 of 11 March 2003 on the Content of *Trans* Fatty Acids in Oils and Fats. IP/A/ENVI/ST/2008-19 Page 1 of 25 PE 408.584

Dhinigra, S.; Kapoor, A. Nutritive Value of Mango Seed Kernel. *J. Sci. Food Agric.* **1985,** *36,* 752–756.

DiRienzo, M. A.; Lemke, S. L.; Petersen, B. J.; Smith, K. M. Effect of Substitution of High Stearic Low Linolenic Acid Soybean Oil for Hydrogenated Soybean Oil on Fatty Acid Intake. *Lipids* **2008,** *43,* 451–456.

Di Vincenzo, D.; Maranz, S.; Serraiocco, A.; Vito, R.; Wiesman, Z.; Bianchi, G. Regional Variation in Shea Butter Lipid and Triterpene Composition in Four African Countries. *J. Agric. Food Chem.* **2005,** *53,* 7473–7479.

Downs, S. M.; Thow, A. M.; Leeder, S. R. The Effectiveness of Policies for Reducing Dietary *Trans* Fat: A Systematic Review of the Evidence. *Bull World Health Organ* **2013,** *91,* 262–269H.

EFSA Panel on Dietetic Products NaAN. Scientific Opinion on Dietary Reference Values for Fats, Including Saturated Fatty Acids, Polyunsaturated Fatty Acids, Monounsaturated Fatty Acids, *Trans* Fatty Acids, and Cholesterol. *EFSA Journal* **2010,** *8*, 1461.

FAO report of an expert consultation on fats and fatty acids in human nutrition. Geneve, 2008. http://foris.fao.org/preview/25553-0ece4cb94ac52f9a25af77ca5cfba7a8c.pdf.

Farr, W. E. Hydrogenation: Processing Technologies. In *Bailey's Industrial Oil and Fat Products,* 6th ed.; Shahidi, F., Ed.; Wiley, 2005; Vol. 5.

Fernandez-Moya, V.; Martinez-Force, E.; Garces, R. Oils from Improved High Stearic Acid Sunflower Seeds. *J. Agric. Food Chem.* **2005,** *53,* 5326–5330.

Floeter, E. Patent WO2003096817A1, 2003.

Garces, R.; Martinez-Force, E.; Salas, J. J.; Bootello MA. Alternatives to Tropical Fats Based on High-Stearic Sunflower Oils. *Lipid Tech.* **2012,** *24,* 63–65.

Graef, G. L.; Miller, L. A.; Fehr, W. R.; Hammond, E. G. Fatty Acid Development in a Soybean Mutant with High Stearic Acid. *J. Am. Oil Chem. Soc.* **1985,** *62,* 773–775.

Gunstone, F. D. Minor Specialty Oils. In *Nutraceutical and Specialty Lipids and Their Co-products;* Shahidi, F., Ed.; CRC Taylor & Francis, 2006; pp 91–126.

Gupta, M. K. Frying Oils. In *Bailey's Industrial Oil and Fat Products,* 6th ed.; Shahidi, F., Ed.; Wiley, 2005; Vol. 4.

Hammond, E. G.; Fehr, W. R. Registration of A6 Germplasm Line of Soybean. *Crop Sci.* **1983,** *23,* 192–193.

Henderson, L.; Gregory, J.; Irving, K.; Swan, G. *The National Diet & Nutrition Survey: Adults Aged 19 to 64 years. Volume 2. Energy, Protein, Carbohydrate, Fat and Alcohol Intake.* Food Standards Agency and the Departments of Health by the Social Survey Division of the Office for National Statistics and Medical Research Council Human Nutrition Research. TSO: London, 2003.

Hsu, N.; Diosady, L. L.; Graydon, W. F.; Rubin, L. J. Heterogeneous Catalytic Hydrogenation of Canola Using Palladium. *J. Am. Oil Chem. Soc.* **1986,** *63,* 1036–1042.

Hsu, N.; Diosady, L. L.; Rubin, L. J. Catalytic Behavior of Palladium in the Hydrogenation of Edible Oils. *J. Am. Oil Chem. Soc.* **1988,** *65,* 349–356.

Hulshof, K. F. et al. Intake of Fatty Acids in Western Europe with Emphasis on *Trans* Fatty Acids: The TRANSFAIR Study. *Eur. J. Clin. Nutr.* **1999.**

Hungary: http://ec.europa.eu/enterprise/tris/pisa/app/search/printable.cfm?fuseaction=pisa_notif_overview&iYear=2013&iNum=371&lang=EN&sNLang=EN. Accessed 1 October 2013.

Iceland: Reglugerð um hámarksmagn transfitusýra í matvælum. No 1045/2010. Regulation on the Maximum Levels for *Trans*-Fatty Acids in Foods Ministry of Industries and Innovation August 1st 2011.

IMACE Code of Practice on *Trans* Fatty Acids—February 2013. http://www.imace.org/files/files/public-website/Europeanx-Margarine-Sector-Code-of-Practice-on-*Trans*-Fatty-Acids.pdf.

IMACE website http://www.imace.org/newsroom/news/the-european-margarine-sector-strengthens-its-commitment-to-healthy-products.html.

Jahurul, M. H. A.; Zaidul, I. S. M.; Norulaini, N. A. N.; Sahena, F.; Jinap, S.; Azmir, J.; Sharif, K. M.; Mohd Omar, A. K. Cocoa Butter Fats and Possibilities of Substitution in Food Products Concerning Coca Varieties, Alternative Sources, Extraction Methods, Composition, and Characteristics. *J. Food Eng.* **2013,** *117,* 467–476.

Kang, K. K.; Jeon, H.; Kim, I. H.; Kim, B. H. Cocoa Butter Equivalents Prepared by Blending Fractionated Palm Stearin and Shea Stearin. *Food Sci. and Biotech.* **2013,** *22,* 347–352.

Karim Zarhloul, M.; Stoll, C.; Lühs, W.; Syring-Ehemann, A.; Hausmann, L.; Topfer, R.; Friedt, W. Breeding High-Stearic Oilseed Rape (*Brassica napus*) with High- and Low-Erucic Background Using Optimised Promoter-gene Constructs. *Molecular Breeding* **2006,** *18,* 241–251.

Kaylegian, K. E.; Lindsay, R. C. *Handbook of Milk Fat Fractionation Technology.* AOCS Press: Urbana, IL, 1995; pp 39–508.

King, J. W.; Holliday, R. L.; List, G. R.; Snyder, J. M. Hydrogenation of Vegetable Oils Using Mixtures of Supercritical Carbon Dioxide and Hydrogen. *J. Am. Oil Chem. Soc.* **2001,** *78,* 107–113.

Knutzon, D.S.; Thompson, G.A.; Radke, S. E.; Johnson, W. B.; Knauf, V.C.; Kridl, J. C. Modification of Brassica Seed Oil by Antisense Expression of a Stearoyl-acyl Carrier Protein Desaturase Gene. *Proceedings of the National Academy of Sciences of the USA* **1992,** 89, 2624–2628.

Kochhar, S. P. Minor and Speciality Oils. In *Vegetable Oils in Food Technology: Composition, Properties and Uses,* 2nd ed.; Gunstone, F. D., Ed.; Wiley-Blackwell: Oxford, U.K., 2011; pp 291–343.

Kodali, D. Vegetable Oil Having Elevated Stearic Acid Content. U.S. Patent 6994882, 2003.

Kontkanen, H.; Rokka, S.; Kemppinen, A.; Miettinen, H.; Hellström, J.; Kruus, K.; Marnila, P.; Alatossava, T.; Korhonen, H. Enzymatic and Physical Modification of Milk Fat: A Review. *Int. Dairy J.* **2011,** *21,* 3–13.

Korver, O.; Katan, M. B. The Elimination of *Trans* Fats from Spreads: How Science Helped to Turn an Industry Around. *Nutr Rev.* **2006,** *64* (6), 275–279.

Lakshminarayana, G.; Chandrasekhara-Rao, T.; Ramalingaaswamy, P. A. Varietal Variations in Content Characteristics and Composition of Mango Seed and Fat. *J. Am. Oil Chem. Soc.* **1983,** *60,* 88–89.

Lalvani, S. B.; Mondal, K. Electrochemical Hydrogenation of Vegetable Oils. U.S. Patent 6,825,367, 2004.

Leth, T.; Jensen, H. G.; Mikkelsen, A. A.; Bysted, A. The Effect of the Regulation on *Trans* Fatty Acid Content in Danish food. *Atheroscler. Suppl.* **2006,** 7 (2), 53–56.

List, G. R.; Mounts, T. L.; Orthoefer, F.; Neff, W. E. Effect of Interesterification on the Structure and Physical Properties of High-stearic Acid Soybean Oils. *J. Am. Oil Chem. Soc.* **1997,** *74,* 327–329.

Liu, Q.; Singh, S.; Green, A. High-oleic and High-stearic Cottonseed Oils: Nutritionally Improved Cooking Oils Developed Using Gene Silencing. *J. Am Coll. Nutr.* **2002,** *21,* 205S–211S.

Majumdar, S.; Bhattacharyya, D. K. *Trans*-free Vanaspati from Palm Stearin and Vegetable Oils by Interesterification Process. *Oleagineux* **1986,** *41,* 235–240.

Männistö, S.; Ovaskainen, M.-L.; Valsta, L. (2003). *The National Findiet 2002 Study.* B3 Publications of the National Public Health Institute: Helsinki, Finland, 2003.

Meremäe, K.; Roasto, M.; Kuusik, S.; Ots, M.; Henno, M. *Trans* Fatty Acid Contents in Selected Dietary Fats in the Estonian Market. *J. Food Sci.* **2012,** *77* (8), T163–168.

Mondal, K.; Lalvani, S. B. A Second-order Model for Catalytic-transfer Hydrogenation of Edible Oils. *J. Am. Oil Chem. Soc.* **2000,** *77,* 1–8.

Narashima-Char, B. L.; Reddy, B. R.; Thirumala-Rao, S. D. Processing Mango Stones for Fat. *J. Am. Oil Chem. Soc.* **1977,** *54,* 494–495.

Nilsson, K.; Flysjö, A.; Davis, J.; Sim, S.; Unger, N.; Bell, S. Comparative Life Cycle Assessment of Margarine and Butter Consumed in the U.K., Germany and France. *The International Journal of Life Cycle Assessment* **2010,** *15,* 916–926.

Ohr, L. M. Following Functional Oils. *Food Tech.* **2009,** *2,* 65–67.

Oomen, C. M.; Ocké, M. C.; Feskens, E. J.; van Erp-Baart, M. A.; Kok, F. J.; Kromhout, D. Association between *Trans* Fatty Acid Intake and 10-year Risk of Coronary Heart Disease in the Zutphen Elderly Study: A Prospective Population-based Study. *Lancet* **2001,** *357* (9258), 746–751.

Opinion of the Scientific Panel on Dietetic Products, Nutrition and Allergies on a Request from the Commission Related to the Presence of *Trans* Fatty Acids in Foods and the Effect on Human Health of the Consumption of *Trans* Fatty Acids. *EFSA Journal* **2004,** *81,* 1–49. http://www.efsa.europa.eu/en/efsajournal/doc/81.pdf.

Ovesen, L.; Leth, T.; Hansen, K. Fatty Acid Composition of Danish Margarines and Shortenings, with Special Emphasis on *Trans* Fatty Acids. *Lipids* **1996,** *31,* 971–975.

Pal, P. K.; Bhattacharyya, D. K.; Ghosh, S. Modifications of Butter Stearin by Blending and Interesterification for Better Utilization in Edible Fat Products. *J. Am. Oil Chem. Soc.* **2001,** *78,* 31–36.

Pedersen, J. I.; Kirkhus, B. Fatty Acid Composition of Post *Trans* Margarines and Their Health Implications. *Lipid Tech.* **2008,** *20* (6).

Petrauskaite, V.; Greyt, W.D.; Kellens, M.; Huyghebaert, A. Physical and Chemical Properties of *Trans*-free Fats Produced by Chemical Interesterification of Vegetable Oil Blends. *J. Am. Oil Chem. Soc.* **1998,** *75,* 489–493.

Pleite, R.; Martinez-Force, E.; Garces, R. Increase of the Stearic Acid Content in High-oleic Sunflower (*Helianthus annuus*) Seeds. *J. Agric. Food Chem.* **2006,** *54,* 9383–9388.

Pot, G. K. ; Prynne, C. J.; Roberts, C.; et al. National Diet and Nutrition Survey: Fat and Fatty Acid Intake from the First Year of the Rolling Programme and Comparison with Previous Surveys. *Brit. J. Nutr.* **2012**, *107,* 405–415.

Precht, D.; Molkentin, J. Recent Trends in the Fatty Acid Composition of German Sunflower Margarines, Shortenings and Cooking Fats with Emphasis on Individual C16:1, C18:1, C18:2, C18:3 and C20:1 *Trans* Isomers. *Nahrung* **2000,** *44* (4), 222–228.

Ramteke, R. S.; Vijayalakshmi, M. R.; Eipeson, W. E. Processing and Value Addition to Mangoes. *Indian Food Industry* **1999,** *18,* 155–163.

Reddy, S. Y.; Prabhakar, J. V. Confectionary Fats from Sal (*Shorea Robusta*) Fat and Phulwara (*Madhuca butyracea*) Butter. *Food Chem.* **1989,** *34,* 131–139.

RSPO: Roundtable on Sustainable Palm Oil. http://www.rspo.org (accessed Aug 2, 2013).

Sanou, H.; Picard, N.; Lovett, P. N.; Dembele, M.; Korbo, A.; Diarisso, D.; Bouvet, J.-M. Phenotypic Variation of Agromorphological Traits of the Shea Tree, Vitellaria paradoxa C.F. Gaertn., in Mali. *Genetic Resources and Crop Evolution* **2006,** 53, 145–161.

Serrano-Vega, M. J., Martinez-Force, E.; Garces, R. Lipid Characterization of Seed Oils from High-palmitic, Low-palmitoleic, and Very High-stearic Acid Sunflower Lines. *Lipids* **2005,** *40,* 369–374.

Shukla, V. K. S. Confectionary Lipids. In *Bailey's Industrial Oil and Fat Products,* 6th ed.; Shahidi, F., Ed.; Wiley, 2005; Vol. 4.

Steingrimsdottir, L.; Thorgeirsdottir, H.; Olafsdottir, A. S. *The Diet of Icelanders. Dietary Survey of the Icelandic Nutrition Council 2002. Main Findings.* Reykjavik 2003.

Stender, S.; Astrup, A.; Dyerberg, J. A *Trans* European Union Difference in the Decline in *Trans* Fatty Acids in Popular Foods: A Market Basket Investigation. BMJ Open 2012; 2.

Switzerland: Ordonnance du DFI sur les huiles et graisses comestibles et leurs dérivés (RS 817.022.105) Federal Office of Public Health (FOPH) 2007

Tarrago-Trani, M. T.; Phillips, K. M.; Lemar, L. E.; Holden, J. M. New and Existing Oils and Fats Used in Products with Reduced *Trans*-Fatty Acid Content. *J. Am. Diet. Assoc.* **2006,** *106,* 867–880.

Temme, E. H.; Millenaar, I. L.; Van Donkersgoed, G.; Westenbrink, S. Impact of Fatty Acid Food Reformulations on Intake of Dutch Young Adults. *Acta Cardiol.* **2011,** *66* (6), 721–728.

Trans *Fatty Acids in Human Nutrition;* Sébédio, J. L., Christie, W. W., Eds.; Oily Press: Dundee, Scotland, 1998; pp 35–58.

Unilever Sustainable Living Plan (USLP) http://unilever.com/sustainable-living/uslp. Accessed 1 October 2013.

Unilever Sustainable Living Plan (USLP)—Progress Report 2012. http://unilever.com/images/USLP-Progress-Report-2012-FI_tcm13-352007.pdf.
United Kingdom Department of Health. Nutrient Analysis of Processed Foods (Including *Trans* Fats), 2013. https://www.gov.uk/government/uploads/system/uploads/attachment_data/file/167938/Summary_Report.pdf.
van Rossum, C. T. M.; Fransen, H. P.; Verkaik-Kloosterman, J.; Buurma-Rethans, E. J. M.; Ocke, M. C. Dutch National Food Consumption Survey 2007–2010: Diet of Children and Adults Aged 7 to 69 Years. 2011. RIVM rapport 350050006.
Wilson, R. F.; Bulton, J. W. Effects of Growth Temperature on Expression of a High Stearic Acid Trait in Soybean. In *Proceedings, World Conference on Oil Seed Technology and Utilization;* AOCS Press: Champaign, IL, 1992; pp 422–429.
Wright, A. J.; Wong, A.; Diosady, L. L. Ni Catalyst Promotion of a *Cis*-selective Pd Catalyst for Canola Oil Hydrogenation. *Food Res. Int.* **2003,** *36,* 1069–1072.
Zhang, H.; Xu, X; Mu, H.; Nilsson, J.; Adler-Nissen, J.; Høy, C; Lipozyme IM-catalyzed Interesterification for the Production of Margarine Fats in a 1-kg Scale Stirred Tank Reactor. *Eur. J. Lipid Sci. Tech.* **2000,** *102,* 411–418.
Zock, P. L.; Katan, M. B. *Trans* Fatty Acids, Lipoproteins, and Coronary Risk. *Can. J. Physiol. Pharmacol.* **1997,** *75* (3), 211–216.

14

Trans Fats Replacement Solutions in South America

Jane Mara Block ■ *Universidade Federal De Santa Catarina, Florianopolis SC, Brazil*

Maria Lidia Herrera ■ *Instituto de Tecnología en Polímeros y Nanotecnología (ITPN), CONICET/University of Buenos Aires, Argentina*

The Hydrogenation Process in Brazil and Argentina

The increase in the degree of saturation of fatty acids by means of hydrogenation has been employed on a large scale since the beginning of the last century. Hydrogenation increases saturated fatty acids and forms *trans* fatty acids (TFAs) containing molecules that can pack together more closely than their corresponding *cis* isomers, resulting in improved functional properties, such as higher melting point, a harder texture, and a longer shelf life (Leth et al., 2003). Recent studies relating *trans* fats in the diet to health have added a new dimension to the practical and technical aspects of oil hydrogenation. What had once been considered a positive effect of hydrogenation (from a technological point of view, *trans* fatty acid formation) is now considered a problem that should be avoided. Besides double bond saturation, other reactions, such as double bond migration and *cis/trans* isomerization, take place during the hydrogenation. The most abundantly formed *trans* isomers during hydrogenation are C18:1 with unsaturation in the 9, 10, and 11 positions. However, small amounts of *trans* C18:2 and C18:3 can also be formed by hydrogenation and deodorization (Leth et al., 2003).

The industrial hydrogenation process is carried out in gas–liquid (hydrogen–oil) phases, which are in contact with a nickel catalyst in a semi batch reactor at 180 °C and 5 bar. Under these conditions, regardless of the catalyst being used, the reaction is strongly limited by the low hydrogen solubility and its mass transfer from the bulk to the catalyst surface. The lack of hydrogen on the catalyst surface has a fundamental importance in the *cis/trans* selectivity, favoring the isomerization and transposition reactions (Piqueras et al., 2008).

In Brazil, hydrogenated vegetable fats and margarines began to be produced in the late 1950s, in order to replace animal fats such as lard and tallow. By the 1970s, fats of vegetable origin modified by partial hydrogenation of oils constituted the type of fat almost exclusively commercialized in the Brazilian market. Until the early 1990s, margarines and table spreads were constituted of water-in-oil emulsions with 60–80% of fat. Currently, products with 25–40% of fat are also available on the market, and most of them are formulated with interesterified fats and are free of *trans* fat. Specialty fats used for specific purposes, such as chocolates, biscuits, bakery products, snacks, soups, and ready meals, among others, are produced especially for the food industry and are the main ingredient in the formulation of most processed foods.

Currently, the modifications of oils and fats used in Brazil include chemical and enzymatic interesterification, partial and total hydrogenation, and fractionation. The fats produced are formulated by blending of oils and/or hydrogenated, interesterified, and/or fractionated fats.

The total amount of fats consumed in Brazil is close to 500,000 t per year, excluding those used in food service. Before industry made the transition to low-TFA fats, soybean oil represented 79% of the raw material used, followed by cottonseed oil, which represented 21% of the market. After this transition, palm oil (which presents more suitable characteristics for the interesterification and fractionation processes) represents 47% of the raw material used, followed by soybean oil (35%), and cottonseed oil (17%). Migration to those raw materials was not uniform; it occurred mainly in the case of fats and margarines used for frying and it was led by larger companies with greater financial resources than smaller ones (ABIA, 2007). Raw materials, including sunflower, corn, canola, palm kernel oil, and babassu, are also used depending on availability and price (Block, 2009).

In Argentina, for the products that do not require solid fat for appropriate texture, most manufacturers replaced *trans* fat with vegetable oils with high oxidative stability, such as high-oleic sunflower oil. When solids are required, animal fat (fat from rendering) is used in the manufacture of margarine, shortening, or widely consumed products such as crackers and cookies. Argentina produces large quantities of fat products that are exported in the form of sebum, crude oils, and refined oils. Although there were studies probing the success of alternatives to conventional hydrogenation processes, the most widespread solution among food industries is replacing the high *trans* fat with a different type of fat having low or no *trans* content, such as animal fat or interesterified fat.

Trans Fat Free Americas

The dietary intake of TFAs produced during hydrogenation and used to make margarines and shortenings has been considered to have a negative impact on cardiovascular health, as well as to contribute to the occurrence of some cancers, among other diseases (Chajès et al., 2008; Chavarro et al., 2008; Willett et al, 1993). Scientific research connecting *trans* fats consumption to an increased risk in the occurrence of such diseases resulted in regulatory changes through legislation and actions of governmental and nongovernmental organizations and health agencies in different countries. With regards to such actions, in 1994, the Food and Agriculture Organization (FAO) and the World Health Organization (WHO) recommended that fats for human consumption contain less than 4% of TFAs. They also encouraged the food industry to reduce the presence of *trans* fats in their products to that level (PAHO, 1994). The Global Strategy on Diet, Physical Activity and Health was approved by the World Health Assembly in May 2004, and it indicated that diet and physical inactivity are the greatest risk factors associated with the increase in the occurrence of chronic diseases. Limiting the consumption of total energy intake from fats, reducing saturated fat intake, increasing the consumption of unsaturated fats, and eliminating TFAs were suggested by the experts in order to achieve a healthier diet for consumers (Nishida and Uauy, 2009; PAHO/WHO, 2007; WHO, 2004).

Different regulatory actions have been taken by different countries to reduce *trans* fats in foods. Among them are mandatory labeling (United States, Canada, Brazil, Chile, South Korea and Taiwan), prohibition (Denmark, Switzerland), prohibition of raw materials containing *trans* fats in restaurants (New York City, Philadelphia, and Boston, and the state of California), and voluntary TFA reduction in certain countries (the UK, the Netherlands, Australia, and New Zealand) (National Conference of State Legislatures, 2011; Oviedo, 2010; Tan, 2009).

In Latin America, the 2003 resolution that makes the labeling of *trans* fats mandatory has been harmonized in Mercosur (Argentina, Brazil, Paraguay, and Uruguay) (Ministry of Health Brazil, 2009; Ribeiro et al., 2007). In Chile, the need to inform consumers of the content of TFAs in a food product became mandatory in November 2006 (PAHO/WHO, 2007). In August of the same year, representatives of the Ministries of Health of Costa Rica, El Salvador, Honduras, Panama, and the Dominican Republic met in Costa Rica and initiated discussions with the objective of implementing regulations for *trans* fats in foods (Murillo, 2006).

In September 2006, in response to concerns of member states about the growing burden of noncommunicable diseases in the Americas, the Pan American Health Organization's (PAHO) 47th Directing Council approved a Regional Strategy and Plan of Action for 2006–2015 on an Integrated Approach to the Prevention and Control of Chronic Non Communicable Diseases (CNCD), which included diet, physical activity, and health. One of its four lines of action, health promotion, includes several initiatives that aim to create environmental conditions that make it easier for individuals to eat healthy diets and engage in active lifestyles (PAHO, 2008a). PAHO, through the Unit of Non Communicable Diseases, convened a task force, *Trans* Fat Free Americas (TFFA), whose members were appointed by the director to serve as PAHO advisers for a two-year period. The TFFA task force was asked to evaluate the impact of TFA in human nutrition and health and to discuss practical ways to phase out TFA from the food supply, including regulatory and voluntary actions and the feasibility of recommending healthier alternative fats. Before the task force, several governments had taken or were considering a wide range of actions to eliminate TFA. In August 2006, the countries that belonged to the Mercosur pact agreement at that time (Argentina, Brazil, Paraguay, and Uruguay) proposed reducing TFA intake in the region. Although these efforts were expected to produce significant benefits, they were not widespread or coordinated at that time. Similarly, the food industry has taken some steps toward eliminating TFA. McDonald's has eliminated TFA in some countries (Denmark, France, Russia, and Argentina) and has substantially reduced TFA in Brazil. Global corporations such as Unilever and Kraft Foods have declared goals to eliminate TFA in all of their products and have started the process. In Argentina and Brazil, some food industries, induced by public health action, have begun to switch from partially hydrogenated oils to nonhydrogenated unsaturated oils at no additional cost to consumers. For example, TFA-free bread and other bakery products have been introduced at similar cost to the previously TFA-laden products (PAHO, 2008a). The first meeting of the PAHO/WHO TFFA task force took place on April 26–27, 2007, in Washington, DC. The task force was composed of expert scientists and public health figures from 11 countries in Latin America and the Caribbean, the United States, and Canada. In addition to the participation of task force members, nongovernmental organizations, research institutes, and consumer associations were invited to attend as observers. The task force concluded that although voluntary actions from industry are welcome, regulatory action is needed to most rapidly and effectively protect population health in the region. The key recommended regulatory measure is to adopt, by legislative action, a threshold limit of less than 2% of total fat as TFA in vegetable oils and soft, spreadable margarines and less than 5% for all other foods (PAHO, 2008a). As part of the PAHO/WHO TFFA initiative, in June 2008, delegates from the subregion's major food companies and industry associations [Brazilian Association of Food Industries (ABIA), Burger King Corporation, Cargill Corporation, Grupo Arcor, Kraft Foods Company, Kellogg Company, McDonald's Corporation, Nestlé, Pepsi Co., SADIA S.A., Watt's S.A., Yum! Brands, Inc.] signed a declaration stating their intention to voluntarily eliminate industrially produced TFAs from the Americas at a meeting in Rio de Janeiro (PAHO, 2008b). Between June and October 2009, the task force and PAHO/WHO invited the food industry delegates to provide information on their reformulations and initiatives to decrease the TFA content of their products. Only 3 of 12 declarants (Pepsi Co., ABIA, and McDonald's Corporation) completed the survey in full. Of the remaining nine companies, Nestlé, Burger King Corporation, and Cargill Corporation responded with a summary statement of their efforts, but without data on specific products. Watt's S.A. stated they were unwilling to participate because they did not carry any of the products detailed in the questionnaire (i.e., baked or fried goods). GrupoArcor, Kraft Foods Company, Kellogg Company, SADIA S.A., and Yum! Brands, Inc. did not respond to up to six requests for data (Monge Rojas et al., 2011). Pepsi Co., ABIA, and McDonald's Corporation have responded that through changing formulations in foods such as fast foods, seasonings, sauces, chocolate candies, cookies, crackers, and chips, it was possible to supply the market with low-*trans* and/or *trans*-free products. The highest amounts of remaining TFA appeared to be in cookies and crackers and in seasonings and sauces. McDonald's Latin American and Caribbean restaurants indicated a shift away from

TFA-containing oils and toward two major substitutes: a blend of cotton, palm, and soybean oils in Brazil and high–oleic acid sunflower oil in the rest of South America. Burger King Corporation indicated that they have used cooking oils with 0 g of TFAs in all restaurants in the Americas and the Caribbean since 2008. Pepsi Co., ABIA, Nestlé, and Cargill Corporation described three key challenges to performing a voluntary transition away from TFAs and toward healthier oils in Latin American and the Caribbean: identification and availability of suitable oils and fats substitutes, the cost of substitution with healthier oils, and concern about consumers' sensory acceptance for some products, especially those requiring "hard" fats, such as cookies and crackers, to maintain the desired mouth feel. According to Monge Rojas et al. (2011), although data from this report suggest a move in the right direction toward TFA reduction, voluntary efforts do not appear to ensure, and certainly do not offer the information to monitor, a major reduction in TFAs in the Latin American and the Caribbean regions. To ensure that there is progress in meeting TFA reduction, the authors recommended implementing regulation in conjunction with systematically and uniformly monitoring the content of TFAs and saturated fatty acids in the food supply.

Besides the intervention via regulation by government agencies and changes in the food industry, there is a need to communicate truthful and consistent messages to the consumer, who must be educated as to the proper consumption and the correct understanding of the information on labels. Governmental agencies should initiate research on how best to communicate this kind of information to consumers.

Regulation of *Trans* Fats in Brazil and Argentina and Intake Recommendation

In Brazil, the regulatory actions coordinated by the Ministry of Health, in association with the National Health Surveillance Agency (Agência Nacional de Vigilância Sanitária [ANVISA]) include the mandatory labeling of *trans* fats, the regulation of food advertising, and the creation of a working group whose goal is to discuss strategies to reduce *trans* fat in foods (Ministry of Health Brazil, 2009).

In December 2003, ANVISA made the labeling of *trans* fats in foods mandatory from July 2006 on. The effective date was extended to July 2007 and the legislation between the countries of Mercosur (Argentina, Brazil, Paraguay, and Uruguay) was harmonized. Since then, foodstuffs with *trans* fat content higher than 0.2% per serving must have a warning about its *trans* fat content on the label. The claim "*trans*-free" or "0% *trans* fat" can be used only for foods with *trans* fat content lower than 0.2% and saturated fat content lower than 2 g per serving (Ministry of Health Brazil, 2003).

In November 2007, a technical cooperation agreement was established between the Ministry of Health, the ABIA, and ANVISA. As part of that agreement, a forum entitled Healthy Eating Forum (Fórum da Alimentação Saudável) was created. Its objective was to find viable alternatives for the industry to replace and reduce the amount of *trans* fats, salt, and sugar in processed foods. The forum was formed by representatives of ANVISA, the Brazilian Agricultural Research Corporation—[Empresa Brasileira de Pesquisa Agropecuária (EMBRAPA), and some universities; they met periodically. The goal established in December 2008 was to reduce the TFA levels in processed foods by the end of 2010, according to the limit recommended by the PAHO and WHO, which is no more than 5% *trans* fat in processed foods and no more than 2% of total fats in oils and margarines (ABIA, 2010; Ministry of Health Brazil, 2009; Oviedo, 2010; PAHO/WHO, 2007)].

In November 2010, ABIA submitted a report to the Ministry of Health with data collected from 135 companies responsible for 73% of food production in Brazil, for the period between March and October 2010. Twelve food categories were studied and the results showed that 94.5% of the companies had achieved the PAHO goal (Table 14.A). According to ABIA, such results correspond to the removal of 230 t of *trans* fats from processed foods (ABIA, 2010).

The decrease of *trans* fats in a great number of processed foods in Brazil is associated with an increase in saturated fat content of such foods. That is the case because in most

Table 14.A Percentage of the Companies Studied that Achieved the PAHO Goal[a] in Brazil

Foodstuffs	Company Type PAHO Goal (%)	Volume Traded in Brazil (%)
Snacks	100	77
Noodles	100	90
Panettones	100	76
Ice creams	99.7	80.8
Bouillons	98.8	78.3
Soups	98.8	84.8
Cakes	98.1	75
Chocolates	97.8	97.5
Oils	96	65.9
Ready meals	91.7	90.7
Cookies	87.7	60.9
Margarines	66.3	66.3
Average	**94.5**	**78.3**

[a]No more than 5% of *trans* fat in processed foods and no more than 2% in oils and margarines (ABIA, 2010).

cases, palm is used to replace partially hydrogenated fats because more saturated fats are needed to obtain a consistency similar to that achieved with partially hydrogenated fats (Aued-Pimentel, 2003, 2009b; Gagliardi et al., 2009; Aued-Pimentel 2009b).

Regarding the reduction of *trans* fats in Brazil, the food service sectors and restaurants were not included in the public policy debate. In the workshop on this topic promoted by ABIA, which took place in the city of São Paulo in 2007 and was supported by International Life Sciences Institute (ILSI) and by the Brazilian Society of Fats and Oils (SBOG), that segment was considered a relevant one to the control of *trans* fat consumption.

Taking into account that restaurant managers may find it difficult to determine when TFAs are added and/or formed during food preparation, Hissanaga et al. (2012) developed the Method for Controlling TFA in Meals (MCTM). The method, which consists of the identification of critical points at which TFAs are added and/or formed, suggests corrective actions in order to avoid TFA formation. Results showed that it may be an effective tool for assisting food services companies in preparing healthier meals.

In March 2010, the proposal of the PAHO task force was accepted, nearly unchanged, by the CONAL (Comisión Nacional de Alimentos—Argentinean National Commission of Foods), which is the government institution in charge of the Argentinean Food Code (ACC—Código Alimentario Argentino) (Dubinsky, 2010). The following rule was added by the joint resolutions 137/10 and 941/10 of the Secretary of Politics, Regulations and Institutes and the Secretary of Agriculture, Livestock and Fisheries on December 3, 2010: According to AFC chapter III, section 155, the content of *trans* fat coming from industrial production in food must not be greater than 2% of the total fats in vegetable oils and margarines intended for direct consumption and 5% of total fats in the other foods. These limits do not apply to the ruminant fats, including milk fat. Based on the adverse effects of *trans* fat, the PAHO/WHO recommended that daily intake must be lower than 1% of total calories (PAHO, 2007). Although AFC code was modified to include the *trans* fat rule, the recommended daily intake value was not included in the legislation.

Trans Fatty Acid Content of Brazilian and Argentinean Foods Before and After Mandatory *Trans* Fat Labeling

Regarding health concerns about fatty acids, some research was undertaken before the *trans* fat rule was issued in Brazil and Argentina. Most dietary TFAs (about 90%) come from the partial hydrogenation of vegetable oils (Okie, 2007; Scheeder, 2007), which also results in the formation of elaidic acid (C18:1 9*t*). The intake of *trans* fats may also come from ruminant fats present in meat, milk, and dairy products. Ruminant fats represent 2–8% of TFAs in the diet. These compounds are formed via biohydrogenation in the rumen of ruminants (cattle, goat, and sheep). In processes such as frying and deodorization (the last step in vegetable oil refining), small amounts of TFAs are formed by a thermally induced mechanism. In frying processes, the TFAs may vary widely depending on the amount of time, the temperature of frying, and on the raw material used (Martin et al., 2007; Sanibal and Mancini Filho, 2002; Schwarz, 2000; Sebedio et al., 1996). Food irradiation can also lead to the formation of *trans* isomers in food (Li et al., 2012).

In the late 1990s, Valenzuela and Morgado (1999) estimated the average consumption of TFAs to be 7–8 g/day/person in developed countries. Allison et al. (1999) estimated TFA consumption at 5.3 g/day. Values between 0.1 and 5.5 g/day were reported in Europe, and in Japan, Semma (2002) reported an intake of 1.56 g/day. The task force of PAHO estimated that consumption of TFA may make up approximately 2–3% of energy (4.5–7.2 grams/day [g/d]) of total calories consumed in the United States, 3% (7.2 g/d) in Argentina, 2% (4.5 g/d) in Chile, and 1.1% (2.6 g/d) in Costa Rica (PAHO, 2007). Because the estimates on the consumption of *trans* fats are not based on databases of nutrient composition with complete data on TFAs, they may not reflect the reality of consumption of those populations (Uauy et al., 2009).

There are no available data about the consumption of TFA in Brazil, but according to the Brazilian Institute of Geography and Statistics (Instituto Brasileiro de Geografia e Estatística, IBGE), increases in the consumption of processed foods (82%) and fat (16%) were observed between 1974 and 2003 (IBGE, 2004).

From the late 1980s to the early 2000s, several studies were carried out in order to determine the levels of TFA in partially hydrogenated fats and in different foods marketed in Brazil. High levels of TFAs were detected in hydrogenated fats and margarines, as well as in potato chips, ice creams, and cookies. Table 14.B shows the TFA contents obtained in some of the studies that were done.

Between 2005 and 2007, Aued-Pimentel et al. (2009a) reported levels between 0.003% and 0.72% of TFAs per serving of 13 ml in samples of soybean, corn, sunflower, and canola oils. Although not listed on their labels, 16 samples of soybean, two of canola, and four of sunflower oil showed levels of TFAs over 0.2 g.

In 2009, the Institute of Consumer Protection (Instituto de Defesa do Consumidor, IDEC) studied 30 samples of cookies and snacks aimed at children. In some of the samples, the results showed high levels of *trans* fat (one sample contained 2.2% *trans* fats and another 4.8%) (IDEC, 2009).

Aued-Pimentel et al. (2009b) reported at least one parameter in disagreement with the information contained on the labels of 12 different foodstuffs, including snacks, potato chips, ice creams, bakery products, dairy beverages, margarines, and noodles. Three of the samples had fat values above the declared total fat (30–58%), 10 samples showed a variation greater than ± 20% for saturated fatty acids, and 7 samples had be-

Table 14.B *Trans* Fatty Acid Content in Different Brazilian Foods before *Trans* Fat Regulation

Food	Range of TFA (%)	Number of Studied Samples	Reference
Hard margarine	25.0–42.9	4	Soares and Franco (1990)
Soft margarine	14.4–31.3	10	
Hydrogenated fats	37.8–42.3	1	
Hard margarines	12.3–38.1	14	Block and Barrera-Arellano (1994)
Soft margarines	15.9–25.1	9	
Hydrogenated fats	0–62	19	
Hydrogenated fats	0–53.9	10	Basso et al. (1999)
Hydrogenated fats	8.9–54.6	12	Azevedo (1999)
Hydrogenated fats	1.3–49.9	15	Grimaldi (2000)
Hydrogenated fats	7.3–40.1	19	Badolato (2000)
Margarines	0–16.1	14	
Ice creams	12.7–45.1	6	Kawashima and Soares (1993)
Potato chips	1.5–21.1	5	Santana et al. (1999)
Ice creams	0.041–1.41	4	Chiara et al. (2003)
Cookies	2.81–5.60	3	

tween 23% and 117% more than the declared content. Values obtained in four samples ranged from 0.3 to 1.8 g per portion, amounts above the limit for the food product to be considered *trans* fat free.

Since June 2006, the American Heart Association recommends an intake of less than 10% for saturated fat and less than 1% of total calories for *trans* fat. On a diet of 1,800 kcal/day, 1% represents 18 kcal, an amount equivalent to 2 g of *trans* fat. Thus, clear information on food labeling and consumer education are necessary so consumers can interpret labels and control the amount of food intake to maintain *trans* fat consumption that is as low as possible (Marcason, 2006). The ingestion of different portions of a product labeled "0 *trans*" throughout the day can lead to the consumption of larger amounts of TFAs than the maximum recommended by health agencies.

Besides, consumers may eat more than the portion that is recommended because they believe the product contains no *trans* fat (Scott-Thomas, 2009). Currently, in Brazil, low-*trans* fats containing from 0 to 8.5% *trans* represent between 30% and 60% of the produced fat. This kind of fat is 15–30% more expensive than partially hydrogenated fats and is used for frying, spraying, ice creams, bakery products, whipped creams, chocolate fillings, topping candies, breads, and processed cheeses. Market research indicates that 65% of the food in Brazil is labeled as "low *trans*," meaning that the product must have less than 0.2% of *trans* fat per serving. *Trans*-free and low saturated fats (less than 30%) are also available for frying, baking (except for fillings and toppings), and dairy products (Block, 2009).

The formulation of *trans*-free fats for application in cookies, chocolate fillings, ice creams, and chocolate toppings is the greatest challenge for the food industry. In these types of applications, the difficulties are related to technological issues and the very high cost of raw materials that could substitute for *trans* fats and that may make the commercialization of the final products not viable (Block, 2009). According to the National Association of Manufacturers of Cookies (Associação Nacional da Indústria de Biscoito, ANIB), 65% of the cookies sold in Brazil in 2007 were free of *trans* fat (Oviedo, 2010).

Despite the reduction in the use of *trans* fats in processed foods in Brazil, there is still a significant portion of foods with high levels of *trans* fats. In addition, there are many problems related to labeling, such as misleading or mistaken information, and uneducated consumers have difficulties interpreting the labels. The public, in general, does not know what *trans* fat is, but they want it out of their foods.

In a market research performed by the IDEC, it was found that, out of 370 products, 37.6% had inadequate labeling with regard to the legal requirement for information about the presence or absence of *trans* fat (IDEC, 2006).

In 2008, research on the labeling of *trans* fat in 10 types of food, including filled cookies, processed cheese, crackers, biscuits, and milk, showed that 43% of the samples had more *trans* fat than was declared on their labels (UNB, 2008).

From the information contained on the labels of cookie packages, Diogo and Maria (2007) calculated: (1) the consumption of cookies necessary for a person to reach the maximum limit of TFA intake (2 g/day) established by the WHO; (2) the amount necessary for a person to have a daily intake of 5 g (an amount related to 25% increased chance of developing a heart disease); and (3) the percentage of *trans* fat in a package. The results showed that in 83% of the samples (34 of 41), the ingestion of 30% of the cookies in a package would be sufficient to achieve the 2 g/day. In two cookie samples (4.8%), the amount of *trans* fat was below 2 g in a serving. In five cookie samples (12.2%), the intake of 30% of the cookies in a package would be sufficient to achieve 5 g/day of *trans* fat. In 28 cookie samples (68.3%), the limit would be reached with the consumption of 30–100% of the cookies. Only four samples (9.7%) did not exceed 0.2 g/portion, which would allow them to be considered *trans* fat free according to ANVISA.

Dias and Gonçalves (2009) studied the labeling of 199 foods, including the labels of cookies, chocolates, ice creams, hamburgers, potato chips, and milkshakes. The results showed the absence of information in 22% of the samples studied. In another study of 2327 food labels, 14 different names to designate the type of fat present in the list of ingredients were reported. Some of the terms/names used did not allow the researchers to know whether the food was formulated with fat containing *trans* isomers, such as the terms *vegetable fat, hydrogenated fat,* and *margarine* (Silveira, 2011).

In Argentina, three studies that provided most of the published data about *trans* fat were selected to exemplify *trans* fat levels in foods before 2006. In these three studies, the food items analyzed were selected according to the results of a survey carried out by the Argentinean National Institute of Statistics and Census (INDEC). This survey showed that over the last 10 years, the consumption of industrial bread had increased two-fold and that of cookies and crackers had increased four-fold (Instituto Nacional de Estadísticas y Censos, 1992). Additional products were selected based on already recognized frequency of use (mayonnaise, oil, margarine, and butter) or because they are used in the manufacture of other products. Representatives of best-selling brands from each product category were selected. Samples of sliced white bread, margarine, butter, cookies, crackers, alfajores (a typical sweet in Argentina, made of two cookies joined with jam), and snacks (potato crisps, cheese curls, cheese-flavored baked sticks) were included. One unit of each brand of each product category was purchased every month for 6 months. Lot numbers were checked to ensure that each unit belonged to a different lot. A pooled sample was prepared by combining portions of each unit and it was divided into two parts: One part was used to quantify total fat, and the other was used to analyze TFAs. Total fat and TFA contents were expressed as wt% of the wet product. Table 14.C summarizes the total fat and TFA contents obtained in three studies (Peterson et al., 2004; Pueyrredón et al., 1999; Tavella et al., 2000). As may be observed, TFAs were found in all samples of cookies and crackers, margarine, butter, and sliced bread. According to these studies, even apparently healthy choices, such as cereal bars, contained partially hydrogenated vegetable oils. On the contrary, TFAs were not found in the processed vegetable oils, mayonnaises, or potato crisps. This is consistent with the use of vegetable oils in the manufacture of the product, as stated on the label, and the fact that manufacturers usually used high-linoleic sunflower oil, which is the most common variety in Argentina. Margarine and butter *trans* fats came from different origins. The former had an industrial origin, while the latter was a ruminant fat. Any type of margarine, regular or light (with reduced content of lipids), had *trans* fatty acid that was greater than the

Table 14.C *Trans* Fat Content of Argentinean Foods before the *Trans* Fat Rule[a]

Food	Total Fat[b]	*Trans* Fat[b]	Total Fat[c]	*Trans* Fat[c]	Total Fat[d]	*Trans* Fat[d]
Hard margarine	85.1	19.0	—	—	—	—
Soft margarine	80.3	14.0	82.0	25.3	83.0	32.6
Light margarine	60.4	9.5	50.0	31.8	50.0	31.8
Crackers	10.5	0.9	12.1	11.1	15.8	4.5
Cookies	12.9	0.5	15.0	7.6	8.5	6.4
Alfajores	11.1	1.1	—	—	18.0	5.5
Light alfajores	3.2	0.1	—	—	—	—
Fast food	34.9	7.9	—	—	—	—
Butter	—	—	85.0	4.6	85.0	4.6
Mayonnaise	—	—	32.0	nd[e]	34.5	nd[e]
Sliced bread	—	—	2.7	0.3	3.0	0.5
Potato crisps	—	—	35.3	0.3	35.0	0.3
Cheese flavored sticks	—	—	38.0	3.7	38.0	10.6
Cheese curls	—	—	38.0	10.6	38.0	3.7

[a]Expressed as wt% of wet product.

[b]Pueyrredón et al. (1999).

[c]Tavella et al. (2000).

[d]Peterson et al. (2004).

[e]nd: Not detected.

saturate fat content. This was in agreement with the fact that, in those years, hydrogenated oils were greatly employed to manufacture margarine in Argentina. To sum up, almost all of the common foods contained TFAs, whereas omega-3 fatty acids were practically absent. When these data were compared to data from countries of the European Union or with food *trans* fat values of the United States, they were similar to *trans* fat values obtained 10 years ago in developed countries. These data showed that, in Argentina, the efforts to reduce *trans* fatty acids in foods were not performed when compared to developed countries (Pueyrredón et al., 1999). According to these authors, it was surprising that products such as light margarine, which contained a high amount of *trans* fat, were called "healthy" simply because they have fewer calories than the regular margarine.

The scientific data from the articles of Pueyrredón et al. (1999), Tavella et al. (2000), and Peterson et al. (2004) were the starting point for the planning of intervention strategies needed to modify the situation observed in Argentina. The first step was to assess whether the agricultural production and the fats and oils industries could provide sufficient quantities of healthy fats and oils to replace TFAs. In 2001, La Plata National University and Dow Agrosciences signed a cooperative agreement to join efforts for this purpose. As a result, four years later, a great variety of TFA-free sunflower oils with high oleic acid content were readily available on the Argentinean market. The properties of these oils, including very high heat resistance and relatively low price, were extremely important in allowing the food industry to replace partially hydrogenated oils (Valenzuela et al., 2004). In addition, product reformulation was actively encouraged by providing a tax bonus to those companies that meet the suggested WHO limit of less than 1% of energy from TFAs in specific food products. The impact of this replacement seems to be substantial; in a very short time, Argentina was able to replace approximately 40% of the 30,000 t of TFAs that were produced annually (L'Abbé et al., 2009).

Alternatives to Reduce *Trans* Fat in Foods

The challenge to agriculturists and food producers in TFA replacement is to examine the issue in a comprehensive way, starting from the breeding of oil seeds and through the production of edible fats and oils, food processing, and final consumption, considering the impact of the changes on human health, on the environment, and on the availability of replacement fats and oils in a particular region. The ultimate goal of TFA elimination is to maximize the benefits and minimize the risks for human health and the environment in a cost-effective way. The actual choices of fats and oils used in many countries are restricted by availability, actual costs of the replacement alternatives, and their capacity to innovate (Uauy et al., 2009).

In assessing approaches to reduce or remove TFA from the food supply in industrialized and developing countries, the experts considered a number of successful public health initiatives adopted by government agencies and public health organizations, in some cases with the collaboration of the food industry. The examples of past and current initiatives reviewed were from Denmark, Canada, United States (New York City), Argentina, India (L'Abbé et al., 2009), and Brazil (ABIA, 2010).

There is a clear need to alert oilseed producers that there will likely be a requirement for an increased supply of substitute oils in order to replace TFA and that this represents an opportunity to expand or develop new oilseed varieties (Valenzuela et al., 2011).

The processes used for modification of fats without the formation of *trans* fat are total hydrogenation, interesterification, and fractionation. Changes in the hydrogenation process used to produce low amounts of *trans* isomers have been reported in the literature. Selective nickel catalysts, palladium, and mixtures of nickel and palladium have been developed as catalyst alternatives for the production of fats containing less than 10% of *trans* fat (Belkacemi et al., 2006; Jackson et al., 2008; Simakova et al.,

2008). Hydrogenation with supercritical carbon dioxide, hydrogen and nickel catalysts, electrochemical hydrogenation (Tarrago-Trani et al., 2006; Wright et al., 2003), or bio-hydrogenation (Carriquiry et al., 2008; Jenkins et al., 2008) have also been studied.

The industrial process commonly used in Argentina is carried out in gas–liquid (hydrogen–oil) phases, which are in contact with a nickel catalyst in a semi batch reactor at 180 °C and 5 bar. Under these conditions, regardless of the catalyst being used, the reaction is strongly limited by the low hydrogen solubility and its mass transfer from the bulk to the catalyst surface. The lack of hydrogen on the catalyst surface has a fundamental importance in the *cis/trans* selectivity, favoring the isomerization and transposition reactions (Piqueras et al., 2008).

According to Rovetto et al. (2003), these problems can be overcome by using a supercritical solvent in which both reactants are soluble. The supercritical fluid increases the hydrogen solubility, eliminating the gas–liquid interface (between H_2 and the substrate and thus creating a homogeneous phase. It also reduces the mass transfer restriction, increasing the diffusion coefficients of both reactants and products. The main role of the supercritical solvent is to get the homogeneous phase in contact with the solid catalyst at the required molar ratio of the reactants. If a single phase is achieved, the various process parameters (temperature, pressure, H_2, concentration, etc.) can be adjusted independently and, as a result, the reaction rate and selectivity are increased. While the conventional hydrogenation process requires high temperatures to increase the hydrogen solubility, the temperature of the single-phase process can be modified without consequences to the composition. This allows working at low temperatures, which have the benefit of improving the selectivity without a conversion reduction. The isomerization reactions, favored by the lack of hydrogen on the catalyst surface, could also be reduced. From the Rovetto et al. (2003) study it can be concluded that the composition of the reaction mixture and the operating process conditions have to be carefully selected in order to ensure single-phase hydrogenation processes. Piqueras et al. (2006) have reported good results in the hydrogenation reactions of sunflower oil using propane as supercritical solvent.

From the point of view of the activity, platinum and palladium are more efficient catalysts than nickel. The former catalysts react at lower temperatures (50–100 °C), thus offering an important energy savings. On the other hand, platinum has been reported as one of the catalysts with better *cis*-isomer selectivity. Piqueras et al. (2008) have studied aluminum, titanium, and platinum catalysts, and their modifications with potassium for the hydrogenation of sunflower oil. An analysis was made of the results of the reactions carried out in conventional and homogeneous conditions using supercritical propane as a solvent. According to their results, an increase in the reaction rate was observed while comparing the homogeneous and conventional processes. Regarding selectivity, the formation of *trans*-isomers was higher in the reaction under conventional conditions, whereas the production of a saturated compound was favored in the homogeneous operation. The homogeneous conditions using supercritical propane as a solvent also showed lower values for *trans*-isomer content, indicating that this kind of process may have applications in the food industry. The Pt-K/TiO_2 catalyst presented a similar specific activity than Pt/TiO_2, although the *cis*-isomer selectivity increased with the alkali addition.

With the technological alternatives to partial hydrogenation currently available, it is not possible to produce partially hydrogenated fats with no *trans* fatty acids without increasing saturated fat and without compromising competitive prices. Therefore, industries produce fully hydrogenated fats, which are free of *trans*-isomers, for subsequent mixture with liquid oils and interesterified fats.

Through chemical or enzymatic interesterification, two different types of fat or oil are interesterified in the presence of an enzyme or chemical, resulting in the rearrangement of fatty acids in the triacylglycerol while keeping the overall fatty acid composition the same, thus changing the melting point, crystal type, and the thermal behavior of interesterified fat. This process does not present the same versatility observed in the hydrogenation process. In order to achieve an adequate solids profile and performance in the final product, it is necessary to use fats with high contents of saturated fatty acids, such as palm oil.

Fractionation is a process in which oils are cooled to partially crystallize, and then are separated into fractions having different melting points; the fractions are called *olein* (the liquid fraction, with a greater content of unsaturated fatty acids with a lower melting point) and *stearin* (a solid fraction, rich in saturated fatty acids with a higher melting point). The process is reversible and does not produce *trans* isomers, but it requires raw materials rich in trisaturated or disaturated triacylglycerols such as palm, milk fat, beef tallow, pork fat, poultry fat, and lauric fats (palm kernel, babassu, and coconut) (Deffense, 1993). Most of these raw materials are not available in Brazil and the fractionation is done exclusively by Agropalma, a company that produces palm oil and other derivatives. Garcia (2011) and Nitatori et al. (2010) developed neural networks using three and five different raw materials, respectively, for the formulation of zero-*trans* fats using interesterified fats. The formulated fats were produced in a pilot plant and used in margarines, filled cookies, cakes, and puff pastries. The results showed that the final products presented similar performance to the products that are typically used (Gandra, 2011; García, 2010; Mattioni, 2010; Scaranto, 2010).

Plant breeding through biotechnology and conventional techniques is also being used to modify TFA in foods and improve its functionality (Kodali, 2005). In Brazil, the main options for new varieties would be high-oleic and high-stearic soybean oil, but those varieties are not commercially available. Importing this kind of raw material would greatly increase the price of the final products. It is estimated that in 5 to 10 years, Brazil will be able to produce genetically modified soybean varieties in adequate quantities and at competitive prices.

The discussion and regulation of *trans* fat in Brazil generated a series of actions by the food industry. For the reformulation of foods, several factors had to be considered, such as the cost and availability of the new raw materials and processes; the physicochemical, sensory characteristics, and performance of the final products; and the labeling. The main challenge for the industry in replacing *trans* fats is to formulate foods with the same performance and cost without a significant increase in the content of saturated fatty acids (Block, 2009).

As part of *trans* fat replacement solutions, in addition to vegetable oils with high oxidative stability, such as high-oleic sunflower oil and bovine sebum when solids are required, other solutions may be applicable to the Argentinean industry. According to Crupkinand Zambelli (2008), one of the best alternatives is stearic acid–rich fats, due to their low impact on consumer health and their plasticity and stability. Available scientific information enables us to confirm with reasonable evidence that when stearic acid is consumed as less than 7% of the total energy, the lipid profile, thrombotic factors, and hemodynamic and cardiovascular risk molecular markers are not modified (Crupkin and Zambelli, 2008; Hunter et al., 2010; Kris-Etherton et al., 2005). This aspect distinguishes stearic acid from other saturated fatty acids present in diets, such as palmitic, lauric, and myristic, regarding cholesterolemic effect since it has similar hypocholesterolemic effect when compared to monounsaturated acid, such as oleic acid, or polyunsaturated acids, such as linoleic acid (Valenzuela et al., 2011). Taking into account stearic acid properties, high stearic acid and high oleic acid/high stearic acid seed oils have been obtained by breeding soybean (Bubeck et al., 1989) and sunflower (Osorio et al., 1995). The Spanish National Research Council (Consejo Superior de Investigaciones Científicas, CSIC), Sevilla, and Advanta Seeds Nutrisun Business Unit in its Biotechnological Center in Buenos Aires Province, Argentina, jointly carried out the development of a new variety of high-stearic/high-oleic sunflower oil (HSHOSFO) coming from seeds obtained through conventional breeding techniques (i.e., nongenetically modified organisms) that are cultivated near Balcarce (a city in Buenos Aires Province, Argentina). Seeds and plants that produce HSHOSFO are so similar to the regular sunflower planted in Argentina that both grains and oils should be produced under identity-preservation schemes through all the value chain steps until final distribution (Dubinsky and Garces, 2011). The main difference between fatty acid profiles of HSHOSFO and regular sunflower oil lies in the stearic content (18% vs. 4%) and oleic content (69% vs. 23%). Furthermore, HSHOSFO displays very low amounts of polyunsaturated fatty acids and about 4% of very long chain fatty acids in the form of arachidic (20:0) and behenic acids (22:0) (Fernández-Moya et al., 2005). It was reported that oils for frying use with high stearic content in the *sn*-1 and *sn*-3 triacylglycerol positions are high-temperature resistant due to their saturated characteristics (Valenzuela et al., 2011). HSHOSFO could be an adequate substitute for partially hydrogenated fats with high contents of TFA isomers that are still used for frying processes in fast food chains (Di Rienzo et al., 2008). For applications that require solids, HSHOSFO can be fractionated to obtain the desired melting point, solid fat content, or appropriate saturated/unsaturated/saturated TAG content when intended for use as a cocoa butter equivalent (CBE). Depending on the fractionation method, different fractions with different physical chemical properties may be obtained. Solvent fractionation is more efficient than dry fractionation and produces a higher enrichment of disaturated TAGs in a single step. This technique is usually applied in the production of valuable fractions used in CBEs or confectionary formulations (Bootello et al., 2012). Dry fractionation is a less specific method, but it is preferred for obtaining fats for baking. The dry and solvent fractionations of HSHOSFO have been investigated in previous works (Bootello et al., 2011; Salas et al., 2011). Recently, the polymorphic behavior of HSHOSFO stearins obtained by dry and solvent fractionation was described (Rincón Cardona et al., 2011, 2012). Stearins showed a complex crystallization behavior, it showed to fractionate and the different solid solutions crystallized in different polymorphic forms. When simple cooling was applied the β_2 and β_1 polymorphic forms were obtained together. Because the β_2 is the one required form for chocolate applications and the β_1 must be avoided since it is the polymorphic form related to blooming, it is probable that stearin might cause difficulties during processing. On the other hand β'_1 form (which is desired for some shortening applications) is very stable, but at several crystallization temperatures it was associated to the β form. These results imply that to use these stearins for food applications, a careful control of processing conditions is necessary.

To extend the use of milk fat in food, pharmaceutical, and cosmetic applications, fractionation may be performed to produce components with specific properties (e.g., melting point). Several applications in which fractionated milk fat performed better than unmodified milk fat have been studied. Milk fat fractions are also blended to give a manufacturer greater flexibility to tailor milk fat as an ingredient to specific functional requirements than could be accomplished with fractionation alone (Kaylegian and Lindsay, 1995). Chemical functionality relies in part on the ratio of saturated and unsaturated fatty acids, which has nutritional as well as flavor implications. Physical functionality includes the crystallization properties and melting properties. One of the most important concerns in the blending of fats is that the crystallization properties of the TAG in the mixture remain compatible. Incompatible TAG in fats can cause retardation or complete lack of crystallization, due to intersolubility effects and formation of eutectic mixtures. As an alternative to hydrogenated vegetable oils in Argentina, modification of high melting point stearins of milk fat by blending with vegetable oils was investigated, since shortenings with appropriate physicochemical properties and good nutritional characteristics that are free of *trans* fatty acids and rich in polyunsaturated fatty acids can be obtained (Cerdeira et al., 2003, 2005, 2006;

Martini et al., 2001, 2002a, 2002b, 2002c, 2004; Puppo et al., 2002). These studies revealed that the blends of both fats have potential as *trans* fat replacements and described the physicochemical properties of milk fat–sunflower oil low-*trans* blends: crystallization behavior, polymorphism, microstructure, and the effect of the addition of emulsifiers in bulk systems. This contribution was recognized by the Senate of Argentina (The Senate of the Argentinean Nation, 2011).

In Argentina, in products that do not require solid fat for appropriate texture, most manufacturers replaced *trans* fat with vegetable oils having high oxidative stability, such as high-oleic sunflower oil. When solids are required, animal fat (fat from rendering) is used in the manufacture of margarine, shortening, or widely consumed products such as crackers and cookies. Argentina produces large quantities of fat products that are exported in the form of sebum, crude oils, and refined oils. Although there were studies probing the success of alternatives to conventional hydrogenation processes, the most widespread solution among food industries is replacing the high-*trans* fat with a different type of fat having low or no *trans* content, such as animal fat or interesterified fat.

References

Allison, D. B.; Egan, S. K.; Barraj, L. M.; Caughaman, C.; Infante, M.; Heimback, J. T. Estimated Intakes of *Trans* Fatty and Other Fatty Acids in the US Population. *J. Am. Diet Assoc.* **1999,** *99,* 166–174.

Associação Brasileira das Industrias de Alimentação (ABIA). *Technical Cooperation Agreement between the Ministry of Health and the Brazilian Association of Food Industries.* Technical Report, Brasília, November 2007.

Associação Brasileira das Industrias de Alimentação (ABIA). *Technical Report: Technical Cooperation Agreement between the Ministry of Health and the Brazilian Association of Food Industries.* Healthy Eating Forum: Reduction of *Trans* Fats in Processed Food, November 2010.

Aued-Pimentel, S.; Caruso, M. S. F.; Cruz, J. M. M.; Kumagai, E. E.; Corrêa, D. U. O. Ácidos Graxos *Trans versus* Saturados em Biscoitos. *Rev. Inst. Adolfo Lutz* **2003,** *62,* 131.

Aued-Pimentel, S.; Silva, S. A.; Kus, M. M. M.; Caruso, M. S. F.; Zenebon, O. *Trans* Fatty Acids in Refined Polyunsaturated Vegetable Oils Commercialized in the City of São Paulo, Brazil. *Ciênc. Tecnol. Aliment.* **2009a,** *29,* 646–665.

Aued-Pimentel, S.; Silva, S. A.; Kus, M. M. M.; Caruso, M. S. F.; Zenebon, O. Evaluation of Total Fat, Saturated and *Trans* Fatty Acids in Foodstuffs with the Claim "*Trans* Free." *Braz. J. Food Technol.,* **2009b,** *VII BMCFB,* 52–57.

Azevedo, C. H. Teores de Isômeros *Trans* em Gorduras Vegetais Hidrogenadas Avaliadas por Diferentes Técnicas Instrumentais. Dissertação, Campinas: Faculdade de Engenharia de Alimentos, Unicamp, 1999.

Badolato, E. S. G. Aspectos Analíticos da Determinação de ácidos Graxos *Trans* em Margarinas e Gorduras Vegetais Hidrogenadas. Dissertação de Mestrado, Universidade de São Paulo, Brasil, 2000.

Basso, R.; Almeida, I. G.; Mancini, J. F. Avaliaçãoqualitativa e Quantitativa dos ácidos Graxos *Trans* em Gorduras Vegetais Hidrogenadas. *Bol SBCTA* **1999,** *33,* 57–63.

Belkacemi, K.; Boulmerka, A.; Arul, J.; Hamoudi, S. Hydrogenation of Vegetable Oils with Minimum *Trans* and Saturated Fatty Acid Formation over a New Generation of Pd-catalyst. *Topics in Catalysis* **2006**, *37,* 113–120.

Block, J. M. Strategies for the Reduction of *Trans* Fat Consumption in Brazil: Current Status and Perspectives. *Inform* **2009,** *20,* 53–55.

Block, J. M.; Barrera-Arellano, D. Produtos Hidrogeados no Brasil: Isômeros *Trans*, Característica Fisico-químicas e Composição em ácidos Graxos. *Arch. Latino Am. Nutr.* **1994,** *44,* 281–285.

Bootello, M. A.; Garcés, R.; Martínez-Force, E.; Salas, J. J. Dry Fractionation and Crystallization Kinetics of High-oleic High-stearic Sunflower Oil. *J. Am. Oil Chem. Soc.* **2011,** *88,* 1511–1519.

Bootello, M. A.; Hartel, R. W.; Garcés, R.; Martínez-Force, E.; Salas, J. J. Evaluation of High Oleic-High Stearic Sunflower Hard Stearins for Cocoa Butter Equivalent Formulation. *Food Chem.* **2012,** *134,* 1409–1417.

Bubeck, D. M.; Fehr, W. R.; Hammond, E. G. Inheritance of Palmitic and Stearic Acid Mutants of Soybean. *Crop. Sci.* **1989,** *29,* 652–665.

Carriquiry, M.; Weber, W. J.; Baumgard, L. H.; Crooker, B. A. In Vitro Biohydrogenation of Four Dietary Fats. *Anim. Feed Sci. Technol.* **2008,** *141,* 339–355.

Cerdeira, M.; Martini, S.; Hartel, R. W.; Herrera, M. L. Effects of Sucrose Esters on Nucleation of Blends of High-melting Milk Fat Fraction and Sunflower Oil. *J. Agric. Food Chem.* **2003,** *51,* 6550–6557.

Cerdeira, M.; Pastore, V.; Vera, L. V.; Martini, S.; Candal, R. J.; Herrera, M. L. Nucleation Behavior of Blended High-melting Fractions of Milk Fat as Affected by Emulsifiers. *Eur. J. Lipid Sci. Technol.* **2005,** *107,* 877–885.

Cerdeira, M.; Martini, S.; Candal, R. J.; Herrera, M. L. Polymorphism and Growth Behavior of Low-*trans* Fat Blends Formulated with and without Emulsifiers. *J. Am. Oil Chem. Soc.* **2006,** *83,* 489–496.

Chajès, V.; Thiébaut, A. C. M.; Rotival, M.; Gauthier, E.; Maillard, V.; Boutron-Ruault, M. C.; Joulin, V.; Lenoir, G. M; Clavel-Chapelon, F. Association between Serum *Trans*-monounsaturated Fatty Acids and Breast Cancer Risk in the E3N-EPIC Study. *Am. J. Epidemiol.* **2008,** *167,* 1312–1320.

Chavarro J. E.; Stampfer, M. J.; Campos, H.; Kurth, T.; Willett, W. C.; Ma, J. A Prospective Study of *Trans*-fatty Acid Levels in Blood and Risk of Prostate Cancer. *Cancer Epidemiol. Biomarkers Prev.* **2008,** *17,* 95–101.

Chiara, V. L.; Sichieri, R.; Carvalho, T. S. F. Teores de ácidos Graxos *Trans* de Alguns Alimentos Consumidos no Rio de Janeiro. *Rev Nutr.* **2003,** *16,* 227–333.

Crupkin, M.; Zambelli, A. Detrimental Impact of *Trans* Fats on Human Health: Stearic Acid-rich Fats as Possible Substitutes. *Comprehensive Rev. Food Sci. Food Safety* **2008,** *7,* 271–279.

Deffense, E. Milk Fat Fractionation Today—A Review. *J. Am. Oil Chem. Soc.* **1993,** *70,* 1193.

Dias, J. R.; Gonçalves, E. C. B. A. Avaliação do Consumo e Análise da Rotulagem Nutricional de Alimentos com Alto Teor de ácidos Graxos *Trans*. *Ciênc. Tecnol. Aliment.* **2009,** *29,* 177–182.

Diogo, V.; Maria, M. Gordura *Trans* na Dieta Infantil Brasileira: Avaliação da Ingestão a Partir dos Teores Declarados na Rotulagem de Biscoitos. *XXIX Jornada de Iniciação Científica, Artística e Cultural/UFRJ,* 2007. http://acd.ufrj.br/consumo/quemsomos/cc_gorduratrans.html (accessed July, 20 2012).

Di Rienzo, M. A.; Lemke, S. L.; Petersen, B. J.; Smith, K. M. Effect of Substitution of High Stearic Acid Low Linoleic Acid Soybean Oil for Hydrogenated Soybean Oil on Fatty Acid Intake. *Lipids* **2008,** *43,* 451–456.

Dubinsky, E. *Trans* Fat Update from Argentina. *Inform* **2010,** *21,* 708–709.

Dubinsky, E.; Garcés, R. High Stearic/High Oleic Sunflower Oil: A Versatile Fat for Food Applications. *Inform* **2011,** *22,* 369–371.

Fernández-Moya, V.; Martínez-Force, E.; Garcés, R. Oils from Improved High Stearic Acid Sunflower Seeds. *J. Agric. Food Chem.* **2005,** *53,* 5326–5330.

Gagliardi, A. C. M.; Mancini Filho, J.; Santos, R. D. Perfil Nutricional de Alimentos com Alegação de Zero Gordura *Trans. Revista da Associação Médica Brasileira* **2009,** *55,* 50–53.

Gandra, K. M. Formulation of *trans* free fats for cookie filling using neural networks. Doctoral Thesis, University of Campinas (UNICAMP). Campinas, Brazil, 2010.

Garcia, R. K. A.; Gandra, K. M.; Block, J. M.; Barrera-Arellano, D. Neural Networks to Formulate Special Fats. *Grasas y Aceites,* **2012,** *63,* 245–252.

Grimaldi, R.; Gonçalves, L. A. G.; Esteves, W. Characteristics of Commercial Brazilian Fats. *Braz. J. Food Technol.* **2000,** *3,* 159–164.

Hissanaga, V. M.; Block, J. M.; Proença, R. P. C. Development of a Method for Controlling *Trans* Fatty Acids in Meals—MCTM. *J. Cul. Sci. and Tech.* **2012,** *10,* 1–18.

Hunter, J. E.; Zhang, J.; Kriss-Etherton, P. Cardiovascular Disease Risk of Dietary Stearic Acid Compared with *Trans,* Other Saturated, and Unsaturated Fatty Acids: A Systemic Review. *Am. J. Clinical Nutrition* **2010,** *91,* 46–63.

Instituto Brasileiro de Geografia e Estatística (IBGE). *Pesquisa de Orçamentos Familiares 2002–2003: Análise da Disponibilidade Domiciliar e Estado Nutricional no Brasil.* Technical Report, Rio de Janeiro, 2004.

Instituto Brasileiro de Defesa do Consumidor (IDEC). Bom Para os Olhos e o Paladar, Ruim para o Coração. Revista do Idec 2006, 103. http://www.idec.org.br/oq_idec.asp (accessed June, 15, 2012).

Instituto Nacional de Estadísticas y Censos (INDEC). Study 20: Encuesta de gastos e ingresos, cantidades consumidas. *Encuesta permanente de hogares.* 1992; SI 10/20.

Instituto Brasileiro de Defesa do Consumidor (IDEC). Além da Conta. *Revista do Idec,* 2009, February. http://www.estadao.com.br/especiais/2009/02/alimentacao_infantil.pdf (accessed June 24, 2012).

Jackson, S. D.; Kelly G. J.; Vass, E. M. Preparation and Catalytic Properties of Cerium Hydride. *Journal of Alloys and Compounds* **2008,** *459,* 113–117.

Jenkins, T. C.; Wallace, R. J.; Moate, P. J.; Mosley, E. E. Recent Advances in Biohydrogenation of Unsaturated Fatty Acids within the Rumen Microbial Ecosystem. *J. of An. Sci.* **2008,** *86,* 397–412.

Kaylegian, K. E.; Lindsay, R. C. Milk Fat and Modifications. In *Handbook of Milkfat Fractionation Technology and Application*; AOCS Press: Urbana, IL, 1995; 1–17.

Kawashima, L. M.; Soares, L. M. V. Gorduras em Sorvetes Nacionais: Conteúdo, Composição de ácidos Graxos e Teor de *Trans* Isômeros. *Ciênc. Tecnol. Aliment.* **1993,** *13,* 194–202.

Kodali, D. *Trans* Fats: Chemistry, Occurrence, Functional Need in Foods and Potential Solutions. In Trans *Fats Alternatives,* Kodali, D. R., List, G. R., Eds., AOCS Press: IL, 2005; pp. 1–25.

Kris-Etherton, P. M.; Griel, A. E.; Psota, T. L.; Gebauer, S. K.; Zhang, J.; Etherton, T. D. Dietary Stearic Acid and Risk of Cardiovascular Disease: Intake, Sources, Digestion, and Absorption. *Lipids* **2005,** *40,* 1193–1200.

L'Abbé, M. R.; Stender, S.; Skeaff, M.; Ghafoorunissa, R.; Tavella, M. Approaches to Removing *Trans* Fats from the Food Supply in Industrialized and Developing Countries. *Eur. J. Clin. Nutr.* **2009,** *63,* S50–S67.

Leth, T.; Bysted, A.; Hansen, K.; Ovesen, L. *Trans* FA Content in Danish Margarines and Shortenings. *J. Am. Oil Chem. Soc.* **2003,** *80,* 475–478.

Li, A.; Wang, F.; Fan, B.; Li, W.; Li, Q.; Zhou H.; Ha, Y. Formation of *Trans* Fatty Acids Induced by Radicals in Irradiated Ground Beef and Liquid Egg. *J. Am. Oil Chem. Soc.* **2012,** *89,* 2207–2213.

Marcason, W. How Many Grams of *Trans*-fat Are Recommended per Day? *J. Am. Diet. Assoc.* **2006,** *106,* 1507.

Martin, C. A.; Milinski, M. C.; Visentainer, J. V.; Matshushita, M. Souza, N. E. *Trans* Fatty Acid-forming Processes in Foods: A Review. *An. Aca. Bras. Ciênc.* **2007,** *79,* 343–350.

Martini, S.; Herrera, M. L.; Hartel, R. W. Effect of Cooling Rate on Nucleation Behavior of Milk Fat Sunflower Oil Blends. *J. Agric. Food Chem.* **2001,** *49,* 3223–3229.

Martini, S.; Herrera M. L.; Hartel, R. W. Effect of Cooling Rate on Crystallization Behavior of Milk Fat Fraction/Sunflower Oil Blends. *J. Am. Oil Chem. Soc.* **2002a,** *79,* 1055–1062.

Martini, S.; Herrera, M. L.; Hartel, R. W. Effect of Processing Conditions on Microstructure of Milk Fat Fraction/Sunflower Oil Blends. *J. Am. Oil Chem. Soc.,* **2002b,** *79,* 1063–1068.

Martini, S.; Puppo, M. C.; Hartel, R.W.; Herrera, M. L. Effect of Sucrose Esters and Sunflower Oil Addition on Microstructure of a High-Melting Milk Fat Fraction. *J. of Food Sci.* **2002c,** *67,* 3412- 3418.

Martini, S.; Cerdeira, M.; Herrera, M. L. Effect of Sucrose Esters on the Crystallization Behavior of Bulk Oil Systems. *J. Am. Oil Chem. Soc.* **2004,** *81,* 209–211.

Mattioni, B. Application of Neural Networks to Formulate Fats for Puff Pastry Based in Soybean and Cotton Interesterified Fats. Masters Thesis, Federal University of Santa Catarina, Florianópolis, Brazil, 2010.

Ministry of Health Brazil. National Health Surveillance Agency. Resolution nº 360, December 23, 2003, Brasilia, DF.

Ministry of Health Brazil. Technical Note: Actions of the Brazilian Government on *Trans* Fat, 2009. http://nutricao.saude.gov.br/documentos/nota_imprensa_gorduras_trans.pdf (accessed September 24, 2012).

Monge Rojas, R.; Colón Ramos, U.; Jacoby, E.; Mozaffarian, D. Voluntary Reduction of *Trans* Fatty Acids in Latin American and the Caribbean Current Situation. *Rev. Panam. Salud Publica,* **2011,** *29,* 126–129.

Murillo, M. Normatización delontenido de ácidos Grasos *Trans* em Alimentos: Experiencia de Costa Rica. Instituto de Nutrición de Centro-América y Panamá, 2006. http://www.incap.org.gt (accessed September 12, 2012).

National Conference of State Legislatures. *Trans* Fat and Menu Labeling Legislation, 2011. http://www.ncsl.org/issues-research/health/*trans*-fat-and-menu-labeling-legislation.aspx (accessed August 25, 2012).

Nishida, C.; Uauy, R. WHO Scientific Update on Health Consequences of *Trans* Fatty Acids: Introduction. *Eur. J. Clin. Nutr.* **2009,** 63, S1–S4.

Nitatori, C. Y.; Gandra, K. M.; Garcia, R. K. A.; Barrera-Arellano, D. Construção e Treinamento de uma Rede Neural para Formulação de Gorduras Especiais a Partir de Gorduras Interesterificadas, Óleos de Soja e Palma. In: XVII Congresso de Iniciação Científica da Unicamp, Campinas, Brazil, 2010.

Okie, S. New York to *Trans* Fats: You're Out! *N. Engl. J. Med.* **2007,** *356,* 2017–2021.

Osorio, J.; Fernández-Martinez, J.; Mancha, M.; Garcés, R. Mutant Sunflowers with High Concentration of Saturated Fatty Acids in the Oil. *Crop Sci.* **1995,** *35,* 739–742.

Oviedo, K. M. M. Análise Comparativa das Experiências de Regulação de Gorduras Trans em Alimentos Processados no Brasil, Canadá, Dinamarca e Estados Unidos. Dissertação de Mestrado, Pontifícia Universidade Católica do Rio de Janeiro, 2010.

Pan American Health Organization (PAHO). *Food and Agriculture Organization of the United Nations, Fats and Oils in Human Nutrition, Report of a Joint Expert Consultation, Food and Agriculture Organization of the United Nations and the World Health Organization.* Food and Nutrition Paper No. 57; 1994.

Pan American Health Organization (PAHO). *Healthy Oils and the Elimination of Industrially Produced Trans Fatty Acids in the Americas: Initiative for the Prevention and Control of Chronic Diseases.* Washington, DC, 2008a.

Pan American Health Organization (PAHO). Trans *Fat Free Americas. Declaration of Rio de Janeiro.* Washington, DC, 2008b.

Pan American Health Organization (PAHO)/World Health Organization (WHO). *Trans Fat Free Americas (TFFA), Conclusions and Recommendations.* Regional Office at the WHO: Washington, DC, 2007.

Peterson, G.; Aguilar, D.; Espeche, M.; Mesa, M.; Jáuregui, P.; Díaz, H.; Simi, M.; Tavella, M. Ácidos Grasos *trans* en Alimentos Consumidos Habitualmente por los Jóvenes en Argentina. Archivos *Argentinos de Pediatría,* **2004,** *102,* 102–109.

Piqueras, C. M.; Fernández, M.; Tonetto, G.; Bottini, S.; Damiani, D. E. Hydrogenation of Sunflower Oil on Pd Catalysts in Supercritical Conditions: Effect of the Particle Size. *Catalysis Communications,* **2006,** *7,* 344–346.

Piqueras, C. M.; Fernández, M.; Tonetto, G.; Bottini, S.; Damiani, D. E. Sunflower Oil Hydrogenation on Pt Catalysts: Comparison between Conventional Process and Homogeneous Phase Operation Using Supercritical Propane. *Catalysis Today,* **2008,** *133–135,* 836–841.

Pueyrredón, P.; Rovirosa, A.; Torres Agüero, M. E.; Uicich, R. Acidos Grasos *Trans*: Actualización y Situación Argentina. *Revista de la Sociedad Argentina de Nutrición* **1999,** *10,* 61–68.

Puppo, M. C.; Martini, S.; Hartel, R. W.; Herrera, M. L. Effects of Sucrose Esters on Isothermal Crystallization and Rheological Behavior of Blends of High-melting Milk Fat Fraction and Sunflower Oil. *J. Food Sci.* **2002,** *67,* 3419–3426.

Ribiero, A. P.; Moura, J. M. L. N.; Grimaldi, R.; Gonçalves, L. A. G. Interesterificação Química: Alternativa pra Obtenção de Gordura Zero *Trans. Quím. Nova* **2007,** *30,* Sept/Oct.

Rincón Cardona, J. A.; Ye, Y.; Martini, S.; Candal, R. J.; Herrera, M. L. *Propiedades Fisicoquímicas de Estearinas de Aceite de Girasol Alto Esteárico Alto Oleico.* 14th AOCS Latin American Congress and Exhibition on Fats and Oils, Cartagena de Indias, Colombia, October 17–21, 2011.

Rincón Cardona, J. A.; Ye, Y.; Martini, S.; Candal, R. J.; Herrera, M. L. *Polymorphic Behavior of Sunflower Oil Stearins.* 103rd AOCS Annual Meeting & Expo, Long Beach, California, April 29–May 1, 2012.

Rovetto, L. J.; Bottini, S. B.; Brignole, E. A.; Peters, C. J. Supercritical Hydrogenation Processes. Experimental Results on the Fluid Phase Behavior of Binary and Ternary Mixtures of Hydrogen, Propane and Tripalmitin. *Journal of Supercritical Fluids* **2003,** *25,* 165–176.

Salas, J. J.; Bootello, M. A.; Martínez-Force, E.; Garcés, R. Production of Stearate-rich Butters by Solvent Fractionation of High Stearic-High Oleic Sunflower Oil. *Food Chem.* **2011,** *124,* 450–458.

Sanibal, E. A. A.; Mancini Filho, J. Alterações Física, Químicas e Nutricionais de óleos Submetidos ao Processo de Fritura. *Food Ingr.* **2002,** 1, 48–54.

Santana, D. M. N.; Marques, M. M.; Rosa, C. A. R. Determinação por Cromatografia Gasosa da Composição em ácidos Graxos e Teor de ácido *Trans* em Algumas Marcas de Batata Frita. *Bol. SBCTA,* **1999,** *33,* 64–69.

Scaranto, B. A. A. Application of Neural Networks to Formulate Fats for Cakes Based in Soybean and Cotton Interesterified Fats. Masters Thesis, Federal University of Santa Catarina, Florianópolis, Brazil, 2010.

Scheeder, M. R. L. About the *Trans*-(hi) Story: How Did *Trans* Fatty Acids Enter the Human Food Chain. *J. Am. Oil Chem. Soc.* **2007,** *18* (2), 133–135.

Schwarz, W., Formation of *Trans* Polyalkenoic Fatty Acids during Vegetable Oil Refining. *Eur. J. Lipid Sci. Technol.* **2000,** *102,* 648–649.

Scott-Thomas, C. Call for More Education on Canadian Nutrition Labeling, 2009. http://www.foodnavigator-usa.com (accessed August 25, 2012).

Sebedio, J. L.; Catte, M.; Boudier M. A.; Prevost, J.; Gradgirard, A. Formation of Fatty Acid Geometrical Isomers and of Cyclic Fatty Acid Monomers during the Finish Frying of Frozen Prefried Potatoes. *Food Res. Int. Barking,* **1996,** *29,* 109–116.

Senate of the Argentinean Nation. *Distinction: Senate Declared of Public Interest the Project "Alternatives to* Trans *Fats" by M. L. Herrera and R. J. Candal.* Resolution VSP-703/11; Buenos Aires, 2011.

Semma, M. *Trans* Fatty Acids: Properties, Benefits and Risk. *J. Health Sci.* **2002,** *48,* 7–13.

Silveira, B. M. *Informação Alimentar e Nutricional da Gordura Trans em Rótulos de Produtos Alimentícios Industrializados.* Dissertação de Mestrado, Programa de Pós-Graduação em Nutrição da Universidade Federal de Santa Catarina, 2011.

Simakova, I. L.; Simakova, O. A.; Romanenko, A. V.; Murzin, D. Y. Hydrogenation of Vegetable Oils over Pd on Nanocomposite Carbon Catalysts. *Ind. Eng. Chem. Res.* **2008,** *47,* 7219–7225.

Soares, L. M. V.; Franco, M. R. B. Níveis de *Trans*-isômeros e Composição de ácidos Graxos de Margarinas e Produtos Hidrogenados Semelhantes. *Ciênc. Tecnol. Aliment.* **1990,** *10,* 57–71.

Tan, A. S. L. A. A Case Study of the New York City *Trans*-fat Story for International Application. *Journal of Public Health Policy,* **2009,** *30,* 3–16.

Tarrago-Trani, M. T.; Phillips, K. M.; Lemar, L. E.; Holden, J. M. New and Existing Oils and Fats Used in Products with Reduced *Trans*-fatty Acid Content. *J. Amer. Diet. Assoc.* **2006,** *106,* 867–880.

Tavella, M.; Peterson, G; Espeche, M.; Cavallero, E.; Cipolla, L.; Perego, L.; Caballero, B. *Trans* Fatty Acid Content of a Selection of Foods in Argentina. *Food Chem.* 2000, *69,* The Truth about *Trans* Fat, 2009. http://www.thetruthabouttransfat.com (accessed in July, 24, 2012).

Uauy, R.; Aro, A.; Clarke, R.; Ghafoorunissa, R.; L'Abbé, M.; Mozaffariam, D.; Skeaff, M.; Stender, S.; Tavella, M. WHO Scientific Update on *Trans* Fatty Acids: Summary and Conclusions. *Eur. J. Clin. Nutr.* **2009,** *63,* S68–S75.

Universidade de Brasilia (UDB). Rótulos São Imprecisos Sobre Gordura *Trans,* 2008, http://www.unb.br/noticias/bcopauta/index2.php?i=285 (accessed August 23, 2012).

Valenzuela, A.; Morgado, N. *Trans* Fatty Acid Isomers in Human Health and in the Food Industry. *Biol. Res.* **1999,** *32,* 273–287.

Valenzuela, A.; Delplanque, B.; Tavella, M. Stearic Acid: A Possible Substitute for *Trans* Fatty Acids from Industrial Origin. *Grasas y Aceites* **2011,** *62,* 131–138.

Valenzuela, A.; Nieto, S.; Peterson, G.; Tavella, M. Comparative Study in Fried Food about the Stability of Different Vegetables Oils. *Fat Oils Magazine,* **2004,** *2,* 22–28.

World Health Organization (WHO). *57th World Health Assembly, Global Strategy on Diet, Physical Activity and Health.* Resolution WHA57.17; Washington, DC, 2004.

Willett, W. C.; Stampfer, M. J.; Manson, J. E.; Colditz, G. A.; Speizer, F. E.; Rosner, B. A.; Hennekens, C. H. Intake of *Trans* Fatty Acids and Risk of Coronary Heart Disease among Women. *The Lancet* **1993,** *341,* 581–585.

Wright, A. J.; Mihele, A. L.; Diosady, L. L. *Cis* Selectivity of Mixed Catalyst Systems in Canola Oil Hydrogenation. *Food Res. Inter.* **2003,** *36,* 797–804.

15

Trans Fats Replacement Solutions in China

Jingyi Zhang, Prakash Adhikari, Tiankui Yang, Shuhua Xia, Peng Hu, Yuanrong Jiang, and Xuebing Xu ■ *Wilmar Global R&D Center, Pudong, Shanghai, China*

Introduction

Naturally occurring *trans* fatty acids (TFAs) are found in small amounts in meat and dairy products as a result of biohydrogenation in ruminants. However, most of the TFAs in human diets are produced from artificial hydrogenation processes, which convert vegetable oils from liquid oils to solid or semisolid fats. Such partially hydrogenated vegetable oils (PHVOs) provided desirable physical properties and prolong the shelf life of foods (Hunter, 2004). Food industries use PHVO in various food products such as margarines, shortenings, bakery products, and processed foods (Mozaffarian et al., 2006). However, numerous metabolic and epidemiological studies confirm that high intake of TFAs is positively associated with the risk of developing cardiovascular disease (CVD). According to China Health Statistical (2012), CVD accounted for approximately 41% of total deaths in 2011. This may indicate that TFA intake is an important issue for the general population.

Due to the rapid social and economic changes in the last 20 years, diet and activity levels of the Chinese population have changed drastically. The Ministry of Health of the People's Republic of China reported that dietary fat contributed more than 35% of Chinese people's total energy intake, which is higher than the recommendation by WHO. Traditional high-carbohydrate diets have gradually been replaced by high-fat diets (Bell et al., 2001). An industrial investigation (CMBF, 2006) revealed the dramatic increase in fast food consumption in the society. The availability of Western-style food products, such as margarines, shortenings, muffins, cakes, cookies, fried potatoes, chips, and so forth, has also been growing very fast (7–9% annually) during the last three consecutive decades. To improve product quality and shelf life, some of the products contain partially hydrogenated fats, which are major source of TFA (Larquéet al., 2005; Tarrago-Trani et al., 2006).

Due to the negative health effects associated with TFA, food industries are using or searching for different technologies to reduce TFA content in oils and fats. Several technologies are already in use to eliminate or reduce TFAs, such as interesterification, fractionation, blending, or a combination of these techniques. In addition, deodorization is very important to control the formation of TFA in cooking oils. Several researchers have focused on production of *trans*-free margarines/shortenings using lipase-catalyzed interesterification (Adhikari et al., 2009, 2010, 2011; Li et al., 2010; Reshma et al., 2008; Zhang et al., 2004). Most of the food industries are using palm oil as main source of hard fat for blending or interesterification.

Labeling and the Regulatory Situation

Amendments to food labeling regulations in Canada in January 2003 and U.S. enforcement of declaration of TFA levels on food labeling in July 2003 have triggered global consideration to reducing TFA in food products. More and more countries are taking steps in enforcing a TFA labeling requirement and/or eliminating the use of TFA. For example, the Danish government passed legislation on March 11, 2003, to prohibit sales of foods containing more than 2% (based on fat) of industrially produced TFAs (artificial TFAs).

According to the National Food Safety Standard for Nutrition Labeling of Prepackaged Foods (published by the Ministry of Health of the People's Republic of China, (2011), labeling of TFAs is not required on all prepackaged foods. However, labeling of TFA content is mandatory when hydrogenated or partially hydrogenated edible oils are used as ingredients (Ministry of Health of People's Republic of China, 2011). *Trans* fatty acid refers to sum of unsaturated fatty acids having one or more unsaturation linkages in the *trans* configuration that are not in a conjugated system. Thus, TFAs from natural sources are not considered *trans* fatty acids in China. *Trans* fat can be labeled either as "*trans* fat" or "*trans* fatty acid" on the nutrition label. The amount should be expressed in grams and rounded to the nearest 0.1 g. Nutrient reference value (NRV) for *trans* fat is not established in China. Thus, "no *trans* fat" or "not containing *trans* fat" can be declared when the food contains no more than 0.3 g of *trans* fat per 100 g (ml) of food.

The Food and Environmental Hygiene Department in Hong Kong requires mandatory labeling of energy and the seven core nutrient contents, including *trans* fat, on all prepackaged food. Similar to China, *trans* fatty acids refers to the sum of all unsaturated fatty acids that contain at least one nonconjugated *trans* double bond. The content of the *trans* fat should be expressed in grams and rounded to the nearest 0.1 g, following the wording "*trans* fat" or "*trans.*" Conjugated linoleic acids (CLAs) are excluded. *Trans* fat within the food should not be more than 120% of the declared value. Like China, there is no NRV established for *trans* fat. The "*trans* fat free" claim can only be used under the following conditions:

- For solid food: (1) Contains not more than 0.3 g of *trans* fat per 100g of food; (2) contains not more than 1.5 g of saturated fat and *trans* fatty acids combined per 100 g of food; and (3) the sum of saturated fat and *trans* fatty acids do not contribute more than 10% of daily energy.
- For liquid food: (1) Contains not more than 0.3 g of *trans* fat per 100 ml of food; (2) contains not more than 0.75 g of saturated fat and *trans* fatty acids combined per 100 ml of food; and (3) the sum of saturated fat and *trans* fatty acids do not contribute more than 10% of energy.

In comparison, in Taiwan, *trans* fats are defined as nonconjugated *trans* fatty acids produced by partial hydrogenation in the edible oil processing. Therefore, natural *trans* fats and CLAs are exempted from labeling. The content of *trans* fat should be expressed in grams and rounded to integer number or to the nearest 0.1 g. Food containing no more than 0.3g of *trans* fat per 100g (ml) of food can be labeled as "0 g/100 g (100 ml)" *trans* fat.

Industrial Responses and Solutions

Specialty Fats

Specialty fats refer to fats developed with specific functionalities, such as plastic fats used in margarine, shortening, and so forth. Fu et al. (2008) investigated the TFA content in 97 products in the Chinese market (88 Western-style products and 9 Chinese-style snacks) (Table 15.A). Only a small number of the products (Western-style products) contained detailed labeling of fat content. Among 35 Western-style products that listed the type of fat, 25 of them contained TFA at greater than 0.5% (w/w) of fat. Five products that were high in TFAs clearly indicated "hydrogenated soybean oil" on the label.

Margarine (about 15 products) contained lower levels of TFAs than those of wafers and pie (Table 15.A). Presence of elaidic acid in pie indicates usage of palm-based hydrogenated fats as raw materials, which contain an average of 39% of oleic acid. In addition, Fu et al. (2008) suggested that the content of TFA in wafers, biscuits, and margarine

Table 15.A Trans Fatty Acids (TFA, w% Fat) Level in Food Products Sold in the Chinese Market

	TFAs			% Products Containing TFAs		
Categories (n)	**Average**	**Min.**	**Max.**	**>0.5%**	**>2%**	**>10%**
Cheese (6)	6.9	5.9	7.9	100	100	0
Chocolate (10)	1.4	0	4.8	60	30	0
Crisps, chips, and fries (10)	2.1	0	8.8	90	50	0
Ice cream (10)	2.7	0	6.7	80	60	0
Margarines (15)	5.1	0	13.2	80	80	20
Pie and cake (10)	12.1	2.4	30.9	100	100	30
Sauces and dressing (8)	2.6	0	4.8	88	63	0
Wafers and biscuits (19)	4.3	0	27.9	53	37	11
Chinese-style snacks (9)	0.8	0	3.7	33	22	0

Source: Fu et al. (2008).

sold in China was comparable to their counterparts sold in the European countries (Aro et al., 1998). Meanwhile, chips and fries, sauces and dressings, and ice cream contained substantially lower levels of TFA than those reported previously by Aro et al. (1998).

Figure 15.1 shows the TFA contents in the selected oil-bearing foods based on a 2012 survey. Cake, bread, pie, and cookies contain more than 1 g TFA per 100 g total fat, and other analyzed samples showed below 1%. None of the samples showed a higher content of TFA.

Compared to 2008, TFA content was drastically decreased in 2012. Cake, bread, and pie contained 12.07% TFA (of total fat) in 2008 and decreased to 1.94% in 2012 (Figure 15.2). Similarly, cookies contained 4.35% TFA (of total fat) in 2008 and decreased to 1.07% in 2012. From these results, it can be concluded that the TFA content in oil-bearing foods decreased significantly. With these data, the overall industrial situation looks very positive for the reduction of TFAs. The oils and fats industry, as well as the food industry, are trying to reduce the TFA content in China following the global trends. The new survey in 2011 concerning products containing higher content of TFA is illustrated in Table 15.B on pages 342–344.

Cooking Oils

Small amounts of TFA isomers are found in refined edible oils due to the high temperatures used in deodorization processes. Refining generally includes degumming,

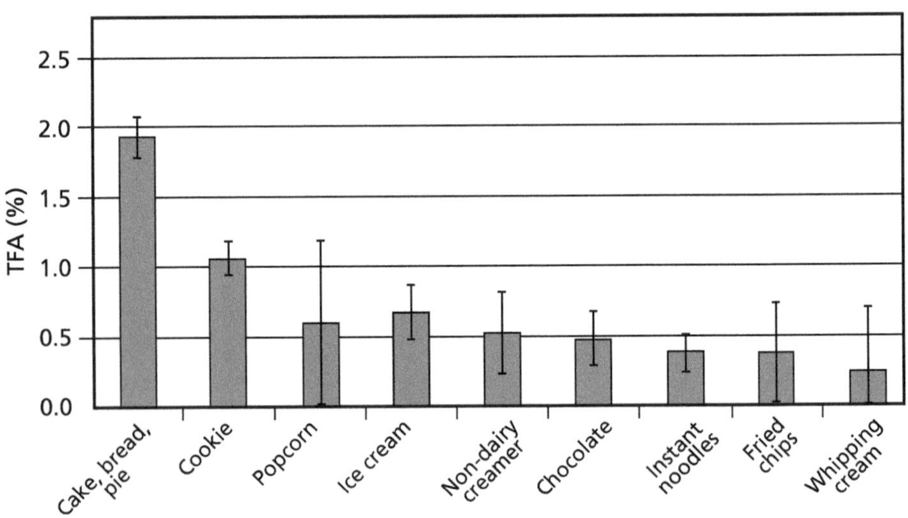

Figure 15.1 TFA content (% based on total fat) in oil bearing food. Data from Jiang et al. (2013).

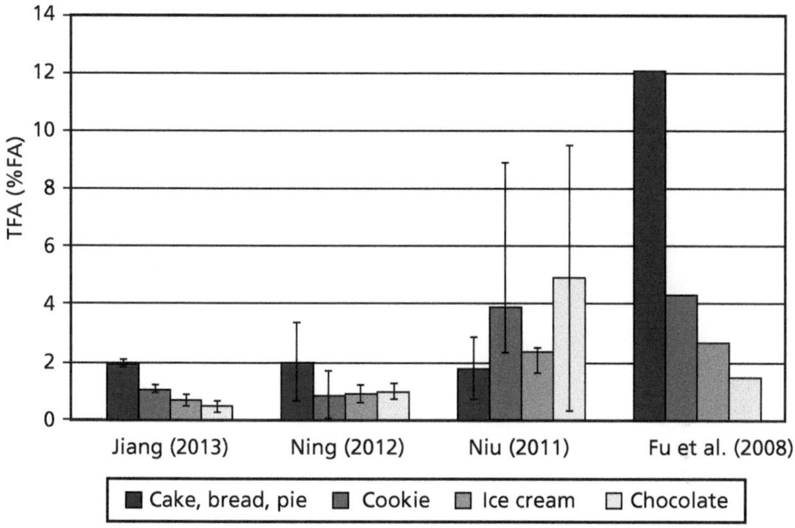

Figure 15.2 Comparison of TFA content in oil-bearing food between 2008 and 2012.

neutralization, bleaching, and deodorization steps. In the refining process, vegetable oils are commonly heated up to 60 °C and 100 °C before deodorization. During the deodorization step, the temperature is increased to 180–270 °C for about two hours, with variation from case to case. According to Tasan and Demirci (2003), the C18:2*trans* content in sunflower oil could increase 13.8-fold after refining steps with normal operation. These values increased even more if the deodorization step was carried out at 230 °C for 2 hours. When the deodorization process was conducted at 265 °C for 1 hour, the C18:2*trans* content was increased by 57.8-fold compared to the crude oil, totaling an increase of 97.4% in TFA production (Tasan and Demirci, 2003). Wolff (1993) studied the deodorization of flaxseed oil in laboratory scale to evaluate the effect of heating time and temperature on isomerization of linoleic and linolenic acids present in vegetable oils. Formation of C18:2*trans* and C18:3*trans* has been shown to strongly depend on these variables, and isomerization starts at around 190 °C. During the deodorization, the critical temperature for isomerization of linoleic acid is above 240 °C, and for α-linolenic acid of canola oils, isomerization occurs between 220 °C and 230 °C. After 4 hours of deodorization at 270 °C, about 80% of the α-linoleic acid was isomerized, while only 13% of the linoleic acid produced TFAs. Figure 15.3 shows the linear relationship between deodorization temperature and TFA content. When the deodorization temperature is increased, TFA content also increases in soybean oil. When the deodorization temperature reaches up to 250 °C, the TFA content also increases from 1.2% to 2.5%.

Table 15.B Food Products Containing High Amounts of TFA (as % of fat)

Category	Food Product	Total Fat	C16:1,9*t*	C18:1,9*t*	C18:1,11*t*	Total TFA Content (%)	TFA/Total Fat (%)
Deep-fried food	Fried bread stick A	39.5	1.27	4.62	2.18	8.08	20.4
	Fried bread stick B	24.8	0.03	0.18	0.06	0.26	1.04
	Fried glutinous rice balls with sesame A	15.3	0.03	0.17	0.05	0.25	1.62
	Fried glutinous rice balls with sesame B	12.5	0.08	0.14	—	0.22	1.76
	Fried fish	21.7	0.05	0.27	0.10	0.12	1.91
Western fast food	Fried chicken A	27.4	0.07	0.39	0.05	0.51	1.85
	Fried chicken B	11.7	0.09	0.15	—	0.24	2.08
	Hamburger	29.9	—	0.25	0.09	0.34	1.13
	Chips	13.4	0.02	0.17	0.04	0.23	1.68
Biscuits	Cookie quality A	29.0	—	0.22	0.07	0.29	1.46
	Cookie quality B	25.8	0.03	0.20	0.072	0.31	1.20
	Cookie quality C	36.7	0.04	0.33	—	0.38	1.02
	Cookie	19.5	0.03	0.20	0.06	0.29	1.46
	Sandwich biscuit A	18.7	0	0.53	1.69	2.22	11.9
	Sandwich biscuit B	18.3	0.21	1.55	0.43	2.19	12.0
	Toughness biscuits A	16.1	—	1.34	0.04	0.23	1.42
	Toughness biscuits B	25.1	—	0.17	0.04	0.21	0.85

Bread	Margarine bread	11.8	—	0.20	0.05	0.25	2.08
	Milk bread A	7.88	—	0.03	—	0.03	0.38
	Milk bread B	29.4	—	0.49	0.02	0.15	0.52
	Shortening bread	9.15	0.095	0.16	0.09	0.35	3.84
Pie/cakes	Chocolate pie	13.3	—	0.29	0.05	0.34	2.57
	Milk pie	21.9	—	0.55	0.09	0.64	2.94
	Birthday cake A	27.1	—	0.43	0.19	0.63	2.31
	Birthday cake B	29.7	—	0.19	0.08	0.27	0.91
	Mousse cake	21.7	—	0.27	0.14	0.41	1.90
	Chocolate cake	18.6	—	0.14	0.02	0.16	0.84
Snacks	Puff	20.1	—	0.26	0.05	0.32	1.57
	Swiss roll	32.1	—	0.09	0.06	0.15	0.47
	Shrimp cracker	12.8	—	0.04	—	0.04	0.29
	Chips A	32.4	—	0.16	0.05	0.21	0.65
	Chips B	14.5	—	0.18	0.10	0.28	1.95
	Chips C	22.5	0.12	0.20	0.09	0.41	1.83
	Shakima A	16.5	—	0.13	0.06	0.19	1.10
	Shakima B	22.1	—	0.11	0.17	0.28	1.27
	French pancakes	7.31	—	0.14	0.08	0.22	3.00

(continued)

Table 15.B *Continued*

Category	Food Product	Total Fat	C16:1,9*t*	C18:1,9*t*	C18:1,11*t*	Total TFA Content (%)	TFA/ Total Fat (%)
Beverage	Coffee mate	13.1	—	—	—	—	—
	Soluble coffee	9.28	0.10	0.08	—	0.18	1.93
	Sesame paste	11.5	—	0.02	0.01	0.03	0.29
	Oatmeal	3.88	—	—	—	—	—
Chocolate	Chocolate A	20.0	—	0.28	0.05	0.33	1.65
	Chocolate B	5.73	—	0.38	0.09	0.47	8.17
Ice cream	Ice cream	6.41	—	0.08	0.07	0.15	2.36
Dairy product	Cream candy	8.38	—	—	—	—	—
	Milk	20.1	—	0.08	0.02	0.10	0.50
Others	Margarine A	62.8	0.23	0.33	0.19	0.75	2.27
	Margarine B	70.9	—	3.26	0.63	3.89	6.39

Source: Niu (2011).

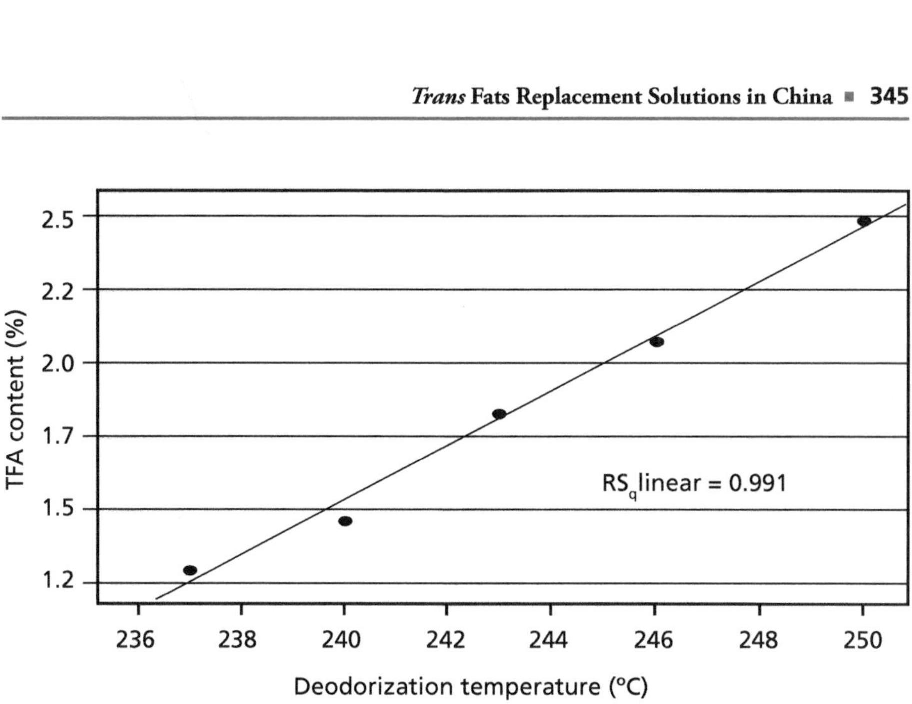

Figure 15.3 The relationship between TFA content and temperature during deodorization of soybean oil.

Hou et al. (2012) analyzed 93 edible oil samples in which 17 samples (18%) showed above 2% TFA content. The number of TFA-positive samples were four (14%) for soybean oil, six (26%) for rapeseed oil, four (18%) for sunflower oil, and three (16%) for maize oil. Earlier studies reported 0.26–0.82 g/100 g in soybean oil and 1.63–3.46 g/100 g in rapeseed oil (Wolff, 1992). Total TFA contents in refined corn, soybean, and rapeseed oils were 1.5%, 4.6%, and 2.4%, respectively (Ferrari et al., 1996). The initial amount of *trans* polyunsaturated fatty acids (PUFAs) (0.1–0.3%) in crude oils may rise up to 5% in refined oils due to higher-temperature deodorization. The formation of TFAs during deodorization may depend on the oil type and the content of PUFAs. For example, deodorization of fish oil above 200 °C under vacuum had the largest amount of *trans* isomer formed (Fournier et al., 2006).

Among 581 collected bottled cooking oils in China, 87.5% contained less than 2% TFA. The range of TFA content in other oils such as soybean, rapeseed, sunflower, blended, maize, and seasoning oils was 1.2–1.9% (Jiang et al., 2013). However, non-refined oils (groundnut, sesame seed, olive, and safflower oil) contained less than 1% TFA (Jiang et al., 2013). Figure 15.4 shows that the contents of C18:1,9*trans,* add total C18:3 *trans,* and total TFA in corn oil were higher than soybean oil, rapeseed oil, and sunflower oil. However, the total content of C18:2*trans* in rapeseed oil and sunflower oil was higher than in soybean oil and corn oil.

The percentages of C18:1*trans* in all samples (soybean oil, rapeseed oil, sunflower oil, and corn oil) were lower than other *trans* isomers (18:2*trans;* 18:3*trans* isomers)

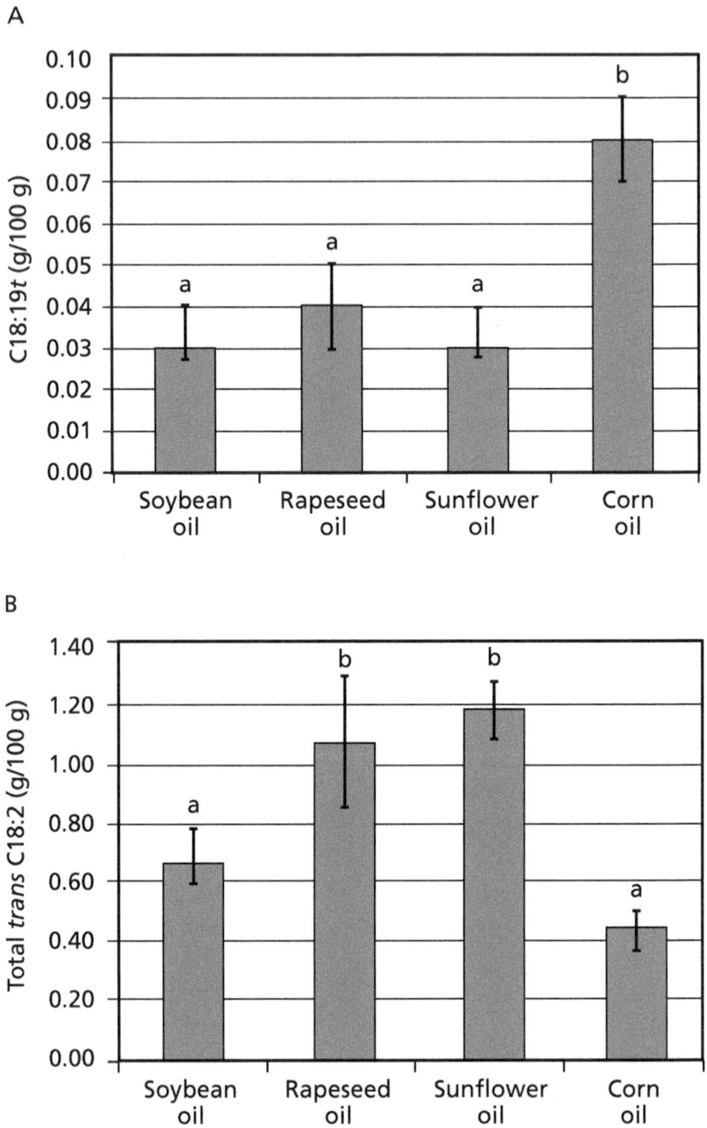

Figure 15.4 The contents of the C18:1,9*trans* acid (A), total *trans* C18:2 acid (B), total *trans* C18:3 acid (C), and total *trans* acids (D) in soybean oil, rapeseed oil, sunflower oil, and corn oil. Means within a column with different letter (a, b) are significantly different ($p < 0.05$).

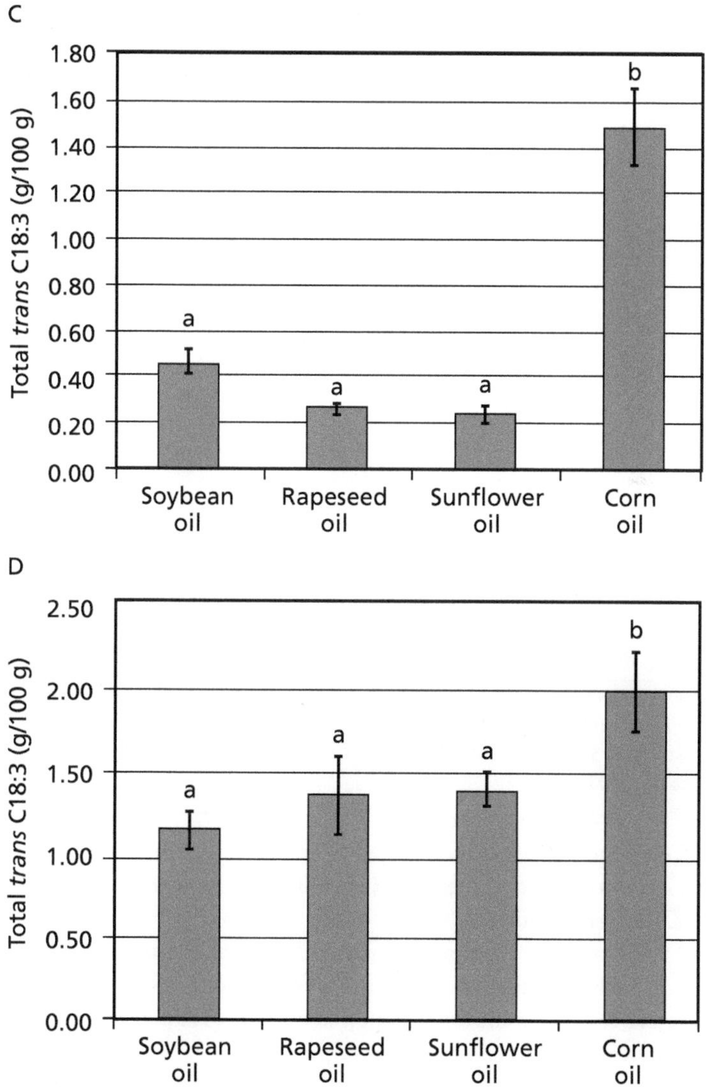

Figure 15.4 *Continued*

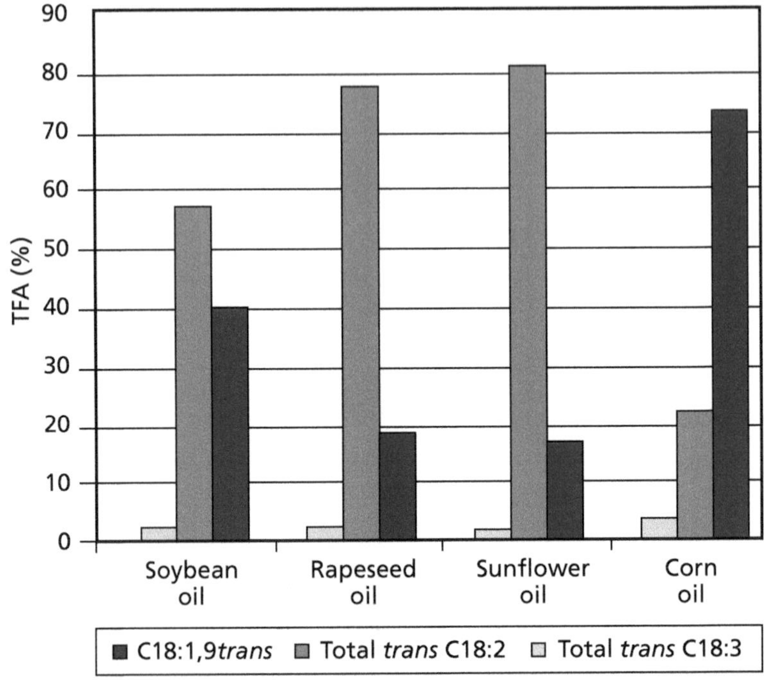

Figure 15.5 The percentage of C18:1,9*trans, trans* C18:2, *trans* C18:3 of the total *trans* fatty acids in soybean oil, rapeseed oil, sunflower oil, and corn oil. Data from Hou et al. (2012).

(Figure 15.5 on page 348). Corn oil showed the highest C18:3*trans* isomer (74.13%) compared to other oils, and soybean oil (57.39%) and rapeseed oil (78.10%) showed the highest C18:2*trans* isomers.

Figure 15.6 shows the comparative study of TFA contents in edible oils in China. Some of the oils had an increase in the TFA content in 2012 compared to that in 2010, whereas other oils showed the opposite. The TFA content in sesame oil was significantly increased in 2012 compared to previously.

Technical Trends in Industry

China began to import palm oil in the 1970s. The amount increased steadily each year and finally reached more than 1 million tons in 1990, reflecting the dramatic expansion of palm oil use in China (Jiang et al., 2010). It is widely used in Chinese food industries, particularly in manufacture of instant noodles, snack foods, milk powder, margarines, shortenings, and so forth. Although palm olein is widely used through-

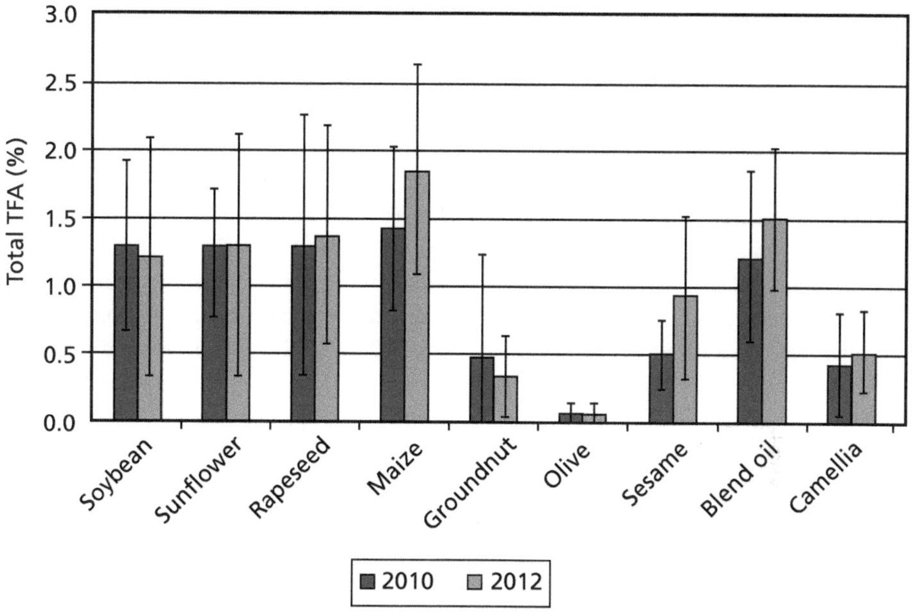

Figure 15.6 Comparative study of TFA content in 2010 and 2012 in edible oils in China.

out the tropics as a cooking oil in household kitchens, its high melting point makes it unsuitable for this purpose in temperate northern regions of China. However, this problem can be solved by blending or interesterification of appropriate proportions of palm olein with other locally available vegetable oils.

Interesterification is also widely used to produce *trans*-free fat (Adhikari et al., 2010, 2012; Fauzi et al., 2013; Reshma et al., 2008) because it improves the melting profile of fats and oils with no TFA formation. Interesterification can be carried out in two ways, enzymatic and chemical. Enzymatic interesterification (EIE) can be carried out using either specific or nonspecific lipases. 1,3-Specific lipases rearrange the fatty acids on the *sn*-1,3 positions, and nonspecific lipases rearrange the fatty acids at all positions. Chemical interesterification (CIE) randomizes all the fatty acids on the triacylglycerol (TAG) backbone. With the strict regulation on imported animal fats, more and more industries are focusing on the use of palm oil or interesterified palm oil mixed with other vegetable oils.

Mayamol et al. (2004) produced a PUFA-rich zero-*trans* shortening using a weight ratio of 50:50 palm stearin:rice bran oil. Similarly, Jennings et al. (2010) produced *trans*-free shortening with palm stearin and rice bran oil structured lipids. They found the properties (i.e., solid fat content, melting and crystallization profile, and crystal forms) to be comparable with existing commercial products. Ming et al. (1999) conducted the enzymatic transesterification of palm stearin and sunflower oils to prepare table margarines. Blends of palm stearin and sunflower oil at 40:60 and 50:50 were found to be suitable for use in table margarine.

Idris et al. (1996) investigated Malaysian *trans*-free tub margarines containing 74% palm oil, 12% palm kernel oil, and 14% soybean oil. Lida and Rahim (1998) analyzed a number of commercial reduced-fat (40–60%) spreads. They found 6.5–11.7% TFA content in tub products and 13.9–20.4% in block products. They investigated blends of sunflower oil with either palm oil or palm kernel olein before and after interesterification. For the ice cream made from vegetable oils, either palm oil or the blend of palm oil with palm kernel oil (60:40 or 80:20) has been used in large-scale manufacture. To prevent oiling off in peanut butter, a hydrogenated vegetable oil is usually added to give sufficient structure to the fatty phase to hold the oil.

Blends of palm stearin with palm kernel oil or palm kernel olein are suitable for confectionary fats after interesterification. Table 15.C lists selected interesterified blends using hard stearins. Recently, an interesterified blend similar to those in Table 15.C has been reported. For the formulation of margarines and spreads, the preparation of an interesterified hardstock is blended with liquid oil to obtain margarine. A number of such hardstocks are shown in Table 15.D.

Remarks and Outlook

Consumption of *trans* fats has adverse effects on health. This is now common sense among the public in China after two years of discussion, particularly in the public me-

Table 15.C Interesterified Blends for Confectionary Fats

	Blend A	Blend B	Blend C
Palm stearin IV[a] 10	25	30	—
Palm stearin IV 8	—	—	25
Palm kernel olein	75	70	37.5
Palm kernel oil	—	—	37.5
MP (°C)	32	34.5	35.9
D20	970	1110	710
D25	275	405	345
D30	20	105	130
D35	15	15	10

[a]IV: Iodine value; MP: melting point; solid contents are based on dilatometry.

Source: Berger and Idris (2005).

Table 15.D Blend Compositions Used by Several Researchers to Make Interesterified Hard Stocks

	A[a]	B[b]	C[c]	D[d]	E[e]	F[f]	G[g]
Palm stearin (soft)	60	—	—	—	60	40	—
Palm stearin (MP 50 °C)	—	—	70	—	—	—	—
Palm stearin (MP 54.4 °C)	—	—	—	—	—	—	50
Palm oil	—	—	—	75	—	—	—
Palm olein	—	75	—	—	—	—	—
Palm kernel oil	—	25	—	—	—	—	50
Fully hydrogenated soybean oil	—	—	—	25	—	—	—
Liquid oil	20	—	30	—	—	—	—
Palm kernel olein	20	—	—	—	40	60	—
Sources	Teah and Ibrahim (1991)	Elias et al. (1996)	Teah et al. (1992)	Zeitoun et al. (1993)	de Man (2000)	de Man (1995)	Ming et al. (1998)

[a]Product A was required to produce the properties of a commercial Japanese soft margarine. Fifty-five parts of the interesterified blend were blended with 45 parts of soybean oil to produce soft tub margarines. Slip MP 34 °C; SFC at 10 °C, 16.0%; 15 °C, 14.0%; 20 °C, 11.0%; 30 °C, 5.9%.

[b]Product B is produced for Russia bulk margarine based on hydrogenated sunflower oil with a trans fatty acid content of 14.1%. Four parts of hardstock were blended with one part of soybean oil.

[c]Three parts hardstock were blended with two parts rapeseed oil for a soft tub margarine with the following solid characteristics: MP 34.4 °C; SFC at 10 °C, 22.3%; 15 °C, 15%; 20 °C, 9.3%; 25 °C, 7.3%; 30 °C, 4.6%.

[d]Product D is described as having good melting and crystallization behaviors and is suitable for blending with liquid oil for margarines and spreads.

[e]Product E is to be diluted with liquid oil.

[f]This interesterified blend is suitable for a soft margarine. MP is 31.7 °C, stable in the β′ form.

[g]Interesterification is carried out using a lipase. The product was stable in the β′ form with SFC at 15 °C, 52%; 20 °C, 39% 25 °C, 27%; 30 °C, 15%. A number of patents have described interesterified hard stocks having as one component palm sterin or fully hydrogenated palm oil and the other component palm kernel stearin or fully hydrogenated palm kernel oil. Selected U.S. patent numbers are 6,117,475; 6,156,370; 6,808,737; and 5,667,837.

dia. As a result, the governments push the regulatory discussion and implementations forward. The TFA contents in foods before this discussion and after this discussion show significantly different levels. The level of TFA content in foods now is very low (2% based on fat) with only a few exceptions, such as fats in formulated milk drinks, certain confectionary products, and so forth. TFAs are mainly produced from partial hydrogenation. Thus, the amount of partially hydrogenated fats in the oils and fats industry has been reduced significantly because the need from the food industry has been quickly reduced. For this reason, the use of palm-based fat materials has replaced partially hydrogenated fats in most shortening and margarine recipes. This replacement occurred during the 2011–2013 period in the oils and fats industry.

The change has left a gap for the oils and fats industry to find solutions for the food industry because replacement brings technical challenges. From public and regulatory aspects, the term *hydrogenation* has been blackened. The use of full hydrogenation to produce needed hard fats is also limited because the term of *hydrogenation* has to be labeled. The challenges raised by the change will stay for some years more before we have all the necessary solutions for the food industry.

References

Adhikari, P.; Shin J.-A.; Lee J.-H.; Hu J.-N.; Hwang K.-T.; Lee K.-T. Enzymatic Production of Trans Free Hard Fat Stock from Fractionated Rice Bran Oil, Fully Hydrogenated Soybean Oil and Conjugated Linoleic Acid. *J. Food Sci.* **2009,** *74,* 87–96.

Adhikari, P.; Yu, F.; Lee J.-H.; Park, H.-K.; Kim, J. W.; Lee, E. J.; Lee, K. T. Comparative Study of *Trans* Fatty Acid Content in 2005 and 2008 Processed Food from Korean Market. *Food Sci. Biotechnol.* **2010a,** *19,* 335–341.

Adhikari, P.; Zhu, X.-M.; Gautam, A.; Shin, J.-A.; Hu, J.-N.; Lee, J.-H.; Akoh, C.C.; Lee K.-T. Scaled-up Production of Zero *Trans* Margarine Fat Using Pine Nut Oil and Palm Stearin. *Food Chem.* **2010b,** *119,* 1332–1338.

Adhikari, P.; Shin, J.-A.; Lee, J.-H.; Kim, H.-R.; Kim, I.-H.; Hong, S.-T.; Lee, K.-T. Crystallization, Physicochemical Properties and Oxidative Stability of the Interesterified Hard Fat from Rice Bran Oil, Fully Hydrogenated Soybean Oil and Coconut Oil through Lipase-catalyzed Reaction. *Food Bioprocess Technol.* **2011.** DOI: 10.1007/s11947-011-0544-4.

Adhikari, P.; Peng, H.; Yafei, Z. Oxidative Stability of Enzymatically Interesterified Fat Containing Conjugated Linoleic Acid. *J. Am. Oil Chem. Soc.* **2012.** DOI:10.1007/s11746-012-2096-9.

Aro, A.; Antoine, J. M.; Pizzoferrato, L.; Reykdal, O.; Poppel, G. V. Trans Fatty Acids in Dairy and Meat Products from 14 European Countries: The *Trans* Fair Study. *J. Food Compos. Anal.* **1998,** *11,* 150–160.

Bell, A. C.; Ge, K.; Popkin, B. M. Weight Gain and its Predictors in Chinese Adults. *Int. J. Obes.* **2001,** *25,* 1079–1086.

Berger, K. G.; Idris, N. A. Formulation of Zero-*trans* Acid Shortenings and Margarines and Other Food Fats with Products of the Oil Palm. *J. Am. Oil Chem. Soc.* **2005,** *82,* 775–782.

China National Centre for Food Safety Risk Assessment. *Risk Assessment of Dietary Trans Fatty Acids Intake in Chinese Population;* China National Centre for Food Safety Risk Assessment: Beijing, 2012.

Chinese Markets for Baked Food (CMBF), 2006. http://data.chinabyte.com/21/2702521.shtml (accessed Nov 30, 2007).

de Man, J. M. *Use of Palm Stearin as a Component of Interesterified Blends.* Meeting of the Society of Chemical Industry, London, Nov 2000.

de Man, J. M.; de Man, L. Formulations for No-*trans* and Low-*trans* Margarines and Shortenings. *Proceedings of 21st World Congress of International Society for Fat Research* **1995,** *3,* 561–563.

Elias, B. A.; Yusoff, M. S. A.; Rasid, M. J. PORIM's Experiments on Low-*trans* Margarine. *Palm Oil Tech. Bull.* **1996,** *6,* 3.

Fauzi, S. H. M.; Rashid, N. A.; Omar, Z. Effect on Chemical Interesterification on the Physicochemical Properties, Micro Structure and Thermal Properties of Palm, Palm Stearin, Palm Kernel Oil and Soybean Oil Blends. *Food Chem.* **2013,** *137,* 8–17.

Ferrari, R. A. P; Schulte, E.; Esteves, W.; Bruhl, L.; Mukherjee, K. D. Minor Constituents of Vegetable Oils during Industrial Processing. *J. Am. Oil Chem. Soc.* **1996,** *73,* 587–592.

Fournier, V.; Juanéda, P.; Destaillats, F.; Dionisi, F.; Lambelet, P.; Sébédio, L. L.; Berdeaux, O. Analysis of Eicosapentaenoic and Docosahexaenoic Acid Geometrical Isomers Formed during Fish-oil Deodorisation. *J. Chromatogr. A* **2006,** *1129,* 21–28.

Fu, H.; Yang, L.; Yuan, H.; Tao, P.; Lo, Y. M. Assessment of *Trans* Fatty Acids Content in Popular Western-style Products in China. *J. Food. Sci.* **2008,** *73,* 383–391.

Hou, J. C.; Wang, F.; Wang, Y. T.; Xu, J.; Zhang, C. W. Assessment of *Trans* Fatty Acids in Edible Oils in China. *Food Cont.* **2012,** *25,* 211–215.

Hunter, J. E. Alternatives to *Trans* Fatty Acids in Foods. *Inform* **2004,** *15,* 510–512.

Idris, N. A.; de Man, L.; Tang, T. S.; Chong, C. L. Chemical Composition and Physical Properties of Soft (Tub) Margarines Sold in Malaysia. *J. Am. Oil Chem. Soc.* **1996,** *73,* 995–1001.

Jennings, B. H.; Akoh, C. C. *Trans*-free Plastic Shortenings Prepared with Palm Stearin and Rice Bran Oil Structured Lipid. *J. Am. Oil Chem. Soc.* **2010,** *87,* 411–417.

Jiang, Y. R.; Xia, S. H.; Zhang, Y. Q.; Yu, J. G.; Yang, H. Present Situation and Production Process Control of *Trans* Fatty Acid in Edible Oil. *J. Chinese Inst. Food Sci. Technol.* **2010,** *4,* 53–58.

Jiang, Y. R.; Xia, S. H.; Zhang, Y. Q.; Yu, J. G.; Hu, P. *Trans* Fatty Acid Content of Foods in China. *J. Chin. Cereals and Oils Assoc.* **2013,** *5,* 112–115.

Larqué, E.; Pérez-Llamas, F.; Zamora, S.; Gil, A. Biochemical and Physiological Effects of Dietary *Trans* Fatty Acids. In; *Trends in Dietary Fats Research;* Nova Science Publishing: New York, Landow, M. V., Ed., 2005; p 51.

Li, D.; Adhikari, P.; Shin, J.-A.; Lee, J.-H.; Kim, Y.-J.; Zhu, X.-M.; Hu, J.-N.; Jin, J.; Akoh, C. C.; Lee, K.-T. Lipase-catalyzed Interesterification of High Oleic Sunflower Oil and Fully Hydrogenated Soybean Oil Comparison of Batch and Continuous Reactor for Production of Zero *Trans* Shortenings Fats. *Food Sci. Technol.* **2010,** *43,* 458–464.

Lida, H. M. D. N.; Rahim, M. A. Physicochemical Characteristics of Palm-based Oil Blends for the Production of Reduced Fat Spreads. *J. Am. Oil Chem. Soc.* **1998,** *75,* 1625–1631.

Mayamol, P. N.; Samuel, T.; Balachandran, C.; Sundaresan, A.; Arumughan, C. Zero *Trans* Shortening Using Palm Stearin and Rice Bran Oil. *J. Am. Oil Chem. Soc.* **2004,** *81,* 407–413.

Ming, L. O.; Ghazali, H. M.; Chiew, L. C. Physical Properties of *Pseudomonas* and *Rhizomucor miehei* Lipase-Catalyzed Transesterified Blends of Palm Stearin:Palm Kernel Olein. *J. Am. Oil Chem. Soc.* **1998,** *75,* 953–959.

Ming, L. O.; Ghazali, H. M.; Chiew, L. C. Use of Enzymatic Transesterified Palm Stearin-Sunflower Oil Blends in the Preparation of Table Margarine Formulation. *Food Chem.* **1999,** *64* (6), 83–88.

Ministry of Health of People's Republic of China. *China Health Statistical;* People's Medical Publishing House: Beijing, 2012.

Ministry of Health of People's Republic of China. *National Food Safety Standard for Nutrition Labeling of Prepackaged Foods;* GB 28050-2011; Ministry of Health of People's Republic of China: Beijing, 2011.

Mozaffarian, D.; Katan, M. B.; Ascherio, A.; Stampfer, M. J.; Willet, W. C. *Trans* Fatty Acids and Cardiovascular Disease. *New Engl. J. Med.* **2006,** *354,* 1601–1613.

Ning, W., Li, Y.; Wang, Y.; Han, W.; Zhang, G.; Yang, C.; Sui, H. The Content of *Trans* Fatty Acids in Instant Food in Yantai, *China. J. Food Hyg.* **2012,** *24,* 74–76.

Niu, C. Determination of *Trans* Fatty Acids in Foods and Assessment of Dietary Intake of Adolescents. MD Thesis, Agricultural University of Hebei, China, 2011.

Reshma, M. V.; Saritha, S. S.; Balachandran, C.; Arumughan, C. Lipase-catalyzed Interesterification of Palm Stearin and Rice Bran Oil Blends for Preparation of Zero *Trans* Shortening with Bioactive Phytochemicals. *Bioresource Technol.* **2008,** *99,* 5011–5019.

Tarrago-Trani, M. T.; Phillips, K. M.; Lemar, L. E.; Holden, J. M. New and Existing Oils and Fats Used in Products with Reduced *Trans*-Fatty Acid Content. *J. Am. Diet Assoc.* **2006,** *106,* 867–880.

Tasan, M.; Demirci, M. *Trans* FA in Sunflower Oil at Different Steps of Refining. *J. Am. Oil Chem. Soc.* **2003,** *80,* 825–828.

Teah, Y. K.; Ibrahim, A. Hydrogenation Is Often Unnecessary with Palm Oil. *Palm Oil Devel.* **1991,** *15,* 9–14.

Teah, Y. K.; Sudin, N.; Kifli, H. Interesterification. A Useful Means of Processing Palm Oil Products for Use in Table Margarine. *Palm Oil Devel.* **1992,** *16,* 6–10.

Wolff, R. L. *Trans*-polyunsaturated Fatty Acids in French Edible Rapeseed and Soybean Oils. *J. Oil Chem. Soc.* **1992,** *69,* 106–110.

Wolff, R. L. Further Studies on Artificial Geometrical Isomers of Alpha-linolenic Acid in Edible Acid-containing Oils. *J. Am. Oil Chem. Soc.* **1993,** *70,* 219–224.

Zeitoun, M. A. M.; Neff, W. E.; List, G. R.; Mounts, T. L. Physical Properties of Interesterified Fat Blends, *J. Am. Oil Chem. Soc.* **1993,** *70,* 467–471.

Zhang, H.; Smith, P.; Adler-Nissen, J. Effects of Degree of Enzymatic Interesterification on the Physical Properties of Margarine Fats: Solid Fat Content, Crystallization Behavior, Crystal Morphology and Crystal Network. *J. Agric. Food Chem.* **2004,** *52,* 4423–4431.

16

Trans Fats Replacement Solutions in Japan

Toshiharu Arishima ▪ *General Manager, Oils and Fats, Processed Foods R&D Center, Fuji Oil Co., Ltd., Tsukubamirai, Japan*

Haruyasu Kida ▪ *Director and General Manager, Food Science Research Institute, Fuji Oil Co., Ltd., Tsukubamirai, Japan*

Introduction

After the development of the hydrogenation process as a processing method to enhance the use of liquid oils, the hydrogenated fats containing *trans* fatty acid (TFA) became part of a variety of different foods. The hydrogenated fats are solidified as a fine crystalline material, stable in the beta-prime form, and show better oxidative stability. The hydrogenation technique was an excellent process for the efficient use of natural liquid oils, and its use spread rapidly among food manufacturers. However, nutritional studies reported that continuous TFA intake of more than 2% of total energy increases the risk of cardiovascular disease (Mozaffarian, 2006). Most of the studies showing a harmful influence on human health were based on the analytical results from Western countries, where the consumption of TFA was higher. Although the effect of TFA on Japanese people (who have a smaller intake of TFA) was not clear, a movement to reduce TFA intake also started in Japan around 2003.

In this chapter, we cover the recent developments on TFA in Japan, especially intake amount, TFA content in various foods, TFA labeling, analytical methods, and various ways to reduce TFA.

Ingested Amount of TFA in Japan

TFA Content of Commercial Products

The Food Safety Commission (FSC) of Japan conducted the comparative investigation on TFA in commercial margarine and spread products between 2006 and 2010. According to the FSC's report (FSC, 2012), the TFA content of the same brand of margarine was decreased from 5.28 g/100 g of product in 2006 to 3.13 g/100 g of product in 2010. The TFA content of the specific brand of shortening was also reduced from 2.48 g/100 g of product in 2006 to 2.01 g/100 g of product in 2010. The average TFA contents of margarine and shortening for food industry use were reduced by one-tenth and resulted in less than 1 g/100 g of product in most products. Although there are a few products showing high TFA content, it is encouraging that Japanese food manufacturers are making solid progress in the reduction of TFA. Saturated fatty acid content of retail margarine products showed no significant increase;

however, the margarine products for food industry use showed 1.4 times higher saturated fatty acid levels, from 29.9 g/100 g of product in 2006 to 40.9 g/100 g of product in 2010. It is suggested that food manufacturers are paying attention to the reduction of both TFA and saturated fatty acids in retail products.

TFA Intake in Japan

Table 16.A summarizes several research studies that estimated the amount TFA intake in Japan either based on TFA production or accumulation. Estimation of the intake amount of TFA in Japan was conducted by the FSC in 2006; by the Ministry of Agriculture, Forestry and Fisheries (MAFF) in 2005 to 2007 and by the Ministry of Health, Labor and Welfare (MHLW) in 2009. Other than these government investigations, there were a few other studies on the TFA intake that are summarized in Table 16.A. They showed same tendencies in TFA intake and as energy percent. In conclusion, the daily energy percentage intake of TFA in the Japanese population was always lower than 1%, which is less than the World Health Organization (WHO) recommendation for *trans* fat intake.

MAFF summarized average intake of each food group and the average TFA content and calculated TFA intake obtained from a total diet study. This is shown in Table 16.B. In the Japanese diet, most TFA came from the fats and oils group, which accounts for 20% of the total, followed by the confectionery group (18%), and the seasoning and spice group (15%).

Table 16.A Estimated Amount of TFA Intake in Japanese Population

Investigated Year	Published Year	Estimated Method	Energy % (g/day)
1998	Okamoto (1999)	Production unit basis	0.7 (1.56)
1999	Zhou (2003)	Accumulation	Male 0.3, Female 0.5
2003	Yamada (2010)	Accumulation	0.75 (1.7)
2006	FSC (2006)	Accumulation	0.3 (0.7)
		Production unit basis	0.6 (1.3)
2005–2007	MAFF (2007)	Production unit basis	0.44–0.47 (0.918–0.962)
2007	MHLW (2007)	Accumulation	0.24 (0.5)

Table 16.B Estimation of TFA Intake from Each Food Group (MAFF, 2012)

Food Group	Average Intake of Food Group (g/day)	Average TFA Content in Food Group (g/100g)	Average TFA Intake from Food Group (g/day)	Intake Ratio of TFA (%)
Grain foods	449.5	0.024–0.025	0.111–0.114	12
Beans	61.5	0.020–0.026	0.0121–0.0159	1
Nuts and seeds	2.1	0.092–0.118	0.0019–0.0025	0
Fish and seafood	82.6	0.064–0.068	0.0532–0.0536	6
Meat	77.9	0.136–0.145	0.106–0.113	12
Egg	34.4	0.028–0.047	0.0095–0.0162	1
Milk	135.4	0.097–0.099	0.131–0.134	14
Fats and oils	10.5	1.770–1.86	0.185–0.195	20
Confectionery	25.6	0.654–0.670	0.167–0.171	18
Seasoning and spice	92.0	0.153–0.155	0.140–0.143	15
Total	971.5	3.038–3.214	0.918–0.962	100

Table 16.C shows energy percent of TFA intake by age bracket and gender line of Japanese as summarized by the FSC. The energy percentage of TFA is higher in the younger generations among both males and females. It was also generally higher in women in the same age brackets.

Specific Ingestion of Linoleic Acid in Japanese

It is necessary to understand that the effects of TFA on serum cholesterol levels is reduced by concurrent ingestion of linoleic acid (Sugano, 2011). In this study on the effect to the serum cholesterol level of a concurrent ingestion ratio of TFA and linoleic acid, it was clearly shown that the serum cholesterol level is reduced with the increased

Table 16.C Energy Percentage of TFA Intake by Age Bracket and Gender Line of Japanese

Age	1–6	7–14	15–19	20–29	30–39	40–49	50–59	60–69	70<	Average
Male	1.02	0.79	0.79	0.74	0.66	0.64	0.58	0.59	0.60	0.70
Female	0.99	0.83	0.82	0.85	0.79	0.76	0.71	0.64	0.62	0.75

Source: FSC (2012).

ingestion of linoleic acid. In the Japanese population, ingestion of linoleic acid is seven times higher than that of TFA, and the ratio of TFA:linoleic acid is 0.14 (Figure 16.1). Serum cholesterol levels of the Japanese are lowered by low TFA intake as described previously, and high ingestion of linoleic acid as compared with other countries.

Production Volume of Hydrogenated Oils

Figure 16.2 shows production volumes of hydrogenated oils, interesterified oils, and fractionated oils in Japan (JMSLIA, 2007, 2011). With regard to TFA reduction, the production volume of hydrogenated oils in 2010 was 31% less than that in 2006. In contrast, interesterified and fractionated oils were increased by 91% and 64% in 2010, respectively. This indicates that interesterified and fractionated oils became alternatives to replace hydrogenated oil.

Response to the TFA Issue in Japan

Risk Management Agencies

Recent investigations on the Japanese TFA intake by MAFF, MHLW, and FSC showed no significant risks because average intake amounts were less than 1% of

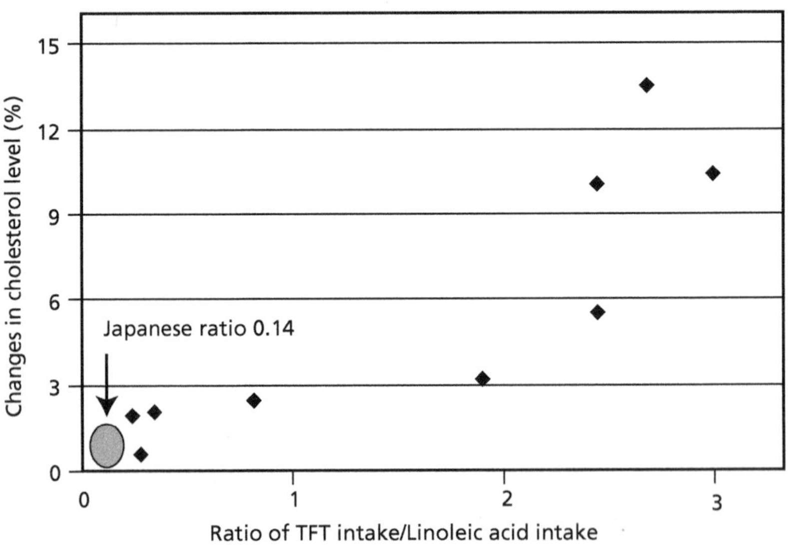

Figure 16.1 Effect on the cholesterol level with the ratio of intake TFA:linoleic acid

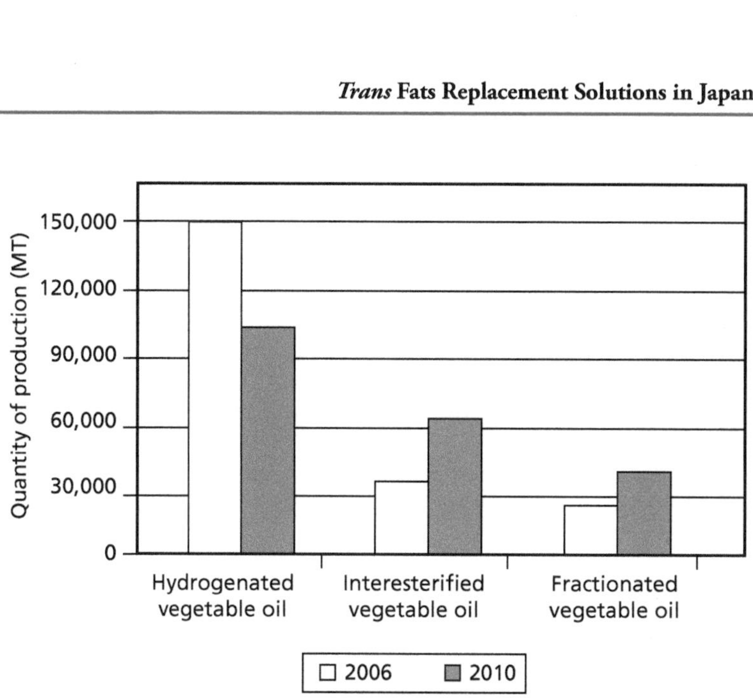

Figure 16.2 Quantities of production of each processed oil in Japan.

energy, which is the targeted value proposed by WHO. These agencies for risk management concluded the risk of TFA to most Japanese is quite low. However, FSC is also expostulating in their fact sheet that people keep a well-balanced ingestion of each nutrient, paying attention to the excess intake of high-fat foods. The health risk of TFA at the current ingestion levels is not a serious situation compared with other harmful chemical substances and food-borne pathogens, and there is no need to take action for managing TFA risk at the present time.

Implementation of Labeling Systems

In the wake of the adoption of labeling systems in foreign countries, the Consumer Affairs Agency (CAA) created tentative guidelines on TFA labeling in 2011 (Figure 16.3.) (CAA, 2011) and promoted the independent disclosure of TFA information by food manufacturers. The institutionalization of this TFA labeling was ultimately shelved due to the low risk of TFA in the Japanese and the increase of the cost for new labeling after hearing public comments.

Retail Distributors

Major retail distributors are making an effort to reduce TFA by switching existing ingredients to the low-TFA oils for frying, cream, and margarine products. They have

Presentation

- *Trans* fatty acid information is expected to be presented on labeling of prepackaged foods offered for sale, at the company's website, and in advertising materials.
- When declaring *trans* fatty acids, basic requirements (i.e., energy, protein, total fat, and carbohydrate) as set out in the Nutrition Labeling Standards as well as saturated fatty acids and cholesterol must be declared.
- Name: *Trans* fatty acids should be listed as "*Trans* fatty acids" within the nutrition labeling table with other nutrients.

Unit

- *Trans* fatty acids should be declared in grams per 100 g/100 ml or per serving, per package, or per reference amount of the food
- Tolerance: Acceptable criterion is plus 20% of the declared value.

  Note: As a general rule, declaring 0 g is only allowed for a food product containing no *trans* fatty acids; however, when the food contains less than 0.3 g/100 g (100 ml for soft drinks), the value can be rounded to 0g.

Nutrient content claim

- Free claim (e.g., free, zero, no, without)
  1. The food contains less than 0.2 g of *trans* fatty acids per 100 g (100 ml for soft drinks) and
  2. The food contains less than 1.5 g of saturated fatty acids (0.75 g per 100 ml for soft drinks) or the food provides less than 10% of energy from saturated fatty acids.
- Reduction claim (e.g., reduced, low, less)

  Declare the name of the reference food as well as the amount or percentage of the reduction.

Methods of analysis

- *Trans* fatty acids should be analyzed using AOCS Ce1h-05 or AOAC 996.06, the major internationally recommended methods of analysis.
- Firms may choose other method equivalent to AOCS and AOAC methods.

Figure 16.3 Summary of guidelines for *trans* fat labeling proposed by Consumer Affairs Agency (2010).

been collaborating with suppliers since 2005. They are considering totally eliminating TFA in their private brand products, but there is much work that would need to be done to achieve this, such as taste change and cost increase. They believe it will be a worthy undertaking due to its long-term significance.

Analytical Method of TFA

Analytical methods of TFA adopted in other countries for labeling regulations were AOAC 996.06 and AOCS Ce 1h-05. Initially, CAA also supported these two methods in the tentative guidelines on TFA labeling; however, AOCS Ce 1j-07 and JOCS-tentative-17 were also recognized as equivalent methods after considering public comment. Maruyama evaluated these four methods using canola, shortening, and butter oil (Table 16.D) and concluded that there was no difference between these methods for the labeling of TFA (Maruyama, 2012). JOCS-tentative-17 is the general method used in Japan and this method has a shorter TFA measurement time.

Reduction Measures of TFA

Technologies for Low TFA

TFAs have various functions and a wide variety of foods were produced by employing these functions. These functions are high oxidation stability, fine crystalline property, high solidification rate, sharp melting behavior, and so forth. Furthermore, as a secondary function, fats and oils containing TFA also give a unique flavor called "hydrogenated smell" to fried food during the frying process. Although it is hard to impart these functions without using TFA, the physical properties can be achieve by replacing TFA with saturated fatty acid by interesterification between fully hydrogenated and nonhydrogenated vegetable oils, fractionation of crystal fraction from

Table 16.D Comparison of Analytical Precision on the TFA Analysis

		AOAC 996.06	AOCS 1h-05	AOCS 1j-07	JOCS T-17-2007
Canola oil	× g/100 g)	0.73	0.74	0.78	0.78
	RSD	2.50	1.60	2.40	2.5
Shortening	× g/100 g)	2.49	2.66	2.73	2.68
	RSD (%)	0.62	0.61	0.71	0.33
Butter oil	× g/100 g)	3.08	3.34	3.45	3.44
	RSD (%)	0.53	0.63	1.00	1.00

Source: Maruyama (2012).

natural semisolid fats, interesterification of semisolid fats, utilization of high melting point emulsifiers and wax, and so on (Sato, 2009; Shiramasa, 2012). Palm oil is becoming widely used as a semisolid fat and has taken over for soybean oils in production volume. In Japan, the overall supplies of soybean oil and palm oil in 2007 were approximately 580,000 t and 530,000 t, respectively. However, in 2011, the overall supply of soybean oil was decreased to 400,000 t, whereas palm oil was increased to 590,000 t (MAFF, 2007, 2011; MFJ, 2007, 2011). The consumption volume was reversed. Besides, flavoring techniques can also be applied to enhance the taste. In lowering the TFA, it is occasionally necessary to combine these techniques to meet the desired outcome.

Low *Trans* Oils and Fats for Margarine and Shortening

The functions required in oils and fats for margarine and shortening are rapid crystallization forming fine crystalline material with high plasticity, high retention capability of liquid oils, and low weakening of hardness against the sheer stress. Generally, the oils and fats used in margarine consist of high melting point hydrogenated oil, mid melting point hydrogenated oil, and liquid oil. To reduce TFA, the high and mid melting point hydrogenated oils can be replaced by interesterified and fractionated oils with which liquid oils are combined. In interesterification, palm and palm kernel oils, or their fully hydrogenated and fractionated oils, and fully hydrogenated soybean and rapeseed oils were used as feedstock. Because interesterified oils have generally low solidification rates, the accelerating technique for solidification is the future challenge. In Japan, extensibility of sheet margarine used in Danishes, spreadability of table margarine, and creaminess in confectionary margarine were already obtained by using low-TFA products.

Low-*Trans* Cocoa Butter Replacer

The chocolate fats containing TFA are in the category called cocoa butter replacers (CBRs). Conventionally, the CBR is produced by hydrogenation or a combination of hydrogenation and fractionation of soybean and palm oils. The TFA content in CBR is normally 30–50%. The functions that are required in CBR are high solidification rate, blooming resistance, high temperature resistance, and sharp melting behavior. In Japan, because cacao mass is always blended in chocolate, even that in which CBR was used, the miscibility of CBR with cocoa butter is also an important function. In producing low-*trans* CBR, interesterification, fractionation, and crystal adjustment technology are also employed. Low-*trans* CBRs generally consist of the combination of symmetric and asymmetric TAGs. When the fractionation process is involved, the efficient use of byproducts needs to be considered in order to cut costs. In addition, there is technology that allows the tempering fats, such as cocoa butter, to be used as nontempering fats by adding seeding agents in the tempering fats.

Future Prospects

In terms of fats intake, it is not just merely overconsumption of TFA alone that contributes to the problem. In the Dietary Reference Intakes of Japanese by MHLW (2009), the desired intake amount of various fats such as total fats, saturated fatty acids, n-6 fatty acids, n-3 fatty acids, and cholesterol are determined. According to the National Nutrition Survey 2008 by MHLW, 20% of adult males and 30% of adult females had energy intake ratios from fats that exceeded the desired amount determined by Dietary Reference Intakes. Recently, the excess ingestion of fats has become a problem, and a well-balanced diet is desirable.

In addition to the survey regarding intake amounts of TFAs, MAFF has also been estimating the intake of saturated fatty acids of Japanese by provisionally checking the concentration of saturated fatty acids in food groups. The average daily intake amount of saturated fatty acids for adult Japanese is estimated at 16.6 g. It is 8.2% of the average in total energy intake (1911 kcal) of adult Japanese and is above the upper limit (7.0% of total energy intake) of the desired amount determined by the Dietary Reference Intakes of Japanese in 2010. This needs to be addressed in the future. In addition to the focus of TFA reduction, it is also found that Japanese might have been excessively consuming saturated fatty acids. This would also induce adult diseases and increase the risks to personal health. Therefore, in addition to maintaining low TFA consumption, it may also be crucial to reduce the intake of saturated fatty acids. However, saturated fatty acids play a very important role in maintaining the texture of foods. To fill the hole left by the reduction of saturated fatty acids, an additional alternative technology involving crystallization will need to be developed.

In addition, discussions about food labeling have been carried out in CAA. Until now, from the experiences of other countries around the world, there is too much information displayed on the food label, which can confuse the consumers. In the future of food labeling, it is necessary to selectively provide information that is helpful to consumers.

References

Consumer Affairs Agency, Government of Japan. Overview: Guidelines for *Trans* Fat Labeling. http://www.caa.go.jp/foods/pdf/syokuhin1112.pdf (accessed Feb 2, 2014).

Food Safety Commission of Japan. Investigative Report of Basic Data for Evaluation of *Trans* Fatty Acids in Food (siyokuhin ni hukumareru toransu sibousan no hyoka kiso siryo tyosahoukokusyo) http://www.fsc.go.jp/sonota/kagaku4-toujitusiryou.pdf (accessed Sept 30, 2012).

Food Safety Commission of Japan (FSC, 2012). *Trans* Fatty Acid Contents in Food (siyokuhinchu no ganyuryo). *Evaluation Document of Newly-developed Food, Trans Fatty Acids in Foods* (Sinkaihatu syokuhin hyokasyo syokuhin ni hukumareru toransu sibosan) **2012,** 11–18.

Japan Margarine Shortening and Lard Industry Association (JMSLIA). Nihon Margarine Kogyokai), Statistical Report of Processed Edible Oils (syokuyo kakoyusi tokei nenpo), 2007.
Japan Margarine Shortening and Lard Industry Association (JMSLIA). Nihon Margarine Kogyokai), Statistical Report of Processed Edible Oils (syokuyo kakoyusi tokei nenpo), 2011.
Maruyama, T. Quantitative Determination of *Trans* Fatty Acid (Toransu Sibosan No Teiryo). *Food Industry for Tomorrow* (Asu no syokuhin sangyo), 2012, **4,** 11–16.
Ministry of Agriculture, Forestry and Fisheries. Investigative Study on the *Trans* Fatty Acids (Toransu sibosan ni kansuru tyosakenkyu) http://www.maff.go.jp/j/syouan/seisaku/trans_fat/t_torikumi/index.html (accessed Sept 30, 2012).
Ministry of Agriculture, Forestry and Fisheries. Performance Research of Oil Production, **2011** http://www.maff.go.jp/j/tokei/kouhyou/oil/index.html (accessed Oct 2, 2012).
Ministry of Finance Japan (MFJ). Statistics of Foreign Trade (Boeki Tokei) http://www.customs.go.jp/toukei/srch/index.htm?M=01&P=0 (accessed Oct 2, 2012).
Ministry of Finance Japan (MFJ). Statistics of Foreign Trade (Boeki Tokei) http://www.customs.go.jp/toukei/srch/index.htm?M=01&P=0 (accessed Oct 2, 2012).
Ministry of Health, Labour and Welfare (MHLW). A Discussion of Details, Lipids. *Dietary Reference Intakes of Japanese.* (in Japanese), **2009,** 77–108.
Mozaffarian, D.; Katan, M. B.; Ascherio, A.; Stampfer, M. J.; Willett, W. C. *Trans* Fatty Acids and Cardiovascular Disease. *N. Engl. J. Med.* **2006,** *354,* 1601–1613.
Okamoto, T.; Matsuzaki, H.; Maruyama, T.; Niya, I.; Sugano, M. Trans-Fatty Acid Content in Hydrogenated Oils and Estimated Intake. *Journal of Japan Oil Chemists' Society* **1999,** *48* (12), 1411–1414.
Sato, K. Structures and Physical Properties of Lipid Crystals. *J. Grad. Sch. Biosp. Sci., Hiroshima Univ.* **2009,** *48,* 77–94.
Shiramasa, H. Reduction of the *Trans*-fatty Acid on the Practical Use. *Journal of Cookery Science of Japan,* **2012,** *45* (3), 223–227.
Sugano, M. Health Effects of Trans fatty Acid (Toransu sibousan no kenkou heno hiyouka nitsuite), In *How do we understand about trans fatty acid and human health?* (Dou Rikaisuru Toransu Sibousan To Kenkou); Japan Oil Chemists' Society (JOCS), Ed.; Nippon Printings, 2011 pp 15–23.
Yamada, M.; Sasaki, S.; Murakami, K.; Takahashi, Y.; Okubo, H.; Hirota, N.; Notsu, A.; Todoriki, H.; Miura, A.; Fukui, M.; et al. Estimation of Trans Fatty Acid Intake in Japanese Adults Using 16-day Diet 144 Records Based on a Food Composition Database Developed for the Japanese Population. *J. Epidemiol.* **2010,** *20* (2), 119–127.
Zhou, B. F.; Stamler, J.; Dennis, B.; Moag-Stahlberg, A.; Okuda, N.; Robertson, C.; Zhao, L.; Chan, Q.; Elliott, P. Nutrient Intakes of Middle-aged Men and Women in China, Japan, United Kingdom, and United States in the Late 1990s: The INTERMAP Study. *J. Hum. Hypertens.* **2003,** *17* (9), 623–630.

17

Trans Fats Replacement Solutions in India

R.B.N. Prasad ■ *CSIR-Indian Institute of Chemical Technology, Hyderabad, India*

K.D. Yadav ■ *Kamani Oil Industries, Mumbai, India*

Introduction

Partially hydrogenated vegetable oil (PHVO), popularly known in India as *vanaspati,* is one of the most important food industries and it has gained immense popularity among the consumers in India. Vanaspati occupies a key position in foods, bakery products, ready-to-eat snacks, deep-fried foods, and so forth. It is not clear how the term vanaspati originated. It was perhaps evolved to emphasize the plant origin of the product as opposed to the animal origin of its more familiar counterpart, clarified butter or ghee. (In Sanskrit, *vana* means forest and *pati* means lord; therefore, lord of the forest.) Vanaspati is made by partial hydrogenation of vegetable oils that converts the liquid oils to a semisolid state, followed by deodorization and addition of vitamins [not less than 25 international units (IU) of vitamin A per gram, and vitamin D is optional]. Vanaspati in India is an all-purpose fat and initially it was used as a butter substitute. It is used not only for cooking and frying, but also for baking, like a Western shortening.

Trans fatty acids (TFAs) are found in PHVO (vanaspati), shortenings, and margarine. TFA levels in vanaspati depend on multiple factors and were as high as 45–50% of total fat content until the legislation recently changed. There is a possibility of *trans* fatty acid formation (up to 1–3%) at the time of processing of edible oils during deodorization, if not monitored properly. *Trans* fats also occur naturally at low levels (generally 2–5% of fat content) in ruminant-based foods such as dairy products and meat. Vanaspati is the main sources of *trans* fats produced in India during typical selective hydrogenation processes of unsaturated vegetable oils.

Typically, depending on the seasonal and local availability of oils and fats and usage patterns, there can be number of variants of vanaspati/bakery shortenings available in the country. However, they can broadly be categorized into: (1) vanaspati/bakery shortening meant for cooking/frying applications, which is a grainy product very similar to desighee (clarified butter) with a texture that consumers prefer, and (2) smooth (grainless) bakery shortenings/margarines for bakery and confectionery industries, which are votated products. These are tailor-made products for specific functional performance applications and specific institutional customers. Smooth bakery shortenings are used for biscuits, cookies, puff pastry, doughnuts, and so forth, and may be aerated or nonaerated depending on the functional requirement. The process of partial hydrogenation maintains the taste and smell characteristics of oils while enabling a longer shelf life for final food products.

Edible oil/fat intake in India is income dependent, and intake in rural and urban poor areas is much lower than the average levels. There are strong regional preferences for the type of edible oil(s). The major edible oils produced in the country are mustard, soya, groundnut, rice bran, cottonseed, sunflower, coconut, sesame, safflower, and linseed. The production of vegetable oils is almost stagnant at about 7.51 million t for the last few years (Table 17.A). The demand for edible oils in India has shown a steady growth, and because of this, the country depends on large amounts of imports. During 2012–2013, about 10.38 million t of oils were imported (Table 17.A) to bridge the demand–supply gap (Solvent Extractors' Association of India, 2013). The growth has been driven by improvement in per capita consumption, which in turn is attributable to rising income levels and living standards. This indicates that India is consuming about 9–10% of total global edible oil production. The current per capita consumption levels of oils and fats in India is about 14 to 16 kg per annum based on different statistical surveys. Compared to the edible oil industry, the Indian vanaspati industry is small—less than 5%, based on 2012–2013 figures.

Hattiangdi (1958) and Madhur (1981) provided a detailed description about the history of the Indian vanaspati industry. The first vanaspati industry was set up by the

Table 17.A Pattern of Vegetable Oil Production and Imports in India (in million tons)

Oil	2007–2008	2008–2009	2009–2010	2010–2011	2011–2012	2012–2013
Mustard	1.51	2.15	2.05	2.28	1.92	2.34
Soya	1.44	1.33	1.28	1.48	1.60	1.65
Groundnut	1.17	0.82	0.61	0.74	0.46	0.29
Rice bran	0.80	0.85	0.80	0.85	0.88	0.90
Cottonseed	1.05	0.90	1.08	1.20	1.20	1.11
Sunflower	0.51	0.40	0.34	0.23	0.22	0.22
Coconut	0.42	0.42	0.43	0.42	0.42	0.39
Sesame	0.16	0.17	0.21	0.18	0.16	0.13
Safflower	0.05	0.05	0.04	0.04	0.03	0.02
Palm	0.06	0.07	0.06	0.06	0.07	0.08
From expelled cakes	0.47	0.41	0.39	0.33	0.28	0.28
Minor oilseeds	0.10	0.10	0.06	0.10	0.10	0.10
Total domestic production	**7.74**	**7.67**	**7.35**	**7.91**	**7.34**	**7.51**
Imported Oils	5.60	8.18	8.82	8.37	9.98	10.38

Source: The Solvent Extractors' Association of India (2013).

Indian Vegetable Product Ltd., Bombay, in 1930, with an installed capacity of 303 t of vanaspati per annum. The present production is about 0.82 million t per annum, although it reached about 1.44 million t during 2001–2002. As in any other country, there are growing concerns about the potential health effects of TFAs, particularly those that are derived from vanaspati. The Indian government and the vanaspati industry have taken several measures to reduce the TFA content in vanaspati, and these efforts are described in this chapter.

History of the Vanaspati Industry in India

Ghee, or clarified butter, is the most widely used milk product in the Indian diet, and it was produced in India as early as 1500 B.C. It is considered a supreme cooking and frying medium for the preparation of sweets and several food items. Ghee is an ideal fat for deep frying because its smoke point is about 250 °C. Ghee is produced in India from both buffalo and cow milk with a little variation in the composition of triacylglycerols (TAGs). Ghee is the pure clarified fat derived solely from milk, *desi* (cooking) butter, or cream, to which no coloring is added. Ghee contributes unique characteristics to the appearance, texture, lubricity, and flavor, and it is a source of energy and several other potential health-promoting components. In its table use, ghee is served in hot molten form and used for garnishing rice or spreading lightly on some food items. Ghee also finds a valuable place in treatment of various diseases in Indian medicine Ayurveda. People believe that ghee provides certain health benefits because it contains anticarcinogens, anti-atherogens, and vitamins. In the Indian diet, ghee is considered as a superior fat over other fats and is preferred for cooking and other food preparations. Ghee is a valuable source of fat soluble vitamins A, D, E, and K. It is a rapid source of energy compared to other vegetable oils because it contains short-chain fatty acids, which are readily absorbed and metabolized (Kanawjia and Makhal, 2005)

During the early 1930s, scarcity of ghee began to be felt in India due to growth of population; conversion of pasture lands into agricultural lands, resulting in reduction in cattle population; development of urban areas and demand for more milk from these areas; the rising standard of living of the people after the First World War, and so forth. Hence, the need for some less expensive substitute for ghee was felt by the people. Thus, the story of vanaspati began in India by importing PHVO from Holland. Its appearance and flavor are similar to that of the traditional ghee, and the fact that it was relatively inexpensive soon made it very popular among the Indian masses. The first factory was set up by the Indian Vegetable Product Ltd., Bombay, in 1930, with an installed capacity of 303 t of vanaspati per annum, followed by four more mills before 1934.

The government of India helped the industry by giving it protection and, due to this, the indigenous production expanded rapidly and the imports became negligible. During 1928–1929, 22,909 t of vanaspati were imported, whereas imports were only 279 t during 1939–1940. During World War II, the industry received further impetus from the increased demand of the defense services. In addition, the desi ghee, which was available at Rs 0.75 paise per pound before the outbreak of the war, was selling at Rs 3 per pound during the war period (Madhur, 1981). Growing urbanization and wartime economic conditions also gave a boost to the demand for vanaspati. The manufacture of vanaspati thus became one of the major food industries in the country. The Indian vanaspati industry got a boost when the government of India began looking for more revenues to meet its deficit budget and imposed a heavy import duty on vanaspati. This enabled the industry to capture the market already established by the importers.

Gradually, vanaspati production exceeded the total installed capacity of all vanaspati factories. There was shortage, and it was felt so intensely that the government of India had to intervene. Thus, the first ever control on the price of vanaspati was im-

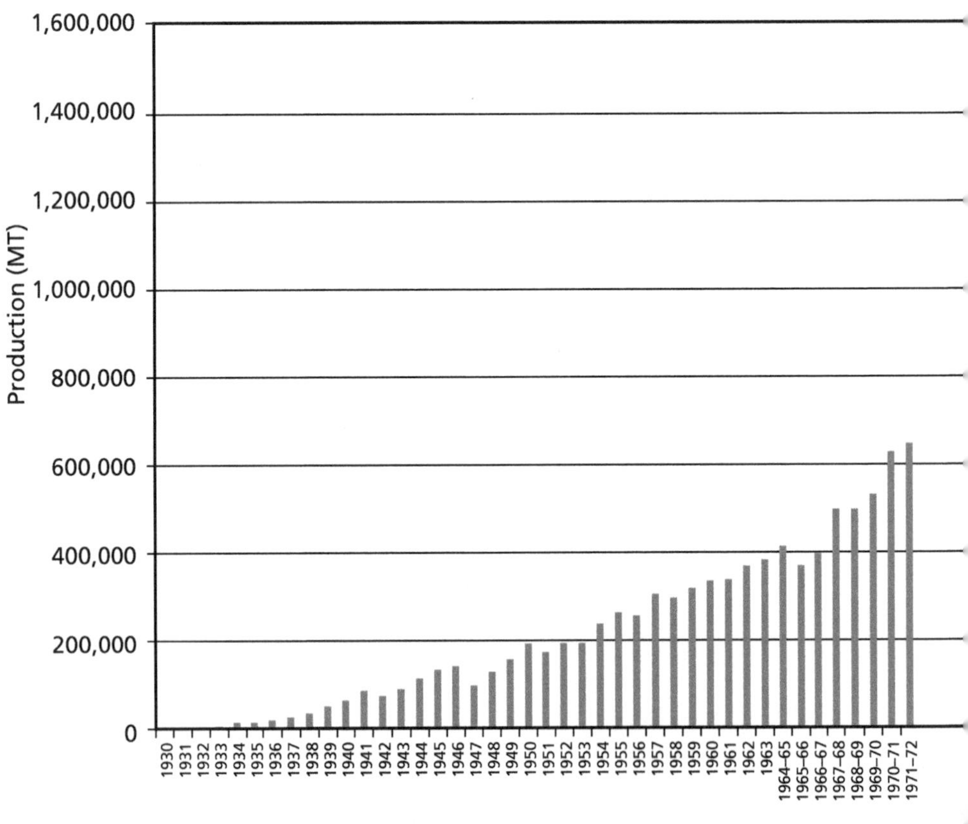

Figure 17.1 Production Figures (metric tons) of vanaspati in India.

posed by the Indian government in 1943. During 1950, vanaspati was recognized as a wholesome food fit for consumption as a fat. The control on vanaspati was removed in 1952. The industry was included in the Schedule of the Industries (Development and Regulation) Act, and regular development of the industry was ensured.

The installed capacity of vanaspati was only 1.2 million t until 1971, but the actual production never went beyond 0.6 million t per year during that time. From 1980 onward, the production figures varied between 0.8 and 1.0 million tons until 1997, and rose to maximum levels of 1.4 million t during 2000–2002. The production figures were between 1.1 and 1.3 million t until 2010. During the 1970s, duty imports on vanaspati from Nepal, Sri Lanka, and Bhutan had crippled the economic viability of the Indian vanaspati industry (Solvent Extractors' Association of India, 2009). Interestingly, during 2010–2011, the production came down to about 1.0 million t and between 2011–2013 it was further reduced to about 0.8 million t (Figure 17.1).

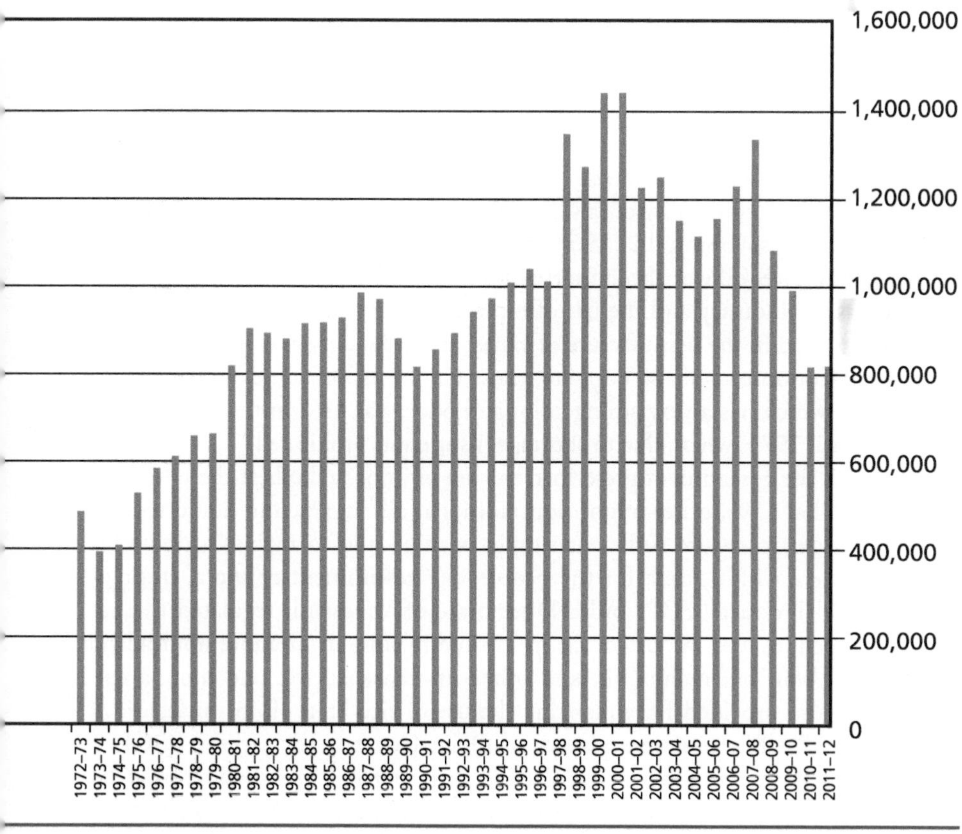

Data from Directorate of Vanaspati, Vegetable Oils and Fats (2009).

According to the 2014 records of Directorate of Vanaspati, Vegetable Oils and Fats (DVVOF), 268 units were registered with a production capacity of 5.8 million t of vanaspati, but the capacity utilization was only 19%, which is a very low figure (Directorate Vanaspati, 2009). In general, the production of margarine and bakery shortening is about 10% of vanaspati production in the country.

Vegetable Oils Used for the Manufacture of Vanaspati

The main qualities of oil that are taken into consideration before making a choice in using it in the production of vanaspati are cost effectiveness and refinable capacity. Initially, groundnut was the major oil used for the production of vanaspati in India (70% in 1966). Sesame oil is added up to 5% as an invisible marker for detecting the presence of vanaspati used for adulterating ghee. It is made in such a way that it has a slip (melting) point of 37 °C, as laid down in the statutory regulations in the initial years. With the gradual acceptance of vanaspati as a common cooking media, and with continuous support from government, there was increase in the demand for vanaspati to meet the domestic (civilian, as well as defense) requirement, leading to acute shortage of groundnut oil. In order to discourage the use of groundnut oil for vanaspati manufacture, the government fixed its use for this purpose at 25%. This measure was taken to save groundnut oil for direct use by consumers. In order to keep the cost under control and ensure availability of raw material for vanaspati, the government of India started importing soybean oil in 1967 and imposed statutory control to use soybean oil. Later, sunflower oil was also imported for use in vanaspati. Thus, with the growth of the vanaspati industry and the use of more and more imported oils up to 50% of the total oils used in the manufacture of vanaspati, dependency on groundnut oil was minimized. Cottonseed oil also began to be used in the manufacture of vanaspati. Even mustard oil, which has a very strong color and odor, was used in the manufacture of vanaspati until 1973, when, due to shortage, its use was prohibited.

In 1978, the government prescribed the use of imported oils at the rate of 75%, cottonseed oil at 15%, other minor nontraditional oils at 5%, and liquid sesame oil at 5%. In order to ensure sufficient supply position and to maintain domestic oil prices that were within reach for the people, the government of India, through its Vegetable Oil Product (VOP) order Directorate of Vanaspati, regulated the use of various indigenous and imported oils from time to time to promote nontraditional oils like rice bran oil, mahua oil, and others in vanaspati. At one time, a special subsidy was also provided for enhancing the use of rice bran oil in vanaspati. After the imports of edible oils were placed on Open Government License (OGL), the industry started sourcing raw material through imports. Presently, imported crude palm oil is major source of raw material in the manufacture of vanaspati in India. Data from Directorate of Vanaspati shows that in 2006, 25% indigenous oil and 75%

imported oils were used for manufacture of vanaspati. It was also made mandatory for vanaspati units to use a minimum 12% of indigenous oils in the manufacture of vanaspati under the VOP Regulation order 1998 (Abbé et al., 2009). Due to this order, vanaspati manufacturers were compelled to use higher priced indigenous edible oils, thereby leading to a higher cost of production. However, with the change in legislation, the availability of imported palm oil, and the fact that palm olein and palm stearin are available at more competitive prices, palm oil and its fractions are being used up to 80% in the vanaspati/bakery manufacture in an effort to bring down the TFA content to less than 10% (FSSAI, 2013).

Fatty Acid Composition of Indian Vanaspati

Early compositional data available on the fatty acid composition of Indian vanaspati (Nanavati et al.,1957; Shenolikar and Subbaram, 1960) indicate that vanaspati contains 30–40% and 40–50% TFA, respectively. A few commercial samples were analyzed at CSIR-Indian Institute of Chemical Technology (Prasad, 2010, 2014) and the results are given in Table 17.B. Jeyarani and Yella Reddy (2005) analyzed nine different brands of commercial vanaspati for their fatty acid composition and reported that the TFA (elaidic acid) content ranged from 5.9% to 30%. Ghafoorunissa (2008) reported that Indian vanaspati PHVO, which is used in Indian cooking and in the preparation of commercially fried, processed, bakery, ready-to-eat, and street foods, generally provides up to 40% TFA, and TFA in biscuits and sweets ranges from 30–40% and 6–26% of total fatty acids, respectively. Abbé et al. (2009) reviewed the global *trans* fat scenario and reported the fatty acid composition of Indian vanaspati across the country; the total TFA content ranged from 4% to 65% of total fatty acids, with elaidic acid being the major *trans* isomer. The lower TFA levels in some brands/batches reflect the use of a higher proportion of palm oil in the mixture of feed oils used for hydrogenation. The Centre for Science and Environment (CSE) analyzed 21 samples of edible oils and 7 samples of vanaspati from the Indian market and reported the ranges of 0.1–3.3% and 9.4–23.7% of TFA, respectively, in these samples (Johnson and Saikia, 2009).

However, according to the new regulation of FSSAI, the TFA content is restricted to less than 10%. Table 17.B clearly indicates this transformation. The commercial vanaspati samples analyzed during 2010 contained about 13.2–25.4% TFA, whereas the samples analyzed in 2014 exhibited less than 10% TFA (Table 17.B).

Vanaspati Manufacturing Process

Hydrogenation is the process by which hydrogen is added to points of unsaturation in the fatty acids at elevated temperature and pressure in the presence of a catalyst

Table 17.B Fatty Acid Composition of Commercial Vanaspati Samples

	Fatty Acid Composition (wt%)										
Commercial Samples	**12:0**	**14:0**	**16:0**	**18:0**	**18:1*t***	**18:1*c***	**18:2*t***	**18:2*c***	**18:3*t***	**18:3*c***	**Total TFA**
Sample 1[a]	—	—	37.6	6.3	22.1	26.7	2.8	1.8	0.5	0.1	25.4
Sampl e 2[a]	—	—	45.8	5.3	10.3	30.5	2.6	3.3	0.4	0.2	13.3
Sample 3[a]	—	—	50.8	4.6	12.2	18.5	0.9	4.8	0.1	0.1	13.2
Sample 4[b]	6.2	3.2	45.6	5.3	2.3	29.8	0.9	6.1	0.4	0.2	3.6
Sample 5[b]	0.4	1.2	44.8	9.1	8.2	32.6	0.8	2.4	0.4	0.1	9.4

[a]Data generated during 2010.

[b]Data generated during 2014.

Source: Prasad (2010, 2014).

(Walter, 2005). Proper selection of starting oils also plays a major role in *trans* formation. Neutralized, bleached, and deodorized oils (either a single oil or an admixture of oils), based on their seasonal and regional availability and cost, are selected according to the stipulated conditions of the Directorate of Vanaspati. The catalyst most widely used is nickel, which is removed from the fat after the hydrogenation processing is completed. The hydrogenation conditions can be varied to meet certain physical and chemical characteristics desired in the finished product. This is achieved through selection of the proper temperature, hydrogen gas pressure, time, catalyst concentration, and agitation. Proper selection of starting oils, its selective or nonselective hydrogenation process, type of catalyst used (like fresh/spent) and temperature, agitation speed, and so forth play a major role in *trans* formation and the end product characteristics and functional properties. Hydrogenation was developed as a result of the need to convert liquid oils to the semisolid form for greater utility in certain food uses and to increase the oxidative stability of the fat or oil by extending its shelf life with lower rancidity and for reusability in deep-fat frying. Hydrogenated fat also adds a certain pleasing mouth feel to the processed food.

Generally, partial hydrogenation of unsaturated oil leads to a higher percentage of *trans* fatty acid formation in the finished product compared to saturated oils under identical hydrogenation conditions. Unlike rest of the world, where there is no melting point limit on hydrogenated vegetable oils, vanaspati in India needed to have a melting point of 31–41 °C until recently, per Indian food legislation. Due to this, the industry was carrying out more selective hydrogenation of oils to restrict the melting point to 41 °C, which results in higher TFA content to get the desired texture in the vanaspati. Consumers prefer and expect vanaspati to be semisolid, even in summer conditions. However, due to the adverse effects of high TFA content in vanaspati so produced, the Food Safety and Standards Authority of India (FASSAI) recently removed the melting point limit in existing law and brought down the TFA content in vanaspati to not more than 10% (FSSAI, 2013). The functional properties that are required in vanaspati for its end application as bakery shortenings, puff margarines, and frying/cooking fat are still maintained.

Trans Fats in the Indian Diet

Vanaspati has several advantages over liquid oils in performance as an edible fat. It is solid or semisolid in most parts of the country most of the year. It does not have a high degree of unsaturation and is therefore more stable during storage, cooking, and frying than liquid vegetable oils. In many instances (e.g., baking or frying of sweets, puris, etc.), the use of harder fat such as vanaspati leads to products with a better texture and taste than when a liquid oil is used. In the kitchen, vanaspati does not go rancid after the tin is opened. For certain kinds of cooking (e.g., baking a cake or making biscuits or to turn out a porous mysore pak [a popular sweet in India]), a liquid oil cannot be used and a hard fat like ghee or vanaspati is necessary.

Vanaspati is the preferred medium for cooking and frying due to its superior palatability and oxidative stability under high temperatures. Apart from its household consumption as an excellent cooking medium, it is widely used in the preparation of commercially fried snacks and ready-to-eat and street foods, which are preferably eaten fresh and hot. The sweet meat industry also uses vanaspati in some of the traditional sweets like laddoo, jilebi, gulab jamun, and so forth. This accounts for approximately 20% of its usage.

Vanaspati and bakery shortening find their major applications in the bakery industry, especially in the unorganized/semiorganized ones where consistency and plasticity of the fat are crucial and of prime importance to get the desired functional performance like puffiness/crispness. Thus, bakery shortening meant for application in biscuits/cookies have to have a steep melting curve and solid fat content (SFC) compared to the shortening meant for puff products, which has to have excellent plasticity, shallow SFC, and slow melting behavior. Of all the bakery shortenings used, biscuit shortenings may account for almost 45–50%, and the remaining 50–55% is the puff shortening. In the recent past, the organized segment of the biscuit/snacks industry is shifting toward palm oil and palm oil–based products, and in unorganized and semiorganized segments, palm/palm olein and vanaspati/bakery shortening are being equally distributed.

Trans Fatty Acid Consumption of the Indian Population

The Vanaspati Manufacturers' Association of India and the Indian Vanaspati Producers' Association took initiative and generated data on the per capita dietary intake of TFAs from various food sources in India at a state level (Frost and Sullivan, 2009).

PHVO (vanaspati, margarines, and bakery shortenings), edible vegetable oils, milk and milk products, and various animal meats were considered the main contributors for the TFAs. The study was based on the secondary sources of information such as the government of India websites, national survey results, WHO, and other Internet databases. The total fat and TFA contents of various foods were estimated based on the fat contents of food items, as described in Table 17.C. India was segmented into 23 states and union territories. The statewide population estimates for 2007–2008 were taken from the Census of India, Government of India. Daily per capita consumption was taken from the National Sample Survey Organization (NSSO). Because NSSO considered only direct consumption of oils and fats, per capita consumption was adjusted for indirect consumption through bakery items and deep-fried food items.

Table 17.D describes the TFA intake (g/day/person) of the statewide population from different sources of fats, namely PHVO, edible vegetable oils, milk, and meat. Punjab and Chhattisgarh have the highest and lowest TFA intake, with 7.89 and 0.59 g/day/person, respectively. The Indian average consumption of fat intake is 43.6 g/day, and Chandigarh consumes the most fat (75.1 g/day) and Jharkhand (23.4 g/

Table 17.C Total Fat Content and TFA Content of Various Food Sources

Food Source	% Fat in Total	TFA as % of Total Fat	Source
PHVO	100	25	Assumed conservatively on higher side of range (9.4%–23.7%) as per CSE Report
Milk and milk products	4.5	5	Assumed conservatively on higher side of range (3.7%–5.3%) as per CSE Report
Edible vegetable oils	100	1	Assumed conservatively on higher side of average (0.3–1.5% ~ avg 0.9%) as per CSE Report
Sheep and goat meat	13	7	Average of range from Internet sources (4.3–9.2%)
Beef and buffalo meat	19	6	Average of range from Internet sources (2.8–9.5%)
Pig/swine meat	13	1	Average of range from Internet sources (0.2–2.2%)
Poultry meat	6	1	Average of range from Internet sources (0.2–1.7%)

Source: Frost and Sullivan (2009).

Table 17.D Statewide per Capita TFA Intake from Various Food Sources for 2007–2008 (g/day/person)

State	PHVO	Edible Vegetable Oils	Milk Fat	Meat	Total TFA Intake
Punjab	6.34	0.12	1.42	0.01	7.89
Chandigarh	3.12	0.32	1.50	0.01	4.95
Haryana	2.55	0.11	1.66	0.03	4.36
Delhi	2.53	0.29	1.17	0.06	4.05
Himachal Pradesh	1.41	0.26	1.12	0.03	2.81
Uttaranchal	1.53	0.20	0.82	0.06	2.62
Jammu and Kashmir	1.03	0.22	1.04	0.31	2.60
Uttar Pradesh	1.07	0.15	0.60	0.13	1.95
Gujarat	0.38	0.42	0.85	0.02	1.67
Rajasthan	0.16	0.20	1.27	0.02	1.65
Maharashtra	0.43	0.53	0.46	0.10	1.52
Madhya Pradesh	0.39	0.25	0.64	0.02	1.30
Karnataka	0.23	0.47	0.49	0.10	1.28
Kerala	0.30	0.22	0.39	0.28	1.19
Andhra Pradesh	0.18	0.46	0.43	0.09	1.16
Tamil Nadu	0.19	0.43	0.45	0.07	1.14
North Eastern States	0.49	0.18	0.22	0.25	1.13
Bihar	0.59	0.14	0.37	0.02	1.13
Jharkhand	0.63	0.14	0.25	0.05	1.08
West Bengal	0.24	0.19	0.24	0.12	0.80
Orissa	0.23	0.24	0.13	0.03	0.63
Chhattisgarh	0.18	0.25	0.15	0.01	0.59
All India	**0.70**	**0.28**	**0.57**	**0.09**	**1.64**

Source: Frost and Sullivan (2009).

day) consumes the least fat (Table 17.E). The data is extrapolated to consumption of TFA from PHVO as a percentage of total energy, and again Chandigarh (2.14%) and Jharkhand (0.17%) are found to be maximum and minimum compared to the Indian average of 0.26%.

India's per capita fat intake of 43.6 g/day is the lowest among other developed and developing nations. India's per capita TFA intake of 1.6 g/day is also lower than most countries. At a national level, India is well below the WHO recommended intake of TFA as a percentage of energy (0.6% compared to the WHO recommendation of

Table 17.E Statewide per Capita Fat and TFA Intake for 2007–2008

State	Per Capita Fat Intake (g/day)	TFA Intake (g/day)	Energy Intake (Kcal/day)	Fat as % of Total Energy	TFA as % of Total Energy	TFA from PHVO as % of Total Energy
Punjab	66.2	7.89	2,664	22.3	2.67	2.14
Chandigarh	75.1	4.95	2,737	24.7	1.63	1.03
Haryana	55.3	4.36	2,697	18.5	1.45	0.85
Delhi	64.0	4.05	2,742	21.0	1.33	0.83
Himachal Pradesh	54.3	2.81	2,623	18.6	0.97	0.48
Uttaranchal	43.9	2.62	2,478	15.9	0.95	0.56
Jammu & Kashmir	52.5	2.60	2,644	17.9	0.88	0.35
Uttar Pradesh	33.4	1.95	2,634	11.4	0.67	0.36
Maharashtra	65.8	1.52	2,287	25.9	0.60	0.17
Gujarat	60.6	1.67	2,576	21.2	0.58	0.13
Rajasthan	46.8	1.65	2,611	16.1	0.57	0.05
Karnataka	59.3	1.28	2,265	23.6	0.51	0.09
Madhya Pradesh	40.0	1.30	2,334	15.4	0.50	0.15
Tamil Nadu	54.2	1.14	2,271	21.5	0.45	0.08
Kerala	36.5	1.19	2,423	13.6	0.44	0.11
Andhra Pradesh	57.2	1.16	2,407	21.4	0.43	0.07
North Eastern States	30.4	1.13	2,507	10.9	0.41	0.17
Bihar	24.3	1.13	2,489	8.8	0.41	0.21
Jharkhand	23.4	1.08	2,498	8.4	0.39	0.23
West Bengal	27.8	0.80	2,459	10.2	0.29	0.09
Orissa	27.9	0.63	2,460	10.2	0.23	0.08
Chhattisgarh	29.1	0.59	2,377	11.0	0.22	0.07
All India	**43.6**	**1.64**	**2,473**	**15.9**	**0.60**	**0.26**

Source: Frost and Sullivan (2009).

less than 1%). Compared to global benchmarks, India's per capita energy, fat, and TFA intakes are the lowest among both developed and developing nations. However, certain states in North India, namely Punjab (2.6%), Chandigarh (1.6%), Haryana (1.4%), and Delhi (1.3%), have high consumption of vanaspati and milk fats and hence have TFA intakes above the WHO recommended level of 1%. Of these, only Punjab and Chandigarh have dietary TFA intake from PHVO as percentage of energy of more than 1%.

Vanaspati Regulations in India

During 1930s, there were no special restrictions on the specifications of the vanaspati and it was made to be an attractive product by using flavors and colors. Vanaspati provided an inexpensive and attractive source of fat to the less well-to-do people in the community, who could not afford more expensive oils or fats like ghee. However, with the increased acceptance of vanaspati, the fears of adulteration of ghee with vanaspati also grew, and some doubts were expressed about the nutritional value and safety of vanaspati.

In order to have effective control over the manufacture, stock, and sale of vanaspati, the government of India promulgated the Vegetable Oil Product Control Order in 1947. However, a new Vegetable Oil Products Control Order was enforced on January 2, 1955, under the Essential Commodities Act of 1955. Under this order, the specifications of vanaspati were fully prescribed. The use of colors and palatable flavors in vanaspati was banned. The maximum limit for the melting point of vanaspati was fixed at 37 °C, with an assumption that the body's temperature is almost identical to this and the product would be easily digested and assimilated in the body. Vitamin A at the level of 700 IU per ounce of vanaspati was also required to improve its overall nutritive value. Addition of sesame oil at the rate of 5% as a marker in the vanaspati manufacture was also required to prevent the adulteration of vanaspati in desi ghee. Adulteration of ghee with vanaspati can readily be detected by a simple chemical test, the Baudouin test, in which Baudouin reagent gives a pink color when it is added to vanaspati. (Sesamolin reacts with furfural solution in the presence of hydrochloric acid and gives a pink color.) It was also suggested, though it is optional, that vitamin D at the rate of 50 IU per ounce of vanaspati should be added. Vanaspati inspectors were introduced for enforcement of control on the quality of vanaspati. Later, it was decided to widen the melting point to a 41 °C maximum, because ghee's melting point is as high as 41 °C and fat does not have to melt completely to be emulsified in the digestive tract, degraded, and ultimately absorbed. Unlike ghee, vanaspati can be specifically made to suit to the consumer requirements and climatic conditions.

Meanwhile, an act to consolidate the laws relating to food and to establish the FSSAI came into existence for laying down science-based standards for articles of food and to regulate their manufacture, storage, distribution, sale, and import; to ensure availability of safe and wholesome food for human consumption; and for matters related to these issues. The FSSAI Act of 2006 went into effect on August 5, 2011, with an emphasis on: (1) food safety and good manufacturing practices (GMP) of manufacturers, (2) product recall and traceability, (3) genetically modified and functional foods, and (4) labeling and communication. With the implementation of the FSSAI Act of 2006, the edible oil industry was governed by FSSAI for issues of licensing, safety, and standard parameters. However, all other issues related to production and procurement of vegetable oils is being administered by Directorate of Vanaspati, Vegetable Oils and Fats under Vegetable Oil Products, Production and Availability (Regulation) Order, 2011.

According to the Food Safety and Standards (Food Products Standards and Food Additives) Regulations, 2011 (FSSAI, 2011), *vanaspati* means any refined edible vegetable oils subjected to a process of hydrogenation in any form. It shall be prepared by hydrogenation from groundnut oil, cottonseed oil, and sesame oil, or mixtures thereof, or any other safe vegetable oils allowed by the government for the purpose. Refined salseed fat, if used, shall not be more than 10% of the total oil mix. Vanaspati shall be prepared from one or more of the following vegetable oils:

Coconut oil, cottonseed oil, dhupa fat, groundnut oil, kokum fat, linseed oil, mahua oil, maize (corn) oil, mango kernel fat, mustard/rapeseed oil, nigerseed oil, palm oil, phulwara fat, rice bran oil, safflower (kariseed) oil, salseed oil (up to 10%), sesame oil, soybean oil, sunflower oil, watermelon seed oil, and vegetable oils imported for edible purposes.

Vanaspati must conform to the following standards:

1. It shall not contain any harmful coloring, flavoring, or any other matter deleterious to health.
2. No color shall be added to hydrogenated vegetable oil unless so authorized by the government, but in no event will any color resembling the color of ghee be added.
3. If any flavor is used, it shall be distinct from that of ghee in accordance with a list of permissible flavors and in such quantities prescribed by government; diacetyl of not more than 4.0 ppm may be added to vanaspati exclusively meant for consumption by the armed forces.
   a. On melting, the product shall be clear in appearance, free from staleness or rancidity, and pleasant to taste and smell.
   b. It shall contain raw or refined sesame (til) oil in sufficient quantity so that when the vanaspati is mixed with refined groundnut oil in proportion of 20:80, the color produced by the Baudouin test shall not be lighter than 2.0 red units in a 1 cm cell on a Lovibond scale.
4. It may contain food additives permitted in these regulations and appendices, provided that imported crude palm oil and fractions thereof shall not be used by the producers other than those who are engaged in manufacture of vanaspati or any other hydrogenated oil product and are equipped in the same location with the facilities for generation of hydrogen gas and hydrogenation of the said imported crude palm oil and fractions thereof with the gas so generated in the manufacture of vanaspati or any other hydrogenated vegetable oil product for edible consumption.

Vanaspati shall also conform to these requirements:

1. Moisture, percent by mass, shall not be more than 0.25.
2. Melting point, as determined by capillary slip method, shall be from 31 °C and 41 °C, both inclusive.
3. It shall not have unsaponifiable matter exceeding 2.0%, but in case of vanaspati in which the proportion of rice bran oil is more than 30% by weight, the unsaponifiable matter shall not be more than 2.5% by weight, provided the quantity of rice bran is declared on the label of such vanaspati as laid down in regulation 2.4.2(8) of packaging and labeling regulations.
4. Free fatty acid (as oleic acid), percent by mass, shall not be more than 0.25.
5. Synthetic vitamin A shall not be less than 25.0 IU per gram at the time of packing and shall test positive when tested with Antimony Trichloride (Carr-Price Reagent) as per IS:5886-1970.
6. Residual nickel shall not be more than 1.5 ppm.
7. The test for argemone oil shall be negative.

Specification for Bakery Shortening: "Bakery shortening" means vanaspati meant for use as shortening or leavening agent in the manufacture of bakery products, that is, for promoting the development of the desired cellular structure in the bakery product with an accompanying increase in its tenderness and volume. This will also confirm to the standards prescribed in regulation 2.2.6(1) except that:

1. The melting point, as determined by the capillary slip method, shall not exceed 41 °C.
2. If aerated, only nitrogen, air, or any other inert gas shall be used for the purpose and the quantity of such gas incorporated in the product shall not exceed 12% by volume thereof.
3. It may contain added monoglycerides and diglycerides as emulsifying agents.
4. The test for argemone oil shall be negative.

FSSAI is adopting an integrated approach by removing the multiple laws being governed by different ministries; ensuring manufacturing, distribution, and sale of safe food to the consumer for the food safety management system; making efforts to harmonize with CODEX and other international laws, depending on the necessity; and adopting a scientific approach with an aim of "innovation through science and technology" because the old Prevention of Food Adulteration Act (PFA) standards were rigid and left a limited scope for product development. The proposal to introduce a regulation for *trans* fat in PHVO was first tabled in 2004 at the Oils and Fats Subcommittee of Central Committee of Food Standards (CCFS). After numerous deliberations on this topic, in the beginning of 2009, the FSSAI expressed a strong intent to enforce a maximum limit on TFA in PHVO and asked the vanaspati industry to conduct in-depth studies and arrive at a feasible recommendation and roadmap. The industry believed that measures adopted to reduce TFA content in PHVO must satisfy consumer requirements of low TFA content with desired consistency across various regions of the country and in different seasons. End products should be heat stable with no oil separation. The solution should be cost effective and allow the flexibility to use various indigenous edible oils. Consumers purchase vanaspati on the basis of physical feel. If the consistency is too soft, then it is not suitable; if it is too hard, it is not workable. India, being a diverse geographical nation, has varied weather (from −10 °C to 50 °C) and therefore the same product will behave differently in summer and winter seasons in the same region and across regions (North–South India) during the same season. As a result, vanaspati manufacturers need to change the consistency of the product according to consumer requirements in different regions of the country. In addition, the PFA regulation at that time mandates a maximum melting point limit of 41 °C. However, CODEX Standards for PHVO do not include an upper limit on melting point. CODEX included hard fractions, such as palm stearin, with melting points of 44–52 °C in a list of edible oils and fats. Countries like Denmark, Canada, the United States, and others that have implemented TFA regulations that follow CODEX standards do not mandate any maximum melting point. PHVO products with low TFA (2–4%) sold in these countries have melting points in the range of 45–54 °C. After several deliberations of the experts in this area, if 10% TFA is the proposed regulation, the TFA intake as percentage of energy is 0.8% and hence below the WHO recommended level of 1%. Based on these points, the government of India issued notifications on June 27, 2013, to amend the Food Safety and Standards Regulations, 2011, related to vanaspati. The following amendments have been made in regulation 2.2 relating to "Fats, Oils and Fat Emulsions":

- Enzymatic process is allowed for manufacture of interesterified vegetable fats.
- Physical, chemical, or enzymatic interesterification is allowed in the process of hydrogenated vegetable oils.
- Palm stearin and vegetable oils imported for edible purposes are permitted for manufacture of vanaspati or interesterified fat.
- The melting point clause has been replaced by the stipulation requiring "*trans* fatty acids, not more than ten percent by weight" for vanaspati, bakery shortening, and margarine.

In addition, the following amendments have been made in subregulation 2.2.2 relating to labeling of prepackaged foods, and also in subregulation 2.4.2 relating to labeling of edible vegetable oils, fats (including hydrogenated vegetable oils), and processed and packaged foods with declared shelf life. All these products will have the following declaration on the label: "Total *trans* fat content not more than . . . percent by weight, and total saturated fat content not more than . . . percent by weight."

Methods to Reduce TFA Content in Vanaspati/Bakery Shortening

Vanaspati with reduced TFA levels meeting consumer expectations can be made by modifying hydrogenation practices. Proper selection of raw materials and modifying the conditions of hydrogenation (e.g., pressure, temperature, and catalyst) result in the reduction of TFA, and properties such as melting point and solid fat content of the oil also change. It is possible to make equivalently performing low-*trans* fats by increasing the degree of hydrogenation, which reduces the level of TFAs but increases the level of saturated fatty acids. The simple substitution of unhydrogenated fats for hydrogenated fats does not work well in baking applications. Low- or zero-*trans* baking fats may have increased levels of stearic acid from the hydrogenation of α-linolenic, linoleic, and oleic acids, and also significant levels of palmitic acid for functionality. An increased level of stearic acid may offer nutritional benefits. With the removal of the melting point limit of 41 °C for vanaspati and bakery shortening by FSSAI, it would be possible to develop a wide range of low-*trans* or *trans*-free products.

Palm stearin was projected as a good feed stock for the production of low-*trans* or *trans*-free products (Bhattacharyya, 1990; Ghosh and Bhattacharyya, 1997; Majumdar and Bhattacharyya, 1986; Shiva Shanker et al., 2012). Because the present regulation permits the use of palm stearin in vanaspati manufacture, this can be used for blending with liquid oils or soft oils to give low-*trans* or *trans*-free products. The interesterification process involves the rearrangement (randomization) of the fatty acid on the glycerol backbone of the fat in the presence of a chemical catalyst or an enzyme. Interesterification modifies the melting and crystallization behavior of the fat, thus producing fats for margarine, spread, and shortening applications with the desirable physical properties of *trans* fats, but without *trans* fats. An unhydrogenated liquid vegetable oil and a fully hydrogenated vegetable oil are mixed and heated in chemical interesterification employing a catalyst, commonly sodium methoxide, and the interesterification process causes a random rearrangement of the fatty acid on the glycerol backbone. In enzymatic interesterification, 1,3-specific immobilized lipase is employed to produce a fat that is partially randomized rather than being completely randomized, as occurs with the use of sodium methoxide. The detailed treatment of enzymatic and chemical interesterification processes are described in other chapters of this book.

Conclusions

The vanaspati industry is facing the toughest time in view of the low capacity utilization (19%) and profitability, thereby threatening the operational viability of the industry. A few years back, the Indian vanaspati industry suffered at the hands of duty-free imported vanaspati from Bhutan, Nepal, and Malaysia. The rapid reduction in the production of vanaspati, from 1.44 million t during 2000–2001 to 0.82 million t during 2012–2013, is due to the shift of biscuit and other similar products to palm oil or its fraction instead of vanaspati. Because the new FSSAI regulation has been introduced with a limit on TFA content to 10% in vanaspati, and there is a possibility of further reduction, the vanaspati industry has to change its strategies in a stipulated timeframe. The industry should replace the present hydrogenation technology with novel hydrogenation methodologies or employ interesterification techniques to produce low- or zero-*trans* vanaspati in the lines of the present regulations by maintaining the characteristic texture, lubricity, moisture barrier, heat transfer, oxidative stability, and flavor. The vanaspati industry also needs to consider introduction of polyunsaturated fatty acids in vanaspati to enhance the nutritional values of the product. The government of India must support the vanaspati industry by helping them in investment and incentives to develop, set up, and operate new technologies for the production of good quality vanaspati.

In addition to vanaspati, refined oils also have been found to contain TFAs up to 1–3%, due to the higher temperatures employed in the deodorization step. Hence, it may be necessary to modify the deodorization step to ensure that TFAs are within minimal specified limits in the refined vegetable oils. The food processing industry should initiate using blends of natural vegetable oils that furnish higher stability to products wherever feasible. For food technological applications that require solid fats, palm oil and its fractions or other suitable saturated-rich oils may also be employed to substitute for hydrogenated fats.

Industry and consumers in India lack awareness regarding the negative health impact of TFAs; therefore, information on the negative health effects of TFAs must be propagated. With the increase in the use of processed, premixed, and ready-to-eat foods, there is a need for educating the consumer to read and understand food labels. A multipronged approach is required to reduce the burden of diet-related chronic diseases by reducing TFAs in Indian diets.

References

Abbé, M. R. L.; Stender, S.; Skeaff, C. M.; Ghafoorunissa, G; Tavella, M. Approaches to Removing *Trans* Fats from the Food Supply in Industrialized and Developing Countries. *European Journal of Clinical Nutrition* **2009,** *63,* S50–S67.

Bhattacharyya, D. K. Palmstearin: An Exclusive Fatty Material for Edible Fat Industry. *Proceedings of the PORIM International Palm Oil Congress (Chemistry and Technology),* **1990,** 139–144.

Directorate Vanaspati. Vegetable Oils and Fats, 2009 http://dfpd.nic.in.2009/20/03/2014.

Food Safety and Standards Authority of India (FSSAI). FSSAI Notification No. 177, June 27, 2013. http://www.fssai.gov.in. 20/03/2014.

Frost and Sullivan, Mumbai, India. Trans *Fat Consumption Trends in India: A Strategic Insight;* The Vanaspati Manufacturers' Association of India & Indian Vanaspati Producers' Association: New Delhi, August 26, 2009.

Ghafoorunissa, G. Role of *Trans* Fatty Acids in Health and Challenges to Their Reduction in Indian Foods. *Asia Pac. J. Clin. Nutr.* **2008,** *17* (Suppl 1), 212–215.

Ghosh, S.; Bhattacharyya, D. K. Utilization of High-melting Palm Stearin in Lipase-catalyzed Interesterification with Liquid Oils. *J. Am. Oil Chem. Soc.* **1997,** *74,* 589–592.

Hattiangdi, G. S.; *The Vanaspati Industry;* Examiner Press: Bombay, India, 1958.

Jeyarani, T.; Yella Reddy, S. Physico-chemical Evaluation of Vanaspati Marketed in India. *J. Food Lipids* **2005,** *12,* 232–242.

Johnson, S.; Saikia, N. *Fatty Acid Profile of Edible Oils and Fats in India.* Report of Centre for Science and Environment, January 2009. http://www.cseindia.org.20/03/2014.

Kanawjia, S. K.; Makhal, S. Ghee—A Functional and Nutraceutical Product. In *Recent Developments in Health Foods and Nutraceuticals,* Lecture Compedium of 18th Short Course Organized by National Dairy Research Institute, Karnal, India, Feb 8–28, 2005. http://www.dairyprocessingcaft.com/wp-content/uploads/2013/03/Recent-Development-in-Health-Foods-and-Nutraceuticals-2005.pdf.20/03/2014.

Madhur, M. M. *Vanaspati Industry in India;* Concept Publishing Company: New Delhi, India, 1981.

Majumdar, S.; Bhattacharyya, D. K. Nutrition of Hydrogenated Vanaspati, and Interesterified Vanaspati Made from Palmstearin and Selective Liquid Oils. *Oleagineux* **1986,** *41,* 393–397.

Mumbai Food Safety and Standards Authority of India (FSSAI). FSSAI, Food Products Standards and Food Additives Regulations, 2011. http://www.fssai.gov.in.20/03/2014.

Nanavati, T. D.; Gupta, S. D.; Aggarwal, J. S. Estimation of *Tran*-iso Oleic Acids in Hydrogenated Fats, *J. Indian Chem. Soc.* **1957,** *34,* 885.

Prasad, R. B. N. Fatty Acid Compositions of Indian Vanaspati Samples. Unpublished data, 2010, 2014.

Shenolikar, I. S.; Subbaram, M. R. *Trans* Fatty Acids in Hydrogenated Oils. *J. Sci. Ind. Res.* **1960,** *198,* 505.

Shiva Shanker, K.; Konda Reddy, K.; Kanjilal, S.; Prasad, R. B. N. Enzymatic Preparation and Characterization of *Trans*-free Fat from Palm Stearin and Natural Vegetable Oils. *J. Lipid Sci. and Tech.* **2012,** *44,* 79–85.

Solvent Extractors' Association of India. Vanaspati Industry. In *SEA Handbook;* Mumbai, 2009; pp 675–696.

Solvent Extractors' Association of India. Production and Import Details of Vegetable Oils in India, 2013. http://www.seaofindia.com.

Walter, E. F. Hydrogenation: Processing Technologies. In *Bailey's Industrial Oil and Fat Products,* Vol. 5, 6th ed.; Shahidi, F., Ed.; John Wiley & Sons: Hoboken, NJ, 2005; pp 385–396.

18

Trans Fats Replacement Solutions in Malaysia

Teng Kim-Tiu and Kalanithi Nesaretnam ■ *Malaysian Palm Oil Board, No 6, Persiaran Institusi, Selangor, Malaysia*

Sivaruby Kanagaratnam ■ *Malaysian Palm Oil Board, and University of Nottingham, Malaysian Campus, Semenyih, Malaysia.*

Introduction

Epidemiological studies have demonstrated convincing evidence on the consumption of *trans* fatty acids (TFAs) in relation to cardiovascular heart disease risk factors and events (Food and Agriculture Organization, 2003). A 2% energy intake of TFAs increases the risk of developing cardiovascular heart disease by 22% (Skeaff and Miller, 2009). TFAs have been reported to increase the concentrations of LDL cholesterol, apolipoprotein A-1, lipoprotein (a), and total:HDL cholesterol ratio. Furthermore, TFAs also have been found to depress the concentrations of HDL cholesterol and apolipoprotein B-100 (Mensink et al., 2003; Mozaffarian et al., 2006). TFAs have also been found to impair endothelial function and provoke a pro-inflammatory state (Baer et al., 2004; Lopez-Garcia et al., 2005). Hence, regulatory measures have been taken globally to eliminate TFAs from the human food chain based on the mounting evidence from in vivo and in vitro studies and human clinical trials (Food and Agriculture Organization, 2003). In Malaysia, the government has also put up regulatory measures in an effort to reduce the TFA content in food products. This chapter will discuss the regulatory measures, TFA content, and alternatives to TFAs in food formulations in a Malaysian scenario.

Regulation of *Trans* Fatty Acids in Malaysia

The food regulation in Malaysia is governed by the Ministry of Health. According to the law gazetted on March 31, 2003, embedded in the Food Act 1983 (Legal Research Board, 2010), the amount of TFAs will be listed whenever they are present in food. Table 18.A shows the allowed nutrient claims for TFAs and other ingredients in the country. The claim of "*trans* fatty acid free" requires that the content be less than 0.1% of the total dietary fat. This nutrient claim is more stringent compared to the regulations enforced by Denmark (less than 2%) and the U.S. Food and Drug Administration (0.5g per serving) (Danish Ministry of Food, 2003; U.S. Food and Drug Administration, 2006). Table 18.B is an example of voluntary food labeling on packaged products adopted by the food manufacturers in Malaysia.

Table 18.A Nutrient Content Claims for *Trans* Fatty Acids in Malaysia[a]

Component	Claim	Conditions
Energy	Low	40 kcal (170 kJ) per 100 g (solids) *or* 20 kcal (80 kJ) per 100 ml (liquids)
	Free	4 kcal p 100 ml or 100 g
Fat	Low	3 g per 100 g (solids) 1.5 g per 100 ml (liquids)
	Free	0.15 g per 100 g (100 ml)
Saturated fat	Low	1.5 g per 100 g (solids) 1.5 g per 100 ml (liquids)
	Free	0.15 g per 100 g (or 100 ml)
Cholesterol	Low	0.02 g per 100 g (solids) 0.01 g per 100 ml (liquids)
	Free	0.005 g per 100 g (solids) 0.005 g per 100 ml (liquids)
Trans fatty acids	Low	1.5 g per 100 g (solids) 0.75 g per 100 mL (liquids) 10% of total energy of the food
	Free	0.1 g per 100 g (solids) 0.1 g per 100 mL (liquids)
Sugar	Low	5 g per 100 g (solids) 2.5 g per 100 ml (liquids)
	Free	0.5 g per 100 g (solids) 0.5 g per 100 ml (liquids)
Sodium	Low	0.12 g per 100 g (solids) 0.06 g per 100 ml (liquids)
	Very low	0.04 g per 100 g (solids) 0.02 g per 100 ml (liquids)
	Free	0.005 g per 100 g (solids) 0.005 g per 100 ml (liquids)

[a]Nutrient content claims is a nutrition claim describing the level of a nutrient in a food product.

Source: Adapted from Legal Research Board (2010), Table 1, Conditions for Nutrient Contents for Use of Nutrition Claims.

Table 18.B Food Labelling on Packaged Food Products[a]

Nutrition Information
Serving size: 26 g
Servings per package: 15

	Per 100 g	Per Serving 26 g
Average composition		
Energy	386 cal	100 kcal
	1621 kJ	422 kJ
	8.0 g	2.1 g
Fat, comprising:		
Monounsaturated fatty acid	3.8 g	0.2 g
Polyunsaturated fatty acid	0.9 g	1.3 g
Saturated fatty acid	5.0 g	0.0 g
Trans fatty acid	0.1 g	2.3 g
Protein	9.0 g	17.1 g
Carbohydrate, including:	68.0 g	13.0 g
Sucrose	31.0 g	8.1 g
Lactose	10.0g	2.6 g
Maltose	6.0 g	1.6 g
Dietary fiber	3.0g	0.8 g
Sodium	200 mg	52 mg
Calcium	500 mg	130 mg
Phosphorus	510 mg	133 mg

[a]Example of food labeling adopted by the food manufacturers in accordance with guidelines from the Food Act of 1983 and Regulations.

Recommended Nutrient Intake for *Trans* Fatty Acids in Malaysia

The Recommended Nutrient Intake (RNI) for Malaysia was set by the National Co-ordinating Committee on Food and Nutrition (2005). Recognizing the detrimental health effects of TFAs, RNI Malaysia (2005) recommended a less than 1% energy intake of TFAs of the total daily diet. This is in accordance with the recommended upper limit intake of TFAs (less than 1% energy) adopted by the World Health Organization/Food Authority Organization (World Health Organization, 2003).

The Malaysian Dietary Guidelines advocate that the public limit the intake of foods containing TFAs. This includes limiting the intake of margarines and shortenings made from hydrogenated or hardened fats, as well as foods prepared with partially hydrogenated or hardened fats, such as french fries, doughnuts, and bakery products (National Coordinating Committee on Food and Nutrition, 2010).

Trans Fatty Acid Content of Malaysian Food Products

In Malaysia, most of the food products containing TFAs are imported products such as margarines, shortenings, vegetable ghee, and bakery products. The country imports most of the dairy products, margarines, and spreads from Australia, New Zealand, and Denmark. Ruminant TFAs (vaccenic acid) are present in dairy products such as milk and butter, as well as meats. Nevertheless, the consumption of dairy products in the Malaysian population is relatively low compared to Western countries.

Cooking Oils

A survey was conducted to determine the levels of TFAs in cooking oils (Tang, 2002). Table 18.C summarizes the TFA content of 113 samples of palm oil and palm kernel oil products obtained from refineries and commercial products in the country. The crude palm oil and crude palm kernel oil contain negligible amounts of TFAs. Refining and deodorization processes slightly elevate the TFA content in refined products. Palm olein and palm stearin displayed similar TFA content (0–0.5%). Refined, deodorized, bleached (RBD) palm kernel oil extracted from the kernel of palm fruits and its fractions demonstrate considerably lower TFA content (0–0.1%) than the liquid fractions of palm oil. Palm kernel oil and its fractions are highly saturated and hence possess better stability to resist isomerization during deodorization and refining processes.

Under the blended palm oil category, palm-based cooking oils demonstrate acceptable levels of TFAs with a mean of 0.5% (and range from 0.3% to 0.7%) (Tang, 2002). On the contrary, non-palm-based cooking oils contain remarkably higher TFA content (0.5–3.8%). The average content of TFAs in vegetable seed oils, namely corn oil, sunflower oil, safflower oil, soybean oil, peanut oil, and canola oil, is 1.4–2.9% (0.5–3.8%). The amount of TFAs found in highly unsaturated vegetable oils in Malaysia is in accordance with the amounts reported for the United States and New Zealand (Ball et al., 1993; Litin and Sacks, 1993). The highly unsaturated nature of vegetable seed oils makes them more susceptible to isomerization during refining and deodorization processes.

A recent survey was conducted to compile TFA claims on packaged commercial cooking oils (Table 18.D). Palm olein and red palm olein were declared as TFA free.

Table 18.C *Trans* Fatty Acid Content of Palm Oil and Palm Kernel Oil Products Sampled from Refineries and Commercially Available Cooking Oils in the Local Markets

Sample	Number of Sample	*Trans* Fatty Acids: C18:1*t*	C18:2 *t* *tc, ct, tt*	C18:3*t* (All *Trans* Isomers)	Total *Trans* Fatty Acids Mean (Range) (%)
Crude palm oil	12	0	0	0	0 (0–0.2)
RBD[a] palm oil	12	0–0.3	0.1–0.4	0.3	0.3 (0.1–0.6)
Liquid palm oil fractions					
RBD palm olein	17	0–0.1	0–0.5	0.3	0.3 (0–0.6)
NBD[b] palm olein	2	0	0.09–0.3	0.2	0.2 (0.1–0.3)
RBD super olein	4	0	0.1–0.4	0.2	0.2 (0.1–0.5)
NBD super olein	1	0	0.2	0.2	0.2
Red palm olein	2	0	0–0.2	0.1	0.1 (0–0.2)
Solid palm oil fractions					
RBD palm stearin	12	0–0.1	0–0.4	0.3	0.3 (0.1–0.4)
NBD palm stearin	1	0	0.2	0.3	0.3
Crude palm kernel oil	8	0	0	0	0
RBD palm kernel oil	7	0–0.7	0	0	0 (0–0.1)
NBD palm kernel oil	1	0	0	0	0
RBD palm kernel stearin	6	0–0.1	0	0.1	0.1 (0–0.1)
RBD palm kernel olein	3	0–0	0.1	0	0 (0–0.1)
NBD palm kernel olein	2	0	0	—	—
Blended palm oil					
Cooking oil, palm-based	9	0–0.1	0.1–0.6	0.5	0.5 (0.3–0.7)
Cooking oil, non-palm-based	14	0–0.1	0.4–2.7	2.0	2.0 (0.5–3.8)
Vegetable seed oils[c]					
Corn oil	4	0–0	0.8–1.5	0.2–0.4	1.6 (1.1–2.0)
Sunflower oil	3	0–0.1	0.6–2.7	0–0.2	1.4 (0.6–3.0)
Safflower oil	1	0	0.7	0.2	0.9
Soybean oil	4	0–0.1	0.4–1.5	1.2–2.7	2.9 (1.6–3.8)
Peanut oil	1	0	0.5	0	0.5
Rapeseed oil (low erucic)	1	0	0.4	2.4	2.8

[a]RBD: Refined, bleached, deodorized

[b]NBD: Neutralized, bleached, deodorized.

[c]The Malaysian cooking oil market is dominated by palm oil and its fractions; vegetable seed oils, however, are also available on the shelf as culinary cooking oils.

Source: Adapted from Tang (2002).

Table 18.D *Trans* Fatty Acid Content of Culinary Cooking Oils in Malaysia[a]

	Number of Sample	*Trans* Fatty Acids (%)	
		Lowest	Highest
Palm oil fractions			
Palm olein	4	0	0
Red palm oil	1	0	0
Vegetable seed oils			
Sunflower oil	6	0	1.1
High-oleic sunflower oil	1	0	0
Canola oil	4	0	0.6
Soybean oil	1	0	0
Corn oil	1	0	0
Rice bran oil	1	0	0
Sesame oil	1	0	0
Grape seed oil	1	0	0
Flaxseed oil	1	0	0
Refined olive oil	3	0	0
Extra virgin olive oil	3	0	0
Blended vegetable oils	8	0	1.1

[a]A survey conducted in the local markets in October 2012 with *trans* fatty acid content from nutrition information panel. Out of 57 cooking oils, a total of 36 cooking oils declared the amount of *trans* fatty acids.

All the vegetable seed oils were labelled with 0% of TFAs (although the zero TFA declaration is voluntary), excluding sunflower oil and canola oil (0–1.1%) and blended vegetable oils (0–1.1%).

Retail Margarines and Spreads

Table 18.E summarises the TFA content of retail spreads and margarines in Malaysia. Out of 21 spreads reviewed, only 14 declared their TFA content on the labels. The range of TFAs in the spreads was 0–3.5%. A total of 11 margarine products were sampled, with 7 reporting TFA content (0.6–2.9%). These margarines and spreads are mostly imported from Australia. The declaration of higher levels of TFAs in the labeling strongly suggests the incorporation of hydrogenated fats or unsaturated soft oils, which contain higher levels of TFAs compared to palm oil fractions (as shown in Table 18.C).

Table 18.E *Trans* Fatty Acid Content of Margarines and Spreads in Malaysia[a]

	Number of Sample	*Trans* Fatty Acids (%)	
		Lowest	Highest
Spread	14	0	3.5
Margarine	7	0.6	2.9

[a]A survey conducted in the local markets in October 2012 with fatty acid composition extracted from nutrition information panel.

Dairy Products

Table 18.F shows the TFA content of dairy products, which are mostly imported. Out of 10 butter products reviewed from the shelves, there were only 3 products with TFAs reported, which ranged from 0% to 4.9%. There were 29 cheese products evaluated with only 13 products declaring the amounts of TFAs (0–5.0%). The TFA content in the labels ranged from 1.1% to 3.9% in the four whipping creams evaluated.

Trans Fat Alternatives

Malaysia is the second biggest palm oil–producing country after Indonesia. The country produced 18.91 million t of crude palm oil in 2011, with 17.99 million t exported to other countries. With a population of 27.6 million people in the country, the consumption of palm oil per capita is estimated to be 22 kg annually. Palm oil is widely used in various food formulations. Palm oil is naturally semisolid at room tempera-

Table 18.F *Trans* Fatty Acid Content of Dairy Products in Malaysia[a,b]

	Number of Sample	*Trans* Fatty Acids (%)	
		Lowest	Highest
Butter	3	0	4.9
Cheese	13	0	5.0
Sour light cream	1	3.9	3.9
Whipping cream	4	1.1	3.4

[a]A survey conducted in the local markets in October 2012 with fatty acid composition extracted from nutrition information panel.

[b]The food labeling indicated that the lowest *trans* fatty acid content of butter and cheese is 0, which is unusual. Further laboratory analysis is needed to verify the information of food labeling found on imported items.

ture and is fractionated into various liquid and solid fractions. Palm olein, the liquid fraction, is widely used as a culinary oil in the country. The use of solid fractions, such as palm stearin, in food formulations does not require hydrogenation. Hence, palm-based products contain negligible amounts of TFAs.

Soft oils are extensively hydrogenated to obtain hardstocks/solid fats for food formulations. Solid fats provide crucial characteristics such as structure, texture, firmness, and oxidative stability. In recent years, natural vegetable fats have gained a pronounced preference in food processing over partially hydrogenated vegetable fats. The limited supply of natural solid fats, coupled with the pressure to replace hydrogenated fats, has driven palm oil to be the natural choice for various food applications.

The continuous advancement in fractionation technology enables production of palm-based fractions with a high degree of selectivity. Fractionation is carried out in a single or multiple steps, giving rise to a wide range of products. The hard solid fractions are subjected to double or even triple fractionations to obtain the palm oil solids with targeted amounts of TAG. These multistage fractionation routes are improvised continuously in producing value-added palm oil fractions (Calliauw et al., 2007). In Malaysia, palm-based fractions are extensively used in the production of shortenings, margarines, confectionary fats, frying fats, milk fat replacers, and ice cream fats that are used in the recipes of breads, biscuits, cakes, cookies, chocolates, ice creams, and pastries (Lai et al., 1998; Ming et al., 1999).

Palm oil fractions are produced and traded based on their melting points. Palm oil has the unique composition of low, medium, and high melting point triacylglycerols. This enables the selective fractionation of palm oil to produce low (melting point below 23 °C), medium (melting point below 37 °C), and high (melting point above 37 °C) melting fractions. The medium and high melting fractions are the key players in the replacement of *trans* fats.

Medium Melting Palm Oil Fractions

The palm-based medium-melting fractions are soft and hard palm mid fractions (melting point below 37 °C). The soft palm mid fractions are obtained through double fractionation of palm olein or palm stearin (melting point 28–32 °C) (Calliauw et al, 2007; Hashimoto et al., 2001; Son et al., 2010). Hard palm mid fractions (melting point 31–32 °C) are obtained through the fractionation of soft palm mid fractions and have a high commercial value (Braipson-Danthine and Gibon, 2007). Hence, these fractions are considered medium melting-fats by the food formulators (Braipson-Danthine and Gibon, 2007; Kellens et al., 2000). These fractions have unique solid fat content profiles that are preferred by the chocolate manufacturers as cocoa butter equivalents (Hashimoto et al., 2001). In addition, these fractions are also blended with exotic fats such as shea, sal, and illipe (source of POS and SOS) to produce fat blends that are compatible to cocoa butter.

High-Melting Palm Oil Fractions

There are three types of palm stearins—soft, hard, and very hard—available on the market. Soft palm stearins (melting point of 40–46 °C) are obtained through single fractionation of palm oil or double fractionation of palm olein (Rashid et al., 2011). These fractions are commonly used as the main components in shortenings and margarines blended with liquid oils. Hard palm stearins (melting point of 52–56 °C) are obtained through single fractionation of palm oil (Chiew Let et al., 2007; Karabulut et al., 2004). These palm stearins are the structural fats that act as the backbone of margarines and shortenings (Jennings and Akoh, 2010; Mayamol et al., 2004, 2009; Reshma et al., 2008; Saadi et al., 2012). The very hard palm stearins (melting point of 59–62 °C) possess the unique solid fat content (above 80% between the temperature range of 25–40 °C) (Lutton et al., 1948; Minato et al., 1996). Hence, small amounts of these fractions (below 5%) are incorporated into margarine formulations to resist deformation of texture by improving stability (Miskandar and Noraini, 2010; Miskandar et al., 2005).

Versatility of Palm Oil Fractions in Food Applications

The margarine and shortening manufacturers in Malaysia have been using palm-based food formulations for more than three decades. The versatility of palm oil fractions in food formulations, coupled with the lower cost, have driven the domination of palm oil in the food sector in Malaysia. The choice of palm oil fractions in food formulations was generally based on their melting points. Table 18.G depicts the melting point and functionality of palm oil fractions used in margarine formulations.

Table 18.G The Main Categories of Palm Oil Fractions Based on Melting Point and Functionality

Palm Oil Fractions	High-Melting Fractions	Medium-Melting Fractions	Low-Melting Fractions/Liquids
Functions	Structural fat that imparts the backbone structure	The main body that imparts the structure, firmness, and texture	Texture modifiers (to modify the solid fat content)
Types of oils	Palm stearin melting point above 52 °C	Palm oil, palm stearin melting point below 45 °C (soft), palm kernel oil, palm kernel stearin, palm mid fractions	Palm olein, palm kernel olein, small amounts of soft oils (soybean, canola, and sunflower)

Table 18.H Palm Oil–Based Blends of Shortening Commonly Produced in Malaysia

	Blend 1	Blend 2	Blend 3	Blend 4
Palm oil	95%	90%	85%	80%
Palm stearin IV 32	5%	10%	15%	20%
Slip melting point (SMP)	38.0	40.5	41.7	43.6
Iodine value (IV)	51.3	50.5	49.3	48.5

Palm-Based Shortenings

In Malaysia, shortenings are mainly used in breads, buns, biscuits, short crust pastries, and cakes. Shortening is usually produced by direct blending of palm oil with palm stearin (Table 18.H) or palm olein with palm stearin without hydrogenation. This common practice of gives the flexibility to produce the desired melting point of the shortening (Miskandar et al., 2011). Figure 18.1 shows the corresponding solid fat content of the blends in Table 18.H.

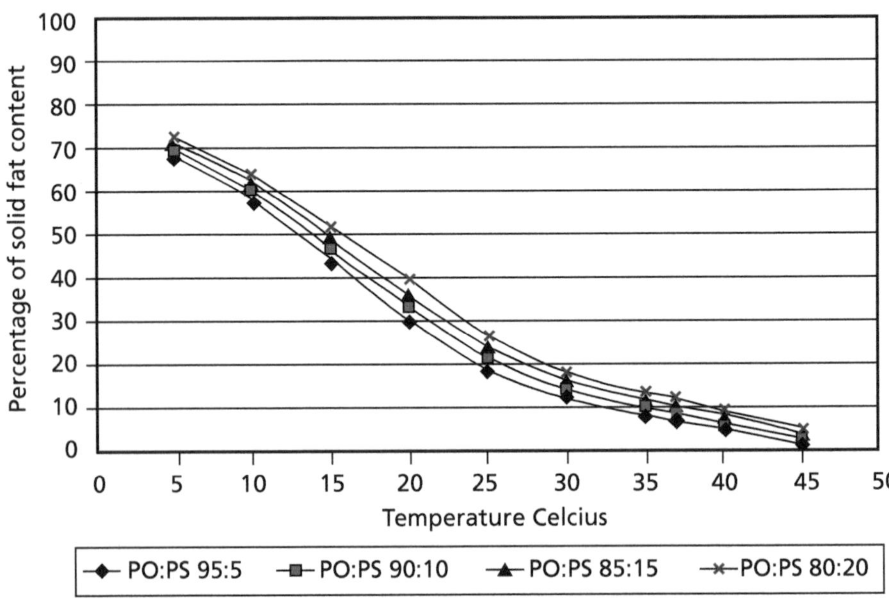

Figure 18.1 The solid fat content of palm oil–based blends of shortening commonly produced in Malaysia.

Palm-Based Margarines

Margarines are produced using various combinations of palm oil fractions without the incorporation of hydrogenated fats. The industrial margarines are selectively developed for specific food applications such as cakes, cookies, pastries, puff pastries, topping creams, filling creams, and multipurpose margarines.

Palm-Based Frying Fats

Palm oil is the preferred industrial frying fat because it exhibits remarkable resistance to oxidation (iodine value of 50–52 I2/100 g) and has a suitable melting point of 36–37 °C. In Malaysia, frying fats are used for frying chips, snacks, and convenience foods such as instant noodles.

Palm-Based Ghee/Vanaspati

The combination of palm oil and palm stearin in the manufacture of palm-based ghee/vanaspati has completely replaced the hydrogenated oil blends that previously dominated this segment. By processing through a series of exclusive cooling programs, palm oil and palm stearin blends are able to produce the desired grainy crystals comparable to the crystals produced by hydrogenated fats.

Other Palm-Based Food Applications

Palm oil and palm oil fractions are also major components in whipped topping and filling fats. Palm fractions have also replaced dairy fats in the non-dairy milk, creamer, and ice cream. Palm oil and its fractions are also ideal raw materials for confectionary fats, cocoa butter substitutes, coatings, and cream filling. These fractions have found their way into caramels, toffees, and fudges (Miskandar et al., 2011). In addition, palm oil and its fractions are also found in local traditional and modern seasonings.

Conclusion

Malaysia, as the second largest producer of palm oil in the world, has adopted palm oil and its fractions into various food applications via extensive research and development. The competitive price of palm oil and its fractions, together with advancements in technology, make it a preferred choice in food applications. Therefore, locally manufactured food products contain negligible amounts of TFAs. However the Ministry of Health should impose a close monitoring on the TFA contents in dairy products, margarines, and bakery products imported into Malaysia. The worldwide enforcement of TFA labeling is a prerequisite to the success of eliminating TFAs from our food chain.

References

Baer, D. J.; Judd, J. T.; Clevidence, B. A.; Tracy, R. P. Dietary Fatty Acids Affect Plasma Markers of Inflammation in Healthy Men Fed Controlled Diets: A Randomized Crossover Study. *Am. J. Clin. Nutr.* **2004,** *79* (6), 969–973.

Ball, M. J.; Hackett, D.; Duncan, A. *Trans* Fatty Acids Content of Margarines, Oils and Blended Spreads Available in New Zealand. *Asia Pac. J. Clin. Nutr.* **1993,** *2,* 162–169.

Braipson-Danthine, S.; Gibon, V. Comparative Analysis of Triacylglycerol Composition, Melting Properties and Polymorphic Behavior of Palm Oil and Fractions. *Eur. J. Lipid Sci. Tech.* **2007,** *109* (4), 359–372.

Calliauw, G.; Gibon, V. R.; De Greyt, W.; Plees, L.; Foubert, I.; Dewettinck, K. Phase Composition During Palm Olein Fractionation and its Effect on Soft PMF and Superolein Quality. *J. Am. Oil Chem. Soc.* **2007,** *84* (9), 885–891.

Chiew Let, C.; Zukarinah, K.; Pierre, L.; Alejandro, M.; Claudie, B.; Michel, O. Thermal and Structural Behaviour of Crude Palm Oil: Crystallisation at Very Slow Cooling Rate. *Eur. J. Lipid Sci. Tech.* **2007,** *109* (4), 410–421.

Danish Ministry of Food AaF. *Executive Order on the Content of* Trans *Fatty Acids in Oils and Fats Etc.;* Danish Veterinary and Food Administration, 2003.

Food and Agriculture Organization. *Fats and Fatty Acids in Human Nutrition: Report of an Expert Consultation,* FAO Food and Nutrition Paper 91; FAO; Rome, 2010.

Hashimoto, S.; Nezu, T.; Arakawa, H.; Ito, T.; Maruzeni, S. Preparation of Sharp-melting Hard Palm Midfraction and Its Use as Hard Butter in Chocolate. *J. Am. Oil Chem. Soc.* **2001,** *78* (5), 455–460.

Jennings, B. H.; Akoh, C. C. *Trans*-free Plastic Shortenings Prepared with Palm Stearin and Rice Bran Oil Structured Lipid. *J. Am. Oil Chem. Soc.* **2010,** *87* (4), 411–417.

Karabulut, I.; Turan, S.; Ergin, G. Effects of Chemical Interesterification on Solid Fat Content and Slip Melting Point of Fat/oil Blends. *Eur. Food Res. Tech.* **2004,** *218* (3), 224–229.

Kellens, M.; Hendrix, M. Fractionation. In *Introduction to Fats and Oils Technology,* 2nd ed*;* O'Brian, R. D.; Farr, W. E., Wan, P. J., Eds.; AOCS Press: Urbana, IL, 2000; pp 194–207.

Lai, O.; Ghazali, H.; Chong, C. Effect of Enzymatic Transesterification on the Melting Points of Palm Stearin-sunflower Oil Mixtures. *J. Am. Oil Chem. Soc.* **1998,** *75* (7), 881–886.

Legal Research Board. *Food Act 1983 (ACT 281) and Regulations;* International Law Book Services: Malaysia, 2010.

Litin, L.; Sacks, F. *Trans*-fatty-acid Content of Common Foods. *N. Engl. J. Med.* **1993,** *329* (26), 1969–1970.

Lopez-Garcia, E.; Schulze, M. B.; Meigs, J. B.; Manson, J. E.; Rifai, N.; Stampfer, M. J.; Willett, W. C; Hu, F. B. Consumption of *Trans* Fatty Acids Is Related to Plasma Biomarkers of Inflammation and Endothelial Dysfunction. *J. Nutr.* **2005,** *135* (3), 562–566.

Lutton, E. S.; Jackson, F. L.; Quimby, O. T. The Polymorphism of the Mixed Triglycerides of Palmitic and Stearic Acids. *J. of the Am. Chem. Soc.* **1948,** *70* (7), 2441–2445.

Mayamol, P.; Samuel, T.; Balachandran, C.; Sundaresan, A.; Arumughan, C. Zero *Trans* Shortening Using Palm Stearin and Rice Bran Oil. *J. Am. Oil Chem. Soc.* **2004,** *81* (4), 407–413.

Mayamol, P. N.; Balachandran, C.; Samuel, T.; Sundaresan, A.; Arumughan, C. Zero *Trans* Shortening Using Rice Bran Oil, Palm Oil and Palm Stearin through Interesterification at Pilot Scale. *Int. J. Food Sci. Tech.* **2009,** *44* (1), 18–28.

Mensink, R. P.; Zock, P. L.; Kester, A. D.; Katan, M. B. Effects of Dietary Fatty Acids and Carbohydrates on the Ratio of Serum Total to HDL Cholesterol and on Serum Lipids and Apolipoproteins: A Meta-analysis of 60 Controlled Trials. *Am. J. Clin. Nutr.* **2003,** *77* (5), 1146–1155.

Minato, A.; Ueno, S.; Yano, J.; Wang, Z. H.; Seto, H.; Amemiya, Y.; Sato, K. Synchrotron Radiation X-ray Diffraction Study on Phase Behavior of PPP-POP Binary Mixtures. *J. Am. Oil Chem. Soc.* **1996,** *73* (11), 1567–1572.

Ming, L. O.; Ghazali, H. M.; Chiew Let, C. Use of Enzymatic Transesterified Palm Stearin-sunflower Oil Blends in the Preparation of Table Margarine Formulation. *Food Chemistry* **1999,** *64* (1), 83–88.

Miskandar, M. S.; Noraini, I. Palm Stearin as Low *Trans* Hard Stock for Margarine. *Sains Malaysiana* **2010,** *39* (5), 821–827.

Miskandar, M. S.; Man, Y. C.; Yusoff, M. S. A.; Rahman, R. A. Quality of Margarine: Fats Selection and Processing Parameters. *Asia Pac. J. Clin. Nutr.* **2005,** *14* (4), 387–395.

Miskandar, M. S.; Karimah, A.; Noor Lida Habi Mat, D.; Wan Rosnani, A. W.; Salmi, Y. S.; Sivaruby, K.; et al. Palm Oil and Palm Kernel Oil for Low *Trans* Food Products. In *Further Advances in Oil Palm Research (2000–2010);* Mohd, B. W., May, C. Y., Eds; Malaysian Palm Oil Board: Kuala Lumpur, Malaysia, 2011; pp 685–720.

Mozaffarian, D.; Katan, M. B.; Ascherio, A.; Stampfer, M. J.; Willett, W. C. *Trans* Fatty Acids and Cardiovascular Disease. *N. Engl. J. Med.* **2006,** *354* (15), 1601–1613.

National Coordinating Committee on Food and Nutrition, Ministry of Health Malaysia. *Recommended Nutrient Intakes for Malaysia: A Report of the Technical Working Group on Nutritional Guidelines;* National Coordinating Committee on Food and Nutrition, 2005.

National Coordinating Committee on Food and Nutrition, Ministry of Health Malaysia. *Malaysian Dietary Guidelines: Technical Working Group on Nutritional Guidelines;* National Coordinating Committee on Food and Nutrition, 2010.

Rashid, N. A.; Let, C. C.; Seng, C. C.; Omar, Z. Crystallisation Kinetics of Palm Stearin, Palm Kernel Olein and their Blends. *LWT—Food Science and Technology* **2011.**

Reshma, M. V.; Saritha, S. S.; Balachandran, C.; Arumughan, C. Lipase Catalyzed Interesterification of Palm Stearin and Rice Bran Oil Blends for Preparation of Aero *Trans* Shortening with Bioactive Phytochemicals. *Bioresource Technology* **2008,** *99* (11), 5011–5019.

Saadi, S.; Ariffin, A. A.; Ghazali, H. M.; Miskandar, M. S.; Boo, H. C.; Abdulkarim, S. M. Application of Differential Scanning Calorimetry (DSC), HPLC and pNMR for Interpretation Primary Crystallisation Caused by Combined Low and High Melting TAGs. *Food Chem.* **2012,** *132* (1), 603–612.

Skeaff, C. M.; Miller, J. Dietary Fat and Coronary Heart Disease: Summary of Evidence from Prospective Cohort and Randomised Controlled Trials. *Ann. Nutr. Metab.* **2009,** *55* (1–3), 173–201.

Son, J. M.; Lee, K. T.; Akoh, C. C.; Kim, M. R.; Kim, M. J.; Lee, J. H. Optimisation of Tripalmitin-rich Fractionation from Palm Stearin by Response Surface Methodology. *J. Sci. Food Agric.* **2010,** *90* (9), 1520–1526.

Tang, T. S. Fatty Acid Composition of Edible Oils in the Malaysian Market, with Special Reference to *Trans*-fatty Acids. *J. Oil Palm Res.* **2002,** *14* (1), 1–8.

World Health Organization. *Diet, Nutrition and the Prevention of Chronic Diseases: Report of a Joint WHO/FAO Expert Consultation.* WHO Technical Report Series No. 916; Geneva, 2003.

U.S. Food and Drug Administration. Division of Nutrition Programs and Labeling OoNP, Labeling, and Dietary Supplements in the Center for Food Safety and Applied Nutrition (CFSAN), 2006.

19

Trans Fats Replacement Solutions in Australia and New Zealand

Amy Logan and Chakra Wijesundera ■ *CSIRO Animal, Food, and Health Sciences, Werribee, Victoria, Australia, 3030*

Introduction

Trans fatty acids (TFAs) are unsaturated fatty acids with one or more double bonds in a *trans* configuration, according to chemical nomenclature. They may be artificially produced through industrial processes, such as partial hydrogenation of oil, or occur naturally in fats from ruminant animals. The process of partial hydrogenation has traditionally been used by the food industry to impart differing functionality to liquid oils, including the textural and melting characteristics of a more solid fat. Not only was this functionality required for the production of margarines and baked goods, it also provided enhanced stability toward oxidative deterioration and is traditionally considered more desirable for frying oil applications.

With increasing evidence to support that TFAs pose a higher risk of coronary heart disease (CHD) compared to saturated fatty acids (SFA) (Brouwer et al., 2010; Mozaffarian et al., 2006; Willett, 2012), nutritional bodies continue to advocate reductions in TFA intake. Although these dietary guidelines do not currently differentiate between industrially produced TFA and ruminant derived TFA, legislative measures introduced by some countries to reduce TFA intake do not apply to food products for which the fat originates exclusively from ruminant sources. This is because no consensus has been reached as to any detrimental effects of ruminant-derived TFA. The effects of ruminant-derived TFA and industrially produced TFA on CHD were initially considered to be similar (Mozaffarian et al., 2009). However, impact of ruminant-derived TFA on CHD has recently been questioned (Bendsen et al., 2011; Gebauer et al., 2011; Tardy et al., 2011), and while the debate continues, a possible role for these acids as a nutraceutical in the prevention of cardiovascular disease (CVD) has been suggested (Wang et al., 2012).

Several countries have introduced legislation aimed at reducing dietary intake of TFAs. Denmark and several other European countries placed limits on the TFA content in foods that can be sold to consumers, while several other countries, including Canada and the United States, required that the TFA content is displayed on the product label if it exceeds a specified amount per serving. More recently, Singapore also has introduced TFA labelling regulations, while China is in the process of introducing legislation that makes it mandatory to declare TFAs on the nutrition label if partially hydrogenated fats have been used in product manufacture. Since the introduction of food labelling regulations, there have been marked declines in the TFA content in the food supplies of both Canada (Ratnayake et al., 2009) and the United States (Rahkovsky et al., 2012), and these reductions have been achieved without causing a significant increase in saturated fats. Australia and New Zealand are yet to introduce any compositional regulatory measures in relation to TFA in the food supply. Instead, the authorities have adopted a position of encouraging the food industry to voluntarily implement strategies to reduce TFA content in the foods they manufacture. This chapter reviews various surveys conducted from 1970 onward on the TFA content of foods in Australia and New Zealand, and discusses measures adopted by regulatory authorities and industry to achieve a reduction in TFA intake by Australians and New Zealanders.

TFA in Foods in Australia and New Zealand

Analytical methodology to identify and quantitate TFAs has continued to improve over the years. The first descriptive reports of TFA content in Australasian foods began to appear in the 1970s. This was the time when margarine, in particular polyunsaturated margarine, was becoming increasingly popular at the expense of butter, due to growing concerns about adverse effects of saturated fats on cardiovascular disease. Although the adverse effects, as we know now, of TFA on human health were not fully appreciated at that time (FAO/WHO, 1977), a possible role of TFA upon the biophysical properties of cell membranes and the desirability of eliminating TFA from margarines were being proposed (Kummerow, 1974, 1975).

In 1976, Parodi published the first comprehensive study on the content of industrially produced TFA in Australian food products. It reported the TFA concentrations of margarines, "hard cube" vegetable oil, animal fat, and blends of vegetable oil and animal fat for products sampled regularly from supermarkets in Brisbane, Australia, from 1973 to 1974. "Table margarine" referred to margarines containing vegetable oil and hydrogenated vegetable oil as the sole or major components, while "polyunsaturated margarine" was defined as a table margarine in which the total fatty acids present contained no less than 40% all *cis*, methylene-interrupted polyunsaturated fatty acids (PUFA) and not more than 20% saturated fatty acids (Parodi, 1976). The average TFA concentrations in the fat component of the products were as follows: polyunsaturated table margarine 17.1% (range 12.9–22.1%), table margarine 14.9% (range 10.8–19%), hard cube polyunsaturated vegetable oil 23.2% (range 21.9–25.1%), hard cube vegetable oil 2.1% (range 0–4.4%), blended vegetable oil and animal fat 5.7% (range 4.6–6.9%), and animal fat 7.8% (range 6.7–8.8%). The average TFA concentration in the Australian margarines was lower than that reported for margarines sold in the United States around the same period (Carpenter and Slover, 1973), where the average TFA concentration was 24.1% (range 14–36%).

Another report on the TFA content of Australian margarines was published by Forgerty et al. (1979) for margarines sampled in 1974 and 1978 from retail outlets in Sydney. The average TFA concentration in the 1974 and 1978 samples was 12.55% (range 5.5–17.2%) and 9.5% (range 0–18.5%), respectively. These values were lower than those reported for margarines sampled in 1973–74 (Parodi, 1976). Another study (Wills et al., 1982) of margarines sampled from supermarkets in Sydney in 1980 reported an average TFA concentration of 11.0% (range 4.0–14%) for polyunsaturated table margarine and zero for table margarine. The data could only be considered representative of margarines on sale in New South Wales, as it was possible that formulations for certain brands varied between different Australian states. However, the total absence of TFAs in table margarines sold in the state of New South Wales suggested the Australian margarine industry had initiated changes in table margarine formulations to exclude hydrogenated oils as early as 1980. These table margarines contained saturated fats at an average concentration of 37.0%. Low levels of lauric acid were present in some samples, indicating the use of coconut or palm kernel oil. Further, a few samples contained cholesterol, showing that animal fats had been used.

The next study of TFAs in Australian margarines was published in 1993 (Mansour and Sinclair, 1993), at a time when concerns about possible detrimental effects of TFAs on human health were beginning to emerge (Lichtenstein, 1993; Mensink and Katan, 1990; Troisi et al., 1992; Willett, 1993). The margarines for this study were sampled from three locations, including Melbourne and Geelong within the state of Victoria. The average TFA concentration in the margarines was 12.1% (range 8–14.5%) (Table 19.A). These values were similar to those found for polyunsaturated margarines sold in Sydney in 1980 (Wills et al., 1982). Although Mansour and Sinclair (1993) did not state whether they deliberately selected polyunsaturated margarines for analysis, all but 2 of the 13 products tested were polyunsaturated margarines, based on their concentration of polyunsaturated (more than 40%) and saturated (less than 20%) fatty acids. By 1992, there were several canola oil–based margarines in the market, in contrast to 1980 when there were none. It was most likely that, by this time, use of interesterified fat was employed as a strategy for achieving the physical characteristics required of margarines. All of the margarines analyzed in 1992 contained interesterified fat at concentrations ranging from 25–100% (average 67.7%). However, there was no apparent correlation between the concentration of TFAs and the amount of interesterifed fats used; the margarine with the lowest TFA content contained 25% interesterified fat, while a margarine with equal highest TFA content contained 100% interesterified fat.

A similar study of New Zealand margarines (Ball et al., 1993), also conducted in 1993, reported an average TFA concentration of 8.5% (range 7.6–9.6%) for margarines widely used by New Zealand consumers and sampled from local grocery

Table 19.A Fatty Acid Classes and Content of Interesterified Fat in Margarines (Coded M1–M13) Tested in 1993

	SAFA[a]	MUFA[b]	PUFA[c]	TFA[d]	IF[e]
M1	28.0	19.8	37.6	14.5	80
M2	19.7	24.8	45.4	11.0	100
M3	19.3	24.2	42.6	13.8	50
M4	19.5	22.4	45.5	12.1	85
M5	19.2	26.2	40.0	14.5	80
M6	15.2	55.8	20.8	8.0	25
M7	20.0	27.4	40.0	11.8	80
M8	13.8	31.4	46.3	8.5	100
M9	20.0	25.0	41.1	14.0	50
M10	14.7	49.4	53.6	9.6	30
M11	20.6	25.5	41.7	12.9	60
M12	13.9	52.5	57.5	14.5	100
M13	20.1	61.8	5.3	12.9	40

[a]Saturated fatty acids (g/100g of total fatty acids).
[b]*Cis* monounsaturated fatty acids (g/100g of total fatty acids).
[c]All *cis* polyunsaturated fatty acids (g/100g of total fatty acids).
[d]*Trans* fatty acids (g/100g of total fatty acids).
[e]Interesterified fat (as a weight percentage of total fat).
Adapted from Mansour and Sinclair (1993).

stores in Dunedin. The margarines tested were generally high in polyunsatured fatty acid (average 35.3%; range 19.8–39.4%) and low in saturated fatty acid (average 23.2%; range 16.5–26.8%), but none of them strictly satisfied the requirements for "polyunsaturated margarine" as stipulated in Australia (Parodi, 1976).

Although these data from two decades ago were restricted to margarines, it is highly probable significant amounts of industrially produced TFA were present in food products other than margarine sold in Australia and New Zealand at the time. However, no published data were available for their concentrations and occurrence in various foods until the Australian Consumer Association survey of 2005. By this time, the detrimental health effects of TFA on cardiovascular health were more firmly established (Hunter, 2006; Korver and Katan, 2006; Mozaffarian et al., 2006) and several countries, including Denmark, Canada, and the United States, had introduced or were preparing to introduce legislations aimed at reducing dietary intake of TFAs. The Australian Consumer Association survey (2005) analyzed over 70 margarines and spreads and over 55 other processed foods sold within supermarkets (such as pies, cakes, biscuits, and confectionery). The products were selected on the basis they were likely made using partially hydrogenated vegetable oils and at the same time would contribute significant amounts of fat to the diet. The margarines and spreads were reported to contain TFA at concentrations averaging 3.2 g/100 g product (range 0–8 g/100 g product). This concentration is considerably lower than the values found earlier (Mansour and Sinclair, 1993), confirming that the Australian industry had implemented effective strategies to reduce TFA in margarines and spreads by 2005. The fat component of 18 out of the 55 processed foods tested was reported to contain TFA concentrations exceeding 2% by weight. However, some of the products included in this category were meat pies, sausage rolls, croissants, crackers, and crisps, in which part or all of the TFA could have been of natural origin (dairy or meat).

The Australian Consumer Association Survey of 2005 was followed by another study a couple of years later (Wijesundera et al., 2007) that also targeted processed foods believed to contain industrially produced TFAs. Dairy products and products containing milk fat as a major ingredient were excluded. Products were sampled from supermarkets or fast food outlets in Melbourne, Victoria, in June 2006. Thirteen categories of foods (103 products) including margarines and spreads were examined, the product selection within each food category being based on the brand or corporate market share to ensure that the most popular products were selected.

Margarines and spreads have been a major contributor to TFA intake by consumers in Europe, Canada, and the United States (Aro et al., 1998; Ratnayake, 2007; Satchithanandam et al., 2004). This was also the case in Australia up to 1993, albeit the intakes were much lower compared with Europe and North America. All but 4 of the 15 margarines and spreads tested in 2006 contained less than 1.0% TFA (Table 19.B), showing that the majority of these products would have been manufactured without using partially hydrogenated oils. By this time, the majority of manufacturers were using virtually TFA-free hardstocks for spreads production using various technologies including full hydrogenation, interesterification, and fractionation. Also, combinations of these technologies were used. Vegetable oils such as canola, sunflower, and soybean oils were probably used, usually in combination with palm oil. Only 3 out of the 15 margarines/spreads tested in 2006 would not have been permitted for sale in Denmark, and 2 would have been compelled to show the TFA content on the product label if marketed in United States. The 2006 study did not measure interesterified fats in the margarines. However, it was most likely that the addition of interesterified fats to impart the physical characteristics required of margarines was still being practiced at that time. The saturated fat concentration of the fats used for manufacturing margarines and spreads ranged from 17% to 30% (g/100 g fat), which is considerably lower than values reported for similar products in Canada (Ratnayake, 2007) and the United States (Satchithanandam et al., 2004). Monounsaturated fatty

Table 19.B Fatty Acid Classes including TFA Content in Selected Australian Foods in 2006

The number of products tested within each category is shown in parenthesis after the product name. Mean values are followed by parenthesis showing the range of values.

	SFA[a] (g/100 g fat)	MUFA[b] (g/100 g fat)	PUFA[c] (g/100 g fat)	TFA[d] (g/100 g fat)	TFA[e] (g/100 g product)	TFA[f] (g/serving)
French fries [ready to eat from fast food outlets (*n* = 6)]	32.1 (8.0–52.0)	49.5 (38.5–67.9)	18.3 (9.5–31.1)	3.7 (1.0–9.5)	0.6 (0.2–1.5)	NA
Frozen french fries and wedges (*n* = 10)	16.8 (7.7–50.1)	58.3 (39.7–66.7)	24.7 (10.2–30.4)	2.6 (0.9–9.8)	0.1 (0–0.7)	NA
Chips [ready to eat, (*n* = 10)]	30.0 (7.9–46.7)	58.7 (39.2–83.2)	11.6 (7.3–23.1)	0.7 (0.3–1.1)	0.2 (0.1–0.4)	0.2
Margarines and spreads (*n* = 15)	23.7 (17.0–30.0)	43.6 (21.9–60.2)	32.6 (22.8–49.1)	1.9 (0.3–8.1)	1.2 (0.2–4.6)	0.3
Household shortenings (*n* = 2)	53.9 (52.8–55.0)	40.4 (38.6–42.3)	5.6 (2.7–8.6)	5.5 (1.7–6.3)	4.0 (1.7–6.3)	0.5
Biscuits and cookies (*n* = 19)	52.9 (12.1–81.1)	36.2 (15.4–60.1)	10.9 (3.5–27.8)	2.3 (0.5–8.3)	0.5 (0.1–2.4)	0.1
Breads (*n* = 10)	16.8 (11.2–25.2)	39.1 (20.4–52.5)	44.1 (36.3–57.2)	1.2 (0–2.6)	0 (0–0.1)	0
Rolls (*n* = 6)	26.0 (21.4–39.5)	23.6 (11.7–38.5)	50.3 (38.9–58.9)	1.7 (0–2.7)	0 (0–0.1)	0
Croissants (*n* = 2)	71.2 (69.6–72.8)	21.6 (19.7–23.6)	7.1 (6.8–7.5)	4.7 (4.1–5.3)	0.8 (0.7–0.9)	0.6
Cakes (*n* = 4)	44.8 (23.8–64.3)	39.0 (25.8–52.4)	11.1 (3.8–20.4)	0.5 (0–1.4)	0 (0–0.1)	0
Cake mixes (*n* = 7)	50.0 (16.9–61.3)	31.8 (17.6–43.4)	18.19 (8.1–65.5)	1.7 (0–8.4)	0.2 (0–1.1)	0.1
Muffin mixes (*n* = 9)	59.6 (47.8–77.3)	29.9 (16.7–44.6)	10.4 (5.2–19.1)	1.9 (0–9.6)	0.2 (0–1.3)	0.1
Cookie mixes (*n* = 2)	61.0 (54.7–67.4)	28.8 (22.1–35.5)	10.1 (9.8–10.5)	0.7 (0.1–1.4)	0.1 (0–0.2)	0

[a]Saturated fatty acids (g/100 g of total fatty acids).

[b]*Cis* monounsaturated fatty acids (g/100 g of total fatty acids).

acid (MUFA) oils were predominantly used, with two thirds of the products containing monounsaturated fats at levels of 45% (g/100 g fat) or greater.

The highest TFA content (6.3%) found in Australian foods in 2007 (Wijesundera et al., 2007) was a household shortening. The relatively high TFA content in this product appeared to be due to the use of animal fat (beef and mutton tallow) rather than partially hydrogenated vegetable oil. Prior to enforcement of mandatory TFA labelling regulations in 2006, the highest (41%) contribution to TFA intake in U.S. adults came from bakery products, where the fat used to manufacture 82% of the biscuits and cookies contained TFAs at a concentration of 20% or more (Satchithanandam et al., 2004). In contrast, 68% of the Australian-made biscuits and cookies tested in 2006 contained less than 0.2 g TFA per serving. Only one product would not have been allowed for sale in Denmark, while all would have qualified for sale as "*trans* free" products in the United States. Out of the other baked products, breads, rolls, and ready-to-eat cakes, all had zero TFA per serving, thus qualifying as them as "*trans* free" products in the United States. None of these products contained more than 5% TFA within the fat component and would have been allowed for sale in Denmark also. Although croissants, on average, contained higher than 0.6 g TFA per serving and 0.8% TFA within the product, this was partly due to the presence of milk fats. Out of the cake, muffin, and cookie mixes, one muffin mix contained higher than 0.5 g TFA per serving, and the same muffin mix and another cake mix contained higher than 5% TFA in the fat used, which would have disqualified their sale in Denmark. Although baked products and ready mixes intended for their preparation were generally low in TFA, it is worthy to note that the fat components of ready-to-eat biscuits and cookies, as well as cake, muffin, and cookie mixes, were composed of saturated fatty acids at levels exceeding 50%.

Around the time the 2006 Australian *trans* fat study (Wijesundera et al., 2007) was conducted, frying oils used for french fries by fast food outlets were a major source of TFA intake in many developed countries, with some popular outlets using oil with TFA content as high as 30% (Slender et al., 2006). The average TFA content in frying oils used in Australia around the same time was only 3.7% (Table 19.B). All but one of the six outlets included in the study appeared to have used nonhydrogenated or minimally hydrogenated oils for frying. However, partially hydrogenated vegetable oil previously used for frying appeared to have been replaced with highly saturated oils, with three out of six outlets tested using oil containing saturated fat in excess of 45%. The high saturated fat content most probably resulted from the use of palm oil or fractions thereof.

Another study published in 2007 (McCarthy et al., 2008) analyzed 92 food items also sampled from retail outlets from Melbourne, Victoria (Table 19.C). In this study, more than half of the food items analyzed contained TFA concentrations greater than 2% of their total fat. The study revealed several food items that contained more than 1 g

Table 19.C TFA Content in Selected Australian Foods in 2008

The number of products tested within each category is shown in parenthesis after the product name. Mean values are followed by parenthesis showing the range of values.

	Total Fat g/100 g Food	TFA g/100 g Fat	TFA g/100 g Food
Hard margarines/cooking fats (4)	90.4 (80.5–100)	3.2 (1.7–4.5)	3.0 (1.7–4.5)
Fries (3)	17.3 (11.7–21.4)	2.1 (1.4–3.4)	0.3 (0.3–0.4)
Crisps (4)	35.3 (18.6–44.1)	1.1 (0.7–1.9)	0.3 (0.3–0.4)
Crackers (5)	18.1 (16.6–21.5)	5.4 (0.8–23.4)	0.9 (0.1–3.9)
Ready popped popcorn (3)	14.4 (4.1–26.8)	1.2 (0.8–1.4)	0.2 (0–0.4)
Microwave popcorn (3)	24.1 (19.5–26.5)	30.0 (28.8–30.7)	7.2 (6.0–8.1)
Chocolate wafer biscuits (4)	23.7 (19.4–27.1)	6.8 (1.0–22.2)	1.7 (0.3–5.7)
Croissants (2)	19.9 (19.1–20.7)	1.6 (1.6–1.7)	0.3 (0.3–0.4)
Croutons (2)	16.6 (6.4–6.8)	3.0 (1.6–4.4)	0.2 (0.1–0.3)
Cinnamon donuts (3)	19.5 (13.5–23.2)	19.7 (0.7–29.8)	3.6 (0.2–6.6)
Blueberry muffins (3)	14.7 (11.5–19.8)	2.8 (1.5–4.9)	0.4 (0.2–0.6)
Breakfast bars (3)	7.3 (6.7–7.9)	1.8 (0.6–3.5)	0.1 (0–0.2)
Meat pies (5)	13.8 (11.4–15.9)	8.8 (7.6–11.9)	1.2 (0.9–1.8)
Sausage rolls/pasties (4)	12.7 (11.0–13.7)	12.5 (6.9–17.4)	1.6 (0.8–2.2)

Adapted from McCarthy et al. (2008).

of TFA per serving. They included meat pie (four brands), sausage roll (one brand), cinnamon doughnut (one brand), and microwave popcorn (three brands). Typically, partially hydrogenated fats are used in microwave popcorn to prevent oiling out in the bag. However, part of the TFA in some of these products, including butter-flavored popcorn, could have been derived from dairy ingredients rather than industrially produced TFA.

The New South Wales Food Authority (2008) analyzed the TFA content in processed and takeaway foods sold within the state of New South Wales and collected data from October 2005 to March 2007. In 2005, 250 samples representing several food categories, including dairy, meat and meat products, soy milk, bakery products, takeaway foods, fats and oils, confectionery, pasta, and snack foods, were tested. In 2006–2007, additional analyses were performed on 114 samples, 11 of which were previously found to contain high concentrations of TFAs. Overall, the TFA content in the processed and takeaway foods was relatively low. Some exceptions included quiche, takeaway fries, sausage rolls, and bakery products. Considering all products tested during 2005–2007, and omitting those products that were known to contain dairy or other ruminant-derived TFAs, 87% of the products contained TFAs at concentrations below 2% in the total fat. Of the remaining products exceeding 2% (g/100 g fat) TFA concentration, 46% contained dairy or other ruminant-derived TFAs.

The New South Wales Food Authority (2009) followed the above survey with another conducted under the "Coordinated Food Survey Plan" with the participation of food regulatory jurisdictions in the Australian states of New South Wales, South Australia, and Western Australia, as well as New Zealand. It analyzed a total of 456 samples collected from a range of supermarkets and takeaway shops from September 2008 to April 2009. Products, specifically those potentially containing partially hydrogenated vegetable oil, were randomly sampled from various chain and independent retailers. The range of products tested included takeaway foods, snack foods, fats and oils including spreads, meat and meat products, bread and bakery products, and others such as dry mix pasta, dry instant soup, and so forth. However, the products were not selected on market share and were not fully representative of binational purchasing trends or intake (Table 19.D).

Omitting the samples likely to contain considerable proportions of dairy or other ruminant TFAs, over 82% of the samples surveyed had TFA levels, on the basis of total fat, equal to or less than 2% (g/100 g fat) (Figure 19.1). Thus, in 2008–2009, the proportion of foods with average TFA levels equal to or less than 2% had increased slightly compared to the proportion found in the 2005–2007 survey (87%). A summary of the TFA results for food categories tested in the two surveys is shown in Table 19.D. While 8 of the 19 food products (chicken nuggets, deep fried fish fillets, hot chips, potato crisps, sausage rolls, cream filled biscuits, savory biscuits, and shelf-stable cakes) showed a reduction in the median TFA content, three products

Table 19.D Changes in the Median TFA Content in the Australia and New Zealand Food Supply from 2005–2007 and 2009.

		2005–2007				2009			
Food Category	**Food Product**	**No. of Samples**	**Min**	**Median**	**Max**	**No. of Samples**	**Min**	**Median**	**Max**
Takeaway foods	Chicken nuggets	10	<0.1	0.35	0.70	26	<0.1	0.10	0.80
	Deep fried fish fillets	5	0.10	0.20	0.70	16	<0.1	0.10	0.80
	Hot chips	20	0.10	0.20	1.60	31	<0.1	0.10	1.40
	Pizza	5	0.20	0.20	0.30	14	0.10	0.20	0.30
Snack foods	Potato crisps	13	<0.1	0.60	1.80	15	<0.1	0.10	1.40
	Extruded snacks	2	<0.1	<0.1	<0.1	4	<0.1	0.10	0.20
	Oil-based dressings	3	0.10	0.20	0.20	9	<0.10	0.20	0.70
	Edible oil spreads	10	<0.1	0.25	2.90	17	0.10	0.50	3.16
Meat products	Meat pies	5	0.20	0.40	0.50	20	0.15	0.60	0.90
	Sausage rolls	5	0.60	1.0	1.0	19	0.09	0.80	2.10
Bakery products	Chocolate biscuits	5	0.10	0.10	0.10	12	<0.1	0.20	0.38
	Cream filled biscuits	6	0.10	0.35	1.40	14	<0.10	0.30	0.80
	Croissants	5	0.30	0.40	0.50	17	0.20	1.00	1.40
	Custard Danish	5	0.20	0.30	0.40	18	<0.1	0.60	1.20
	Donuts	22	<0.1	0.30	8.70	23	<0.1	0.50	1.27
	Prepared pastry	5	0.10	0.90	1.40	19	0.02	1.35	2.80
	Savory biscuits	5	0.10	0.20	0.20	12	<0.1	0.10	1.60
	Shelf stable cakes	15	0.10	0.30	2.30	7	<0.1	0.20	0.60
Others	Muesli bars	5	<0.1	<0.1	<0.1	9	<0.1	<0.1	0.20

Adapted from Food Standards Australia and New Zealand (2009).

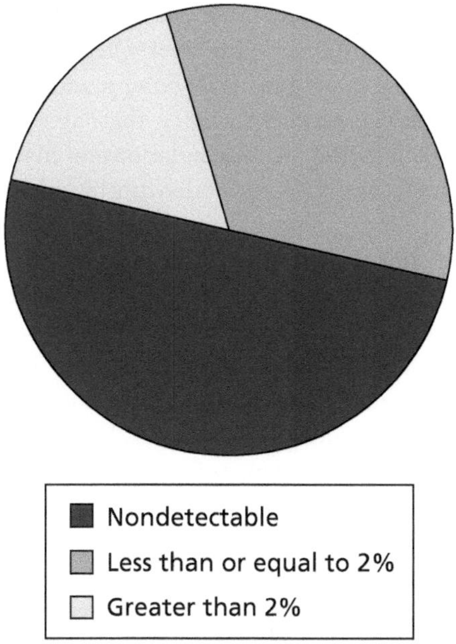

Figure 19.1 Proportion of samples containing different ranges of industrially produced TFA in the Australia and New Zealand food supply (2009). Adapted from FSANZ (2009).

(pizza, oil-based dressings, and muesli bars) remained similar, and the remainder (extruded snacks, edible oil spreads, meat pies, chocolate biscuits, croissants, custard Danish, doughnut, and prepared pastries) showed an increase. It must be pointed out that, of the eight products showing an increase in the median TFA content, four (meat pies, croissants, custard Danish, and prepared pastries) were likely to contain natural (ruminant) TFAs or a mixture of natural and industrially produced TFAs. The increase in the TFA content in prepared pastries was despite a significant reduction in the total fat content, whereas total fat contents remained the same for croissants.

Trans Fat Regulations in Australia and New Zealand

The primary responsibility for the development of domestic food regulatory policy and the development of policy guidelines for setting domestic food standards in Australia and New Zealand lies with the Legislative and Governance Forum on Food Regulation (the Forum). Prior to December 2011, it was known as the Australia and New Zealand Food Regulation Ministerial Council. The Forum also has the capacity to adopt, amend, or reject standards and to request that these be reviewed. The membership of the Forum comprises a minister from New Zealand and the health ministers from the Australian states and territories or other ministers from related portfolios (Primary Industries, Consumer Affairs, etc.) where these have been nominated by their jurisdiction, and the Australian Government (http://www.health.gov.au/internet/main/publishing.nsf/Content/foodsecretariat-anz.htm). Food Standards Australia New Zealand (FSANZ) is a binational government agency that, among other responsibilities, develops food standards and makes recommendations on matters pertaining to labelling for both packaged and unpackaged foods with regard to policy guidelines set by the Forum.

By 2007, several Western countries, including Denmark, Canada, and the United States, had introduced regulatory measures aimed at reducing dietary intake of TFAs. However, the Australia New Zealand Food Standards Code prevailing at the time did not require manufacturers to label TFAs unless a nutrient claim was made related to cholesterol, saturated fats, monounsaturated fats, polyunsaturated fats, TFA, omega-3 fatty acids, omega-6 fatty acids, or omega-9 fatty acids. Voluntary labelling of TFAs was permitted, and many oil producers and manufacturers of edible oil spreads declared TFA content on the product label (FSANZ, 2009). In 2007, FSANZ conducted a formal scientific review of TFAs in the food supply (Food Standards Australia and New Zealand, 2007). From the results of this study, FSANZ estimated that natural and industrially produced TFAs, taken together, contributed on average 0.6% and 0.7% of total energy intake in Australia and New Zealand, respectively. These figures met the goal of 1.0% maximum proposed by the World Health Organisation (WHO/FAO, 2003) and were comparable to or lower than intake estimates from some countries overseas. The Ministerial Council (as it was at the time) endorsed the findings of the FSANZ Review Report (FSANZ, 2009) and came to the conclusion that immediate regulatory intervention was not required and that nonregulatory measures to further reduce the levels of TFAs in the Australian and New Zealand food supply would be the most appropriate action.

The Australia New Zealand Collaboration on *Trans* Fats was established in 2007 to assist in reducing levels of TFAs in foods in Australia and New Zealand. Representatives included the National Heart Foundation of Australia, the National Heart Foundation of New Zealand, the Dietician's Association of Australia, the Australian Food and Grocery Council, the New Zealand Food and Grocery Council, the New Zealand Food Safety Authority, and FSANZ. The primary aim of this group was to work cooperatively with industry in reducing the amount of TFAs in the Australian and New Zealand food supply without increasing the amount of saturated fats (FSANZ, 2009).

The 2007 FSANZ review (FSANZ, 2007) also recommended that a reassessment of TFA in foods and dietary intake would commence in early 2009, and this was approved by the Ministerial Council. The review would measure the effectiveness of the nonregulatory measures aimed to reduce industrially produced TFA content in the food supply. The 2009 review found that, since 2007, intake of industrially produced

TFAs in the Australian and New Zealand population had declined by around 24–25%, reflecting changes in industry practice to reduce TFA concentrations in foods manufactured in Australia and New Zealand. The mean industrially produced TFA intake was estimated at 0.4 g/day or less for Australians and 0.6 g/day or less for New Zealanders. The mean total intake of both natural and industrially produced TFAs was estimated to be 0.5–0.6% of total energy, with more than 90% of Australians and 85% New Zealanders having TFA intakes below 1.0% of energy. These figures indicated that Australia and New Zealand continued to meet the WHO population goal for TFA intake (FSANZ, 2009). Equally important, FSANZ concluded that the reductions in industrially produced TFAs in Australia were not accompanied by increases in saturated fat intake, which remained steady at around 29–32 g/day calculated using both pre- and post-2007 data (FSANZ, 2007). TFA intake data from a more recent (2011–2012) Australian Health Survey, will reveal if there have been further reductions in TFA intake by Australians since 2009.

Pre-2007 studies showed that foods served at quick service restaurants (QSR) contributed significantly to the TFA intake of Australians and New Zealanders (FSANZ, 2007). In 2007, FSANZ set up a QSR roundtable, comprising the major fast-food and restaurant chains operating in Australia, as part of a management strategy to monitor TFA in the Australian food supply. It comprised the following broad categories of food: pizza, burgers, chicken, pasta, and snack foods. The roundtable also included representatives of the oil industry. A similar QSR was established in New Zealand by the New Zealand Food Safety Authority (NZFSA). Questionnaires were sent out to QSR members seeking information on their plans to reduce TFAs in their foods.

In Australia, questionnaires were sent to 16 QSR members and 13 responses were received. Seven reported that their companies had active plans and strategies to either manage TFA in their products or to work with the food industry to reduce TFA levels in foods. Some of these plans had been in place for three to four years, indicating that the industry had been proactive in reducing TFA levels in foods. Four companies advised that they did not have a plan in place because all products were "virtually TFA free" (less than 0.5 g TFA/100 g food) or at minimum levels, except for those products in which the TFA was of natural origin from ingredients such as cheese and meat. However, three of these restaurants reported active plans to investigate alternative blends of cooking oils that would reduce the levels of saturated fats in their products. The other two respondents indicated that they had fully implemented their TFA plans, and considered no further reductions in TFA possible (FSANZ, 2009).

In New Zealand, the NZFSA sent out questionnaires to 28 QSR sector stakeholders as well as to New Zealand participants of the Australian-New Zealand Trans Fat Collaboration, which included the National Heart Foundation of New Zealand and the New Zealand Food and Grocery Council. Nineteen QSR sector stakeholders responded and five reported having plans that were at different stages of implementation. Some had been implemented since 2003, resulting in much lower TFA levels in their products. Others were reported to be still in the planning stages, but no targets or timelines were provided in the follow up responses. However, a number of QSRs reported implementing significant changes to their frying media, as well as to the fats used in bakery products, resulting in lower TFA levels in products. Oil suppliers who responded reported that they are currently modifying their product ranges to lower TFA levels, and that the drive for that reduction had come from the QSRs themselves. However, it was also pointed out that the higher price of TFA-reduced frying media compared to oils conventionally used was an impediment to expanding the use of lower TFA frying media, particularly in difficult economic climates. NZFSA was unable to conclude whether the nonregulatory initiatives had been successful in achieving a reduction in TFA content in the New Zealand food supply based on the QSR survey, as only 19 out of 30 stakeholders responded. The survey had highlighted that during times of economic downturn, New Zealand may see voluntary initiatives such as TFA plans not being prioritised (FSANZ, 2007).

Overall though, based on the 2009 TFA review, FSANZ recommended that the status quo (i.e., the nonregulatory approach) be maintained. This recommendation took into consideration that the intake of industrially produced TFAs had declined in the Australian and New Zealand population by around 25–45% since 2007, which is equivalent to a population average of 0.1% of total energy intake reduction. This was taken as evidence that Australia and New Zealand met the WHO population goal for TFA intake of less than 1.0% of total energy. Furthermore, for a small group of Australians whose total TFA intake is above 1.0% of total energy, pastry products, sausages and luncheon meats, and creamery style pasta dishes, as well as cheese, popcorn, doughnuts, and takeaway style fish products made a disproportionate contribution to TFA intake. A significant proportion of TFA in these products would have resulted from the use of dairy and meat ingredients, and there was no evidence of average daily industrially produced TFA intakes exceeding 0.5 g, as had been reported for some countries.

Despite this declining trend in the TFA levels in the Australian and New Zealand food supply, a recent editorial published in the *Medical Journal of Australia* still called for mandatory labelling in order to inform individuals whose intake may not fall within that of the normal population (Kaur et al., 2012). The authors were of the opinion that mandatory labelling would safeguard Australian consumers from high TFA products imported from countries where there are no TFA regulations. A recent review of labelling by a panel of experts, appointed at the time by the Ministerial Council, recommended that mandatory declaration of all TFA above an agreed threshold be introduced in the nutrition information panel if industrially produced TFAs have not been phased out of the food supply by January 2013 (Commonwealth of Australia, 2011).

Strategies for *Trans* Fat Replacement

For many years now, margarines and spreads manufactured in Australia and New Zealand have generally been virtually free of TFAs. For example, none of the spreads manufactured by a major fats and oils manufacturer in Australia contained TFAs in excess of 0.6 g/100 g (http://www.peerlessfoods.com.au). These low levels have been achieved by use of interesterified fats to obtain the physical properties required for manufacture of margarine (R. Smith, personal communication). However, two of the company's pastry margarines contained 7.6 and 14.6 g/100 g of product, respectively. Furthermore, three out of the four cake margarines supplied by the company contained TFA concentrations in the range 10.8–11.5 g/100g. The pastry shortenings supplied by the same company were low in TFAs (<1%) but very high in saturated fatty acids (>70%), while the solitary doughnut shortening contained high concentrations of industrially produced TFA (38.3 g/100 g) as well as saturated fat (51.4 g/100 g). Even after allowing for tallow, which was listed as a component in some of these products, these values indicate that significant amounts of industrially produced TFA are still present in these products. We can only assume that the same applies to shortenings and pastry and cake margarines supplied by other Australian manufacturers. Thus, although most manufacturers have introduced low-TFA versions of cake and pastry margarines and shortenings, products high in industrially produced TFA continue to be manufactured in Australia, potentially contributing to TFA intake by Australians through consumption of bakery products. Average TFA content information published in the literature for margarines and spreads between 1973 and 2008 shows a general decrease in TFAs over time (Figure 19.2).

The 2009 Australia and New Zealand QSR industry survey (FSANZ, 2009) suggested that a number of strategies had been or were being employed by these industries to reduce TFA levels in foods. Some QSRs reported reengineering of vegetable oil based shortenings and bakery margarines to achieve low-TFA products, without providing details of the strategies used. One oil supplier who participated in the survey claimed that all partially hydrogenated vegetable oils (16g/100g TFAs) had been replaced with interesterified oils (<1g/100g TFAs) in spreads, margarines, and pastry fats.

With regard to eliminating TFAs from deep-frying oils, strategies reported by some QSR participants were: use of low-TFA vegetable oil blends for both frying and par-frying, use of straight vegetable oils (e.g., canola) for par-frying potato products, and use of oven-baking rather than deep-frying techniques during manufacture of retail products. Other replacements of "heavily hydrogenated oils" (mostly canola oil based) include partially hydrogenated canola, "long life" nonhydrogenated canola, or other nonhydrogenated alternatives, such as rice bran oil (FSANZ, 2009).

In September 2004, McDonald's Australia moved away from a tallow-based frying medium to a liquid oil canola blend. Stage two of this initiative was completed

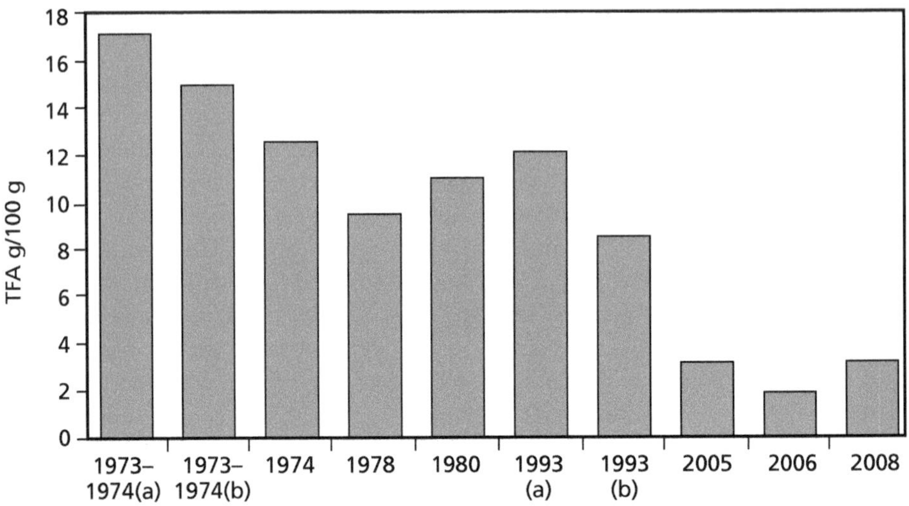

Figure 19.2 Average TFA content in Australian margarines and spreads between 1973 and 2008. A historical perspective of results in the literature, as follows: 1973–1974, Parodi (1974, 1976); Fogerty et al. (1979, 1980); Wills et al. (1982, 1993a); Mansour and Sinclair (1993, 1993b); Ball et al. (1993, 2005); Australian Consumer Association Survey (2005, 2006); Wijesundera et al. (2007, 2008), McCarthy et al. (2008).

in November 2006, when levels of TFA and saturated fat were further decreased. This involved a nationwide roll out of liquid frying oil comprising a blend of canola and high oleic sunflower oils, which contained 85% less TFAs than the previous canola oil blend (media release 27th October 2006 "McDonalds Australia launches virtually *trans* free oil"). More recently, Yum! Restaurants, owner of the KFC and Pizza Hut brands, confirmed that all Australian KFC restaurants have switched from imported palm oil to high oleic canola oil, which is entirely sourced from Australian farmers. This move reduced the saturated fat content in frying oil from as high as 50% (palm oil) to less than 8% (canola oil). According to a recent "current affairs" television program, some of the other major fast food chains in Australia have also switched to TFA-free vegetable oils. Hungry Jacks now uses canola oil, Nandos uses cottonseed oil, and Red Rooster uses a blend of canola and palm oil (*Today Tonight,* 2012).

In a study conducted in 2009, the Australian consumer association "Choice" found high concentrations of TFAs (29.4%, g/100 g fat) in Krispy Kreme doughnuts sold in Australia (Choice, 2009). This led to Krispy Kreme Australia being pressured by both government and consumer groups to follow in the footsteps of their U.S. counterpart to reduce levels of TFAs within their products. Nutritional information currently available on the Australian Krispy Kreme website (http://www.krispykreme.com.au/) indicates levels of TFA are now between 0.92–1.56% of the total fat content. This has been achieved by using shortenings made from sunflower, palm, and canola oils.

Conclusion

Although a number of countries have introduced legislation aimed at reducing levels of TFAs, both Australia and New Zealand currently rely on a self-monitoring model to maintain low levels within the diet. This approach has been successful in further reducing already low levels, as the majority of products and foods currently available on the supermarket shelf or from QSRs contain no or low TFAs. Further, those products that do contain TFAs, for the most part, are well within guidelines implemented by other countries, and historical data suggest that the TFA content of foods in Australia and New Zealand is generally lower than that in either the United States or Europe. There are a few exceptions, such as pastry products, sausages and luncheon meats, creamery style pasta dishes, popcorn, and doughnuts. However, a significant proportion of TFAs within those listed food items would have resulted from the use of dairy and meat ingredients, rather than industrially produced TFAs. Recently, a federal government review has a made a recommendation that mandatory declaration of TFAs above an agreed threshold be introduced in the nutrition information panel by January 2013. The outcome of these recommendations will become apparent over the coming years.

References

Aro, A.; Amelsvoort, J. V.; Becker, W.; van Erp-Baart, M. A.; Kafatos, A.; Leth, T.; van Poppel, G. *Trans* Fatty Acids in Dietary Fats and Oils from 14 European Countries. *Journal of Food Composition and Analysis* **1998,** *11,* 137–149.

The Australian Consumer Association survey (2005).

Ball, M. J.; Hackett, D.; Duncan, A. *Trans* Fatty Acid Content of Margarines, Oils and Blended Spreads Available in New Zealand. *Asia Pac. J. Clin. Nutr.* **1993,** *2,* 165–169.

Bendsen, N. T.; Christensen, R.; Bartels, E. M.; Astrup, A. Consumption of Industrial and Ruminant *Trans* Fatty Acids and Risk of Coronary Heart Disease: A Systematic Review and Meta-analysis of Cohort Studies. *Eur. J. Clin. Nutr.* **2011,** *65,* 773–783.

Brouwer, I. A.; Wandes, A. J.; Katan, M. B. Effect of Animal and Industrial *Trans* Fatty Acids on HDL and LDL Cholesterol Levels in Humans—A Quantitative Review. *PLoS One,* **2010,** *5,* e9434.

Carpenter, D. L.; Slover, H. T. Lipid Composition of Selected Margarines. *J. Am. Oil Chem. Soc.* **1973,** *50,* 372–376.

Choice. Hidden Danger—*Trans* Fat in Foods, 2009. http://www.choice.com.au/reviews-and-tests/food-and-health/food-and-drink/nutrition/trans-fats-in-foods.aspx (accessed November 2012).

Commonwealth of Australia. Labelling Logic, Review of Food Labelling Law and Policy, 2011. http://www.foodlabellingreview.gov.au/internet/foodlabelling/publishing.nsf/content/48C0548D80E715BCCA257825001E5DC0/$File/Labelling%20Logic_2011.pdf (accessed November 2012).

FAO/WHO Joint Expert Consultation Group. *The Role of Dietary Fats and Oils in Human Nutrition.* FAO Food Nutrition Paper 3; Rome, 1977.

Food Standards Australia and New Zealand (FSANZ). Review Report: *Trans* Fatty Acids in New Zealand and Australian Food Supply, 2007. http://www.foodstandards.gov.au/_srcfiles/Transfat%20report%202007.pdf (accessed November 2012).

Food Standards Australia and New Zealand (FSANZ). Intakes of *Trans* Fatty Acids in New Zealand and Australia. Review Report—2009 Assessment, 2009. http://www.foodstandards.gov.au/_srcfiles/TFAs_Aus_NZ_Food_Supply.pdf (accessed November 2012).

Forgerty, A. C.; Svoronos, D. Composition of Some Australian Margarines: A Correction. *CSIRO Food Research Quarterly* **1980,** *40,* 33–34.

Forgerty, A. C.; Ford, G. L.; Pearson, J. A. Composition of Some Australian Margarines. *CSIRO Food Research Quarterly* **1979,** *39,* 38–43.

Gebauer, S. K.; Chardigny, J. M.; Jakobsen, M.U.; Lamarche, B.; Lock, A. L.; Proctor, S. D.; Baer, D. J. Effects of Ruminant *Trans* Fatty Acids on Cardiovascular Disease and Cancer: A Comprehensive Review of Epidemiological, Clinical, and Mechanistic Studies, American Society of Nutrition. *Adv. Nutr.* **2011,** *2,* 332–354.

Hunter, J. E. Dietary *Trans* Fatty Acids: Review of Recent Human Studies and Food Industry Response, *Lipids* **2006,** *41,* 967–992.

Kaur, G.; Cameron-Smith, D.; Sinclair, A. Are *Trans* Fats a Problem in Australia? *Med. J. Aust.* **2012,** *196* (11), 666–667.

Korver, O.; Katan, M. B. The Elimination of *Trans* Fat from Spreads: How Science Helped to Turn an Industry Around. *Nutr. Rev.* **2006,** *64,* 275–279.

http://www.krispykreme.com.au/ (accessed November 2012).

Kummerow, F. A. Current Studies on Relation of Fat to Health. *J. Am. Oil Chem. Soc.* **1974,** 255–259.

Kummerow, F. A. Lipids in Atherosclerosis. *J. Food Sci.* **1975,** *40,* 12–17.

Lichtenstein, A. *Trans* Fatty Acids, Blood Lipids and Cardiovascular Risk: Where Do We Stand? *Nutr. Rev.* **1993,** *51,* 340–343.

Mansour, M. P.; Sinclair, A. J. The *Trans* Fatty Acid and Positional (sn-2) Fatty Acid Composition of Some Australian Margarines, Dairy Blends and Animal Fats. *Asia Pac. J. Clin. Nutr.* **1993,** *2,* 155–163.

McCarthy, J.; Barr, D.; Sinclair, A. Determination of *Trans* Fatty Acid Levels by FTIR in Processed Foods in Australia. *Asia Pac. J. Clin. Nutr.* **2008,** *17,* 391–396.

Mozaffarian, D.; Katan, M. B.; Ascherio, A.; Stampfer, M. J.; Willett, W. C. *Trans* Fatty Acids and Cardiovascular Disease. *New Eng. J. Med.* **2006,** *354,* 1601–1613.

Mozaffarian D.; Aro A.; Willet, W. C. Health Effects of *Trans*-Fatty Acids: Experimental and Observational Evidence. *Eur. J. Clin. Nutr.* **2009,** *63* (Suppl. 2), S5–S21.

The New South Wales Food Authority. *Trans* Fatty Acids Survey, May 2008. http://www.foodauthority.nsw.gov.au/_Documents/corporate_pdf/trans-fatty-acid-survey--FI037–0902.pdf (accessed November 2012).

The New South Wales Food Authority. Report on 2009 *Trans* Fatty Acid Survey—Analytical Results. A Survey Conducted under the Coordinated Food Survey Plan with Participation from Food Regulatory Jurisdiction in NSW, SA, WA and NZ. Food Standards Australia New Zealand, 2009. http://www.foodstandards.gov.au/_srcfiles/TFA_survey_analytical_2009.pdf (accessed November 2012).

Parodi, P. W. Composition and Structure of Some Consumer-Available Edible Fats. *J. Am. Oil Chem. Soc.* **1976** *53,* 530–534.

http://www.peerlessfoods.com.au/catalogue/bakery/ (accessed 9 November 2012).

Rahkovsky, I.; Martinez, S.; Kuchler, F. *New Food Choices Free of Trans Fats Better Align, U.S. Diets with Health Recommendations;* EIB-95; U.S. Department of Agriculture, Economic Research Service: 2012.

Ratnayake, W. M. N. *Trans* Fatty Acid Content of Canadian Margarines Prior to Mandatory Trans Fat Labelling. *J. Am. Oil Chem. Soc.* **2007,** *84,* 817–825.

Ratnayake, W. M. N.; Abbe, M. R. L.; Farnsworth, S.; Dumais, L.; Gagnon, C.; Lampi, B.; Casey, V.; Mohottalage, D.; Rondeau, I.; Underhill, L. *Trans* Fatty Acids: Current Content in Canadian Foods and Estimated Intake Levels for the Canadian Population. *J. AOAC Int.* **2009,** *92,* 1258–1276.

Satchithanandam, S.; Oles, C. J.; Spease, C. J. Brandt, M. M.; Yurawecz, M. P.; Rader, J. I. *Trans,* Saturated, Unsaturated Fat in Food in the United States Prior to Mandatory *Trans*-fat Labelling. *Lipids* **2004,** *39,* 11–18.

Smith, R. (personal communication).

Strapnel, W. S.; Calvert, G. D.; Nestel, P. J.; Truswell, A. S. Diet and Coronary Heart Disease. *Med. J. Austr.* **1992,** *156* (Suppl.), S9–S16.

Tardy, A. L.; Morio, B.; Chardigny, J. M.; Malpuech-Brugere, C. Rumaninat and Industrial Sources of *Trans*-fat and Cardiovascular Diabetic Diseases. *Nutr. Res. Rev.* **2011,** 1–7.

Today Tonight. [Television program.] Hot Chips; August 20, 2012.

Troisi, R.; Willett, R.; Weiss, S. T. *Trans* Fatty Acids in Relation to Serum Lipid Concentrations in Adult Men. *Am. J. Clin. Nutr.* **1992,** *56,* 1010–1024.

Wijesundera, C.; Richards, A.; Ceccato, C. Industrially Produced *Trans* Fat in Foods in Australia. *J. Am. Oil Chem. Soc.* **2007,** *84,* 433–442.

Willet, W. C. Intake of *Trans* Fatty Acids and Risk of Coronary Heart Disease among Women. *The Lancet* **1993,** *341,* 581–585.

Willett, W. C. Dietary Fats and Coronary Heart Disease. *J. Int. Med.* **2012,** *272,* 13–24.

Wills, R. B. H.; Myers, P. R.; Greenfield, H. Composition of Australian Foods 14. Margarines and Cooking Fats. *Food Tech. Austr.* **1982,** *34,* 240–244.

Yang, Y.; Jacome-Sosa, M. M.; Proctor, S. D. The Role of Ruminant *Trans* Fat as a Potential Nutraceutical in the Prevention of Cardiovascular Disease. *Food Res. Int.* **2012,** *46,* 460–468.

Index

FSC
www.fsc.org
MIX
Papier | Fördert gute Waldnutzung
FSC® C083411

Kolibri 360 GmbH
Ferdinand-Jühlke-Straße 7
99095 Erfurt, Deutschland
produktsicherheit@kolibri360.de